Understanding the Principles and Practice of Legal Oncology

Understanding the Principles and Practice of Legal Oncology

EDITORS

Tony S. Quang, MD, JD, FCLM
President and Gold Medalist
American College of Legal Medicine
Attending Physician
VA Puget Sound Health Care System
Associate Professor of Radiation Oncology
University of Washington School of Medicine
Adjunct Associate Professor of Law
University of Washington School of Law
Seattle, Washington

Michelle S. Taft, JD
Partner
Johnson, Graffe, Keay, Moniz & Wick, LLP
Seattle, Washington

Sushil Beriwal, MD, MBA, FASTRO, FABS
Professor and Academic Chief
Department of Radiation Oncology
Allegheny Health Network
Pittsburgh, Pennsylvania

New York   Chicago   San Francisco   Athens   London   Madrid   Mexico City
Milan   New Delhi   Singapore   Sydney   Toronto

Understanding the Principles and Practice of Legal Oncology

1 2 3 4 5 6 7 8 9   LCR   27 26 25 24 23 22

ISBN 978-1-260-47407-7
MHID 1-260-47407-0

This book was set in Chaparral Pro Regular by KnowledgeWorks Global Ltd.
The editors were Jason Malley and Christie Naglieri.
The production supervisor was Richard Ruzycka.
Project management was provided by Nitesh Sharma, KnowledgeWorks Global Ltd.
The cover designer was W2 Design.

This book is printed on acid-free paper.

Names: Quang, Tony S., editor. | Taft, Michelle S., editor. | Beriwal, Sushil, editor.
Title: Understanding the principles and practice of legal oncology / editors, Tony S. Quang, Michelle S. Taft, Sushil Beriwal.
Description: New York : McGraw Hill, [2021] | Includes bibliographical references and index. | Summary: "For the busy clinician, this is the authoritative handbook with easy-to-follow clinical vignettes and relevant legal principles to master in their day-to-day practice to avoid common medico-legal pitfalls, whether the clinician is a physician, surgeon, nurse, researcher, medical physicist, or technician. Knowing a few commonly litigated and settled legal cases and appreciating the principles underlying the causes of action can fortify a clinician's confidence in what they are doing. Being empowered by this knowledge and understanding will mitigate their anxiety of having to do unnecessary exhaustive work ups and documentations. The benefits not only include reducing health care cost and increasing better patient access, but will also allow clinicians to practice like a pro where they think like a lawyer but care for patients like a clinician."— Provided by publisher.
Identifiers: LCCN 2021031381 | ISBN 9781260474077 (hardcover) | ISBN 9781260474084 (ebook)
Subjects: MESH: Medical Oncology—legislation & jurisprudence.
Classification: LCC RC263 | NLM QZ 21 | DDC 616.99/4—dc23
LC record available at https://lccn.loc.gov/2021031381

This textbook is dedicated to the memory of Professor Daniel E. Koshland, Jr, who instilled in me the love of science; to the memory of Dr. Luther W. Brady, MD, who inspired me to master clinical oncology and to appreciate the art of humanity; and Professor Steve P. Calandrillo, my law school professor, who takes every opportunity to support and encourage me to explore the intersection of law and medicine. Most important of all, I dedicate this textbook to my patients and US Veterans, who have taught me so much all these years so that I can use the knowledge gained to improve the delivery of cancer care that is high quality, equitable, and provided with compassion.

— Tony S. Quang, MD, JD, FCLM

This textbook is dedicated to my parents, Pam and Craig Taft, who instilled in me the intellectual curiosity and work ethic necessary to pursue my academic and professional dreams; my husband, Max Mannisto, who loves and supports me personally and professionally every day; my colleagues at Johnson, Graffe, Keay, Moniz & Wick, LLP for their professional mentorship and friendship; my law school classmate and friend, Tony S. Quang, MD, JD, FCLM who cajoled me into editing this medical-legal textbook and kept me on track even when I was up to my eyeballs in work; and to all of my clients, whose deep passion for quality patient care inspires me to lead a life of compassion and service to others.

— Michelle S. Taft, JD

This textbook is dedicated to all my mentors who inspired me to work harder and be focused on patient care. I also dedicate this to my wife, Shilpa Beriwal, who supported me through all ups and downs of life. Last but not the least, I dedicate this book to all my patients who trusted me to care for them.

— Sushil Beriwal, MD, MBA, FASTRO, FABS

Table of Contents

Contributors

Timothy Craig Allen, MD, JD
Professor and Chair, Department of Pathology
The University of Mississippi Medical School
The University of Mississippi Medical Center
Jackson, Mississippi
Chapter 9

Christopher Anderson, MA, JD
Managing Attorney
Cultiva Law
Seattle, Washington
Chapter 18

Becky Bye, DDS, JD, FCLM
Associate General Counsel
Cue Health Inc.
Denver, Colorado
Chapter 15

Randall Y. Chan, MD
Associate Professor of Clinical Pediatrics
Keck School of Medicine of the University of
    Southern California
Los Angeles, California
Chapter 8

Glen Cheng, MD, JD, MPH
Chief of Occupational Medicine
VA Pittsburgh Healthcare System
Pittsburgh, Pennsylvania
Chapter 21

Sarah Diekman, MD, JD, MS, FCLM
Chief Resident of Occupational and
    Environmental Medicine
Johns Hopkins Bloomberg School of Public
    Health
Baltimore, Maryland
Chapter 28

David Edul Dryburgh, JD
Legal Research Assistant
University of Washington School of Law
Seattle, Washington
Chapter 12

Ana E. Dvoredsky, MD, MJ
Consultant in Graduate Education, DVK
Seattle, Washington
Chapters 2 and 26

Sarah Fagan, MPH, MA
Medical Student
Touro University Nevada College of
    Osteopathic Medicine
Las Vegas, Nevada
Chapter 17

Kristen Fishler, MS, CGC
Munroe-Meyer Institute for Genetics and
    Rehabilitation
University of Nebraska Medical Center
Omaha, Nebraska
Chapter 12

Michelle Francis, JD, MPH
Senior Corporate Counsel
Microsoft
Redmond, Washington
Chapter 20

Viney Hardit, MD, JD
Fellow, Department of Pediatric
  Hematology/Oncology
University of Miami/Jackson Memorial
  Hospital
Miami, Florida
Chapter 8

C. William Hinnant, Jr., MD, JD, FCLM
Adjunct Associate Professor of Public
  Health Sciences
Clemson University
Instructor in Health Law
Limestone University
Anderson, South Carolina
Chapter 4

Jessica Huening Poppenk, JD
Director, Office of Research Integrity and
  Compliance
Ann & Robert H. Lurie Children's Hospital
  of Chicago
Chicago, Illinois
Chapter 20

Aarthi B. Iyer, JD, MPH
Associate General Counsel
Dartmouth-Hitchcock
Lebanon, New Hampshire
Chapter 20

Cindy Jacobs, RN, JD
Partner, Jacobs Riggs Legal & Business
  Services
Affiliate Faculty, University of Washington
  School of Law
Consultant, Drug and Device Advisory
  Committee, University of Washington
  School of Medicine Institute for
  Translational Health Sciences
Seattle, Washington
Chapter 22

Mudit Kakar, PhD, JD
Partner, Choi Capital Law, PLLC
Seattle, Washington
Chapter 13

Richard Harlin Knierim, MD
Pathologist
Swedish Medical Center
Seattle, Washington
Chapter 9

Quynh La, JD
Legal Research Assistant
University of Washington School of Law
Seattle, Washington
Chapter 8

Danial Laird, MD, JD
Director, Flamingo Medical Clinic PLLC
Owner, Laird Law PLLC
Las Vegas, Nevada
Chapter 17

Hamid R. Latifi, MD, JD, MA, FCLM
Founder and Nuclear Radiologist, Avicenna
  Consulting, PLLC
Attorney at Law, Latifi Law, PLLC
Dallas, Texas
Chapter 11

Deni Malavé-Huertas, MD
Fellow of the American Congress of Obstetrics
and Gynecology
Vero Beach, Florida
Chapter 14

Rebekah J. Maloney, JD
Managing Associate
Sidley Austin, LLP
Dallas, Texas
Chapter 11

Taylor G. Maloney, MD
Diagnostic and Interventional Radiology
Resident
Baylor University Medical Center
Dallas, Texas
Chapter 11

Melissa Mariano, DO
Resident Physician, Department of Medicine,
Mount Auburn Hospital/Beth Israel Lahey
Health
Cambridge, MA
Clinical Fellow of Medicine, Harvard Medical
School
Boston, Massachusetts
Chapter 29

Michelle L. McGowan, PhD
Research Associate Professor, Ethics Center
Cincinnati Children's Hospital Medical Center
Departments of Pediatrics and Women's,
Gender & Sexuality Studies
University of Cincinnati
Cincinnati, Ohio
Chapter 12

Claire E. Murphy, MD
Pathologist
Pathology Consultants
Eugene, Oregon
Chapter 9

William J. Pao, MD, JD, FACR
Radiation Oncology Associates Ltd.
Mequon, Wisconsin
Chapter 24

Benjamin Pardue, JD
Editor, Washington Law Review
University of Washington School of Law
Seattle, Washington
Chapter 9

Amirala S. Pasha, DO, JD
Assistant Professor of Medicine
Mayo Clinic
Rochester, Minnesota
Chapter 19

Joseph D. Piorkowski, Jr., DO, JD, MPH, FCLM
Founding Partner, The Piorkowski Law
Firm, PC
Adjunct Professor of Law, Georgetown
University Law Center
Washington, District of Columbia
Chapter 5

Markus Ploesser, MD, LLM
Assistant Clinical Professor, Department of
Psychiatry and Neurosciences, University of
California Riverside
Forensic Psychiatry, Department of
Psychiatry, Faculty of Medicine, The
University of British Columbia
Vancouver, British Columbia
Chapter 16

Lauren Price
Medical Student
Touro University Nevada
College of Osteopathic Medicine
Henderson, Nevada
Chapter 17

Cody Miller Pyke, MD, JD, LLM, MSBe
Baylor College of Medicine
Houston, Texas
Chapter 25

Tony S. Quang, MD, JD, FCLM
President and Gold Medalist
American College of Legal Medicine
Attending Physician
VA Puget Sound Health Care System
Associate Professor of Radiation Oncology
University of Washington School of Medicine
Adjunct Associate Professor of Law
University of Washington School of Law
Seattle, Washington
Chapter 27

Archie L. Rich II, Esq.
Principal, LawMD, Chartered Law Firm
Commissioner, District of Columbia Board of
    Medicine
Washington, District of Columbia
Chapter 1

Santos Ruiz-Cordero, MD, JD, FCLM
Compassionate Medical Center Inc.
Zayas and Ruiz Immigration Attorneys LLC
    Fort Pierce l
Ronin Police Defensive Tactics
Winter Heaven, Florida
Chapter 14

Kenji Saito, MD, JD, FACOEM
Chief Medical and Science Officer, LiveWell
    WorkWell, a MedLaw Limited Liability
    Company
Clinical Assistant Professor, Dartmouth
    College Geisel School of Medicine
Clinical Assistant Professor, University of
    New England
Adjunct Faculty, University of Pennsylvania
    Perelman School of Medicine
Augusta, Maine
Chapters 12 and 29

**Bruce H. Seidberg, DDS, MScD, JD, DABE,
FCLM, FACD**
Former Associate Professor, State University
of NY at Buffalo, School of Dentistry
Past President, American College of Legal
    Medicine
Past Chairman, NYS Board for Dentistry
Retired Endodontist
Syracuse, New York
Chapter 15

Eric E. Shore, DO, JD, MBA, FCLM
Attorney at Law
Shore Legal Group, LLC
Bala Cynwyd, Pennsylvania
Chapter 23

Michelle S. Taft, JD
Partner, Johnson, Graffe, Keay,
    Moniz & Wick, LLP
Seattle, Washington
Chapters 3 and 27

Thanh T. Ton, DDS, MS, MPH
Associate Professor of Clinical Dentistry
Herman Ostrow School of Dentistry of the
    University of Southern California
Los Angeles, California
Chapter 15

Veling W. Tsai, MD, JD, FCLM
Clinical Assistant Professor, Department of
  Head and Neck Surgery
University of California Los Angeles
David Geffen School of Medicine at UCLA
Los Angeles, California
Chapter 7

Michael Vinluan, MD, JD, FCLM
Medical-Legal Consultant
Fellow and Governor, American College of
  Legal Medicine
Baltimore, Maryland
Chapters 1 and 27

Mary J. Wall, MD, JD, FCLM, FAALM, DABR
Director, Nuclear Medicine
Bon Secours Ohio Mercy Health
Toledo
Chapter 10

Terry J. Wall, JD, MD
Attorney
TRI, PA
Shawnee Mission, Kansas
Chapter 6

Victor Waters, MD, JD, FCLM
Chief Medical Medical Officer Dignity Health
  Central Arizona and West Valley Market
Dignity Health, St Joseph Hospital and
  Medical Center
Phoenix, Arizona
Chapter 30

Jenny L. Wong, DMD, MD
Lecturer, UCLA School of Dentistry
University of California, Los Angeles
Adjunct Clinical Assistant Professor of
  Medical Education, Keck School of
  Medicine of USC
University of Southern California
Los Angeles, CA
Private Practice
Claremont, California
Chapter 15

Johnson Wong, DO
Resident Physician, Department of Internal
  Medicine
Kirk Kerkorian School of Medicine at
  University of Nevada, Las Vegas
Las Vegas, Nevada
Chapter 14

Matthew H. H. Young, MD, JD, MBA, CMQ, FCLM, Esq.
Founder & Executive Director
Patient Advocacy Organization and
  Resource, Inc.
Philadelphia, Pennsylvania
Chapter 1

Junying Zhao, PhD, PhD, MPH, MBBS
Assistant Professor, Department of Health
  Administration and Policy
The University of Oklahoma Health Sciences
  Center
Oklahoma City, Oklahoma
Chapter 21

Preface

Over the past decade, science and technology have advanced the field of oncology. In the era of precision medicine, treatments that were not otherwise readily available are now accessible to patients. Molecular testing coupled with the advent of immunotherapy, radiation therapy, chemotherapy, and surgery brings new hope for the cure of cancer.

In the meantime, the health care delivery system has gone through an enormous amount of transformation, making the delivery of cancer care complex; in addition, cancer care represents a significant portion of total US health care spending. Approximately $183 billion was spent in the United States on cancer-related health care in 2015, and this amount is projected to grow to $246 billion by 2030—an increase of 34%. Cost containment while maintaining a high level of quality care is of paramount importance.

In this high-stakes system, it is easy for a clinician, such as a radiation oncologist, medical oncologist, surgeon, primary care physician, pharmacist, social worker, nurse, or other specialist involved in cancer care, to make mistakes. Such mistakes come at great costs not only to individual clinicians and patients but also to the entire system; in addition, it is distressing when a clinician is named in a lawsuit or when a patient is harmed as a result of medical malpractice, resulting in pain and suffering. Therefore, it behooves a clinician to have basic familiarity with the legal aspects of clinical medicine. It is no longer adequate for clinicians just to know medicine. They must be versed in the various issues in the interface of law and medicine so that they have a road map to practice medicine effectively, economically, and safely. As a specialty, oncology pervades all medical specialties, and understanding law and medicine through the lens of cancer care is a provocative and prudent proposition.

Furthermore, just as clinicians should learn about law and medicine, other stakeholders such as health care attorneys, hospital CEOs, office managers, public health officials, social workers, entrepreneurs, and those who work in health care should also find the various topics invaluable to their understanding of the complexity of health care administration. In fact, there is no better time to start to learn than when they are students. Therefore, medical students, residents, MHA students, MPA students, law students, and MBA students would greatly benefit from reading this treatise as they progress into their careers and leadership positions.

This textbook explores the intersection of law and medicine, focusing on an array of topics specific to the field of oncology and its nexus to other specialties. It is divided into 3 sections: Section I (Chapters 1 to 5) dives into the fundamentals of law with respect to how the legal system operates on cancer care. Section II (Chapters 6 to 16) speaks to the different specialties where law and medicine manifest most prominently in cancer care. Section III (Chapters 17 to 30) explores cogent topics that are relevant to cancer care. Illustrative examples via clinical vignettes in Sections II and III reinforce the legal relevance to the clinician's day-to-day practice. Case laws alert the reader to mistakes that have been made and how these mistakes have been borne out in the legal system. The reader should use them as learning tools. Key points are practical recommendations at the end of the chapter for the reader as take-away pearls.

Each chapter is authored by expert specialists, almost all of whom have both a medical or dental and legal background, in particular fields of law and medicine. Their treatise reflects their own research, experience, and professional opinions. While each chapter provides a general discussion of its intended topic, laws and regulations vary by jurisdiction. The reader is therefore encouraged to review the laws, regulations, and standards of care specific to the reader's jurisdiction and field of practice as they relate to the issues discussed in these chapters.

We hope you enjoy this first-of-its-kind textbook for the understanding of the principles and practice of legal oncology.

Tony S. Quang, MD, JD, FCLM
Michelle S. Taft, JD
Sushil Beriwal, MD, MBA, FASTRO, FABS

PART I

Introduction to Legal Oncology

CHAPTER 1

Medical Malpractice

Michael Vinluan, MD, JD, FCLM, Archie L. Rich II, Esq., and
Matthew H. H. Young, MD, JD, MBA, CMQ, FCLM, Esq.

INTRODUCTION: MEDICAL ERROR VERSUS MEDICAL MALPRACTICE

A team from Johns Hopkins Medicine estimated that a quarter of a million people die each year as a result of a medical error.[1] The study ranks medical error as the third leading cause of death in the United States (250,000 deaths), next to heart disease (650,000 deaths) and cancer (600,000 deaths).[2] To put it in perspective, the study suggests that more people die each year from medical errors than from accidents/unintentional injuries (170,000 deaths), chronic lower respiratory disease (160,000 deaths), or stroke (150,000 deaths).[2,3]

Another team from Johns Hopkins Medicine estimated that, each year, up to 12 million diagnostic errors occur, resulting in 80,000 preventable deaths.[4] Such medical errors include misdiagnosis and delayed diagnosis. The team identified three major disease categories that account for serious harms: vascular events, infections, and cancers.[5]

A medical error, however, is not the same as medical malpractice. A medical error is based on the science of medicine, whereas medical malpractice is the legal consequence of the medical error. As discussed later in this chapter, not all medical errors are considered medical malpractice.

This chapter provides a snapshot of relevant concepts in medical malpractice litigation. While it does not cover all legal principles and rules encountered in litigation, it does provide need-to-know information meant for cancer care physicians and clinicians in general, whether as a defendant in a case, as a nonparty treating physician, or as an expert witness.

NEGLIGENCE

Medical malpractice falls within our civil justice system in an area called tort law and is based on the legal definition of negligence. Negligence, as defined by the law, is failure to provide reasonable care. It has four necessary elements: (1) a duty to provide reasonable care; (2) a breach of that duty or, in medical malpractice, a violation of the standard of care; (3) the violation of the standard of care was the actual and proximate cause of the injury; and (4) resulting damages. Each of these four elements must be proven. Like a four-legged table that needs all four legs, a medical malpractice lawsuit must have all four elements of negligence to stand in court.

DUTY

A duty to provide reasonable care is the first prerequisite to establish negligence. Without duty owed to another person, the subsequent elements of negligence need not be established. For example, an Olympic gold medalist swimmer strolling by the beach happens to see a person drowning and pleading for help. This champion swimmer could just pull up a beach chair and watch the person drown without any risk of being sued for negligence. He might rightly be considered a despicable person in this situation, but he had no legal duty to rescue the drowning person.

Similarly, a medical doctor cannot be held liable for an alleged injury unless he or she had a duty in the first place to provide reasonable care to the patient at the time of the alleged malpractice. This duty is typically created when there is a doctor-patient relationship. This legal relationship is established through a contract, formal or implied, or any conduct that indicates the medical doctor is a clinical participant in the patient's diagnosis or treatment.

Curbside and informal consults

When a physician provides general advice as a mere professional courtesy to a colleague, a doctor-patient relationship is not necessarily established, and the consulted physician typically does not have a duty to the patient.[6] The consulted colleague may not have examined the patient, may not have read the chart, and may not have billed for the consultation. The use of general advice such as "for patients with ____ condition, the current guideline is ____" may be employed, rather than specific directions, such as "for this patient, I would recommend ____." The latter may present as being almost a participant in the diagnosis or treatment of the patient at issue and points toward establishing a doctor-patient relationship.

A lack of a doctor-patient relationship, however, may not protect a medical doctor from malpractice. A medical malpractice case in Minnesota involved a hospitalist who was consulted on the phone by an outside clinic nurse practitioner about a patient complaining of fever and abdominal pain, who had an elevated white blood cell count. The hospitalist, who was not affiliated with the clinic, did not recommend sending the patient to a hospital, and the patient died three days later from sepsis from untreated *Staphylococcus* infection. The patient's son sued the nurse practitioner as well as the hospitalist. The case reached Minnesota's highest court, which held that duty exists despite not having an established physician-patient relationship if (1) there is sufficient evidence to conclude that the consulted physician knew or should have known that the advice given would be relied on by the provider who sought consultation and (2) it is foreseeable that the patient could be harmed by a violation in the standard of care of the consulted physician.[7]

On-call physicians

In general, when an on-call physician receives information about a patient and takes affirmative action to treat the patient, a doctor-patient relationship is established.[8] On-call obligations are based on a contractual relationship between the hospital (or clinic) and the physician. An on-call physician who fails or refuses to appear within a reasonable period of time may also be sanctioned for Emergency Medical Treatment and Labor Act (EMTALA) violations.[9]

However, an on-call physician may not even be aware of the requested consult and be sued for malpractice. Consider the following scenario. A head and neck cancer patient presented incidentally to the emergency room with abdominal pain of two days in duration, and a subsequent computed tomography scan revealed an abdominal aortic aneurysm with a possibility of rupture or leak. The on-call vascular surgeon was called multiple times but never returned the call. The patient was transferred to another hospital and ultimately had several cardiac arrests before going to the operating room (OR). Postoperatively, he was found to have an anoxic brain injury and died after a few days. The wife argued that had the patient been taken to the OR sooner, he would not have died from the aneurysm. The on-call vascular surgeon who never returned the call and his employer were named as defendants. The wife argued that the vascular surgeon had a duty to provide treatment because of his existing contractual relationship with the hospital.

Supervising physicians and residents/fellows

A supervising physician has a duty to provide care to the patient being cared for by his supervised resident or fellow and to adequately supervise residents or fellows. In medical malpractice cases, the supervising physician can be held liable under the so-called "borrowed servants" doctrine, where residents and fellows are temporary "borrowed" employees of the supervising physician who has authority over them. Thus, a negligent act committed within the scope of their residency or fellowship training can be imputed to the supervising physician. Another legal basis for liability is called the "captain of the ship doctrine." This legal theory is traditionally seen in OR cases where the surgeon is regarded as the ultimate person responsible for the outcome of the surgery. Despite these theoretical applications, the borrowed servant doctrine and captain of the ship doctrine are not universally applied in all states or medical malpractice suits.

Under the duty to supervise, a supervising physician may also be liable for negligent conduct of residents and fellows through negligent supervision. Here, the supervising physician's own failure to provide proper supervision is the actual violation of the standard of care.

Physicians and nonphysician practitioners

The scope of practice of nonphysician practitioners such as physician assistants and nurse practitioners varies by state. In general, if a physician has control or oversight of the nonphysician provider's clinical decisions or actions related to the negligent conduct at issue, the physician may be held liable under negligent supervision. In addition, if the physician is the employer of the nonphysician practitioner, the physician may also be liable under the legal doctrine called vicarious liability, as long as the nonphysician practitioner was acting within the scope of his or her employment at the time of his or her alleged misconduct. Negligent supervision and vicarious liability will be discussed further in this chapter.

Note, however, that in general, the negligent conduct of a nursing staff is not imputed to the attending physician unless the conduct resulted from direct or standing orders of the attending physician.

Independent medical examinations and third-party evaluations

Independent medical examinations (IMEs) and third-party evaluations historically do not put the physician at risk for medical malpractice lawsuits because it is well known that no doctor-patient relationship is established during these activities. To express such lack of relationship, patients typically sign a disclaimer clearly stating that no doctor-patient relationship is established.

In a case in Arizona, however, an occupational health medicine physician who conducted an IME on a workers' compensation claimant was sued by the injured worker.[10] The IME doctor reported to the worker's compensation carrier that the injured worker did not need supportive care, did not need work restrictions, and was medically able to perform unrestricted work. Relying on this report, the carrier terminated the benefits. However, the injury progressed, and eventually, the worker needed a spinal cord decompression and later died of accidental overdose of narcotic pain medications. The court held that the IME doctor owed a duty of reasonable care to the injured worker when he provided an evaluation of the injury and treatment recommendations. The court, however, did not hold that every IME physician has a duty of care in every situation. To determine if duty exists, the court explained that the following factors should be considered: whether the doctor was in a unique position to prevent harm, the burden of preventing harm, the degree of certainty of the harm, whether the patient relied on the IME doctor's diagnosis, and the closeness of the connection between the IME and the injury.

Termination of duty versus abandonment

Termination of duty in the clinical setting means formally ending the doctor-patient relationship and the duty owed to the patient due to various nondiscriminatory reasons. Termination must be done under specific requirements, such as (1) not terminating during a time when the patient needs the continuous care being provided, (2) giving reasonable notice of such termination, (3) providing general guidance on how to find subsequent medical care, and (4) giving records and relevant information to the new doctor. Abandonment arises if these conditions are not met. As such, without proper termination, duty still exists.

Oncologists should be mindful that cancer patients need continuous care; thus, termination should not be attempted during a time when the cancer patient needs critical treatment. The typical 30-day notice may also not be sufficient for cancer patients to find another oncologist, depending on the location of the patient. Likewise, telling cancer patients to contact their insurance company or primary care provider to find a new cancer doctor may not be prudent for those needing immediate chemotherapy. Under these "constructive abandonment" situations, the oncologist puts the cancer patient in a difficult, if not life-threatening, position and puts the oncologist at risk for medical malpractice.

BREACH

Central to medical malpractice lawsuits is the breach of duty or violation of the standard of care. Standard of care is defined as what a reasonably prudent medical doctor with similar training and background would or would not do under the same or similar situation. The "reasonably prudent medical doctor" standard is akin to the "average medical doctor," and it does not require the knowledge and skill of a preeminent medical specialist who does cutting-edge research on the specialty at issue. It simply requires, for example, what a typical oncologist of ordinary prudence would do or would not do under the same situation, that is, under the same set of facts and circumstances. The "same situation" means in the same clinical setting.

Most states follow the national standard of care because training and certifications are based on national standards. However, some states (Arizona, Arkansas, Idaho, and New York) still follow the locality rule, where the standard of care may slightly vary between rural and urban physicians. Thus, there might be a slight variation in the standard of care between a small rural clinic or hospital and a university medical center.

Thus, a violation of the standard of care is failure to provide the kind of care that an average doctor would have or should have provided under the same situation. Other language commonly used is "deviation from the standard of care" or "breach in the standard of care." As with all medical malpractice cases, both the patient and defendant-doctor retain experts in the specialty at issue who will educate the jury about what the standard of care is and whether the defendant-doctor violated this standard of care. Although the jury is composed of lay people who typically do not have a background in medicine, the jury decides which expert testimony makes more sense and is more credible. Intuitively, one may ask why jurors who are far from being experts in medicine get to decide whether the standard of care was violated. However, the right for a jury trial in civil cases is preserved by the Seventh Amendment of the US Constitution.

For example, a 50-year-old woman with a history of vulvar cancer who underwent vulvectomy followed by radiation therapy came in for a chronic, nonhealing ulcer in the perirectal area. A wound care doctor performed debridement for a few months until he finally decided to perform a punch biopsy. Biopsy results showed the patient had an invasive squamous cell carcinoma. Subsequently, the patient underwent an exenteration followed by plastic surgery and now lives with a permanent colostomy bag. She alleged that, had a biopsy been done much sooner, all she would have needed was a wide excision of the new cancer.

On the question of standard of care, would an average wound care doctor under the same set of facts and circumstances diagnose this nonhealing wound as a side effect of radiation and perform repeated debridement? Or would an average wound care doctor initially perform a biopsy to rule out cancer recurrence? As is the case in all medical malpractice litigation, both the patient and defendant-doctor would present multiple experts to argue their case. If during litigation the patient fails to prove that an average wound care doctor would have done an initial biopsy prior to debridement, then despite the diagnostic error that likely led to the catastrophic outcome, the defendant-doctor will more likely prevail on the merits. As in this case, it does not matter if there was a catastrophic outcome or if the patient died as a result of the medical error; if the plaintiff-patient fails to prove that the defendant-doctor deviated from what an average wound care doctor would have done under the same or similar situation, then the doctor prevails despite a diagnostic error. Thus, a medical error can occur with catastrophic outcomes but without medical malpractice as long as there was no violation in the standard of care.

As discussed earlier in this chapter, negligent supervision is a distinct liability theory that concerns itself with a person or entity's duty to hire, train, and manage its workforce in a manner that does not create unreasonable risks of harm to persons or property. While this theory may be used to hold individual defendants accountable, most often, negligent supervision is claimed against institutional, rather than individual, defendants. In the clinical setting, these institutions are most often hospitals, clinics, nursing homes, and other care facilities in which substantial elements of care delivery are systematized or administrative in nature.

Generally speaking, breaches giving rise to negligent supervision claims most often arise in the nature of system failures as opposed to a clinician's mistake at the instance of treatment. However, it is usually an individual mistake that premises the negligent supervision claim. For example, if a hospital hires a nurse who is, by her training, unqualified to safely perform procedures, such as putting in a portacath or peripherally inserted central catheter (PICC) line to which she is assigned, when that unqualified nurse botches the procedure, substantially because she is unqualified, the hospital may be liable for the injury to the patient for negligently hiring an unqualified nurse. In the same instance, the nurse may herself be liable for negligently and injuriously botching the procedure. The duty to supervise reasonably to prevent harm to patients begins with screening and hiring the employee (including contractors and agents) and extends to include a duty to train and manage the employee according to what is reasonable under the circumstances to prevent foreseeable harm to patients. What is important to remember about negligent supervision is that negligence in the supervision must be proven, independent from the injurious act itself as inflicted by an individual provider.

Another important legal doctrine within medical malpractice litigation, as mentioned earlier, is called vicarious liability. Unlike negligent supervision claims, vicarious liability requires no wrongdoing at all by the institutional actor. Liability of the institutional defendant, that is, the hospital, can be established because its employee or agent was negligent. It is the employer-employee or principal-agent relationship itself that cements liability for a hospital if the physician delivers negligent care to a patient, while acting on behalf of the hospital within the scope of that employment. Vicarious liability also cements liability of the actual employer in cases where the physician is employed by a physician practice group or health care system.

Hospital liability also exists even if the physician is not an employee of the hospital and is not subject to the control of the hospital. Under a legal doctrine called apparent agency, if a patient perceives the physician to be an employee or agent of the hospital, the hospital can be sued for actions of this nonemployee physician. Apparent agency applies typically in cases involving emergency physicians, radiologists, hospitalists, and other hospital-based physicians who are not employed by the hospital at issue.

CAUSATION

After establishing that a doctor or provider breached an applicable standard of care, it is next required to prove the breach was the legal cause of injury. Breaches of a standard of care alone are legally insufficient to establish the basis for a legal claim. An injury must result from the breach, or any related claim is without legal merit. If a patient is able to prove that there was a violation of the standard of care but cannot prove that the violation was the cause of the alleged injury, the patient will not win the case.

Causation is a legal term that has deep roots in our justice system.[11] For purposes of medical malpractice litigation, causation simply means that the violation of the standard of care was (1) an actual cause and (2) a proximate cause of the alleged injury. For a violation of the standard of care to be an actual cause of the harm, the patient must prove that the alleged injury would not have occurred *but for* the violation of the standard of care. In the nonhealing ulcer case discussed earlier, the patient would have to prove that *but for* the failure to biopsy the ulcer, she would not have needed exenteration.

In addition to being an actual cause of the alleged injury, the violation of the standard of care must also be a proximate cause of the alleged injury. The patient would have to prove that the alleged injury was a type of injury that is a "foreseeable" result of the violation of the standard of care. Going back to the earlier nonhealing ulcer case, was exenteration a foreseeable result of the failure to biopsy? Assuming the patient developed a wound infection and died of sepsis, would the patient's family be able to prove that sepsis was a foreseeable result of the failure to biopsy?

Importantly, legal causation in the majority of state jurisdictions can be established even in the presence of other contributing causes of the claimed injury. For example, a doctor who negligently fails to administer an antibiotic to address an infection that was caused by conditions created by a different person or circumstance may be liable for the injurious worsening of the infection. The legal test for legal causation in most jurisdictions is what is widely referred to as the "substantial factor" test. Under this test, as long as the breach was a "substantial factor" in causing the injury, the breaching doctor may be fully liable for the resulting injury to the patient. Establishing legal causation in oncology cases is often far more critical to a determination of liability than is establishing breach. It is also often the most challenging for the patient to establish. Unlike causation in many medical malpractice cases, the doctor does not cause the harm: the physician can rarely be identified as a causative agent of a patient's cancer. Instead, these claims against doctors most often pertain to acts of omission, rather than acts of commission, focusing on the provider's failure to timely and appropriately diagnose or treat a cancer, prior to its metastasis, that the provider had no role in causing.

The wide variability between types of cancers in the relative ease or difficulty to diagnose the cancer prior to metastasis correlates with disparities in the numbers of successful legal claims among the variable types. In many instances, by the time a patient experiences symptoms within the differential for pancreatic cancer, it has already progressed beyond the point that a physician's intervention can make a difference in the patient's outcome. Consequently, successful claims regarding failure to diagnose pancreatic cancer are rare.

On the opposite end of the spectrum, successful claims regarding failure to diagnose lung cancer are far more common, principally because there is far more time and opportunity from the onset of symptoms in the diagnostic differential for the clinician to intervene with effective, lifesaving treatments for the patient. Cancers vary in how many symptoms support a clinical suspicion for malignancy, and some cancer symptoms are shared with more common, less concerning conditions. The early stages of ovarian cancer, for example, rarely produce symptoms. In advanced stages of ovarian cancer, the patient may experience nonspecific symptoms, such as nausea, stomach aches, and lower back pain, which are easily mistaken for more common benign conditions. Thus, if a clinician is judged to be negligent in failing to suspect ovarian cancer after numerous office visits in which the patient has complained of these symptoms, the patient would still have to prove that at the time the clinician should have suspected cancer and intervened, the intervention would have prevented the adverse outcome.

In failure-to-diagnose cancer cases, very often the interpretive results of the radiologist are at the heart of the breach, such as an instance where the radiologist misses or misidentifies a carcinoma on the film. In other instances, the radiologist correctly identifies a concerning structure and recommends the treating doctor order an ultrasound to better visualize a suspected carcinoma. When, in the latter instance, the treating doctor fails to perform the ultrasound and the undetected malignancy predictably advances to an untreatable stage of cancer, it is the doctor's, not the radiologist's, breach that provides the basis for the ensuing lawsuit. Yet, despite the clean logical sequence of these two patterns leading, alternatively, to liability for the radiologist or the treating doctor, legal causation in either case may not yet be provable. In both cases, the plaintiff would still have to prove that the patient's injurious or fatal outcome could have been avoided if the radiologist or treating doctor had not breached the applicable standard of care.

Determining legal causation in a cancer case is often very difficult because of the many variables that must be considered. It is sometimes impossible to state with clinical certainty that a patient would have survived if the doctor had not breached the standard of care in treating the patient. Thus, in many jurisdictions, the causation question is framed in terms of whether the doctor's breach of the standard of care caused the patient to lose an important chance to improve.

The prior ovarian cancer example leads to a legal principle where a patient's chance of survival decreased because of the alleged delay in diagnosis. Traditionally, when a patient has a greater than 50% chance of dying from the pre-existing condition even without the alleged negligence, the defendant-doctor may not be found liable for negligence. The pre-existing cancer, for example, is the cause of death, not the delay in cancer diagnosis.

Some states, however, have relaxed this legal principle and created what is known as the "loss of chance" doctrine. Loss of chance theory considers the value of the patient's lost chance of recovery or survival due to a delay in diagnosis or treatment. The loss of chance doctrine essentially states that a patient can still prove causation as long as he or she is able to prove that the alleged violation of the standard of care reduced the patient's chance of survival, even if that chance of survival was less than 50% to begin with. For example, a pancreatic cancer patient whose chance of survival is 40% even absent negligence can still prove causation as long as he or she can prove that the alleged violation of the standard of care reduced that chance of survival. In this case, the physician who violated the standard of care is liable for 40% of the patient's harm because he or she deprived the patient of 40% of the chance of survival. Many states, however, have not adopted the loss of chance doctrine.

Similar to standard of care experts, most cases involve causation experts. Often, the standard of care expert in a cancer case is also selected to provide the expert opinion on legal causation because the qualifications of a good standard of care expert are sometimes closely matched with those of a good causation expert in a particular case. However, in many instances, it is the primary care doctor who misses the differential in a cancer case, and the breach was the primary care doctor's failure to refer the patient to a cancer specialist. In these instances, the standard of care expert and the causation expert may share very few qualifications apart from their foundational medical training.

Here, it is important to note that the "standard of proof" or threshold in proving causation is "preponderance of evidence." While it may sound like a high threshold, it simply is not. All it requires is that the weight of evidence "more likely than not" favors the argument. To put it in mathematical terms, "more likely than not" simply means there is a 51% chance that the argument is true. This is a sharp contrast to the weight of evidence in criminal cases, where the standard of proof is "beyond reasonable doubt." In the earlier nonhealing ulcer case, the causation argument would be something like "more likely than not, if biopsy was done during the initial consult, the patient would not have needed exenteration." Would the patient still have needed exenteration even if a biopsy was done during the initial visit? Possibly, but if the patient's expert is able to prove that there was a 51% chance that she would not have needed exenteration if the biopsy was done sooner, then the patient has established causation.

On the contrary, if the outcome would have been the same despite the alleged violation of the standard of care, the patient will not win the case. For example, a radiologist recommended in her report a pelvic ultrasound. The treating doctor, however, did not order the ultrasound. After about three months, the patient was diagnosed with an advanced-stage ovarian cancer and needed surgery and chemotherapy. Assume that the failure to order the pelvic ultrasound is a violation of the standard of care. In this case, the defendant-doctor can still win the case if the patient is not able to prove by preponderance of evidence that the treatment needs, outcome, and prognosis would have been better but for the defendant-doctor's failure to order the ultrasound at issue.

DAMAGES

Because medical malpractice falls within the civil law system and not the criminal law system, the remedy provided is meant to compensate the injured person rather than punish the wrongdoer. As such, the remedy is payment to the injured person rather than jail time to the wrongdoer. This payment is based on a damages category called compensatory damages and is divided into two general categories: economic and noneconomic damages.

Economic damages include (1) cost for past, present, and future medical treatment and (2) loss of income and loss of earning capacity. When presenting the cost for past medical expenses to the jury, typically, one of the patient's experts would testify that the charges are reasonable and necessary.

Due to a legal doctrine called the collateral source rule, in most states, evidence of any health insurance payments related to the alleged injury is not admissible. Thus, the jury is prevented from knowing and considering whether or not the patient had medical insurance. Likewise, the patient is not allowed to tell the jury that the doctor has malpractice insurance that will pay for any resulting damages.

Note, however, that the health insurer of the patient will have a right to get all their money back, in the form of a medical lien. Health insurance providers are entitled to this repayment as long as the expense was related to the injury at issue and only if the patient recovers any money from the case. In most cases, however, plaintiff attorneys are able to request a lien reduction, especially if the settlement or award is not significantly higher than the lien.

As to future medical expenses, plaintiffs often have a life care planner who provides a report as to the future needs of the patient, including medical treatment and supplies, caregiver needs, and household modifications. An economist is also often retained to place a dollar value, adjusted to yearly inflation, to these future needs.

Noneconomic damages, on the other hand, include payment for pain and suffering. They also include payment for physical disfigurement, mental anguish, and poor quality of life. There is no formula to calculate for pain and suffering damages, and the amount is typically an arbitrary amount set by the jury to reasonably compensate for the alleged pain and suffering. Noneconomic damages also include damages claimed by a family member, typically the spouse, under what is called a loss of consortium claim. Loss of consortium simply means deprivation of benefits of the relationship because of the injury suffered by the patient. This loss of relationship includes loss of affection, intimacy, and support.

In many states, noneconomic damages are capped by statutory laws to a certain maximum amount. Thus, even if the jury awards millions of dollars for pain and suffering, if the statutory cap is $250,000, the court will reduce by law the noneconomic damages award to the maximum cap. Recently, however, some state courts have held that caps for noneconomic damages violate certain constitutional rights and thus have eliminated these limits.[12] Most states do not cap economic damages.

In addition to the compensatory damages described earlier, there is another category of damages called punitive damages. While compensatory damages are meant to compensate for the injuries suffered by the patient, punitive damages are meant to deter the wrongdoer's conduct. In rare cases that involve actual malice or willful misconduct, punitive damages may be awarded to the plaintiff. Similarly, in cases that involve gross negligence or extreme indifference or reckless disregard to patient safety, a patient may also be awarded punitive damages. Although rarely awarded, most states allow punitive damages in medical malpractice. Moreover, cases involving willful misconduct or willful disregard for the safety of others may be brought in to the criminal court system.

OTHER CAUSES OF ACTION: SURVIVAL ACTION AND WRONGFUL DEATH

A survival action is brought by the personal representative of the estate of the decedent, on behalf of the decedent. In this action, the estate seeks to recover damages that the decedent would have brought had he or she survived the alleged injury. Therefore, this cause of action includes damages for medical expenses and loss of income of the patient while still alive, causally related to the alleged negligence. It also includes any alleged pain and suffering while the patient was still conscious, causally related to the alleged negligence.

A wrongful death action is brought by the next of kin of the decedent and seeks to recover damages related to the death of the patient. Unlike a survival action, the damages sought here are damages for the loved ones of the decedent, not for the decedent himself or herself. Damages here typically include pain and suffering; loss of care, affection, and companionship; loss of consortium; and loss of financial support to the family.

Both survival action and wrongful death causes of action are typically filed together in lawsuits where a patient's death is allegedly caused by medical malpractice.

CONCLUSION

While no patient or medical doctor wants to be a party in a medical malpractice suit, our justice system ensures that there is a forum to hear complaints based on the rule of law. In summary, medical malpractice is based on the law of negligence, where the plaintiff must prove four elements: (1) a duty to provide reasonable care; (2) a breach of that duty, specifically, a violation of the standard of care; (3) the violation of the standard of care was an actual and a proximate cause of the injury; and (4) resulting damages. Duty is typically created when there is a doctor-patient relationship. A violation in the standard of care is the failure to provide the kind of care that an average doctor with similar training and background would have or should have provided under the same situation. After establishing that a doctor or provider breached an applicable standard of care, it is next required to prove the breach was the legal cause of injury. And lastly, there must be damages that resulted from the breach of that duty, including economic and noneconomic damages.

References:

1. Makary MA, Daniel M. Medical error: the third leading cause of death in the US. *BMJ* 2016;353:i2139.
2. Deaths and mortality. Centers for Disease Control and Prevention, National Center for Health Statistics. https://www.cdc.gov/nchs/fastats/deaths.htm. Accessed August 5, 2021. Numbers are rounded.
3. Provisional mortality data—United States 2020. Centers for Disease Control and Prevention. https://www.cdc.gov/mmwr/volumes/70/wr/mm7014e1.htm. Accessed August 5, 2021.
4. Center for Diagnostic Excellence. Armstrong Institute for Patient Safety and Quality, Johns Hopkins Medicine. https://www.hopkinsmedicine.org/armstrong_institute/centers/center_for_diagnostic_excellence/index.html. Accessed August 5, 2021.
5. Johns Hopkins Medicine researchers identify health conditions likely to be misdiagnosed. Johns Hopkins Medicine. July 11, 2019. https://www.hopkinsmedicine.org/news/newsroom/news-releases/johns-hopkins-medicine-researchers-identify-health-conditions-likely-to-be-misdiagnosed. Accessed August 5, 2021.
6. See, for example, *Mead v Legacy Health System*, 352 Ore 267 (2009). Merely providing advice to a colleague about that colleague's patient does not give rise to a physician-patient relationship.
7. *Warren v Dinter*, 926 NW2d 370 (Minn App 2018). Holding that a physician who was on a call with a nurse practitioner seeking advice can be sued for malpractice because he knew or should have known that his decision regarding whether or not to admit a patient would be relied on by the nurse practitioner.

8. *Majzoub v Appling*, 95 SW3d 432 (Tex App 2002). When a physician undertakes an affirmative action to treat a patient, the physician's consent to establish a physician-patient relationship may then be implied. See also *Anderson v Houser*, 240 Ga App 613 (1999). The key question in determining the existence of a doctor-patient relationship is whether the physician has knowingly accepted such individual as his patient.

9. Emergency Medical Treatment and Labor Act, 42 USC § 1395dd(d)(1).

10. *Ritchie v Krasner, MD, et al.*, 211 P3d 1272 (Ariz Ct App 2009). But see *Hafner v Beck*, 185 Ariz 389 (1995), explaining that a doctor is not liable for medical malpractice where a doctor conducts an examination of an injured employee only for the purpose of evaluating disability for the insurance carrier and the doctor neither offers nor provides treatment to the injured worker.

11. See, for example, *Palsgraf v Long Island Railroad Co.*, a US Supreme Court case in 1928 about the scope of liability in negligence cases. The Palsgraf case involved a woman standing on a railroad platform who was injured when a passenger, attempting to board a train in haste and who was pushed by a guard to help him, dropped a package containing fireworks. The explosion caused some scales at the platform to fall and injure the woman. The justices analyzed whether the railroad company's alleged negligence proximately caused her injuries.

12. See, for example, *North Broward Hospital District v Kalitan*, 219 So 3d 49 (2017), holding that Florida caps on personal injury noneconomic damages in medical negligence actions violated the constitution's equal protection law because the statutory caps arbitrarily reduced damage awards to plaintiffs with the most drastic injuries.

CHAPTER 2

Informed Consent

Ana E. Dvoredsky, MD, MJ

INTRODUCTION

Consent is a phenomenon that happens every day in social transactions. In a tacit and often unaware manner, people defer to someone else's choice to determine their own conduct ("Here are clothes for you to change into before your x-ray."—"Sure!" or "Take this pill every morning."—"I will!"). There are many assumptions in those interactions: that shirt or pants will fit and size is the only variable in question or that the person is able to swallow pills. Because of the many unknown parameters, the result of an interaction where an unaware consent has been given ranges from an enthusiastic "I understand" to an irritated "I don't like this." It is important to remember that whenever people consent to someone else's choices, they are providing an *active* giving up of control of the decision.

Between 2015 and 2017, US courts heard 916 cases dealing with medical informed consent. Notably, about two-thirds of these cases were unreported,[1] meaning that they replicated previous cases or used two or three courts for the same case. But this is just the tip of the iceberg because the majority of legal conflicts are resolved through conversation, direct payment, negotiation, legal mediation, insurance company intervention, or simply abandonment by the affected party.[2] None of these out-of-court methods provide a learning experience to other practitioners because they do not result in a published, public judicial opinion. Thus, the number of published cases does not reflect the significant physician, attorney, and court time that is used to resolve problems regarding informed consent, and the need for informed consent is still often treated by most practitioners as an irritation.

Legal conflict regarding informed consent is considered to be a type of medical malpractice claim.[3] Because most of these cases are resolved privately in mediation[4] and most legal decisions are not published, only a tiny fraction of this unpleasant legal experience is used to teach peers in order to improve their medical practice. Practitioners could do well by learning from others' errors and improving their own methods of obtaining informed consent.

INFORMED CONSENT IN MEDICAL CARE

Informed consent deals with a specific subarea of consent, where certain terms of the verbal or written exchange between doctor and patient are clearly specified because it is thought that such terms are important ("Here are clothes for your x-rays. Are you very cold?" — "Yes, I need a blanket."; "Take this pill every morning. Can you swallow pills?" — "No, I choke on them. Do you have the medicine available in a syrup?").

In the health care environment, such as cancer care, any consent *must* be made open and explicit rather than tacit and implicit. The reason for the extra care is that the cost of misunderstanding in health care settings is too high because it may result in the patient's death. Before the 20th century, clinical terminology did not appear as an element in legal conflicts between patients and physicians.[5] But once patients began to resort to the courts in situations fraught with misunderstandings, the law stepped in, assisting medical care by forcing physicians gradually to make consent obvious when necessary and providing structure to its steps. Rather than looking at the courts as the enemy, one might see them as assisting physicians by defining components precisely when the medical profession was not able to do it by itself.[6-15]

INFORMED CONSENT IN MEDICAL CARE FROM THE LEGAL POINT OF VIEW

Informed consent means that a patient agrees to a clinician's idea or proposal while possessing reliable knowledge upon which to base that agreement.[16] But it also requires that this "sufficient knowledge" must be obtained *with a sound mind*. Therefore, under the law, informed consent does not exist without the patient's **competency** ("Take this medication every morning. Sir, do you know what this medication is for?"). This is an important additional factor. While clinicians often remember the need to ensure that the patient is an active participant in decisions that affect their well-being, courts have helped us remember that it is essential to *ensure and document* that the patient is **competent**. Competency is *the mental ability to understand problems and make decisions*.[17] This ability needs to be evaluated and documented *at the time the decision is made*. The treating physician is able to make this evaluation with some simple tools that help document that the patient is alert, oriented, aware of the environment, and cognizant of the staff around them, the illness, and the treatment. Not included in this definition, but equally important from a legal point of view, is the patient's physical ability to make a decision. This is called *capacity*, or "the ability to do the job." Both competency and capacity are abilities that a physician may be called to assess in a legal determination.[18]

Physicians need to be aware that patients who are cognitively compromised may oscillate in their state of awareness and display changes in alertness throughout the day or around medication dosing. The patient may appear aware at some hours of the day and not at others, and the interview may give different results depending on the patient's current state of consciousness. A metastatic colon cancer patient may just have taken a large dose of morphine for her bone pain or she may be sun downing. Should there be any question about the patient's alertness and competency and if the treating physician is not able or confident to make the diagnosis of competency, a consultant should be engaged. A psychiatrist or neuropsychologist would be most helpful in this situation.

If the patient is not competent to consent to treatment, decisions must be reviewed with someone who has been given a power of attorney to make such choices (such as a relative or friend) because any decisions made by the patient in an incompetent state will not be legally enforceable and will place the physician in a vulnerable position. An incompetent patient cannot consent to chemotherapy, radiation therapy, or surgery. The physician or surgeon needs to work very closely with the patient, understand the wishes of the patient, and gain a clear sense of the family's or significant other's support in order to enforce consent at the proper time.

INFORMED CONSENT IN RESEARCH ACTIVITIES

Medical research is ahead of the clinical setting in terms of its demands for informed consent.[19-21] This may be due to governmental intervention as a result of the allocation of research grants or the extensive joint participation of research bodies.[22] Informed consent requirements for subjects participating in research are exact, specific, and under the control of institutional research boards (IRBs) in the organizations where the research is carried out.

In 2003, a study of 113 US medical school research groups evaluated the forms for readability and found that they scored at the 10th-grade level according to one scale and the 12th- to 13th-grade level according to another.[23] Federal law requires that research informed consent forms must be set at basic readability levels.[24] Readability is considered to be a safety standard,[25] and courts have determined repeatedly that consent, to be considered *informed* by legal standards, must be legible and understandable and include all information the patient needs.[14,26] The principal research physician is ultimately responsible for the correct completion of this process.

Informed consent for research activities must be reviewed and approved by an organization's IRB. There are many sources from which to model informed consent forms for research; the most reliable is the National Institutes of Health (NIH) website. Significant assistance regarding informed consent forms can be found at the NIH and PubMed websites, as well as by consulting a local IRB. While legal support may be provided by the IRB, it is good practice to always ensure that the readability of the consent forms is at the sixth-grade level to confirm that patients or research subjects truly understand that to which they are consenting. This is required by law and is also a condition of funding in many grants.

THE COMPONENTS OF INFORMED CONSENT

Elements that constitute a proper understanding and provide consent have been discussed since the late 1970s. After multiple legal challenges, with the support of the courts, the legal definition of informed consent now includes the following elements[12-15]:

- A patient must have obtained knowledge and understanding of:
  a. The disorder
  b. The natural course of the illness without any treatment
  c. The treatment proposed by the team
  d. The benefits and risks of the proposed treatment
  e. The benefits and risks of alternative available treatments
- The physician or team must answer any questions the patient has.

It is important to remember that informed consent is *part of the physician-patient relationship*, not just a legal requirement. Sometimes this portion of clinical care gets lost in the modern practice of medicine, where everything happens fast and so much of medicine is completed in digital form. A clinician needs to keep in mind that this phase of care may be emotionally laden. It should focus on the patients, their needs, and their particular concerns ("You are an athlete and will be confined to a chair for 3 months") and should be at a level of literacy that is consistent with their education. All these aspects need to be discussed *before* the patient undergoes treatment and must be documented at the time the conversation is held.

WHO IS RESPONSIBLE FOR OBTAINING INFORMED CONSENT?

Legally, informed consent is part of the care provided by the attending physician. Most states will have clarified this responsibility in a law, which can be found under the state's public health law statutes. The wording will involve terms similar to the following: "the person providing the professional treatment or diagnosis."[27] Residents, nurses, and other assistants will be considered to be "individuals acting in place of the treating physician," but ultimately, it is the treating physician who will maintain responsibility and liability. Whatever the mechanics of the paperwork at the site of care, the physician must always keep in mind that ensuring a patient's understanding of the illness and its treatment is a critical part of the clinician-patient relationship.

Any time a physician delegates this responsibility to another member of the treatment team, it is important that the physician in charge keep track of the place where informed consent was obtained and the wording and conditions of the consent because the responsibility will always ultimately remain in the treating physician's hands. For instance, Dr. Jesse Crump, a 63-year-old practicing physician, began to show polyuria, nocturia, and confusion. A magnetic resonance imaging (MRI) scan and other tests revealed an ectopic germinoma near the pituitary gland. A neurosurgeon was to do the surgery; his resident took the history, performed the physical exam, and obtained the informed consent. Dr. Crump suffered surgical complications, with visual sequelae. He claimed liability for injuries and lack of informed consent. Although the neurosurgeon clarified that his resident obtained the informed consent, the court dismissed the resident from the case as a defendant. The court ruled that the resident's failure to obtain proper informed consent imposed liability on the neurosurgeon, who was ultimately in charge of treatment, but no liability on the resident or the hospital.[28] Liability always remained with the neurosurgeon because he was the physician who performed the treatment.

INFORMED CONSENT IN THE CLINICAL CHART

Data that physicians and hospitals collect about a patient may legally belong to the patient, but the documents themselves belong to the providers of care (not necessarily the health professional). A bureaucracy has been created to ensure that data are obtained, maintained, selected, and transmitted according to protocol. There are new professionals who ensure that records are created according to legal standards and procedure, under the purview of the health care provider, records professionals, and attorneys. Physicians need to become familiar with the geographic situation of the forms in every setting where they work. When providing care, physicians are best served by reviewing consent forms obtained and filed by assistants and other professionals because the physicians will ultimately be responsible for those records.

IF IT'S ALL SO CLEAR, WHY DO LEGAL DISPUTES ARISE ABOUT INFORMED CONSENT?

Informed consent has been on the minds of practicing physicians throughout the ages, always deferential to therapeutic outcomes, within the social norms of the times. As time and customs have changed, so has the practice of obtaining informed consent. What used to be a very personal, private process between the physician and patient,[29-31] who had formed a long relationship where both parties knew each other fairly well, has changed. In modern health care, physicians have new concerns of which they need to be aware.

Take, for example, Arthur, who is going for a routine colonoscopy. He has seen the physician in the office for 15 minutes and scheduled the procedure with the associate for three weeks later. Tests have been obtained and cleared, and nurses have examined him. On the day of the procedure, Arthur has been premedicated and is ready to undergo the procedure. As the physician comes into the procedure room, fully masked and putting on his gloves, and as the nurse anesthetist places the IV cannula into Arthur's left arm, the operating room nurse places a board with a paper in front of Arthur's face and a pen in his right hand and tells Arthur he needs to sign a consent form prior to anesthesia. Would this consent procedure survive a legal challenge from Arthur? *Keep in mind the purpose of informed consent: it is the process through which the patient comes to learn and understand the illness and possible treatment and finally agrees or rejects the proposed course of action. The form is simply an objective proof of that process. We know Arthur signed a form, but did he provide informed consent?*

A variety of different events may give rise to legal concerns about a patient's informed consent.

Informed consent was not obtained

If an informed consent is not obtained at all, all procedures are unwarranted. This rule was first enunciated in the *Mohr* case in 1905,[6] and it still holds true: "the free citizen's first and greatest right – which underlies all others – the right to himself . . . If it was unauthorized, then it was . . . unlawful." This concept was later confirmed by Justice Cardozo in 1914[8] in simple words: "Every human being of adult years and sound mind has a right to determine what shall be done with his own body, and a surgeon who performs an operation without the patient's consent commits an assault." There is no shortcut to this rule.

Informed consent was incomplete

Sometimes a clinician sees a case as so clear and obvious that he or she neglects to discuss alternative diagnoses or possible options with the patient. In fact, the treating physician may also downplay complications with the assisting staff to the extent that care is compromised. Physicians need to keep in mind all alternative options, even in these times of supposedly superb diagnostic tools. One must recall that pathologic exams still provide surprises, and there is no such thing as certainty before treatment. In addition, new therapeutic options always provide the possibility of long-term effects currently unknown to medical science. These concepts should be shared with the patient and documented in the chart.

For example, Jerry Canterbury, a young man, suffered from back pain. Following an abnormal myelogram, his neurosurgeon suspected a ruptured disk and suggested a laminectomy. After a complex operatory and post-operatory period, many complications ensued, terminating in paralysis that affected the patient's life forever. He brought legal action against his physician for negligence. Mr. Canterbury felt that the surgery had been represented to him as a simple, low-risk procedure but then found himself in a situation that had not been presented to him in a clear manner. He claimed he would not have agreed to the surgery had he known of the possibility of paralysis.[12] His lawsuit became a landmark case, both for lawyers and physicians, because the court helped define the components of informed consent.

Informed consent does not include significant parts of the illness or complications

The physician is not always sure about how much of their clinical reasoning should be shared with the patient, including their alternative hypotheses and doubts. This is a very valid point. In addition, while physicians are explaining their reasoning, patients may not be able to follow along, even if they are seemingly agreeing to what is being said. Sometimes the patient may be unable to comprehend the information at that particular time because of emotional factors. At times, there may be more than one professional providing care, or the patient may receive care in more than one setting. All of these variables highlight the need to ensure that informed consent conversations occur and are documented.

For example, Timothy Keogan, a 37-year-old man, consulted his physician due to chest pain. The physician suspected angina but had no actual test proof. He did not tell Mr. Keogan of his hypothesis or schedule follow-up with angiography, treadmill test, or nitroglycerin test. Instead, the physician indicated decreased activities and follow-up, with some alternative diagnoses. Apparently, Mr. Keogan was resistant to the thought that he might have cardiac disease at his age. In the following week, his symptoms worsened; he collapsed and was taken to the emergency room, where poor communication resulted in complications and he died of a myocardial infarction on that same day. Legal action was brought by his wife and estate.[32]

The court in this case clarified the principles of informed consent in difficult situations. The language was very clear and should be easy to remember by physicians:

1. Inconclusive symptoms should not prevent the physician from providing enough information to obtain informed consent. It is the physician's duty to tell a patient all possible diagnoses, especially if there is a potentially fatal disease in the differential.

2. A review of diagnostic hypotheses with the patient, prior to any diagnostic tests, is essential in creating informed consent. Without a review of all possible diagnoses, the patient is unable to weigh all testing and therapeutic options.

3. Informed consent *must include any unpleasant arguing with the patient* regarding diagnoses the patient does not want to hear about. It is true that sometimes physicians avoid those conversations with patients when bad news or issues the patient does not want to hear are involved. But it *is* part of the job to speak about difficult topics with difficult patients. This is another step in the path to partnership in patient health care.

The requirement to obtain informed consent is activated *any time it becomes necessary for the patient to do something specific* to confirm or refute a diagnosis.

Options were not discussed

Every single option must be provided to the patient in the case of treatment. In fact, it is suggested that, after all alternatives and possible findings are considered, the physician should raise the possibility of unknown findings or consequences. This is of particular importance in oncology, where there is an abundance of new treatments and some effects are not known for years. In fact, it was in this area that legal cases resulted in the rule that *all possible outcomes be revealed, including all information available at the time of treatment*.[13,14]

For example, Irma Natanson was diagnosed with a cancerous tumor; the tumor was excised, and she received cobalt radiation treatment. After treatment, the remaining tissue showed no cancerous cells, but she suffered radiation burns. The court found that although she had been properly treated, she had not been properly informed of the full risks of the treatment, as the radiation burns had not been addressed.[10]

RESULTS OF LEGAL ACTIONS

Court cases of medical malpractice for any reason, including incomplete or absent informed consent, are extremely unpleasant. Physicians and patients who previously worked in cooperation are placed on opposing sides in bitter disputes. Ultimately, it becomes a "he said–she said" situation. Statements made by patients are considered to be facts. While the patient, as the plaintiff in the case, has the burden of proof, physicians are required to prove their positions, which they most often do through documentation, as well as through opinions of colleagues and other processes.

Often, the parties will present statements that appear as if two separate realities occurred at the same time. This may be the truth, as both parties may have been using language that was interpreted differently by each other. Until the late 1970s, the courts accepted what was known as "standards of care" for informed consent. This meant that a physician was expected to tell the patient what most practitioners would tell a patient under the same circumstances. Gradually, the emphasis changed. Physicians are now expected to tell patients what they need to know in order to make an adequate choice.[13] This is quite different. Now, the critical factor to the courts is not whether the information was given in a manner acceptable to any *physician*, but whether the *patient*, any patient, would understand the information provided.

HOW TO BEST OBTAIN CONSENT

Obtaining informed consent is a process; merely asking the patient to sign a form is not enough. Likewise, it is not sufficient to have a good relationship with the patient. There are some landmark cases where the patient liked the physician very much but was quite unhappy with some specific result of the treatment.[13] Clear communication of goals and expectations must be included in the process. A number of well-designed studies carried out since the 1970s show that, despite the best attitudes and broadest efforts by medical staff to share information, it is quite likely that patients will not remember the data provided by the health care providers, and sometimes, they will not even remember that someone talked to them.[19,20,33–35] A proper informed consent, acceptable under the law, will not be obtained as long as the attitude among professionals and patients alike is that *informed consent is just a ritual obligated by the lawyers to protect the physicians*. Informed consent is far more than a ritual. It is a method by which the patient learns about the illness and options to manage it and arrives at a decision in a shared process with the treating physician. This shared decision-making process is essential to the patients and to the courts, and it cannot be bypassed.[26]

Wanting to share information with a patient is also not enough. Information must be shared in language that is easy to understand by patients, and the same is true for consent forms. The treating clinician should ensure that patients understand the content of what they are being told. Informed consent forms written by attorneys using technical legal and medical jargon are mostly unreadable to the average individual. These forms can become more accessible to a patient if a staff member assists the patient by explaining the meaning of the words. Still, it is essential that the patient actually understands all elements of informed consent, as delineated earlier, and that such understanding be documented in the chart.[13,26]

Health literacy has been accepted as an effective part of daily patient treatment for over 20 years, and its effects on patient recovery have been proven repeatedly. Numerous publications show the positive effects of patient education, as well as the variety of education methods available.[35–39] These positive effects include better patient recollection of important elements of the illness and treatment options, increased patient participation in decision making and in activities that improve outcome, and patient acceptance of limitations. Today, the concept of *health literacy* includes many of the elements previously sought to be fulfilled in the brief encounter known as "obtaining informed consent," with the exception of the conversation with the physician. A clinician can use available methods to provide health literacy to enhance the patient's understanding of the illness and management, as required in the informed consent legal requirements, and document in the chart that such steps have been taken.

For example, Elizabeth is a 25-year-old woman who has been recently diagnosed with breast cancer. She is married and has a two-year-old child, but she always dreamt about having at least three children. Her husband is very supportive and will remain with her throughout her treatment. Some serious decisions need to be made regarding her treatment, not immediately but urgently. Her oncologist begins by referring her to a health educator from the clinic, gives her reading material to evaluate, and offers her a referral to a counselor and a follow-up appointment in a week to discuss all treatment alternatives. At the next appointment, the oncologist evaluates the level of health literacy Elizabeth has obtained and realizes that, although she and her husband have learned a great deal about her cancer, they are still unclear about the various treatment options.

At this point, one should obtain feedback from the counselor. Consider Elizabeth's need to receive personal instruction from specialists through consultation for each treatment option, as well as referral to a survivor's group. It is important to document each step in the chart and not make final decisions until the couple appears to fully understand the illness and treatment options and the consequences of each.

CONCLUSION

Modern medicine sees informed consent as a necessary step in most medical activities where "something must be done," not only for medical and surgical procedures, but also for medical, surgical, and genetic testing, as well as therapies and interventions that will affect future generations. Diagnoses that involve family members, including descendants, collaterals, and spouses, open a significant and most interesting new door for future need for informed consent. As is true in all sciences, the sophistication of the methodology will come far sooner than the wisdom of those using it. Informed consent is not simply a matter of autonomy and sharing of information. A certain modicum of insight and prudence is necessary, which the courts will need to keep in mind.

The informed consent should involve a session between the clinician and the patient that should occur once the patient has achieved health literacy in their illness and treatment, and this session should be dedicated to discussing any particular questions the patient might have regarding their own situation.[40]

One must always keep in mind that the goal is not to have a signed form, but to protect the patient's engagement in the care process, as that is the only way to become a decision partner in care. The signed form only documents that the process took place.

Further Readings

Alahmad G. Informed consent in pediatric oncology: a systematic review of qualitative literature. *Cancer Control.* 2018;25(1):1073274818773720.

Berg J, Appelbaum P, Lidz C, Parker L. *Informed Consent. Legal Theory and Clinical Practice.* 2nd ed. Oxford, United Kingdom: Oxford University Press; 2001.

Federman DD, Hanna KE, Rodriguez LL, eds. *Responsible Research: A Systems Approach to Protecting Research Participants.* Washington, DC: National Academies Press; 2002.

French MG, Wojtowicz A, eds. *Health Literacy in Clinical Research: Practice and Impact: Proceedings of a Workshop.* Washington, DC: National Academies Press; 2020.

Gillies K, Duthie A, Cotton S, Campbell MK. Patient reported measures of informed consent for clinical trials: a systematic review. *PLoS One.* 2018;13(6):e0199775.

Grisso T, Appelbaum PS. *Assessing Competence to Consent to Treatment.* Oxford, United Kingdom: Oxford University Press; 1998.

Miller F, Wertheimer A. *The Ethics of Consent.* Oxford, United Kingdom: Oxford University Press; 2010.

Nathe JM, Krakow EF. The challenges of informed consent in high-stakes, randomized oncology trials: a systematic review. *MDM Policy Pract.* 2019;4(1):2381468319840322.

References:

1. An unpublished opinion is a court decision that is not available for citation as precedent by future courts or lawyers because the court deemed the case to have insufficient precedential value.
2. Lexis-Nexis search performed on December 12, 2018.
3. DeWolf DK, Allen KW. *Tort and Law Practice*. 4th ed. Washington Practice Series. Vol 16. New York, NY: Thomson Reuters; 2013.
4. Holbrook JR. Negotiating, mediating, and arbitrating physician-patient conflicts. *Clin Obstet Gynecol*. 2008; 51(4):719–730.
5. Westlaw search performed on December 15, 2018.
6. *Mohr v Williams*, 95 Minn 261 (1905).
7. *Pratt v Davis*, 224 Ill 300, Sup Ct Ill (1906).
8. *Schloendorff v Society of New York Hospitals*, 211 NY 125, 126, 105 NE 92, 93 (1914).
9. *Salgo v Leland Stanford Jr University Board of Trustees*, 154 Cal App 2d 560 (1957).
10. *Natanson v Kline*, 186 Kan 393 (1960).
11. *Wilkinson v Vesey*, 110 RI 606 (1972).
12. *Canterbury v Spence*, 464 F2d 772 (1972).
13. *Archer v Galbraith*, 18 Wash App 369 (1977).
14. *ZeBarth v Swedish Hospital*, 81 Wash 2d 12, En Banc (1972).
15. *Truman v Thomas*, 27 Cal 3d 285 (1980).
16. Garner B, ed. *Black's Law Dictionary*. 10th ed. New York, NY: Thomson Reuters; 2014. "A voluntary yielding to what another proposes or desires, agreement, approval or permission regarding some act or purpose, especially given voluntarily by a competent person."
17. Garner B, ed. *Black's Law Dictionary*. 10th ed. New York, NY: Thomson Reuters; 2014.
18. Bisbing SB. Competency and capacity: a primer. In: Sanbar SS, Gibofsky A, Firestone MH, et al., eds. *Legal Medicine*. 4th ed. St. Louis, MO: Mosby; 1998:32–43.
19. Cassileth BR, Zupkis RV, Sutton-Smith K, March V. Informed consent: why are its goals imperfectly realized? *N Engl J Med*. 1980;302:896–900.
20. Hutson MM, Blaha JD. Patients' recall of preoperative instruction for informed consent for an operation. *J Bone Joint Surg Am*. 1991;73(2):160–162.
21. Bergler JH, Pennington AC, Metcalfe M, Freis ED. Informed consent: how much does the patient understand? *Clin Pharmacol Ther*. 1980;27(4):435–440.
22. Informed Consent, DHEW Publication No. CFR 45-46.103. Washington, DC: Government Printing Office; 1976.
23. Paasche-Orlow MK, Taylor HA, Brancati FL. Readability standards for informed-consent forms as compared with actual readability. *N Engl J Med*. 2003;348:721–726.
24. Health literacy. US Department of Health and Human Services. https://www.ahrq.gov/topics/health-literacy.html. Accessed August 2, 2021.
25. Weiss BD. *Health Literacy and Patient Safety: Help Patients Understand*. 2007. American Medical Association. http://www.hhvna.com/files/Courses/HealthLiteracy/Health_Literacy_Manual_AMA_Revised.pdf. Accessed August 2, 2021.
26. King NMP. Consent and the courts: the emergence of legal doctrine. In: Faden R, Bauchamp T, eds. *A History and Theory of Informed Consent*. Oxford, United Kingdom: Oxford University Press; 1986:124.
27. New York Public Health Law § 2805–d(1).
28. *Crump v Patterson*, US District Court, WL 437692, No 92 Civ 871 (HB) (Not Reported in F. Supp. 1995).
29. Garrison FH. *An Introduction to the History of Medicine*. Philadelphia, PA: W.B. Saunders; 1966.
30. Dunn PM. Maimonides (1135-1204) and his philosophy of medicine. *Arch Dis Child Fetal Neonatal Ed*. 1998;79:227–228.
31. Rush B. *On the Vices and Virtues of Physicians*. Philadelphia, PA: Bradford and Innskeep; 1745.

32. *Keogan v Holy Family Hospital*, 95 Wash 2d 306, Supreme Court of Washington, En Banc (1980).

33. Robinson G, Merav A. Informed consent: recall tested postoperatively. *Ann Thorac Surg.* 1976;22(3):209–212.

34. Morrow G, Gootnik J, Schmale A. A simple technique for increasing cancer patients' knowledge of informed consent to treatment. *Cancer.* 1978;42:793–799.

35. Mazzuca S. Does patient education in chronic disease have therapeutic value? *J Chronic Dis.* 1982;35(7):521–529.

36. Lorig KR, Mazonson PD, Holman HR. Evidence suggesting that health education for self-management in patients with chronic arthritis has sustained health benefits while reducing health care costs. *Arthritis Rheum.* 1993;36(4):439–446.

37. Rimer B, Jones WL, Keintz MK, Catalano RB, Engstrom PF. Informed consent: a crucial step in cancer patient education. *Health Educ Q.* 1984;10(suppl):30–42.

38. Greenfield S, Kaplan S, Ware J. Expanding patient involvement in care: effects on patient outcomes. *Ann Intern Med.* 1985;102(4):520–528.

39. Koelling TM, Johnson ML, Cody RJ, Aaronson KD. Discharge education improves clinical outcomes in patients with chronic heart failure. *Circulation.* 2005;111:179–185.

40. Dvoredsky AE. *Rashomon Revisited. Informed Consent in Medical Care* [master's thesis]. Seattle, WA: University of Washington School of Law; 2020.

CHAPTER 3

Depositions

Michelle S. Taft, JD

INTRODUCTION

Law and medicine have long been among the most highly regarded and most impactful fields chosen by professionals. As these two fields have evolved to become both more inclusive and more highly specialized in the late 20th and early 21st centuries, so too have they become inexorably intertwined. With this evolution, patient advocacy and patient responsibility for medical care have also grown, and lawsuits against physicians involving their care as treating providers and/or requiring physician expert testimony are common. As such, young physicians are often warned that they will likely one day become involved in a lawsuit, as a treating physician, an expert witness, or a defendant themselves.

Regardless of the physician's role in the litigation, the most important task that the physician will perform outside of the trial itself is to give a deposition. The purpose of a deposition is to allow the lawyers for the parties to ask questions of the physician relating to that physician's care and treatment of the patient if the physician is a treating provider or a defendant, or to ask for the physician's expert opinions following a review of the records and documents relating to the case. Deposition testimony is given under oath, can be used at the time of trial, and may have long-term consequences for the physician, regardless of whether the physician is a treating provider, an expert witness, or a defendant. It is therefore imperative that physicians understand their rights and responsibilities when giving depositions in order to provide clear, honest testimony and to avoid unintended consequences of poor deposition testimony.

The idea of a deposition is often daunting for physicians, especially those who have never been deposed before. This is not helped by the media's portrayal of the deposition process as an opportunity for lawyers to verbally attack and intimidate the person they are deposing. However, if approached with thorough preparation and representation by a lawyer, if desired, a deposition does not need to be intimidating or scary. Rather, the deposition is an opportunity for physicians to explain the facts they know, the facts they do not know, and the care they provided.

FORMAT OF A DEPOSITION

A deposition is sworn testimony taken orally in a question-and-answer format. Depositions typically occur when the parties engage in the discovery phase of a lawsuit, which is the time during the lawsuit that the parties exchange documents and information before the case goes to trial.

Lawyers use depositions for two primary purposes: (1) to learn information that may be relevant for their case and (2) to obtain sworn testimony that may later be used to help their case or hurt the other side's case. In addition to providing valuable information to the parties during the discovery process, depositions may be relied upon by expert witnesses and used at trial for the purpose of showing prior inconsistent testimony of a witness. Depositions may also be taken via video to preserve testimony of a witness who is unavailable to testify during trial. These "preservation" depositions are then shown to the jury in the place of the witness's live testimony.

In federal cases, Rule 30 of the Federal Rules of Civil Procedure permits parties to depose any person, including a party, without leave of the court except in very specific circumstances, by sending a legal document called a subpoena to the witness and the other parties.[1] State courts typically have their own version of Rule 30 that governs depositions in their jurisdiction. State court deposition rules are often similar to the federal rules, and many states have adopted the Uniform Interstate Depositions and Discovery Act, which authorizes parties in a lawsuit in one state to take the deposition of a witness located in another state.[2]

Depositions usually occur in person, although they are sometimes taken telephonically or via videoconference. A deposition can be noted (requested) by any party who wishes to examine the witness under oath. The deposition is attended by a court reporter, a lawyer for each party, the witness, and the witness's lawyer, if the witness is represented. A videographer may also attend if the deposition is being video recorded. The court reporter's role is to swear in the witness and write down a verbatim transcript of the deposition. To be "sworn in" means that the witness swears to tell the truth under the penalty of perjury. Once the witness is sworn in, each lawyer has an opportunity to ask the witness a series of questions. The other lawyers may state objections between a question and an answer in order to make a written record for the judge to review and rule on before the deposition is used at trial. Because everything is being recorded in real time, it is important for the witness to pause after listening to the whole question and before answering so that the lawyers can make their records without talking over the witness. Typically, a witness must answer a question unless instructed not to answer by their lawyer.

PURPOSE OF A DEPOSITION

The purpose of a deposition is to allow parties to discover relevant, factual information and opinions from witnesses that may be used to evaluate the strength or merits of the case, analyzed by other witnesses, and presented to the jury at trial. Depositions of defendant-physicians and treating providers are particularly important to both experts and attorneys. For example, expert witnesses may rely on deposition testimony from a party or treating provider as the basis for their opinions, even when the party or treating provider is not called to testify at trial.[3] Attorneys also often consider the strength of defendant-physician and treating provider testimony when determining whether to settle a case or proceed to trial.

Treating providers are often considered "unbiased" because they are not hired by either side to analyze the case and testify as an advocate for that side at trial. Therefore, where a treating provider has specialized knowledge of the patient's course of care that may be relevant to the issues in the case, the attorneys for the parties will often want to depose the treating provider. This knowledge may include interactions with other providers whose care is at issue in a medical malpractice case; treatment provided after an injury-producing event, such as oncology treatment following a cancer diagnosis caused by carcinogen exposure; and knowledge of the patient's past injuries or future disabilities caused by the injury-producing event or medical care. In such instances, the provider's deposition will allow both sides to analyze the strength of their theory of the case and determine what factual issues they will need to navigate as the case proceeds. The deposition may also allow the parties to analyze the monetary value of the case, in particular relating to past and future medical care for the injury. It is therefore essential that a physician provide direct, honest testimony during his or her deposition.

ROLE OF THE PHYSICIAN DURING A DEPOSITION

Physicians involved in a lawsuit typically fall into one of three categories: a treating health care provider, a defendant, or an expert witness. This chapter focuses on the roles of treating providers and defendant-physicians. The physician's role, whether as a treating provider or as a defendant, is simple; it is to listen to each question and answer honestly unless instructed not to answer by their lawyer.

The American Medical Association Code of Medical Ethics Opinion 9.7.1 states that "physicians have an obligation to assist in the administration of justice" and provides guidance to physicians who serve as witnesses.[4] Physician witnesses must accurately represent their qualifications, provide honest testimony, and not allow their testimony to be influenced by financial compensation.[4] Opinion 9.7.1 prohibits physicians from accepting compensation that is contingent on the outcome of the lawsuit and from testifying in matters that could affect the patient's medical interests absent consent or a legal requirement to testify. Opinion 9.7.1 also advises physicians whose testimony may place the physician and patient in adversarial positions to transfer care of the patient to another physician.[4] Where a physician is a defendant in the lawsuit, it is especially important to consider transferring care early in the litigation in order to avoid conflicts of interest and because any communications between the patient and the physician could be explored during the physician's deposition and would be admissible at trial.[5]

As treating health care providers who are otherwise uninvolved in a lawsuit, some physicians will feel pressure to be an advocate for one side or the other during their deposition. A physician may feel pressure from their patient, their patient's family, or their patient's lawyers to criticize other providers or entities or to dramatize the patient's negative outcome. Conversely, a physician may feel pressure from their employer or their colleagues to defend medical care rendered by others, even where the physician does not have the qualifications or factual knowledge to defend that care. Physicians care deeply about their patients and their profession, so these conflicting pressures are understandable. However, the decision to become an advocate for one side can open a treating provider up to criticism from the other side, potentially lead to the provider being brought into the lawsuit as a defendant, and discredit the provider, especially if the provider is not in possession of the complete facts of the case or criticizes a provider of a different specialty. This is especially true in oncology cases where patients are often treated by physicians from a multitude of different specialties.

A physician is typically not qualified to comment on or criticize the care of a physician of another specialty absent the training, knowledge, and experience specific to the other specialty.[6] Therefore, where a physician is deposed as a treating provider, it is important for the physician to avoid commenting on care provided by other providers, especially providers of other specialties. Missed or delayed cancer diagnosis cases are common in medical legal oncology cases and often involve providers of various specialties.[7] Often, the oncologist is a treating provider whose care occurs after the patient is diagnosed and, therefore, after the allegedly negligent care occurred and was discovered. Rarely will treating oncologists or defendants know all the facts or allegations of the lawsuit when they are deposed. Yet, they may be asked to criticize their own care or the care of others. This may result in the treating oncologist being used as an expert witness in the lawsuit even though the oncologist has not agreed to serve as an expert witness.

Similarly, while uncommon, lawyers may ask questions of the treating oncologist that are intended to coerce the oncologist to admit that he or she was negligent, could have done better, or somehow contributed to the patient's bad outcome. Without counsel, it is unlikely that an unrepresented oncologist will know the purpose of these questions or be prepared to testify in a manner that deflects them. Testimony that inadvertently causes the oncologist to appear negligent may result in the oncologist being added to the lawsuit if the statute of limitations has not passed. Negligent testimony may also result in a report and investigation by that state's medical licensing board. While it is important to answer questions honestly, no physician is obligated to admit their own liability or negligence, criticize their own care, or criticize the care of another provider.

ROLE OF A LAWYER DURING A DEPOSITION

While defendants in criminal cases have a constitutional right to a lawyer, that constitutional right does not extend to civil litigants.[8] Therefore, whether a party, including a physician whose care is at issue, has legal right to counsel in a civil case will vary by state law. Regardless, health care institutions and liability insurers typically have contracts and procedures in place to hire a lawyer to represent a physician who receives a deposition subpoena or who is named as defendant in a lawsuit. The lawyer's role is to defend that physician's care, prepare the physician for their deposition, and, to the extent possible, prevent that physician from giving testimony that would amount to an admission of liability or result in the physician being brought into the lawsuit or investigated by the state department.

Most physicians are not lawyers and often have little or no experience with the deposition process before they are deposed. Depositions are not like natural conversation, and it can often be difficult for witnesses who have never been deposed before to get used to the question-and-answer format. Many physicians find it helpful to have their own lawyer prepare them for their deposition, including practicing deposition questions and answers so that the physician enters the deposition knowing what to expect and how to avoid testimony that will get them into trouble.

A personal lawyer can also confidentially answer the physician's questions, provide guidance, and protect the physician from being contacted by other lawyers in the case. When a physician has their own lawyer, the communications between the lawyer and physician are protected by the attorney-client privilege and strictly confidential.[9] Therefore, absent a court order, the physician never has to disclose what questions they asked their lawyer, the advice given, or anything else the physician and their lawyer discussed. Lawyers are also ethically precluded from contacting a physician who they know is represented by a different lawyer.[10] This prevents the lawyers for the parties from contacting or pressuring the physician outside the presence of the physician's lawyer. In fact, in some states, the physician-patient privilege completely bars defense lawyers from contacting a treating physician who was not involved in the allegedly negligent care outside of a formal deposition.[11] The treating physician's lawyer can help the physician determine who, if anyone, is allowed to speak to the physician outside of a formal deposition and monitor those conversations if the physician is willing to have them.

Because the deposition is sworn testimony, there are several risks that providers should be aware of and prepared to address before giving a deposition. First, if the statute of limitations has not passed, a treating provider can be brought into the lawsuit as a defendant based on his or her sworn deposition testimony. Second, deposition testimony can open a provider up to investigation by his or her medical licensing board or state health department if the testimony does not comport with the standard of care. This is true regardless of whether the statute of limitations has passed.

Moreover, whether testimony is written or given via deposition, problematic testimony may open a physician up to investigation by that physician's professional accrediting board or academy. For example, in *Graboff v Colleran Firm*, an orthopedic surgery expert witness in a medical malpractice case wrote a report that violated the American Academy of Orthopedic Surgeons (AAOS)'s Standards of Professionalism on Orthopedic Expert Witness.[12] The defendant in the medical malpractice case filed a grievance with the AAOS asserting that the report was based on incomplete medical information. The AAOS investigated, conducted several hearings, and found that the orthopedic surgeon had violated its professional standards. As a result, the AAOS suspended the orthopedic surgeon's membership for two years and published the suspension in its monthly periodical on its website. The orthopedic surgeon then sued the AAOS for defamation and tortious "false light" invasion of privacy based on the AAOS's publication. The case went to trial, and he was awarded money damages. The AAOS appealed, and the Third Circuit Court of Appeals affirmed the judgment.[13] While the orthopedic surgeon had a claim against the AAOS due to the *way* it published its findings, the fact that the AAOS suspended his membership in the first place was not an issue.

The *Graboff* case serves as an example of the power of an accrediting body or medical academy to govern its members and the risks associated with giving medical opinions or testimony that may violate a professional organization's ethical standards. State medical boards and licensing bodies have even greater power to investigate a provider's license and suspend or revoke it where appropriate.[14] It is therefore extremely important for the lawyer to investigate the basis of the lawsuit, explore any problematic care with their client before the deposition, and prepare the physician to answer questions about their testimony in a way that minimizes the risk that they will be brought into the lawsuit as a defendant or investigated by their accrediting body or state medical licensing board.

The lawyer should prepare the physician for the deposition by helping the physician focus on important information in his or her records and teaching the physician techniques to give clear and straightforward answers while simultaneously avoiding problematic testimony. A thorough lawyer will ensure that the physician is very familiar with his or her own records. The lawyer will teach the physician that he or she has the right to understand every question before answering it. Most lawyers are not health care providers and therefore do not have the breadth and depth of medical knowledge equal to the physicians they depose, sometimes resulting in questions that do not make sense from a medical perspective. These questions can be awkward and inartful. When this happens, and indeed any time a physician does not understand a question, a physician has a right to ask the lawyer to clarify or rephrase the question before answering so that the physician understands what is being asked.

A physician's lawyer should also remind the physician that he or she has the right not to guess or speculate when he or she does not know or does not recall an answer to a question. If the lawyer asking the question pushes for an answer, the physician has a right to say, "I don't remember" or "I don't know," or to tell the lawyer that any answer would be speculation or a guess.

Most importantly, a physician has a right not to be bullied into giving a certain answer just because the lawyer asking the question wants it. Lawyers are advocates. Their goal is to position the case in the most favorable light for their client. Sometimes this involves obtaining specific deposition testimony that can be used to bolster their case or hurt the other side's case at trial. However, a physician giving a deposition is under no such obligation. The physician's only obligation is to answer honestly and to the best of their ability. Sometimes lawyers will re-ask or rephrase the same question or will become more aggressive toward the physician because they do not like the physician's answer to a question. This tactic is nothing more than an attempt to push a physician to change their answer. The physician has a right to stand by their answer and to request a break if the lawyer questioning them becomes disrespectful or too aggressive. The physician's lawyer should prepare them for these types of questions and give them tools to respectfully resist bullying during the deposition. A skilled lawyer will also redirect any bullying at the deposition away from the physician. For these reasons, if a physician receives a deposition request, the physician should ask their employer or malpractice insurer to hire a lawyer to assist them through the deposition process.

Within the field of oncology, medical-legal cases often involve delayed or missed cancer diagnoses and/or product liability from cancer-causing agents. While oncologists are not always the target of the lawsuit, their care and deposition testimony may be important to the lawsuit. The following clinical vignettes demonstrate several instances where an oncologist's deposition testimony may be essential to the outcome of the litigation and/or where poor deposition testimony may result in the oncologist being brought into the case as a defendant. The following is a case of delayed diagnosis.[15]

For instance, patient John Davis presented to his internist for a routine physical, during which a chest x-ray was taken. Because Mr. Davis did not properly fit the x-ray and because the x-ray revealed an area of questionable haziness, he was referred to a radiologist for follow-up imaging. The internist told the radiologist that Mr. Davis had been a four- to five-pack-a-day cigarette smoker for many years but failed to mention a shadow on the first x-ray. The radiologist informed the internist that follow-up imaging was negative. One month later, Mr. Davis collapsed and was taken to a local emergency department, where additional imaging revealed lung cancer that had metastasized to his brain. Mr. Davis underwent radiation and chemotherapy treatment but ultimately died. Mr. Davis's estate sued the internist and the radiologist for failing to timely diagnose his metastatic lung cancer, causing a delay in diagnosis and treatment and reducing his chance at survival. Mr. Davis's treating oncologist was deposed and testified that the metastases were likely present at the time of the first x-ray. However, she could not say whether an earlier diagnosis would have led to different treatment or changed Mr. Davis's likelihood of survival. Because Mr. Davis's estate did not provide any physician testimony to show that the delayed diagnosis proximately caused a reduced chance of a better outcome, the case was dismissed.

This case demonstrates that even where an oncologist is not a hired expert, his or her testimony may determine the outcome of the case, especially on the issue of causation. A patient in a medical malpractice case is required to demonstrate that, but for the alleged negligence, his or her poor outcome would not have occurred; in a delayed diagnosis case, the patient must show that the negligence caused an increased risk of harm or an increased risk of the poor outcome.[16] Because the oncologist could not say that she would have treated her patient differently with an earlier diagnosis or that her patient would have had a greater chance of survival with earlier treatment, the patient did not have sufficient causation evidence to support his claim. Had the oncologist testified differently, the outcome of the case may have been in the patient's favor. This demonstrates how the treating oncologist's deposition testimony may determine the outcome of the case, highlighting the importance of clear and honest deposition testimony.

Another example is patient Mary Miller who was a 45-year-old breast cancer patient undergoing chemotherapy. Due to breakthrough pain, her oncologist prescribed a transdermal fentanyl patch. At a follow-up visit, Ms. Miller presented with mild dysarthria. Due to her age, a lack of any other neurologic symptoms, and dysarthria being a rare but known side effect of transdermal fentanyl, Ms. Miller's oncologist attributed her mild dysarthria to the transdermal fentanyl. Ms. Miller's dysarthria did not improve, so she went to a local hospital's emergency department (ED), where she was evaluated for a stroke. A brain magnetic resonance imaging (MRI) scan showed mild evidence of an ischemic stroke, but the radiologist read the MRI as negative, so she was sent home. Four days later, Ms. Miller returned to the ED because her symptoms still had not improved, at which point she was diagnosed with a stroke. Her stroke caused a permanent speech impairment.

Ms. Miller sued the hospital and radiologist. During discovery, the oncologist was required to give a deposition. The oncologist had been deposed before, so he did not contact his malpractice insurer to request a lawyer to represent him for his deposition. During the deposition, he was asked whether dysarthria is a known symptom of stroke, to which he answered "yes." He was also asked whether he had considered a stroke in his differential and why he did not refer Ms. Miller to the ED for an immediate stroke workup. He testified that given a lack of other neurologic symptoms and Ms. Miller's age he did not consider stroke in his differential and therefore did not think she needed to be referred to the ED, although in retrospect, he "probably should have" because Ms. Miller had never before shown any speech problems. Based on this admission, Ms. Miller decided to add the oncologist as a defendant to the lawsuit, alleging that his failure to consider and refer her to the ED for a stroke workup contributed to the delay in her diagnosis and treatment. The case ultimately settled before trial, and the settlement was reported to the National Practitioner Databank.[17] This caused the oncologist's state medical board to investigate his care. It determined that he had breached the standard of care, and a settlement was reached in which the oncologist was required to pay a fine and take continuing medical education classes relating to stroke diagnosis in order to avoid restrictions on his license. The settlement was also made publicly available on the state medical board's website.

This example illustrates the unintended consequences of deposition testimony. Even when an oncologist believes that his or her care is not the target of a lawsuit, it is possible to be brought in as a defendant based on poor deposition testimony, which can have insurance and licensing implications. Had the oncologist requested an attorney, he would have been prepared to defend his care and may have avoided being brought into the lawsuit.

Lastly, Dr. Amy Smith is an oncologist, whose patient, Katie Anderson, is a 55-year-old postmenopausal female recently diagnosed with breast cancer. Ms. Anderson originally developed symptoms ten months ago, including right breast pain and inflammation. Due to her busy schedule working full time as a floor supervisor at an airplane manufacturing plant and raising her three minor children with her husband, Ms. Anderson chose to have a telemedicine appointment with her primary care provider (PCP) to address her symptoms. Ms. Anderson's PCP, a family medicine physician, diagnosed her with an infection and prescribed antibiotics but did not recommend a mammogram to rule out cancer. The antibiotics did not help, and Ms. Anderson continued to live with her pain for another ten months until her pain and inflammation began to extend into her right armpit and arm. Ms. Anderson then returned to her PCP, this time in person. The PCP ordered a mammogram, which showed a tumor in Ms. Anderson's right breast. A biopsy and follow-up imaging revealed stage IV metastatic breast cancer that had metastasized to Ms. Anderson's lymph system, liver, and right hip. Ms. Anderson was referred to Dr. Smith for oncologic care.

Unfortunately, given the progression of Ms. Anderson's cancer, even with aggressive treatment, her five-year projected survival rate was less than 20% based on current available literature. Based on the literature and the likely progression of Ms. Anderson's disease, if she had been diagnosed ten months earlier, her five-year survival rate would most likely have been between 60% and 75%. Dr. Smith informed Ms. Anderson of these facts and presented her with her treatment options, which included surgery, radiation, chemotherapy, and nontreatment. Dr. Smith informed Ms. Anderson of the risks and benefits of each option, and Ms. Anderson chose to undergo radiation and chemotherapy but not surgery. Treatment slowed the spread of her cancer but caused extreme fatigue and nausea that rendered Ms. Anderson unable to work. The Anderson family lost Ms. Anderson's $50,000 per year income, and Mr. Anderson was forced to reduce his hours working as a customer service representative in order to take Ms. Anderson to her many medical appointments and take on the majority of the couple's child care and domestic responsibilities, costing the couple an additional $10,000 in wages lost per year.

Due to the financial and emotional hardships caused by Ms. Anderson's cancer, the Andersons decided to file a medical malpractice lawsuit against Ms. Anderson's PCP and the PCP's clinic. They alleged a medical negligence claim against the PCP, arguing that the PCP's failure to order a mammogram when Ms. Anderson first reported her symptoms breached the standard of care of a reasonably prudent family medicine physician and reduced her likelihood of survival. They also alleged that the clinic was vicariously liable for the negligence of the PCP.

Ms. Anderson's attorney sent Dr. Smith a letter informing her that Ms. Anderson had filed a lawsuit against the PCP and that Dr. Smith may be called to testify as a witness. Upon receipt of the letter, Dr. Smith contacted her clinic administrator, who worked with the clinic's insurer to retain an attorney for Dr. Smith. Dr. Smith did not want to get dragged into the lawsuit as an expert witness and was not comfortable testifying on the standard of care of a physician of another specialty. She was also worried that she would inadvertently testify in a way that could bring her care into the case. Dr. Smith explained her reservations to her attorney, who taught her how to avoid standard of care and expert-type questions, helped her explain her care clearly and succinctly, and taught her techniques to defend against any criticisms of her care.

Dr. Smith's deposition was requested several months later. During the deposition, Dr. Smith explained that she was not a family medicine physician and would not be testifying on the standard of care for a family medicine physician. Her testimony was therefore limited to her knowledge as Ms. Anderson's treating oncologist. Dr. Smith testified that Ms. Anderson's five-year survival was less than 20% and that her 5-year survival rate with the earlier diagnosis would have been 60% to 75%. Without radiation and chemotherapy, Ms. Anderson was unlikely to survive another year, but Dr. Smith believed that radiation and chemotherapy would most likely give Ms. Anderson an additional one to three years with her family. She testified that she had informed Ms. Anderson of these facts and that Ms. Anderson had thus chosen to undergo radiation and chemotherapy. Dr. Smith also testified that Ms. Anderson was no longer able to work due to her radiation and chemotherapy treatments and the physical requirements of her job.

Dr. Smith came across as credible and unbiased, in large part because she limited her testimony to her area of medical expertise and the facts of which she had direct knowledge. Defense counsel felt that given Dr. Smith's credible testimony and the facts of the case, the best outcome for his clients would be an early settlement. The parties therefore attended early mediation, which resulted in a favorable settlement for the Andersons. Ms. Anderson and Dr. Smith also continued to have a positive physician-patient relationship following the lawsuit.

This clinical vignette demonstrates the importance of proper deposition preparation and the value of clear, honest testimony by a treating provider. By thoroughly preparing with her attorney, Dr. Smith was not turned into an unwilling expert or brought into the case as a defendant. While harmful to the defense's case, Dr. Smith's testimony was also valuable to the defense because it allowed the PCP's attorney to evaluate the strength of the Andersons' case and advise his clients accordingly. This led to an early settlement that avoided significant defense costs, the stress of trial to the PCP, and the risk of a large verdict against the PCP and the clinic. Ultimately, Dr. Smith's testimony was useful to both sides.

CONCLUSION

Depositions are important to the litigation process, and it is possible that an oncologist may be required to give a deposition at some point in his or her career. This is especially true when a patient suffers from cancer following a delay in diagnosis or exposure to cancer-causing agents. Deposition testimony can have serious consequences for the litigation and the oncologist. Even if an oncologist has been deposed before, it is wise to request legal representation and be well prepared prior to the deposition.

References:

1. Fed R Civ P 30(a); Fed R Civ P 45.
2. *Yelp, Inc. v Hadeed Carpet Cleaning, Inc.*, 770 SE2d 440, 444 (Va 2015); see also *Matter of Roche Molecular Sys., Inc.*, 60 Misc3d 222 (NY 2018); *BlueMountain Credit Alternatives Master Fund L.P. v Regal Ent. Grp.*, 465 P3d 122 (Colo App 2020); and *Catalina Mktg. Corp. v Hudyman*, 212 A3d 997 (NJ Super Ct App Div 2019).
3. Fed R Evid 703.
4. Code of Medical Ethics Opinion 9.7.1. American Medical Association. https://www.ama-assn.org/delivering-care/ethics/medical-testimony. Accessed August 5, 2021.
5. Fed R Evid 801(d)(2).
6. Fed R Evid 702; "the general rule . . . is that a practitioner of one school of medicine is not competent to testify as an expert in a malpractice action against a practitioner of another school of medicine"; 85 ALR2d 1022 (originally published in 1962).
7. See, for example, *Hayden v Gordon*, 91 AD3rd 819 (NY App Div 2012) and *Claudet v Weyrich*, 662 So 2d 131 (La Ct App 1995).
8. US Const amend VI; US Const amend XIV, § 2.
9. Model Rules of Prof'l Conduct R 1.6.
10. Model Rules of Prof'l Conduct R 4.2.
11. See, for example, *Loudon v Mhyre*, 756 P.2d 138 (Wash 1988).
12. *Graboff v Colleran Firm*, 744 F3d 128, 132-133 (3d Cir 2014).
13. *Graboff v Colleran Firm*, 744 F3d 128, 140-141 (3d Cir 2014).

14. See, for example, *North Dakota State Board of Medicine Examiners-Investigative Panel B v Hsu*, 726 NW2d 216 (ND 2007).

15. Example based generally on *LaBieniec v Baker*, 526 A2d 1341 (Conn App Ct 1987).

16. See, for example, *Herskovits v Grp. Health Co-op. of Puget Sound*, 664 P2d 474 (Wash 1983).

17. Reporting medical malpractice payments. National Practitioner Databank website. Updated October 2018. https://www.npdb.hrsa.gov/guidebook/EMMPR.jsp. Accessed May 28, 2021.

CHAPTER 4

Trial Practice

C. William Hinnant, Jr., MD, JD, FCLM

INTRODUCTION

If war is the ultimate failure of diplomacy, trial is the ultimate failure of negotiation. In the 21st century, civil and criminal processes are largely driven by mechanisms promoting settlement, or entry of a plea agreeable to the parties, to the exclusion of trial itself. Indeed, there are barriers precluding trial in most jurisdictions until alternative dispute resolution (ADR), generally mediation, has been attempted.

Attorneys, once focused from the time they are retained on gathering evidence for trial preparation, are now forced on a continuous basis to evaluate the merits, the relevant contingencies, and the potential value of the claim, in preparation for civil settlement. In the criminal context, the focus at all times is on the risk of conviction. Indeed, in many cases, counsel does not enter "trial mode" until ADR (or in the criminal context, plea bargaining) has failed.

In the contest of administrative process, jury trial is not generally available in most jurisdictions, but hearings before administrative tribunals are common, many considered quasi-criminal as opposed to civil. There, the tribunal itself serves as the jury, with appellate process available thereafter. In certain administrative matters, fact finders must have specialized knowledge not necessarily available to the lay jury pool, ergo why the tribunal itself must serve as the "jury." Such is true in the cases of state medical, nursing, and pharmacy boards.

In civil and criminal matters, expert witnesses may be called to assist the fact finder in reaching conclusions that will likely require specialized knowledge and opinion testimony prior to deliberation and the rendering of a verdict. In the context of oncology, the lay public clearly has little specialized knowledge, whereas physicians in general, specialists providing cancer care and radiation and medical oncologists themselves, compose the graduated knowledge cohort that may be required to render factual findings, conclusion of law, a verdict, and finally, a penalty. Needless to say, oncologists' specialized knowledge base and the standards of care applicable to the many patients with literally hundreds of varying tumor histologies, grades, and clinical stages are best evaluated by other oncologists, but our legal system makes no such accommodation.

This chapter will explore trial practice, theoretically in all of the above arenas, those processes preceding trial, the pretrial process, trial itself, and the posttrial and appellate processes thereafter. Emphasis is placed on specific scenarios likely to affect oncologists.

LITIGATION IN LEGAL ONCOLOGY

Trials and hearings in general

The term *trial* typically is applied only in the civil and criminal context and denotes a process governed by rules, whereby a fact finder (a judge or jury) renders a verdict for or against a party or parties based on evidence and guided by an authority as to matters of law, generally a judge.

Hearings may also be before judges but, particularly in the administrative context, may alternatively be before a tribunal, commission, or board. Such would be the case in the context of provider licensure, workers' compensation, provider panel credentialing matters, medical boards, and Social Security disability, all potentially implicating oncologic matters.

All of the above includes graduated appellate mechanisms generally involving administrative law courts, jurisdictional trial courts, and the state's intermediate appellate and supreme courts. In such appellate cases, the scope of evidence allowed generally is the existing record from the administrative tribunal, with the appellate judges in such matters solely reviewing for errors of law, although in some scenarios, so-called "de novo review" may be available. The standard of review will be dictated by statute, regulation, or local rule.

Civil issues facing oncologists

Medical malpractice

Medical malpractice actions involve allegations of medical negligence, which has 4 discrete elements: (1) a legal duty; (2) a breach in that duty (in the context of health care, known as the standard of care); (3) causation, both in fact and proximate; (4) leading to damages.

Health care providers owe a duty by statute or common law (the latter derived from judicially derived case law and applied under the doctrine of *stare decisis*, the legal principle of determining points in litigation according to precedent). That duty requires that such professionals diagnose and treat patients within the applicable standard of care, which is defined as what a reasonably prudent practitioner would do in the same or similar circumstances.

In the past, standards of care could be deemed local or national; however, recent case law has generally supported only one national standard that does not vary with jurisdiction. To establish the standard of care, as well as causation, both proximate and in fact, expert testimony is required. Expert witnesses are those whose education, training, and experience will generally mirror those of the defendant and will entitle them to render opinion testimony under Rule 702 of most jurisdictions' Rules of Evidence.

In the context of oncology, the more common bases for allegations of professional negligence include unexpected injury, failure to diagnose or treat, errors in medication administration (including failure to consider drug interactions), failure to follow safety procedures, poor documentation of patient education, and lack of informed consent.[1] Improper targeting of external beam radiotherapy is always problematic for radiation oncologists, particularly as targeting errors must be reported to the Nuclear Regulatory Commission, or its state designee,[2] where they are available via a Freedom of Information Act request by any potential plaintiff.

Fraud and abuse and *qui tam* actions

In the United States, the ability to file and collect claims made to the federal payers Medicare, Medicaid, Tricare, and the Federal Employees Health Program is integral to oncology practice. Indeed, financial survival requires participation in these provider panels. Claims are filed electronically in virtually all cases using a Centers for Medicare and Medicaid Services (CMS)-1500 form, wherein Current Procedural Terminology (CPT) codes populate each claim line correlating to an applicable International Classification of Diseases (ICD), 10th edition, diagnosis code. The filing entity certifies the accuracy of each claim to the relevant payer.

The False Claims Act (FCA; 31 USC § 3729 et seq) prohibits "knowingly" presenting or causing to be presented to the United States any false or fraudulent claim for payment for which the government may recover 3 times the amount of damages it sustains and a civil monetary penalty of between $5500 and $11,000 per claim. There is also a substantial risk for provider exclusion, generally a death knell for a provider. Many states have parallel provisions. Plaintiffs in *qui tam* actions are known as "relators."

Express false claims include those for procedures not performed, claims upcoded to include fraudulent dosing, or unbundling wherein, for instance, chemotherapy premedications such as antiemetics, steroids, sedatives, and hematopoietic stimulators are coded as separate infusions when, in reality, they were given in a single mini-bag or by way of a single slow intravenous (IV) push. In contrast, implied false claims may include claims actually filed accurately but wherein the provider did not meet all compliance standards associated with that claim, possibly by certifying as accurate certain other claims that were in fact fraudulent. A claim can be deemed false for purposes of liability under the FCA based on an implied representation that the provider or supplier who submitted the claim is in compliance with all applicable statutes, regulations, or government contract provisions.[3]

This is known as the implied certification theory of liability—that providers were impliedly certifying to compliance with laws associated with the claim when it was submitted, such that any claim, even an accurate one, was impliedly false. Given the thousands of such requirements that apply to providers, the scope of implied certification theory is incredibly broad and poses a quandary for oncologists whose billing is generally more complex than many specialties, including evaluation and management services, procedures, frequently laboratory services, chemotherapy and premedication provision and administration, and hospital care.

Until 2015, circuit courts were split as to their acceptance of implied certification theory, until the Supreme Court, in *Universal Health Services, Inc. v United States Ex Rel. Escobar* (136 S Ct 1989, 195 L Ed 348 [2016]), upheld implied certification. However, in light of the broad range of potential impliedly certified false claims, the court imposed a demanding materiality standard, actually giving providers a new and very effective defense. In finding that omissions that create a misleading representation give rise to FCA liability because of its bar on "false or fraudulent" claims for payment or approval, the court held that liability did not require such a misrepresentation be expressly designated as conditions of payment, rather that it must be material to the government's decision to pay the claim. Such materiality must be pled with particularity and proven to prevail in a *qui tam* action.[4]

Medical oncologists must also comply with the provisions of the Prescription Drug Marketing Act of 1987,[5] with its implementing regulations at 21 CFR §§ 203, 205. Chemotherapy medications provided to patients by third parties such as patient assistance programs or foundations cannot be reduced to claims submitted to insurers. Irregularities in payment for chemotherapy are common fodder for disgruntled former employees or, in some cases, patients' families who question an explanation of benefits (EOB) they receive.

Such FCA actions may be brought by the government of its own initiative but are more commonly brought by so-called "relators," commonly former employees or associates of the provider entity who are essentially whistleblowers. Those individuals file a federal complaint under seal and concomitantly serve the local US attorney's office as well as the office of the attorney general with that pleading and the relator's disclosure. The government then has a minimum of 60 days to elect to investigate and intervene, although consent orders to extend the seal are commonly granted on motion by the government. In consideration of their contribution, relators are entitled to a "bounty" of 15% to 20% of the recovery in the event of intervention or 25% to 30% in the event of nonintervention and a successful settlement or judgment when the relator proceeds, individually. Further, if relators suffer a retaliatory discharge as a result of their disclosure of the fraud, they are entitled to additional damages, including a salary multiple and equitable relief under 39 USC § 3730(h).

Peer review and credentialing

During the pendency of the seminal case of *Patrick v Burget* (486 US 94, 108 S Ct 1658 [1988]), wherein peer review was held not to be state action, certain medical staff members were held liable for antitrust violations related to their peer review of another physician. In response, Congress passed the Health Care Quality Improvement Act of 1986 (HCQIA)[6]; its purported purpose was to prevent incompetent physicians from migrating from state to state and to provide qualified immunity from damages to those physicians engaging in effective professional peer review.

In short, for those involved to be qualifiedly immune from damages being assessed, a professional review action must be taken:

1. in the reasonable belief that the action was in the furtherance of quality health care,
2. after a reasonable effort to obtain the facts of the matter,
3. after adequate notice and hearing procedures are afforded to the physician involved or after such other procedures as are fair to the physician under the circumstances, and
4. in the reasonable belief that the action was warranted by the facts known after such reasonable effort to obtain facts and after meeting the requirement of paragraph (3). A professional review action shall be presumed to have met the preceding standards necessary for the protection set out in section 411(a) [42 USCS § 11111(a)] unless the presumption is rebutted by a preponderance of the evidence.[7]

Virtually all oncologists know that peer review is an inherently political process in that hospital-based sanctions are not necessarily meted out fairly to all medical staff members. Further complicating truly nonbiased peer review today is the fact that most medical staffs are composed primarily of health system–employed physicians, with others serving on the medical staff as independent contractors. Nonetheless, all medical staff need to do to be qualifiedly immune from damages in any lawsuit related to the peer review process is meet the minimum requirements of the previously discussed four-prong test. Further, there is a presumption that those peer reviewers have met the necessary standard unless it is rebutted by a preponderance standard. Virtually all jurisdictions have set a low bar for such immunity, the same affirmed generally at the appellate level.

Many lawsuits challenging peer review have been brought in federal court, and a review of each federal judicial circuit's related case law shows that virtually all of these cases are dismissed at summary judgment in the health system's favor when the involved physician simply cannot meet his burden in rebutting the statutory presumption. To the dismay of involved physicians, the HCQIA, which was intended to provide qualified immunity for those involved in good faith peer review, has been extended to the point of virtual absolute immunity through its interpretative case law.

Poliner v Texas Health Systems[8] was a landmark case that clarified the legal protections provided both to peer reviewers and doctors undergoing review. After ten years of litigation in the federal courts, a favorable trial court verdict finding that the defendants had failed to meet their obligations under HCQIA's due process provisions, and an award in the amount of $360 million, the Fifth Circuit Court of Appeals reversed the judgment of the district court and ordered judgment for the defendants, vacating all monetary awards. Later, Poliner appealed this decision to the US Supreme Court, which declined to consider his petition.

In its holding, the appellate court further broadened HCQIA immunity offering 5 guiding principles: (1) a failure to comply with hospital bylaws does not defeat a peer reviewer's right to HCQIA immunity from damages if the health care entity complies with the statutory provisions; (2) the good or bad faith of the peer reviewer is irrelevant to the HCQIA immunity standard (although Poliner had offered evidence of anticompetitive motives, the court found ample objective evidence for concern about Poliner's medical competence); (3) actions of peer reviewers should be judged based on whether those actions were objectively reasonable, based on facts available at the time and not whether they are later proved right or wrong; otherwise, any physician unhappy with the peer review process could defeat HCQIA immunity by presenting testimony of other doctors who have a differing viewpoint from that of the peer reviewers; (4) peer reviewers must conduct a reasonable, not necessarily perfect, investigation (under the totality of the circumstances, the operative question is whether a reasonable jury could find that the defendants had failed to make a reasonable effort to obtain the facts); and (5) despite HCQIA, peer review actions are still open to legal challenges for declaratory or injunctive relief (i.e., equitable damages could still apply, even though the peer reviewers are shielded from money damages). For physicians caught in the crosshairs of a hostile peer review process, harsh and seemingly unfair outcomes may occur, but Congress saw this as an acceptable balance between encouraging peer review and discouraging misuse of the process. Nonetheless, the process is commonly misused, generally aimed at the expulsion of the accused from the medical staff.

Peer review hearings generally exclude strict compliance with relevant rules of evidence or civil procedure. They are generally governed more by doctors than by lawyers, and under some so-called hospital "fair hearing plans," actual participation by attorneys is not allowed, although an attorney, usually a hospital-aligned attorney, may serve as the hearing officer. Peer review committees make a final determination as to the involved practitioner, which may be appealable, albeit to the medical executive committee and then to the hospital board, both with the usually predicable result of affirming the peer review committee's findings.

Involved physicians are encouraged to engage counsel and seek some compromise, even if it involves resignation under investigation and a move to "greener pastures." Rarely are remedial schemes offered, underscoring again the general objective of the hospital simply seeking to rid itself of the involved practitioner. Regardless of the merits, suspensions lasting more than 30 days, revocation of privileges, and resignations while under investigation are all reportable to the National Practitioner Data Bank (NPDB); however, in the context of making a "clean break," physicians under review can usually negotiate neutral language for such reports and potentially even neutral references. NPDB entries may be disputed administratively, though generally not successfully, and involved practitioners may enter individual statements made available to those querying the data bank.

Employment matters

Oncologists may employ individuals in the operation of their offices, including nurses actively involved in patient care as well as clerical personnel. Conversely, oncologists may be employees themselves, usually of a health system, with some element of oversight over those co-employees with whom they work to optimize patient care.

Employed oncologists are generally expressly contracted by their employer, provided a salary usually with an incentive component and relative value unit (RVU) methodology, and provided benefits including health insurance, disability insurance, payment of malpractice insurance premiums, vacation time, and provisions to assist in meeting relevant continuing medical education (CME) requirements. While employment in most states is considered at will, that is, the employee and employer can terminate their relationship unilaterally at any time for any reason, in the case of a contractually employed physician, the contract will control. Nonemployed physicians on the medical staff are independent contractors yet may receive compensation for call coverage or other services they provide at a health care entity's request or as a condition of medical staff membership.

The general rule is that an individual is an independent contractor if the payer has the right to control or direct only the result of the work and not what will be done and how it will be done. The earnings of a person who is working as an independent contractor are subject to self-employment tax unless they are paid by way of a business association such as a corporation, professional association, or limited liability partnership or company.

If you perform services that can be controlled by an employer (when and what will be done and how it will be done), you are not an independent contractor. This applies even if you are given freedom of action. What matters is that the employer has the legal right to control the details of how the services are performed. Employers usually provide tools of the trade to employees, while independent contractors provide their own tools.

Whether applicable to the oncologist as employee or as employer, public policy issues supersede contract rights or the employment at will doctrine in the event of employment discrimination based on sex, disability, failure to pay equal wages, religion, nationality, and age, with the recent addition of sexual preference.[9] In all these cases, in the context of employment by an entity with 15 or more employees, the Equal Employment Opportunity Commission (EEOC) has exclusive jurisdiction over such claims for a minimum of 6 months after they arise.[10]

The EEOC will investigate all discrimination claims on the merits and has an active mediation program wherein the parties, usually with the assistance of counsel, seek a mutually acceptable resolution to their disagreement. Alternatively, in the event of an impasse, the EEOC will issue a right to sue letter, after which the employee/claimant may file an action in federal court, the latter with exclusive jurisdiction over employment discrimination claims. State agencies may have concurrent jurisdiction to investigate such claims.

In the event of an employee's termination, unemployment compensation will be available to such an employee only in the event that the termination was not for cause. If there is a dispute as to the latter, an administrative hearing mechanism is generally available through the state to determine whether payment of compensation is proper.

Criminal issues facing oncologists

While oncologists are just as susceptible to common criminal charges such as driving under the influence, criminal domestic violence, assault and battery, or burglary as the general population, there are certain criminal matters to which they are more likely exposed based on their profession.

Controlled substances act violations

The Controlled Substances Act of 1970 (21 USC § 801 et seq) regulates the manufacture, importation, possession, use, and distribution of certain substances. It establishes five schedules of controlled substances, all very familiar to physicians; establishes licensure standards for their prescription; and penalizes the unauthorized possession, diversion, manufacture, and distribution of controlled substances. Its provisions affect physicians, pharmacists, and physician extenders, in addition to low-level drug offenders and so-called traffickers.

Oncologists commonly prescribe narcotics to patients with malignancies, particularly those with metastases or undergoing diagnostic or therapeutic interventions such as bone marrow biopsies or surgical procedures. They are best served to avoid the dispensing of such substances from their offices or clinics as there are strict requirements as to invoice and inventory management and dispensing and administration logs, the violation of which can lead to costly civil administrative penalties or, in some cases, criminal prosecution, the latter generally reserved for gross abuses in record keeping and/or dispensing.

Unfortunately, physicians occasionally become involved in illegal individual sales or conspiracies to distribute controlled substances. While such matters may be prosecuted under state law, because there is commonly involvement by the Drug Enforcement Administration or, alternatively, some interstate nexus, particularly in drug distribution conspiracies, jurisdiction is usually federal. Such matters involve arrest, arraignment before a federal magistrate judge, detention or the setting of bond, and then a period of trial preparation wherein the government either on motion or under a standing discovery order provides the fruits of its investigation—the so-called "discovery"—to the defendant and his counsel. After extensive review of the findings, a decision is made as to whether the defendant should enter a guilty plea or face trial.

The federal government's investigative resources are vast, and its skill with electronic discovery is unparalleled by any state. More than 95% of federal criminal matters progress to entry of a guilty plea rather than trial on the merits. In addition, the US Department of Justice, on motion, may "sweeten the pot" by offering defendants who enter a guilty plea and provide substantial assistance to law enforcement a downward departure under the Federal Sentencing Guidelines, potentially leading to a significant reduction in sentencing. The Sentencing Reform Act of 1984 authorizes a sentence below the statutory minimum for certain nonviolent, nonmanagerial drug offenders with little or no criminal history.[11] No motion by the government is necessary, only the satisfaction of certain criteria. On motion, Rule 35(b) of the Federal Rules of Criminal Procedure affords a sentencing court comparable latitude to those already sentenced who provide substantial assistance.

If a guilty plea is entered, the US Probation Office prepares a presentencing report (PSR) documenting the defendant's criminal history category and base offense level, and that information is plugged into the Federal Sentencing Table for calculation of a guidelines sentencing range. Departures either upward or downward depending on aggravating or mitigating circumstances are applied as the PSR is prepared, and the defendant and government are both given an opportunity to object to the contents of the PSR, with any objections provided to the sentencing judge.

The US Sentencing Guidelines replaced a nonuniform system of federal sentencing wherein the district judge had considerable discretion within the relevant statutory framework and were mandatory when initially implemented in the 1980s. District judges were bound to use the Sentencing Guidelines' sentencing framework until the Supreme Court ruled in *United States v Booker*.[12] In this cases, the court ruled that the Sixth Amendment right to jury trial required that, other than a prior conviction, only facts admitted by a defendant or proved beyond a reasonable doubt to a jury could be used to calculate a sentence exceeding the prescribed statutory maximum sentence, whether the defendant has entered a guilty plea or been convicted at trial. In addressing the constitutional infirmity of mandatory guidelines, yet respecting Congress's clear intent to achieve uniformity in sentencing, the court held the Sentencing Guidelines advisory only, yet "maintain[ed] a strong connection between the sentence imposed and the offender's real conduct—a connection important to the increased uniformity of sentencing that Congress intended its Guidelines system to achieve."[12]

Sentencing judges must consider those factors enumerated in the Federal Sentencing Statute,[13] which may potentially increase or decrease the ultimate sentence imposed by the judge, and those sentencing factors generally briefed by defense counsel for review by the judge.

Unless the defendant has agreed to an appellate waiver as a component of a plea agreement, any convicted defendant can appeal to the jurisdictional federal circuit court of appeals. Even in the face of an appellate waiver, those convicted may still appeal as to issues of prosecutorial misconduct or ineffective assistance of counsel. Appeals from the federal circuit court may be appealed to the Supreme Court; however, review there is discretionary, requiring a writ of certiorari from a three-justice panel, which is granted generally only when there are splits as to matters of law among the relevant federal circuit courts or when matters clearly have significant public policy relevance.

Sexual misconduct

With the exception of matters involving child pornography, sexual misconduct is virtually always prosecuted under state law. Oncologists clearly may face such allegations given their need to perform thorough physical examinations including of the genitalia and female breasts in some cases. The need to always have a chaperone present during the physical examination of sensitive areas and particularly for patients who show any level of apprehension in undergoing such an examination cannot be overemphasized.

In the context of oncologic practice, allegations typically include inappropriate touching, possibly pled as civil assault and battery or, in the criminal context, criminal sexual conduct. Patients are generally poorly versed in the intricacies of physical examination and can misinterpret perfectly acceptable and necessary examination techniques as inappropriate.

State civil assault and battery allegations made in the context of a physical examination undertaken as a part of medical practice may be covered by the accused physician's professional liability insurance, with the carrier immediately notified upon service of a complaint alleging assault. Negligence is an unintentional tort, while civil assault and battery is not; however, a patient alleging intentional inappropriate touching may actually be misinterpreting a perfectly acceptable portion of the physical examination, with the relevant malpractice carrier possibly reserving its rights under the policy, but nonetheless providing a defense. Needless to say, during the discovery process, the defendant's chaperone, usually an employee, will be deposed and hopefully testify as to the appropriateness of the examination as performed. Bear in mind that, in such a scenario, the plaintiff-patient likely contacted law enforcement first, which elected not to further investigate, leaving the patient only a civil remedy; however, many attorneys will instruct such a patient to file a medical board complaint, essentially allowing the board investigator to conduct an interview and investigate the allegations as to sexual misconduct and then electing not to proceed further civilly unless the investigator finds merit as to the patient's accusations.

If the jurisdiction's authorities elect to prosecute allegations of criminal sexual conduct against a practitioner, that professional will initially be arrested and then arraigned with consideration given to bond, allowing the professional to be released either on their own recognizance or subject to a surety's guaranteeing their court appearance subject to forfeiture of the bond amount. The general criteria requiring deliberation prior to setting bond are the defendant's potential danger to the community and their risk for flight. Such an accused will frequently be required to surrender their passport and, in some cases, may be required to have their location monitored by way of GPS technology.

While the defendant is released on bond, defense counsel will request discovery material from the district attorney prosecuting the case allowing counsel to review witness statements and frequently photographs and/or video relevant to the case. Forensics, including a sexual assault evaluation performed by a qualified practitioner, will also be included, as will the indictment issued by the grand jury, the latter presenting the facts and evidence collected by investigators as indicia of probable cause to charge and arrest. Counsel will advocate for the defendant with the district attorney, seeking dismissal or alternatively a plea agreement, potentially to a lesser-included offense. Those prosecuted and convicted of criminal sexual conduct in most cases will be placed on that jurisdiction's sex offender's registry, potentially precluding medical practice and affecting such an accused's living arrangements and, in some cases, requiring notice of such a designee's neighbors. All of the above, however, only become material following the service of a significant term of imprisonment.

State criminal liability

Oncologists, like all citizens, face potential state criminal liability for common criminal charges such as driving under the influence, criminal domestic violence, simple possession of marijuana or other illicit drugs, or receipt of stolen goods. More unusually, they may be accused of burglary, robbery, or crimes of violence such as assault and battery or murder. In the latter circumstances, physicians will be treated no differently than their fellow citizens, with all of the listed charges, with the likely exception of simple possession of marijuana, necessitating arrest, arraignment with potential bond, and then a period of discovery followed by consideration of dismissal, a plea agreement, or trial. Practitioners must avoid the use of excessive alcohol and of any illicit drugs because the collateral consequences (discussed later) of these vices will potentially be worse than the criminal penalty. In purchasing items from private individuals, if the price seems too good to be true, it probably is, and such items are frequently the fruits of theft. Although there is a "knowingly" component of receiving stolen goods, that degree of culpability could be implied if the cost of whatever item is purchased is simply unreasonably inexpensive.

Domestic violence is a serious problem in the United States that also has significant potential collateral consequences, in some cases worse than any associated criminal penalty. However, many jurisdictions permit conditional discharge of first offense domestic violence and simple possession of marijuana charges upon completion of an educational requirement and/or community service. Additionally, many states (and the federal government) have embraced drug courts, wherein with judicial guidance and oversight, a first-time offender may have more serious drug charges conditionally discharged upon completion of drug education, community services, and counseling with periodic negative drug screens.

Collateral consequences

Non–professionally licensed citizens generally face only the criminal consequence of their illegal actions; however, those licensed to practice medicine, law, pharmacy, nursing, or other professions also face the administrative consequences potentially imposed by their licensing authorities, including penalties progressing from letters of caution and public reprimand to temporary license suspension or even licensure revocation.

Administrative discipline is considered quasi-criminal, but the most severe penalty in virtually all cases will be permanent licensure revocation. Unless a memorandum of agreement or stipulation of the facts can be reached, state prosecutors present evidence to the licensing authority (a board in the case of health care professionals or court in the case of attorneys), which then renders a sanction appropriate to the degree of the respondent's professional misconduct.

In the case of substance abuse, virtually all jurisdictions have established programs for addicted professionals to enter professional health programs involving counseling, strict adherence to sobriety with random drug screening, and mentorships in consideration of a respondent's being able to continue to practice. Professionals who successfully complete those programs may be reprimanded or, in some cases, be required to have a supervising mentor as they graduate back to independent practice but will not suffer licensure revocation. Bear in mind that these sanctions will generally become a part of the public record and, in the case of health care providers, will be memorialized forever in the NPDB (and in the case of physicians, the Federation of State Medical Boards). Once listed in any database, a practitioner may face sanction from certain credentialing third-party payers or from professional societies such as their respective certifying board, the latter potentially revoking their certification and further thereby damaging their ability to contract with third-party payers.

Administrative issues facing oncologists
Medical licensure complaints
Medical licensure investigations generally arise most commonly from patient complaints or those of disgruntled employees, although state and/or federal regulatory authorities may commonly involve licensing authority investigators when drug diversion, criminal activity, sexual misconduct, or issues of billing fraud are alleged.

Health professional licensing boards are composed generally of either elected or appointed licensees, in many cases, with lay, politically appointed members as well. Board composition, members' tenure, and their respective scopes of authority and ability to sanction are outlined in a state's professional practice act, whether governing physicians, nurses, pharmacists, or other professionals. A medical license is held in most jurisdictions to be a constitutionally protected property interest subject to strict Fourteenth Amendment scrutiny, with medical board holdings subject to appeal to either an appellate administrative law court or directly to the statutorily delegated appellate courts of the given state. Such appeals solely address errors of law, and the standard of review at the appellate level may be strictly and narrowly limited. Health care professionals are not trained jurists and are particularly unaccustomed to dealing with criminal matters involving licensees.

Health care regulatory complaints
The general public, patients, and in some cases disgruntled employees frequently contact state or federal agencies regarding concerns over excessive billing; prescribing, storage, and drug dispensing practices; office cleanliness; and employment matters. Agency investigators have jurisdiction over state matters, whereas, federally, the Office of the Inspector General of the Department of Health and Human Services and the Drug Enforcement Administration (DEA) will be the most

likely entities to address billing and drug issues, respectively. Additionally, regional Medicare administrative contractors, through employed investigators, may be involved when there are allegations of overpayment to a provider.

When allegations involving prescribing practices arise, the DEA, state drug authority, and medical board investigators descend upon the practitioner's office usually with administrative subpoenas for various documents, medical records, drug invoices, and prescribing logs. Such subpoenas are authorized by statute but lack the requirement of judicial authorization and generally do not have probable cause requirements, thereby frequently provoking critics concerned with Fourth Amendment search and seizure requirements being compromised. Clearly, this is a possible defense to compliance with such subpoenas that might be grounds for delay in the search; however, judges will virtually always enforce such subpoenas if they are obtained per the allowed statutory scheme.

Paper and electronic records are commonly sought, and practitioners, by counsel, should request a timely return of all materials seized once inspected or copied by investigators. Investigators will present their evidence to the US Attorney's Office in the case of federal investigations or to the state attorney general or disciplinary counsel in state cases, which may thereafter potentially generate complaints requiring adjudication. Penalties generally include a significant civil monetary penalty, remedial measures with an enforcement mechanism, and in the case of the DEA or state drug authority, a request to forfeit DEA licensure as to all controlled substances. The latter should not be voluntarily forfeited because the DEA has an administrative mechanism including a hearing procedure whereby the practitioner can defend his or her licensure before an administrative law judge. Respondents refusing to voluntarily surrender licensure will be queried by the DEA as to the forfeiture recommendation and moved to a hearing docket wherein they can defend their DEA licensure.

Medicare audits, overpayments, and statistical extrapolation

Medicare was established in 1965 under Title VIII of the Social Security Act and is now administered by the CMS, a component of the Department of Health and Human Services, to provide health insurance to those over 65 years of age, the disabled, and those with end-stage renal disease and amyotrophic lateral sclerosis. It pays 80% of its maximum allowed charge for evaluation and management services and clinical procedures, all entered electronically on CMS-1500 forms using CPT codes. The program's conditions of participation require that the health care delivered be medically necessary and that the level of service billed match the requirements of the CPT code billed. In cases where services are not medically necessary, where services are billed but not actually performed, or where the level of service billed does not actually encompass that level of service performed, an overpayment from Medicare to the provider will occur. The program has a right to recoup such an overpayment.

Medicare generally approaches potential overpayment to a practice initially by the local Medicare administrative contractor (MAC) performing an audit of medical records. These are requested from the practice and should be timely provided. The MAC's auditors identify potential overpayments and forward them to the regional recovery audit contractor (RAC), which reviews the MAC's audit and, if recovery of overpayment is indicated, will request that payment from the practice. In many cases, the RAC will apply statistical extrapolation to the claims alleg-edly overpaid to the universe of claims during the corresponding time frame, greatly increasing the practice's financial liability to the program. Such statistical methodology can increase the repayment necessary from thousands to hundreds of thousands of dollars. In such scenarios, counsel for the practice must work to invalidate the statistical extrapolation.

Historically, contractor extrapolation was permitted when there was a sustained or high level of payment error or when educational intervention had failed to correct payment errors. As there was no universal indicator of what constituted a "sustained or high level of payment error," the practice was literally left at the contractor's discretion. The 2020 revisions to the *Medicare Program Integrity Manual* make it clear that statistical sampling is appropriate only after documented educational intervention has failed to correct the payment error. This guidance is significant because it suggests that sampling may only be permissible if documented education has not led to improvement. Further, the same guidance provides some clarification of what may or may not be a sustained or high level of payment error and alternative avenues a contractor may use to determine a sustained or high level of error, including prior history of noncompliance, information from law enforcement investigations, and audits conducted by the Office of the Inspector General (OIG). Contractors are also required to employ the services of a qualified statistician to review the extrapolation methodology, the sample utilized, and its accuracy, providing the practice another avenue to question the overall amount due to the contractor.

Overpayment matters follow a five-level appeals process progressing from the initial review by a Medicare contractor, to a qualified independent contractor, to the Office of Medicare Hearings and Appeals (OMHA), to the Medicare Appeals Council, and finally, to the federal district court.

Provider panel expulsions

The ability to submit and have claims paid by the federal payer programs is a must to remain solvent in medical practice in the United States. To be expelled from a federal payer provider is the death knell of a practice, and the grounds for expulsion to the Medicare program are speci-fied in the Code of Federal Regulation (CFR).[14] Clearly, expulsion can be a collateral consequence of criminal activity, fraudulent or abusive billing, inappropriate prescribing practices, medical licensure actions, or failure to pay a federal debt (such as a student loan).

Program expulsion is appealable, but there is a significant backlog in the dockets of CMS administrative law judges, and the same is the case in Medicare overpayment appeals, particu-larly at the level of the OMHA. For that reason, negotiation may be an option to consider, par-ticularly if the facts do not in any way mitigate expulsion as an appropriate sanction. CMS applies a first-time reenrollment bar to any expelled practitioner lasting from one to ten years, except in cases of noncompliance with, or remediation of, problematic provider enrollment requirements. Given the delay in getting a hearing, negotiation of a sanction including the shortest possible reenrollment bar is always worth consideration. A history of prior expulsion can carry a reenroll-ment bar of up to 20 years. In all cases, once Medicare expulsion has occurred, Medicaid, Tricare, and private insurers quickly follow suit.

JURISDICTION AND VENUE

Jurisdiction under state and federal law

Jurisdiction refers to the inherent authority of a court to hear and dispositively address a dispute between the involved parties, which include at least two legal persons in the case of civil matters and a legal person and the government in a criminal matter.

State jurisdiction turns largely on a court's being granted statutory authority to hear that type of case. That court must have subject matter and personal jurisdiction; that is, the court must have statutory authority to hear the type of case and the court must properly be authorized to decide matters of a particular defendant (*in personam* jurisdiction) or an item of property (*in rem* jurisdiction).

Federal jurisdiction has two components. District courts have "original jurisdiction" of all civil actions arising under the Constitution, laws, or treaties of the United States.[15] They also have jurisdiction of all civil actions where the matter in controversy exceeds the sum or value of $75,000, exclusive of interest and costs, and is between citizens (or permanent residents) of different states, foreign states, or a foreign state and a citizen or permanent resident, so-called "diversity jurisdiction."[16]

Venue under state and federal law

Venue refers to the location where an action can be heard by a court of competent jurisdiction.

Venue in state court generally lies in the county of the state where the defendant resides or where the acts and/or omissions encompassing the cause of action occurred. Federally, an action may be heard (1) in a judicial district in which any defendant resides, if all defendants are residents of the state in which the district is located; (2) in a judicial district in which a substantial part of the events or omissions giving rise to the claim occurred or a substantial part of property that is the subject of the action is situated; or (3) if there is no district in which an action may otherwise be brought as provided by law, in any judicial district in which any defendant is subject to the court's personal jurisdiction with respect to such action.[17]

CIVIL AND CRIMINAL PROCEDURE

Federal and state civil procedure

Civil procedure governs disputes between parties and is governed by rules promulgated by the relevant jurisdiction's legislature, usually with input from its judiciary, state or federal. State rules of civil procedure generally closely mirror the federal rules and govern the filing of pleadings, their amendment, their service, how a served party must respond, subpoenas, procedures for the filing of motions (requests for orders of the court), and in-depth guidance as to discovery (the sharing of information relevant to the case by the parties). Civil rules also dictate the various issues of timeliness in filing and in responding to adverse parties, the conduct of trial including jury matters, entry of judgment, posttrial motions and procedure, seizure, and final remedies.

Parties seeking appeal of an adverse judgment do so under the jurisdiction's rules of appellate procedure, generally specifying procedures for notice of the appeal, its scheduling, the provision of the trial court transcript, and procedures for briefing the matters of law at issue in the appeal, both directly and in opposition to any briefing filed by the adverse party.

Federal and state criminal procedure

Criminal matters in state and federal court are also governed by rules promulgated by the jurisdiction's legislature and again with judiciary input. Rules of criminal procedure govern the issuance of warrants and the affidavits used to obtain them, bonds, and the return of executed search warrants. All these related materials must be provided to the clerk of court and prosecutor's office for later disclosure to defense counsel. The criminal rules also govern the issuance of subpoenas and motions, including those for continuance and for directed verdict (of acquittal). They also govern trial procedure including jury matters and instructions, expert witnesses, and preservation of objections.

Federal and state administrative procedure

Administrative process is governed generally by statute, commonly a state's administrative procedures act. On the federal side, administrative process is generally described in the CFR and will vary with the involved agency. In the case of health care licensure boards, hearing procedures are generally governed by the relevant state practice acts for doctors, nurses, and pharmacists.

Administrative procedure, generally to meet Fourteenth Amendment due process requirements, grants an opportunity for an evidentiary hearing prior to any controversy's disposition. The rules for such a hearing are established by statute or regulation and usually do not require strict adherence to the relevant jurisdiction's rules of civil procedure or evidence. Appellate process is generally through a state administrative law court or the state's appellate court system. Whichever route is taken, the administrative law court or the appellate court system will have its own rules governing practice.

INITIATION OF HEALTH LITIGATION

Filing of civil matters

Filing of a civil action generally requires production of a complaint, which is submitted to the clerk of court with an accompanying fee and usually a summons, the latter providing instructions and a timeline for responding to the complaint. The signature of an attorney admitted to practice in that jurisdiction is required on both documents, although recently, filings have largely transitioned to an online process with electronic signatures and credit card payments. The filed documents are generally stamped, indicating the filing date and assigning a docket number, and then served on the opposing party by a so-called process server, which provides an affidavit of the service time and date to the party retaining it to perform service of process. Once respective counsels have noticed their appearance, service is generally deemed as perfected when a document is published via the relevant electronic filing system.

Depending on the jurisdiction, in cases of alleged medical malpractice, the complaint or some notice of intent to file such a complaint must be accompanied by the affidavit of a qualified expert in whatever subject matter may be at issue in the complaint. That expert must meet certain requirements generally specified by statute as to their education, training, experience, and board certification and whether they are actively practicing or teaching. The expert's curriculum vitae may be a filing requirement, as may responses to certain standard preliminary discovery. Other jurisdictions solely require certification of counsel that they have verified the merits of the case with such an expert to be later named.

Again, as to medical malpractice, depending on jurisdiction, such a complaint or notice thereof may also necessitate early mediation or the consideration of the case's merits by a panel of professionals similarly licensed who must then attest merit prior to the case moving forward. These preliminary requirements generally emerged in the 1990s and early 2000s to eliminate frivolous filings and control rising medical malpractice insurance premiums.

Initiation of criminal matters

Criminal matters begin by way of the filing of a criminal complaint or an indictment in the federal system. A criminal complaint is essentially a statement of the facts alleging probable cause to charge and arrest a defendant. It must be approved by a federal magistrate judge in the federal system, whereas in state systems, a warrant must be approved by a low-level state court judge, sometimes known as a magistrate or small claims judge. In both cases, affidavits from law enforcement must attest to probable cause to arrest. An indictment requires a grand jury proceeding wherein prosecutors present affidavits and preliminary evidence attesting to probable cause, with the grand jury then voting to issue a formal true bill indictment in the event of finding probable cause or a no true bill in the case of evidence insufficient to indict.

Following arrest on a complaint, warrant, or true bill of indictment, a defendant is held for arraignment or appearance before a judge who recites the charges, in some cases entering an initial plea of guilty or not guilty and then setting a bond amount to assure that defendant's appearance at subsequent proceedings. Bond will turn on whether the defendant is determined to be a flight risk or whether he or she is a danger to the community. Should neither be the case, the court must determine a reasonable bond to impose, whatever that amount may be, to be either paid in full by the defendant or pledged as bond based on the value of real estate owned by the defendant, or a bond in that amount may be provided by a surety such as a bonding company. In the latter case, the defendant pays only a small, nonrefundable portion of the bond amount to the surety and is released, in some cases to be monitored by GPS.

Administrative matters

Administrative matters generally are initiated by an investigation, in some cases beginning with an unannounced visit by investigators with an administrative subpoena or search warrant. In serving such a document, investigators search the premises for potential evidence of use to the agency in proving its allegations against the practitioner. Thereafter, the involved agency may issue a formal complaint or, in some cases, if the facts are not in dispute, request a memorandum of agreement wherein the facts are stipulated, the latter requiring the agreement of the respondent. Such a memorandum obviates the need for the prosecuting agency to otherwise prove the facts relevant to the investigation. At that point, the memorandum or complaint is adjudicated before a panel, board, hearing officer, or judge; respondents in administrative matters generally are not entitled to a jury trial, at least until the agency's action is appealed. The facts thereafter are not at issue, and the agency or appellate court need only concern itself with an appropriate penalty, if any.

Service of process and notice

Adequate notice is fundamental to Fifth and Fourteenth Amendments due process.[18] The Sixth Amendment also specifically guarantees the right of a criminal defendant to be notified of the charges and their grounds.

In the context of civil actions, the US Supreme Court held that notice must be "reasonably calculated, under all the circumstances, to apprise interested parties of the pendency of the action and afford them an opportunity to present their objections."[18] Unless there is consent to the contrary, in-person service of civil complaints is essential, with the process server virtually always executing an affidavit certifying service and indicating the person to whom the complaint was served, the date, and the time service was effected.

In the context of criminal actions, service of a warrant is generally accompanied by arrest followed by detainer, arraignment, and an opportunity to post bond. When a warrant has been obtained, relevant law enforcement serving the warrant return it indicating the date and time it was served.

Legal representation

The Sixth Amendment Assistance of Counsel Clause grants criminal defendants the right to be assisted by counsel.

Despite precedent to the contrary,[19] in *Gideon v Wainwright*[20] and its progeny, the Supreme Court held that criminal defendants unable to afford an attorney must be provided a public defender in all trials posing the possibility of imprisonment. The Assistance of Counsel Clause includes five distinct rights: the right to counsel of choice, the right to appointed counsel, the right to conflict-free counsel, the effective assistance of counsel, and the right to represent oneself *pro se*.

Plaintiffs in civil matters may also proceed *pro se* and frequently do in small claims, eviction, and traffic cases. In major civil actions, however, counsel is necessary to ensure a well-pled complaint, timeliness as to all deadlines, prior trial experience, and familiarity with jury research and ADR.

Doctrines of privilege and protection

The attorney-client privilege is among the oldest common law privileges and encompasses a "client's right to refuse to disclose and to prevent any other person from disclosing confidential communications between the client and his attorney."[21] "The purpose of the attorney-client privilege is to encourage full and frank communication between attorneys and their clients and thereby promote broader public interests in the observance of law and administration of justice. The privilege recognizes that sound legal advice or advocacy serves public ends and that such advice or advocacy depends upon the lawyer's being fully informed by the client."[22]

The attorney-client privilege is not without exceptions. Communications must be made solely in the presence of client(s) and their attorney(s) involved in the operative case. It does not apply when third parties are included, when the communication was for the purpose of committing a crime or fraud, or when the client has waived the privilege expressly or constructively by public disclosure.

The work product doctrine protects materials prepared in anticipation of litigation from discovery by opposing counsel.[23] In 1947, the US Supreme Court, affirming the Third Circuit Court of Appeals, excluded oral and written statements made by witnesses to a defendant's attorney from discovery.[24] Since 1970, after recommendation by the Advisory Committee of the Judicial Conference, the Supreme Court enshrined the doctrine as Rule 26(b)(3) of the Federal Rules of Civil Procedure, protecting trial preparation materials. Most states have a similar rule in their respective civil practice rules.

Much like the attorney-client privilege, most, if not all, jurisdictions also recognize a physician-patient privilege wherein evidence at trial or another legal proceeding may be excluded on the basis that any information disclosed by a patient to a doctor for the purpose of diagnosis or treatment is confidential (unless the patient consents to disclosure). Just as is the case with exceptions to the attorney-client privilege, there are also exceptions to the physician-patient privilege, most notably, perhaps, the Tarasoff doctrine wherein many jurisdictions impose a common law duty upon a provider to warn anyone potentially at risk of harm by a patient. Such a duty usually arises in the context of mental health providers and mentally ill patients; however, all providers acquiring knowledge of any intent to harm a third party should in all cases alert law enforcement and the patient's family.[25]

Also notable is the spousal communications privilege applicable in civil and criminal cases, but most commonly exercised in the latter. Both the accused spouse and the witness spouse have the privilege, and either may invoke it to prevent testimony as to confidential communication made during the marriage. It does not apply to premarital communication or that following divorce but may be evoked after divorce when the communication occurred during the marriage.

Diversion in criminal matters

Over the past 20 years, first-time criminal defendants, particularly drug offenders and those committing certain misdemeanors, have been given diversionary options in lieu of imprisonment or a term of probation. Qualification for such diversion will vary with jurisdiction, but if available, those arrested for simple possession of marijuana can receive a conditional discharge in consideration of drug education and community service. Drug courts have also become popular, incorporating drug and addiction education, periodic drug screening, and community service, in many cases under the direct supervision of the presiding judge.

Those qualified for conditional discharge or drug court must generally enter a plea of guilty and then enter into the program, be monitored, complete certain educational and behavioral milestones, remain drug free, and then successfully graduate. Thereafter, their charges and entry of a guilty plea are expunged, leaving their records untarnished.

Certain jurisdictions also allow pretrial diversion for certain lower-level offenses. In this case, the defendant is not required to enter a guilty plea; instead, the prosecutor formally elects to proceed *nolle prosequi* (without prosecution). Those defendants must generally pay a supervisory fee and complete a term of community service, and once those requirements are met, their arrest records are destroyed and their criminal records are expunged of the offense.

THE PLEADINGS

Complaint

Civil actions concerning oncologists as defendants or plaintiffs begin with the filing of a complaint, which must include a caption naming the parties, the relevant court wherein the action was filed, a statement as to the basis of jurisdiction and venue, a statement of the facts entitling the party to relief, and individual claims including each and every element of the civil action whether established by common law or statute. The same necessities apply to a counterclaim when a defendant pleads a civil action against the plaintiff (usually pled in combination with the answer) who originally filed, with both of these pleadings generally concluding with a so-called "wherefore" clause, which recites the relief requested by the pleading party.

Answers

The response to a complaint is termed an *answer* or, in the case of a counterclaim, a *reply*. The timeline and instructions for responding to a complaint or counterclaim are specified in an accompanying summons; a period of 30 days is the general time limit to respond to a complaint in state court, with 21 days being the time wherein an answer must be filed and served in federal court. These time limits may be altered by consent of the parties or when the defendant waives formal service of a summons.

Generally, per Rule 12 of most jurisdictions' rules of civil procedure, all defenses to a claim must be asserted in a responsive pleading addressing the facts of the claim as pled; however, certain defenses may be asserted by motion, including (1) lack of subject-matter jurisdiction; (2) lack of personal jurisdiction; (3) improper venue; (4) insufficient process; (5) insufficient service of process; (6) failure to state a claim upon which relief can be granted; and (7) failure to join a party.

Counterclaims, cross-claims, and third-party claims

As previously referenced, a defendant may file a counterclaim against a plaintiff, file a so-called cross-claim against another defendant, or implead a third party in a third-party complaint. The defendant's factual pleading and defenses will outline the bases of those claims, again with the claims requiring all elements of the civil causes of action pled. Those parties implied through these types of claims must all answer and, in all cases, may also counterclaim. A summons must be included with any counterclaim, cross-claim, or third-party claim.

Amending the pleadings

A party may amend its pleading generally at any time prior to the receipt of a responsive pleading as a matter of course and without leave of court. Under the federal rules, the pleadings may be amended up to 21 days following receipt of the responsive pleadings or any motion from the defendant. State rules generally provide similarly but may allow a longer period of time to amend.

Pleadings may be supplemented on motion and with notice as to any transaction, occurrence, or event that happened after the date of the pleading to be supplemented. Further, an amendment will relate back to the date of the original pleading's filing if the applicable statute of limitations allows relation back, the amendment asserts a claim or defense that arose out of the original conduct pled, or the amendment changes the party named against whom the claim is asserted, provided the latter has not and will not be prejudiced and knows or should have known that, but for mistake concerning the proper party's identity, the action would have been brought against it.

Once a responsive pleading has been filed or the federal deadline thereafter has lapsed, leave of court by way of a motion is necessary to amend, and if a scheduling order is in place, there is a good cause requirement to amend.

Motions on the pleadings

Demurrer was the common law term for a defense asserting that even if all the factual allegations in a complaint are true, they are insufficient to establish a valid cause of action. The precise basis for a demurrer, more commonly now termed a *motion on the pleadings* or a *12(b)(6) motion* (named for the usual jurisdictional civil rule applicable), can vary, with some examples being a failure to state a claim for which relief can be granted, failure to meet a procedural predicate, failure to plead with requisite particularity, or pleading under an allegedly unconstitutional statute.

When the pleading fails to state a claim for which relief can be granted, the usual remedy is to amend the pleading to meet the necessary pleading requirements. Rule 9(b) of the Federal Rules addresses matters requiring particularity in pleading, specifically in cases of fraud (including health care fraud), mistake, or special damages. In the context of health care fraud, pleading materiality of the fraud to the government's decision to pay the involved claim(s) is a necessity to overcome a motion on the pleadings, with such a motion now almost a given in any health care fraud case. The materiality requirement, described by the Supreme Court as "rigorous" and "demanding," frequently forces whistleblowers to have an in-depth knowledge of the specifics of the fraud, which is usually very difficult because the offending party commonly makes every effort possible to conceal the mechanism of the fraud.[26]

Criminal matters

Pleadings is a term not commonly utilized in the context of criminal prosecution or defense. Pleadings include the indictment, the information, and the pleas of not guilty, guilty, and *nolo contendere* (no contest).[27]

In a federal white-collar criminal case, an *indictment*, an *information*, and a *complaint* all serve to initiate a criminal case and notify the defendant of those charges against him or her. Additionally, they ensure that a prosecutor has probable cause that a crime has been committed. Like an indictment, an information is a formal charging document describing the criminal charges and their factual basis. Unlike an indictment, an information does not require a grand jury's vote. Instead, the information is presented generally to a federal magistrate judge, who, after review, decides whether there is probable cause that a crime occurred.

A complaint is simply a statement of the essential facts of the offense to be charged, made under oath by a law enforcement official. The purpose of the complaint is to establish probable cause, which will allow an arrest warrant to be issued.

Virtually all federal white-collar criminal offenses, including those involving health care fraud, are felonies and thus require an indictment under the Fifth Amendment; however, some white-collar felonies can begin with an information or a complaint, while (in the case of a complaint) additionally preserving time under the Speedy Trial Act of 1974.[28] A complaint or information can be filed far more quickly than a grand jury indictment can be obtained, so if prosecutors must move quickly in making an arrest, they may file a complaint or information. After the arrest, the government must obtain a grand jury indictment, unless the defendant chooses to waive and proceed solely by information. Constitutionally, a felony case cannot go forward on the basis of a complaint alone; the framers of the Constitution (under the Fifth Amendment) intended for the grand jury—a body of ordinary citizens—to serve as a buffer against overzealous prosecution.

The Speedy Trial Act of 1974 regulates the time in which a trial must begin to ensure that criminal prosecutions are not unduly delayed. The act requires a trial to begin within 70 days of the filing of information, an indictment, or the initial appearance of the defendant. The initial filing of a criminal complaint thereby provides additional investigative time, although defendants commonly waive their right to a speedy trial, with the only requirement being the court's making specific findings supporting such a waiver's serving the ends of justice.[29]

Realistically, indictment requirements present a very low hurdle to criminal prosecution; prosecutors control the evidence the grand jury sees, instruct the grand jury on the law, and write the indictments. Under those circumstances, it is no surprise that it is frequently said that prosecutors "can indict a ham sandwich."

THE DISCOVERY PROCESS

Paper discovery

Rules 26 through 37 of most jurisdictions' rules of civil procedure cover discovery, with all but Rule 37 (which covers sanctions) covering its substantive aspects. So-called "paper discovery" is addressed in Rules 33, 34, and 36, covering interrogatories, requests for production of documents, and requests for admission. Interrogatories are essentially questions to be answered by the party served; requests for production of documents requires the served party to produce documentary evidence relevant to the allegations in the complaint, whereas requests for admission address factual issues the served party is requested to admit. Rule 34 also covers the production of electronically stored information, as well as a party's entering land or a premises for inspection or photography, whereas Rule 35 allows a party to obtain a mental or physical examination (including blood typing) upon motion and a showing of good cause. There are deadlines for responding to each of these discovery tools, all potentially extended by agreement; however, requests for admission are unique in that they are deemed admitted if the served party does not respond within the statutory deadline (usually 30 days).

Responses to discovery must be truthful and timely. Following a certified attempt to obtain relevant disclosure or discovery without court action, the party may file a motion to compel. If such a motion is granted, payment of the movant's attorney fees may be ordered, subject to the nonmovant being given an opportunity to be heard. Failure to respond to an order compelling discovery is subject to the court's contempt power, leading to potentially more severe sanctions absent good cause in not responding.

Depositions

Governed by Rule 30 of most jurisdictions' rules of civil procedure, a deposition is no more than an examination of a witness under oath, generally by counsel opposing the party disclosing the witness. Depositions may be obtained for discovery or trial purposes, in the case of the latter, usually with video recording, particularly when the availability of such a witness for trial may be problematic or costly.

Depositions are noticed by the party taking the deposition, with the opposing party noticed and invited to attend. A verbatim transcript is prepared by a court reporter, with the deponent being given the opportunity to read, sign, identify, and correct errors in the transcript or to waive review. Depositions are generally obtained as a discovery tool but can be used for impeachment purposes at trial. A discovery deposition may be read at trial by consent of the parties, whereas trial depositions on video are played for the jury and the video is then entered into evidence and available for the jury's review. Expert witnesses are commonly examined under oath, with a trial deposition on video then played at trial to save costs otherwise necessary for the expert to travel to the trial location. Depositions may also be obtained upon written questions to the deponent.

Rules govern the conduct of depositions and vary by jurisdiction. Under the federal rules, a deposition is limited to a maximum of seven hours in one day. Need for clarification as to questions posed to a deponent must generally be directed to the deposing attorney. Further, failure of a party, either individually or by counsel, to attend its own noticed deposition or to subpoena a nonparty deponent, who thereafter fails to attend, can subject it to sanctions by the court, including payment of the not-at-fault party's attorney fees.

Motion practice

Motions are no more than a request for an order of the court filed by a party to a lawsuit. They may seek orders changing venue, compelling discovery, requiring a bill of particulars or a more definitive statement, granting leave to amend a pleading, or even dismissing the action under certain circumstances.

One of the more common dispositive motions heard by a court is a motion for summary judgment. Governed by Rule 56 of most jurisdictions' rules of civil procedure, summary judgment may be granted if the movant shows that there is no genuine dispute as to any material fact and the movant is entitled to judgment as a matter of law. Subject to certain deadlines in many jurisdictions, motions for summary judgment commonly are filed either at or near the conclusion of discovery.

Summary judgment is appropriate only if the movant shows that there is no genuine dispute as to any material fact and the movant is entitled to judgment as a matter of law. When a court considers a summary judgment motion, the evidence of the nonmovant is viewed as truthful, and all justifiable inferences are to be drawn in his or her favor. Moreover, the judge does not weigh the evidence and determine the truth of the matter but, instead, determines whether there is a genuine issue for trial. The court's role in deciding a motion for summary judgment is to identify factual issues, not to resolve them. By definition, no findings of material facts that were in genuine issue are possible in granting summary judgment.

In the health care context, motions for summary judgment are common, particularly when an expert fails to identify a breach in the standard of care applicable to the defendant.

ALTERNATIVE DISPUTE RESOLUTION

Since the 1990s, virtually all jurisdictions have progressively incorporated ADR as a means of civil docket management and as an alternative to trial to facilitate settlements when possible. In many cases, depending on the jurisdiction, ADR to impasse is required prior to a civil action being placed on the trial docket. Mediation and arbitration are the most commonly used forms of ADR used in trial practice.

Mediation

Mediation is a nonbinding private process where a neutral third person called a mediator helps the parties discuss and try to resolve the dispute. Decision makers, including insurance adjusters, as applicable, must be present. The parties have the opportunity to describe the issues; discuss their interests, understandings, and feelings; provide each other with information, including damages analysis; and explore ideas for the resolution of the dispute. While courts can mandate that certain cases go to mediation, the process remains "voluntary" in that the parties are not required to come to agreement. The mediator does not have the power to make a decision for the parties but can help the parties find a resolution that is mutually acceptable. The only people who can resolve the dispute in mediation are the parties themselves.[30]

Following opening statements in a joint session, the parties more often than not move to separate rooms to caucus. Mediation generally includes a volley of demands and offers from the plaintiff and defendant, respectively. The parties voice what they see as strong points of their respective positions and discuss differing theories on liability, the true value of the plaintiff's damages, whether causation as espoused is realistic, and possibly jury research. The mediator works to control the parties' emotions and focuses on finding consensus on as many points as possible and then on placing a value on the case upon which the parties can agree. Once the parties reach a bracket range of valuation wherein settlement is possible, the process intensifies in hopes of settlement. The mediator generally can never be compelled to testify for either party at trial.

If the parties reach an agreement, the mediator may help reduce the agreement to writing, which may be enforceable in court. If no agreement is reached and impasse is declared, the mediator generally must file a report to that effect with the clerk of court, allowing the matter to move to the trial docket, although the parties could still settle of their own accord.

Arbitration

Arbitration is typically a binding process (although it may be nonbinding) that replaces the full trial process with multiple (often three) arbitrators to serve essentially as judges. The arbitrators make decisions about evidence, hear testimony, and give written opinions. Although arbitration is sometimes conducted with one arbitrator, the most common procedure is for each side to select an arbitrator. Then, those two arbitrators select a third arbitrator, at which point the dispute is presented to the panel. Decisions are made by majority vote.

Arbitration is commonly used in business and contractual disputes, in many cases mandated by an existing contract that will describe the arbitration procedure and rules. It is typically not mandated by any jurisdiction's local rules or by statute as a prerequisite to trial. It can be utilized as an alternative to trial but typically only by mutual consent of the parties.

PRETRIAL PROCEDURE

Should negotiation fail and the dispute reach the trial docket, pretrial procedure will begin informally, generally becoming more intense in the weeks prior to the trial date, to fully inform the parties of what to expect and to prevent "trial by ambush."

In a criminal matter, the state and defense counsel will exchange witness and exhibit lists, motions *in limine* (motions to be heard outside the presence of the jury), *voir dire* questions to be posed to potential jurors, and proposed jury instructions. Should the court require, respective counsel may also be asked to submit pretrial briefs and agree to the issues in a statement of the case. The process in civil matters will be very similar.

The motions *in limine*, usually addressing evidentiary issues, will be ruled upon, and the parties will prepare proposed jury instructions, with the court considering the latter and generally accepting those instructions agreed upon by consent of the parties. If the parties cannot agree on the instructions, the court will fashion some amalgam of their requested instructions and give those instructions to the jury at the closure of the parties' cases, just prior to the jury's beginning deliberations.

TRIAL

The venire

Venire is a general term referring to the jury pool in a given locality. State court jury pools are generally drawn from the county wherein venue is proper, whereas federal juries are drawn from the federal judicial district wherein venue is proper. When a given federal judicial district is subdivided into divisions, the jury pool is drawn from those counties zoned to that particular federal division. Federal juries are therefore typically more diverse than those drawn from a single county.

Qualifying and choosing a jury

To qualify as a juror in both state and federal court, a potential juror must be a US citizen of at least 18 years of age, residing primarily in the county or judicial district for a minimum of one year. Jurors must be adequately proficient in English to satisfactorily complete the juror qualification form and understand the proceedings and have no disqualifying mental or physical condition. Jurors cannot currently be subject to felony charges punishable by imprisonment for more than one year and cannot have been convicted of a prior felony unless their civil rights have been legally restored, generally by way of pardon.

Members of the armed forces on active duty, members of professional fire and police departments, and "public officers" of federal, state, or local governments who are actively engaged full time in the performance of public duties are exempt from service on federal juries. While requirements vary from state to state, many states exempt or excuse senior citizens, those with documented health conditions precluding their service, those subject to undue hardship, those who have recently served as jurors, and those whose presence is so essential at a place of employment that it would by necessity affect the business's operation.

Voir dire refers to the preliminary examination of a witness or a juror by a judge or counsel. Potential jurors and alternates are initially asked general questions to ascertain their competence to serve and generally later questioned as to any biases or opinions they may hold that could impact one or both of the parties. Certain jurors may be stricken for cause if they are clearly materially biased toward either party, with each party additionally able to peremptorily strike any juror for no particular reason. Such peremptory strikes must be race neutral.[31]

Opening statements

Opening statements by the party's respective attorneys occur following the seating of the jury and essentially paint their respective themes and theories of the case. The party that has the burden of proof will be the first to open, which is the plaintiff in a civil matter and the state in a criminal matter. Opening statements should not be argumentative and are not evidence; the judge usually instructs the jury as to the latter prior to the opening statements proceeding. Objections, while allowed during opening statements, generally do not occur except in the case of egregious overreaching by the other party.

An opening statement will summarize the case's facts in the light most favorable to that party and can allude to the evidence (of any type) a party intends to enter to prove its case. It can refer to expert opinion evidence and will usually conclude with the respective party explaining why the jury should find for that party.

Plaintiff's and defendant's cases

As is the case with opening statements, the party that holds the burden presents their case first. This will include their calling each witness to the stand, where the clerk will administer the oath. Once under oath, direct examination by counsel for the party calling the witness is followed by cross-examination by opposing counsel, followed by re-direct examination and then re-cross-examination, if appropriate. The scope of re-direct examination and re-cross-examination is limited to questions arising solely from the opposing counsel's prior line of questioning.

Documentary and physical evidence must be authenticated prior to entry, that is, proven to be genuine and not a forgery. Evidence may be authenticated by the testimony of a witness that a document is what it is claimed to be, as in the case of a witness testifying that a photograph accurately depicts the subject matter therein. Health care professionals or clerical staff can authenticate a patient's medical records. Certain documents are self-authenticating, including newspaper articles, public or business records or certified copies thereof, governmental publications, trade inscriptions, and commercial papers.

Once authenticated, the party proffering the exhibit into evidence moves for its admission by sequential numbering, with opposing counsel being given an opportunity to object. All objections voiced must state a reason for the objections, and the court either sustains or overrules the objection. Certain sustained objections may be overcome by simple rephrasing of a question, such as in a nonleading or noncompound manner, whereas others may require withdrawal and a change in direction to another line of questioning or asking the witness a question that does not evoke hearsay.

Following the completion of the initial party's case, the opposing party will present its case, including its witnesses and the introduction of its evidence for the jury's consideration. The rules of criminal or civil procedure and evidence apply equally to both parties, with the party presenting its case first being required to present evidence by way of testimony and exhibits that, in the civil context, proves the defendant's liability by a preponderance standard; in contrast, in the criminal context, the state must prove its case beyond a reasonable doubt. The court recesses after the party with the burden of proof rests, and the jury is temporarily excused.

Types of evidence

There are many types of evidence, some of which have no relevance to trial and cannot be utilized therein. The most common types of evidence introduced at trial include the following:

1. **Testimonial evidence:** This is one of the most common forms of evidence and consists of either spoken or written evidence given and authenticated by a witness under oath. It can be gathered in court, at deposition, or through an affidavit.

2. **Demonstrative evidence:** Demonstrative evidence directly demonstrates a fact usually through an object or document. It includes, for example, photographs, video and audio recordings, and charts.
3. **Documentary evidence:** Documentary evidence includes letters or wills and is most commonly considered to consist of written forms of proof. It can also include media, such as images or video or audio recordings.
4. **Digital evidence:** This includes any digital file from an electronic source such as e-mails, text messages, GPS information, instant messages, files and documents extracted from hard drives, electronic financial transactions, audio files, and video files.
5. **Direct evidence:** Direct evidence requires no inference and is the most reliable and powerful type of evidence. It alone is the proof and includes the testimony of a witness who saw an incident firsthand.
6. **Character evidence:** Testimony or a document used to prove that someone acted in a particular way based on the person's character is termed character evidence.
7. **Physical evidence:** This includes tangible objects, such as a firearm, fingerprints, a knife, a pill bottle, rope, tire casts, or a foreign body recovered at surgery.
8. **Forensic evidence:** Scientific evidence, such as DNA, trace evidence, fingerprints, or ballistics, that can provide proof to establish a person's guilt or innocence constitutes forensic evidence. It is generally considered to be strong and reliable, helping to convict criminals; in other cases, it helps to exonerate the innocent.
9. **Circumstantial evidence:** This is indirect evidence used to form an inference based on facts separate from the fact an argument seeks to prove and is not considered strong evidence. It requires a deduction of facts from other facts that can be proven.
10. **Exculpatory evidence:** This is evidence that can exonerate a defendant in a criminal case. Prosecutors are required to disclose any exculpatory evidence they find or risk having the case dismissed.[32]
11. **Hearsay evidence:** This evidence consists of statements made by witnesses who are not available for examination at trial. Although hearsay evidence is generally not admissible in court, there are numerous exceptions that can be useful at trial.[33]

Expert witness testimony

Fact witnesses, such as the plaintiff, his family, other consulting physicians, pharmacists, therapists, nurses, and/or durable medical equipment providers, provide no opinion testimony, only evidence establishing the facts of the case and explaining them to the jury. At all times, the judge rules on matters of admissibility of evidence, qualification of experts, questions of law, and any motions brought by either party outside the presence of the jury, so-called "motions *in limine.*"

A jurisdiction's rules of evidence govern the use of expert witnesses at trial.[34] With the exception of opinions related to individual perception, an opinion necessary to understand a witness's testimony or to determine a fact in issue, or an opinion not based on scientific, technical, or specialized knowledge, only qualified experts may express their opinions at trial.[35] The testimony of expert witnesses for the plaintiff supports liability of the defendant through his or her breach in the applicable standard of care, whereas the testimony of the defendant's experts supports his or her compliance with the standard of care, thus supporting that he or she is not liable.

A witness who is qualified as an expert by knowledge, skill, experience, training, or education may testify in the form of an opinion or otherwise if (1) the expert's scientific, technical, or other specialized knowledge will help the trier of fact to understand the evidence or to determine a fact in issue; (2) the testimony is based on sufficient facts or data; (3) the testimony is the product of reliable principles and methods; and (4) the expert has reliably applied the principles and methods to the facts of the case.[36]

Under federal law, the *Daubert* standard is a rule of evidence regarding the admissibility of expert witness testimony. Under the *Daubert* standard, the factors that may be considered in determining whether the methodology is valid are (1) whether the theory or technique in question can be and has been tested; (2) whether it has been subjected to peer review and publication; (3) its known or potential error rate; (4) the existence and maintenance of standards controlling its operation; and (5) whether it has attracted widespread acceptance within a relevant scientific community.[37]

Some state jurisdictions rely upon the older *Frye* standard as to the admissibility of expert testimony.[38] Generally, the difference between the *Daubert* and *Frye* standards is the broadened approach of the latter. Whereas *Frye* essentially focuses on one question—whether the expert's opinion is generally accepted by the relevant scientific community—*Daubert* offers the previously discussed five-factor test focusing on the relevance and reliability of the expert's testimonial evidence.

A *Daubert* motion is a specific type of motion *in limine* raised before or during trial to exclude the presentation of unqualified evidence to the jury. The Supreme Court's *Daubert* holding requires that trial judges act as the gatekeeper to determine the scientific validity of evidence before admitting it. The judge's ruling will determine whether the expert's testimony is admissible.

If a judge excludes or questions the admissibility of an expert's testimony, the judge may, *sua sponte* or through motion by the affected party, allow the expert to proffer testimony outside the presence of the jury for consideration on appeal, should the latter occur.

TRIAL MOTION PRACTICE

In additional to *Daubert* motions and other motions *in limine*, at the conclusion of the plaintiff's case in a civil action or the close of the state's case in a criminal action, the opposing will virtually always move for a directed verdict in favor of the defendant or for acquittal, respectively. In the civil context, these motions allege that the plaintiff has failed to produce evidence adequate to prove liability on the part of the defendant, whereas in the criminal context, they allege that the state has failed to produce evidence adequate to prove its case beyond a reasonable doubt. These motions are generally perfunctory and seldom successful but are important to place on the record.

Motions to strike certain testimony in the civil context and those to exclude evidence perhaps obtained in violation of the Fourth Amendment's prohibition against unlawful search and seizure in the criminal context are also common and important to preserve in the record should appeal be necessary.

Rebuttal witnesses

At the conclusion of the defendant's case, the plaintiff or state can present rebuttal witnesses or evidence to refute evidence presented by the defendant. This may include evidence not presented in the case initially or a new witness who contradicts the testimony of the defendant's witnesses. The opposing party can cross-examine these witnesses and is keenly aware that their testimony must solely address rebuttal of testimonial evidence they presented. As a result, rebuttal is generally very limited in scope and very brief.

Closing statements/summations

Counsels' closing arguments or summations discuss the evidence and those inferences properly drawn therefrom. Issues outside the case or about evidence that was not presented are excluded. Generally, the judge will have reviewed the proposed jury instructions with the parties prior to closing arguments such that those instructions can be related specifically to the evidence presented.

Counsel for the plaintiff or state closes first, summarizing and commenting upon the evidence in a light most favorable for their client, showing how it proved the elements necessary to prevail in the case. The defense then presents its closing, usually addressing statements made in the plaintiff's or government's argument, pointing out deficiencies in its case, and summing up the facts favorable to their client.

Because the plaintiff or government has the burden of proof, counsel for that side is entitled to make a concluding argument, sometimes called a rebuttal. This is a chance to respond to the points made in the defendant's closing and make one final appeal to the jury. If the defense chooses not to make a closing statement, the plaintiff or government loses the right to make a second argument.

Jury charge, deliberation, and verdict

The jury charge is the judge's instructions to the jurors on the law that applies to a case's relevant subject matter and definitions of the relevant legal concepts in layman's terms. These instructions, always mutually agreed upon by the respective parties, are drawn from the relevant applicable statutes and case law, may be complex, and are often pivotal in a jury's deliberations.

After receiving the charge, the jury retires to the jury room for deliberation, usually receiving a verdict form agreed upon by the parties. Jurors are instructed to not discuss the case at hand with anyone until they actually retire to the jury room, with all the admitted evidence in hand to deliberate and render a verdict. Generally, their first task is to elect one of the jurors as the foreperson, who will preside over discussions and votes of the jurors and often deliver the verdict. In some jurisdictions, the jury may take the exhibits introduced into evidence and the judge's charge into the jury room. After an initial poll of the jurors, deliberations continue until, hopefully, a verdict is reached; the verdict is then provided to the bailiff, who informs the judge. The judge then reconvenes with the parties to announce the verdict. The bailiff's job is to ensure that no one communicates with the jury during deliberations, although jurors may direct questions to the judge through the bailiff, if necessary. Communication from the judge to the jury will be shared with respective counsel or done in their presence.

Jurors may be sequestered (i.e., housed in a hotel and secluded from all contact with other people, newspapers, and news reports) until they are able to reach a verdict. In most cases, however, the jury will be allowed to go home at night. In all cases, the judge will instruct jurors not to read or view reports of the case in the news. They are also instructed to not consider or discuss the case while outside of the jury room.

Generally, the verdict in a criminal case must be unanimous. In some states, a less than unanimous decision is permitted in civil cases. All federal cases require a unanimous verdict.

Mistrial

When a trial is not successfully completed, a mistrial occurs. The trial is declared void before the jury returns a verdict or the judge renders his or her decision in a bench trial.

Mistrials occur for many reasons, such as juror misconduct or an impropriety in the drawing of the jury discovered during trial, death or incapacitation of a juror or attorney, or a hopelessly deadlocked jury that is unable to reach a verdict.

Often, the first time a jury reports being deadlocked, the judge will issue further instructions and encourage them to continue deliberating in an attempt to reach a verdict. This instruction may be referred to as an Allen charge, an Allen instruction, or, in the vernacular, a "dynamite charge."[39] The judge will admonish those jurors in the minority to give due deference to the majority and consider their duty to reach a verdict, heeding the majority if at all possible. Courts should not deliver such charges in a way that has a coercive effect; however, there is clearly some element of coercion inherent in such a charge. If no verdict can be reached after reasonable effort, a mistrial may be declared. Such a declaration is without prejudice to the plaintiff, who may request another trial.

On occasion, a fundamental error prejudicial to the defendant that cannot be cured by appropriate instructions to the jury (such as the inclusion of highly improper remarks in the prosecutor's summation) can lead to a mistrial. Either side may make a motion for a mistrial. The judge will either grant the motion and declare a mistrial, or he or she will not grant the motion and the trial will go on. If the case ends in mistrial, it may be tried again at a later date before a new jury, or the plaintiff or government may decide not to pursue the case further.

POSTTRIAL MATTERS AND APPEAL

Should a party suffer an adverse verdict or bench decision at trial, it can file a posttrial motion to correct such an error. Examples would include a motion for a new trial based on an error in the jury verdict or the jury's charge or if the jury finds a defendant liable but fails to award damages despite the plaintiff's evidence supporting damages. In the absence of obvious error, however, judges give significant deference to juries and are unlikely to overrule them.

The same applies to posttrial motions for a judgment notwithstanding the verdict (JNOV); however, a judge who has heard the evidence might be inclined to grant a JNOV if the jury's verdict clearly flies in the face of the weight of the evidence presented.

In the case of appeal, the adversely impacted party must generally notice the appeal within 30 days of the entry of judgment and order the trial transcript, which may be included in a joint appendix to be provided to the appellate court. The appellant then prepares and files an opening brief citing the error or errors at issue on appeal, followed by a response brief to be filed by the appellee. The appellant may then file a reply brief, addressing issues addressed initially in the appellee's response brief.

JUDGMENT

The decision of the jury does not take effect until the judge enters a judgment on the decision (i.e., an order that it be filed in public records).

In a civil suit, the judge may have the authority to increase (additur) or decrease (remittitur) the amount of damages awarded by the jury or to modify the judgment before it is entered. In criminal matters, the judge usually has no authority to modify the verdict. In most jurisdictions, it must be accepted or rejected (e.g., by granting a motion in arrest of judgment).

If the defendant does not pay the damages awarded to the plaintiff in a civil case, the plaintiff may request an execution of the judgment. In the latter case, the clerk of the court will deliver the execution to the sheriff, commanding him to take and sell the property of the defendant and applying that money to pay the judgment.

CONCLUSION

Trial practice is complex and requires in-depth investigation, frequent legal research, a firm and detailed grasp of the case's facts, and a knowledge of discovery techniques and the rules of civil and criminal procedure.

Occupationally, oncologists are most frequently exposed to trial law in the context of medical malpractice, either as a party or expert witness, but also occasionally are drawn into court based on domestic, criminal, employment, regulatory, and health care fraud and abuse scenarios. In each of these cases, an experienced attorney, or group of attorneys, with some knowledge of health law and significant trial practice experience is of significant benefit.

References:

1. Peckham C, Grisham S. Medscape Medical Malpractice Report: 2015. https://www.medscape.com/features/slideshow/malpractice-report-2015/oncology#page=3. Accessed August 5, 2021. See also Marshall D, Tringale K, Connor M, Punglia R, Recht A, Hattangadi-Gluth J. Nature of medical malpractice claims against radiation oncologists. *Int J Radiat Oncol Biol Phys.* 2017;98(1):21–30.
2. Ganesh T. Incident reporting and learning in radiation oncology: need of the hour. *J Med Phys.* 2014;39(4):203–205.
3. See *US Ex Rel. Thompson v Columbia HCA Healthcare Corporation*, 125 F.3d 899 (1997) and *Universal Health Services, Inc. v US Ex Rel. Escobar*, 136 S Ct 1989, 195 L Ed 348 (2016).
4. See Rules 8(a) and 9(b), Fed R Civ P.
5. Pub L 100-293, 102 Stat 95.
6. 42 USC § 11101 et seq.

7. 42 USC § 11112(a).

8. *Poliner v Texas Health Systems*, 537 F3d 368 (5th Cir 2008), cert denied 555 US 1149, 129 S Ct 1002, 173 L Ed 2d 315 (2009).

9. *Bostock v Clayton County*, 590 US ____ (2020).

10. 42 USC §§ 2000e-5(b), 2000e-5(e) (1982).

11. 18 USC § 3553(f).

12. *United States v Booker*, 543 US 220 (2005).

13. 18 USC § 3553(a).

14. 42 CFR § 424.535.

15. 28 USC § 1331.

16. 28 USC § 1332.

17. 28 USC § 1391.

18. *Mullane v Central Hanover Bank & Trust Co.*, 339 US 306 (1950).

19. *Betts v Brady*, 316 US 455, 62 S Ct 1252, 86 L Ed 1595 (1942).

20. *Gideon v Wainwright*, 372 US 335, 83 S Ct 792, 9 L Ed 2d 799 (1963).

21. Garner BA. *Black's Law Dictionary*. 10th ed. St Paul, MN: Thomson West; 2014:1391.

22. *Upjohn Co. v United States*, 449 US 383, 386, 101 S Ct 677, 681 (1981).

23. Black HC, Garner BA. *Black's Law Dictionary*. Abridged 7th ed. St Paul, MN: West Group; 2000:1298.

24. *Hickman v Taylor*, 329 US 495, 67 S Ct 385; 91 L Ed 451 (1947).

25. See *Tarasoff v Regents of the University of California*, 17 Cal 3d 425, 551 P2d 334, 131 Cal Rptr 14 (Cal. 1976).

26. See *Universal Health Services, Inc. v US Ex Rel. Escobar*, 136 S Ct 1989, 195 L Ed 348 (2016).

27. See Rule 12, Fed R Crim Proc.

28. 18 USC §§ 3161-3174.

29. See 18 USC § 3161(H)(8).

30. Mediation. American Bar Association. https://www.americanbar.org/groups/dispute_resolution/resources/DisputeResolutionProcesses/mediation/. Accessed August 5, 2021.

31. *Batson v Kentucky*, 476 US 79, 106 S Ct 1712, 10 L Ed 2d 215 (1986).

32. See *Brady v Maryland*, 373 US 83, 83 S Ct 1194 (1963).

33. See Rule 803, Fed R Evid.

34. See generally Rules 701-706, Fed R Evid.

35. Rule 701, Fed R Evid.

36. Rule 702, Fed R Evid.

37. *Daubert v Marion Merrell Dow Pharmaceuticals*, 509 US 579, 113 S Ct 2786; 125 L Ed 2d 469 (1993).

38. *Frye v United States*, 293 F 1013 (DC Cir 1923). States still using the *Frye* standard at the time of this text's publication include California, Illinois, Maryland, Minnesota, New Jersey, New York, Pennsylvania, and Washington.

39. *Allen v United States*, 164 US 492 (1896).

CHAPTER 5

Expert Testimony

Joseph D. Piorkowski, Jr., DO, JD, MPH, FCLM

INTRODUCTION

The objectives of this chapter are two-fold. The first objective is to familiarize readers who have not previously been involved with the overall process of civil litigation with the basics of that process. The second objective is to aid the reader in navigating the process by providing practical guidance about serving as an effective expert while protecting oneself and steering clear of ethical pitfalls.

THE ROLE OF AN EXPERT WITNESS IN LITIGATION

Over the past two decades, expert witnesses ("experts") have played an increasingly important role in litigation. The outcomes of cases involving complex scientific concepts often come down to "a battle of the experts." Physicians serving as experts provide an important service to the community and to the legal system by helping to ensure that litigation outcomes are based on scientific facts and principles. Experts who are good communicators can assist a judge or jury in understanding difficult and complex scientific concepts by breaking them down into comprehensible pieces, in much the same way an oncologist might explain the complexities of a cancer diagnosis and treatment plan in understandable terms to a patient.

Physicians with expertise in oncology have been involved primarily in three types of litigation: (1) medical malpractice cases alleging that a physician failed to comply with the standard of care in diagnosing or treating a patient; (2) product liability cases involving allegations that exposure to a particular chemical or medication was the cause of plaintiff's injury; and (3) intellectual property cases involving patent disputes. There is no limitation, however, on the types of cases in which an expert can get involved.

Importantly, unlike the attorneys, who must be advocates for their clients, experts are supposed to be objective, impartial, and unbiased, with a commitment to being fair to both sides. Ultimately, of course, an attorney would not call an expert to testify if that expert's opinions on balance are not helpful to the attorney's case. The responsibility of the expert, though, is to provide a candid, unbiased review of the case as opposed to simply telling the attorney what he or she wants to hear. When a case review is ultimately "favorable" (i.e., supporting the position of the party on whose behalf the expert was retained), there are still likely to be some aspects of the case that are challenging. An expert's review is most useful when it provides a candid assessment of not only the strengths of the party's case but also the weaknesses.

Even a case review that is ultimately "unfavorable" provides value. For example, it is important for a plaintiff's attorney to know when, from a scientific vantage point, his or her case is relatively weak or lacking in merit. Ultimately, that knowledge may prevent the attorney from devoting a lot of financial resources to a case that has limited value. Conversely, from the vantage point of a defense attorney, it would be valuable to know that the defense of a case would be challenging from a medical standpoint; such knowledge might persuade the attorney to seek early resolution of the matter instead of putting forth a vigorous defense.

Fact witnesses versus experts

For the purposes of this chapter, the terms *expert* and *expert witness* refer to a physician who is specially retained by a party and who is generally compensated for his or her time with the expectation that, if the expert's opinions after reviewing the case are favorable to the retaining party, he or she would testify at the trial of the case.

Physicians who have special expertise in a discipline such as oncology can also be hired to work as confidential consultants who are not expected to file an expert report or to testify at deposition or trial. Typically, these expert consultants work behind the scenes to assist attorneys with a variety of tasks such as evaluating the potential merits of a case, reviewing and interpreting the medical literature, and preparing to take the depositions of important fact witnesses or the opposing side's experts. These consulting relationships are almost always confidential and not subject to discovery by the opposing party. Although some of the considerations discussed in this chapter may be applicable to such consultants (e.g., the need to have clear agreement regarding compensation), this chapter is focused on experts who may testify at trial.

Physicians who provided care and treatment to patients who later become involved in litigation are sometimes asked to testify about their observations and their findings, either at a deposition or at trial. For example, a treating oncologist might be asked to testify about the cause of the plaintiff's cancer or the plaintiff's prognosis. Although such physicians are certainly "experts" in their field, they are not "experts" in the sense that this term is used in this chapter. That is, they have not been retained specifically for purposes of the litigation and, therefore, would not be subject to many of the requirements of litigation experts (e.g., submitting a written report).

GETTING INVOLVED IN THE LITIGATION PROCESS

Attorneys or members of their staff will often reach out to physicians who, based on their curriculum vitae, websites, or LinkedIn pages, appear to be promising prospective experts for their case. Sometimes this communication will be by e-mail or sometimes by telephone call to the physician's office.

Expert witness services

There are a variety of expert witness services that assist attorneys in identifying and retaining prospective experts for their cases. These services attempt to facilitate pairing together experts who are interested in getting involved in litigation with attorneys who are looking for experts to staff their cases. A variety of business models are used; many of these companies also handle billing and invoicing for the experts. These services make money through a finder's fee and/or by adding on a supplemental charge to the expert's usual hourly billing rate.

For an expert who is interested in getting involved in litigation consulting, affiliation with one of these companies may be worthy of consideration. Before deciding to do so, however, the expert should ensure that he or she has a complete understanding concerning billing arrangements (who is responsible for payment). Also, it is important to know whether the service advertises and, if so, whether the prospective expert would be specifically identified in any marketing or promotional materials.

PRERETENTION CONSIDERATIONS

Initial contacts

Whether the initial contact comes directly from an attorney or from an expert witness service, it should be understood that agreeing to have a preliminary discussion with an attorney about a case does not obligate an expert to undertake a review of the case. Rather, the purpose of the initial contact is generally informational. It is useful to have a general understanding of the subject matter of the case to ensure it is within the expert's area of expertise. It is important to understand what party or parties the attorney contacting the expert represents. In addition, as discussed later, it is also prudent to obtain a list of interested parties and/or potential witnesses to determine if there is any conflict of interest or relationship that might affect the expert's ability to conduct an objective and unbiased evaluation of the case. If the expert is being asked to undertake a case review, then he or she should ensure that the attorney has an understanding of the expert's hourly billing rate for this assignment, as well as an understanding that payment of the expert's fee does not depend on the outcome of the review (i.e., if the expert's opinion upon reviewing the case is not favorable, the attorney is still required to pay the expert for time spent). Memorializing this in an e-mail may avoid potential disagreements down the line.

Finally, the expert should have an understanding as to whether the attorney is potentially looking to the expert to testify at trial or whether the attorney is simply looking for a confidential case review to assess the strength of his or her case. It is prudent to ask the attorney about the anticipated time commitment for the engagement. If the attorney ultimately may want the expert to testify, then before agreeing to take the case, the expert should review the timetable for key events such as due dates for submission of expert reports, depositions, and trial to ensure that his or her schedule can accommodate the attorney's needs.

Conflicts

Before agreeing to review a case, the expert should ensure that there are no actual or perceived conflicts and nothing that would affect the expert's partiality or ability to offer unbiased testimony in that particular case.

Generally, it is useful to ask the attorney at the outset of the matter to provide a list of the physicians, other health care providers, institutions, and/or companies who are involved in the case.

One of the clearest conflicts would be if an expert was being asked to testify in a case in which one of the expert's patients was a plaintiff on the opposing side. Some courts have held that the sanctity of the physician-patient privilege prevents a physician from doing so, even if the issue in the litigation is not directly related to the subject of the physician's care and treatment.

A potential expert also needs to consider other matters that could affect his or her partiality or ability to provide an impartial and unbiased review. If one of the key treating physicians in the case was the expert's college roommate, for example, the expert would need to consider whether that personal relationship would affect his or her judgment, positively or negatively. If the defendant physician is someone held in high esteem in the expert's specialty and testifying against him or her could adversely affect the expert's standing in medical organizations in which both the expert and the defendant physician participate, that potential conflict should be identified on the front end. If the expert served previously as a consultant to a company the safety of whose product is being called into question in the current case, the expert would need to evaluate his or her ability to fairly evaluate the evidence in light of that relationship. There are endless additional examples; the bottom line is that each expert needs to determine, fairly and honestly, whether he or she is capable of conducting an objective review in the particular case.

To be clear, an expert need not refrain from getting involved just because he or she knows one of the parties or the key witnesses. The expert does, however, need to ask himself or herself whether the relationship with this person or entity would affect his or her judgment. If there are any questions in this regard, it is best to discuss them with the attorney at the outset.

Baggage

It is important for attorneys to know early in the process of working with an expert whether the expert has any "baggage" that would detract from the expert's credibility. It is critical for attorneys to avoid the type of scenario depicted in the movie *A Time to Kill*, in which the defense psychiatry expert, Dr. Willard Tyrell Bass, is effectively destroyed on cross-examination when he is confronted with a prior statutory rape conviction of which the defense counsel was unaware. Most attorneys will conduct background checks on experts at some point in the process, so it is best to discuss any potential baggage on the front end.

Baggage can take a lot of forms, and it can be either professional or personal in nature. Professional baggage includes things ranging in seriousness from not passing board exams on the first attempt or having some substantive negative online patient reviews to having been previously (or currently) sued for medical malpractice, medical license suspensions or terminations, or a history of having been fired from a professional position. Treatment for substance abuse is increasingly seen among professionals, including physicians.

Personal baggage can range from a rude or insensitive comment posted on a social media site to a record of DUI (driving under the influence) or a domestic violence complaint to an arrest and/or conviction for a more serious offense.

Most of this information probably would not be admissible at trial, but it would be fair game for inquiry at deposition. A good policy is for the expert to be up front about these issues with the attorney with whom he or she is working, to allow the attorney to make an informed decision as to whether the baggage in question would be disqualifying and, if not, to best prepare the expert to handle questions about these matters at deposition.

Communications with counsel

Experts should be sure to discuss with the attorney with whom they are working whether communication between the expert and the attorney is privileged or whether such communication is subject to discovery by the opposing party. The rules concerning the confidentiality of both written and verbal communications between expert and attorney vary widely from jurisdiction to jurisdiction. Until about 2010, the prevailing rule in federal courts and in the vast majority of state courts was that any and all communications between an attorney and expert were fair game for discovery. The federal rule changed such that most communication, with the notable exception of communications involving fees and payments, is privileged.[1] Many states have adopted discovery rules that are consistent with the current federal rules, although many others have not. It is important from the outset to understand the ground rules about communications between an expert and the attorney with whom the expert will be working.

Communications with third parties

Although communications between an expert and the attorneys with whom he or she is working are considered confidential in the federal courts and in many states, generally there is no confidentiality attached to an expert's communications with third parties. So, for example, if an expert discusses the facts of the case with a colleague who is not involved in the case, that conversation would not be privileged, and the opposing attorney could ask about that conversation during a deposition or at trial. Accordingly, attorneys typically instruct experts not to have any substantive communications about the case with any third parties, including spouses or partners.

Compensation

One important preliminary matter is agreeing on the fee schedule for the services to be provided as a litigation expert. The most common practice is for experts to bill for their time at an agreed-upon hourly rate. Typically, experts charge the same hourly rate for activities such as reviewing medical records, reviewing and/or conducting a search of the scientific literature, meetings with counsel, and preparing a report, if one is required.

Experts should ask the attorney with whom they are working in advance about the level of detail they would like to see in the expert's invoices. Some attorneys and their clients prefer a lot of detail because it provides them with assurance that they are getting good value for their money. More typically, because invoices are generally discoverable by the opposing side, lawyers prefer for invoices to be very general with respect to the description of work performed because they do not want the opposing counsel to have a roadmap of how the expert approached the case. The expert should take guidance about this from the attorney with whom he or she is working.

Experts should set an hourly rate that is reasonable based on their education, experience, and position. Experts who are new to litigation often try to set their rates as high as the client is willing to pay, although this is not advisable for a couple of reasons. First, attorneys have a responsibility to ensure that their clients are receiving good value, and if one expert has a billing rate that is excessive in comparison to other options, the attorney will often divert work to the less expensive alternative. Most doctors who engage in expert consulting would prefer to have a steady stream of work at $500 per hour rather than a few hours of work at $700 per hour. Second, attorneys prefer to avoid calling experts at trial whose compensation is so large that the jurors' jaws will drop. The greater the hourly rate and the more out of step it is with that of other experts in the case, the more susceptible the expert is to the suggestion that he or she is "just doing it for the money."

One strict prohibition in terms of expert work involves being compensated on a contingency basis. If the expert's compensation depends on the outcome of the case, the expert has a vested financial interest and, by definition, cannot be viewed as objective and unbiased. The American Medical Association (AMA) Code of Medical Ethics Opinion 9.7.1 states the following: "Whenever physicians serve as witnesses they must: . . . (c) Not allow their testimony to be influenced by financial compensation. Physicians must not accept compensation that is contingent on the outcome of litigation."[2]

The vast majority of an expert's fees are paid by the party retaining the expert. Depositions, however, are generally an exception, and the opposing party usually pays for the expert's time.[3] Some experts have separate billing practices for giving deposition testimony. For example, many experts will use separate half-day or full-day rates (e.g., $4000 per day). The reason for this is that, because they are required to take a block of time out of their clinical schedule during which they would otherwise be seeing patients, they should be compensated for the time they are losing, even if the attorney taking the deposition ends up not utilizing the full time allotted. Similarly, some experts use cancellation policies (e.g., the full deposition fee is due if cancellation occurs <72 hours prior to the scheduled deposition) for the same reason, given that patients generally cannot be rescheduled to fill the void on such short notice.

Because appearing at trial involves many of the same considerations as depositions, experts will often use daily rates (in lieu of hourly rates) and include cancellation policies. Because trials may occur in a different location than where the expert works or resides, one other important consideration to work out in advance is how travel time will be handled. Often travel time during which an expert is not actively working on the case is compensated at a discounted hourly rate or sometimes is wrapped into the flat daily rate. In any event, it is important to have an understanding about this question from the outset. Generally, travel expenses are reimbursed, but it would be prudent to discuss the details of this in advance.

Retention agreements

Some attorneys prefer to have formal retention agreements with experts, and others do not. Whether an expert signs a formal retention agreement or not, there should be some written documentation (e.g., e-mail exchange) that outlines the key terms of the working relationship between the expert and the attorney including the fee schedule, the timeliness of payments (e.g., payments due within 30 days of receiving invoice), and an understanding of who is responsible for the payment (i.e., the attorney or the client whom the attorney represents).

EXPERTS IN THE LITIGATION PROCESS

Initial review of materials

Once a prospective expert agrees to review a case, the first step is typically for the attorney to provide the expert with a set of materials to review. In a medical malpractice case or products liability case, this generally will involve the plaintiff's medical records, depositions of the parties, and/or depositions of treating physicians.

One helpful practice is for the expert to ask the attorney to provide him or her with a complete copy of the medical records rather than a subset of records that the attorney selects as being relevant. This helps to insulate the expert from later claims that his or her opinion was based on an incomplete review and that the expert relied exclusively on selected records that were "spoon fed" to the expert by the attorney.

Most states have provisions to protect the confidentiality of a patient's medical records, even when the patient's medical care and treatment are at issue in litigation. The expert may be asked to sign an agreement to maintain the confidentiality of documents the parties have designated as "confidential," which is a fairly standard practice.

Literature searches

In addition to reviewing the plaintiff's medical records, most cases also require a review of the relevant scientific and/or medical literature addressing the specific issues in the case.

Often, the attorney's staff will have already compiled a collection of relevant literature applicable to the case. Such collections are often shared with experts and can be an efficient mechanism to avoid having each and every expert in the case needlessly spend dozens of hours separately downloading the same studies.

It is important, however, for an expert to be able to demonstrate that his or her review of materials was not limited to those provided by the attorney. There is no more effective way to undermine an expert's credibility than to show that the expert relied entirely on the materials provided by the attorney with whom he or she was working. Rather, an expert wants to be able to show the jury that he or she conducted a comprehensive, independent review of the literature to identify all relevant studies, regardless of which party's position such studies actually support. It is useful for experts to conduct such a search as an initial step (and if possible to keep track of the search terms used) and then to compare the results of that medical literature review to whatever collection was compiled by the attorneys.

Preparation of expert reports

In the majority of state courts and in all cases that are filed in federal courts (regardless of the state in which the federal court is located), experts who are expected to testify at trial are required to provide a written report summarizing the opinions the expert intends to offer at trial.[4] In lieu of a written report authored by the expert, a minority of states require an expert "designation," which is a statement written by an attorney summarizing the anticipated testimony of that side's experts.[5] A small number of states require neither expert reports nor substantive expert designations.

Purpose of expert reports

The primary purpose of expert reports is to provide notice to the opposing party regarding the substantive opinions that each expert is prepared to offer at trial. In cases that require expert testimony (e.g., medical malpractice cases), the expert report or designation is a critically important milestone in the case; it is the point at which the parties are required to define with specificity what they are claiming and what the issues are in the case.

Because of a practice referred to as "notice pleading," a plaintiff can generally file an action that includes only vague and conclusory allegations that provide little detail about the specific claim(s) the plaintiff is making. For example, in a malpractice case, the complaint might allege that the defendant doctor failed to comply with the standard of care in evaluating, diagnosing, and treating the plaintiff's breast cancer, and that because of the defendant's violations of the standard of care, the plaintiff has incurred pain, suffering, and emotional damage in addition to economic damages. Such a general description, of course, provides no meaningful information about key questions in the case; these question might include the following: (1) In what way did the defendant allegedly violate the standard of care? What did the defendant do or fail to do specifically that was outside the standard of care? (2) How did these alleged violations cause the plaintiff's alleged injuries? Would not many of these injuries have occurred in any event? (3) In what ways was the plaintiff damaged (e.g., loss of earnings, loss of chance of survival, additional medical expenses)?

The serving of the plaintiff's expert report(s), therefore, usually represents the first time in a civil action that the defendant has notice of the specific contentions that a plaintiff is making in a case. Conversely, the serving of the defense expert report(s) usually represents the first time in a case that the plaintiff receives notice about the specific positions that the defendant is taking with respect to these same issues as well as the details of any affirmative defenses.

Notice is critically important in the litigation process because it prevents "trial by ambush," a situation in which a party is hearing for the first time at trial a new position that the opposing party is taking. Trial by ambush is regarded as fundamentally unfair as it does not provide a meaningful opportunity to prepare for cross-examination or the opportunity for a party to prepare his or her own experts to address the issue. Judges, regardless of their backgrounds or political leanings, are fairly consistent on this point. They do not want an expert to state an opinion at trial as to which the opposing party has not had sufficient advance notice, particularly given the complex nature of medical and scientific testimony.

Accordingly, in preparing an expert report, it is important to ensure that all the major opinions that the expert intends to offer at trial are included in the report. If they are not, there is a reasonable chance that the judge may preclude the expert from offering such opinions at trial. Some states are very strict about this requirement. Pennsylvania, for example, uses what is referred to as the "4 corners" test (i.e., if the opinion is not clearly set forth somewhere within the "4 corners" of the expert report, the expert will not be permitted to offer it at trial). Some courts are more lax depending on additional circumstances. For example, if the expert gave a deposition and, in response to questioning, offered an opinion that was not contained in his or her report, a court might allow the expert to offer that opinion at trial, reasoning that the opposing party had both advance notice of the opinion before trial as well as an opportunity to explore the basis for the opinion at deposition. The judge's decision ultimately will turn on whether the party against whom the expert's testimony is being offered had fair notice of the opinion and a reasonable opportunity to respond. If not, the previously undisclosed opinion probably will be precluded. The prudent course of action, therefore, is to ensure that all of the expert's major opinions are included in his or her report; if additional opinions are later formulated that were not included in the original report, the expert should talk with the attorney with whom he or she is working about the need to file a supplemental report.

Requirements of expert reports

The specific requirements concerning what information needs to be included in an expert's report vary somewhat from jurisdiction to jurisdiction. The Federal Rules of Civil Procedure, which set forth the standards for civil actions in federal courts, however, provide a good overview and are consistent with the practice in many state courts.

The Federal Rules of Civil Procedure require expert reports to include the following: "(i) a complete statement of all opinions the witness will express and the basis and reasons for them; (ii) the facts or data considered by the expert in forming them; (iii) any exhibits that will be used [at trial] to summarize or support them; (iv) the witness's qualifications including a list of all publications authored in the previous ten years; (v) a list of all other cases in which, during the previous four years, the witness testified as an expert at trial or by deposition; and (vi) a statement of the compensation to be paid for the study and testimony in the case."[6]

Although many states have adopted requirements similar to the federal rules, there is tremendous variability with respect to the requirements for expert reports in individual states. As noted earlier, some states have expert designations in lieu of expert reports. It is important to take guidance from the attorney with whom the expert is working about the specific requirements in the venue in which the case is filed.

Process of report preparation

A few frequent questions, particularly asked by novice experts, are as follows: What is the appropriate role of the lawyer in completing and preparing the expert's report? Is it okay for the attorney to edit my report? Is it appropriate for the attorney to suggest that additional opinions be added or that certain opinions be deleted?

The rules of civil procedure in both federal and state courts are essentially silent on these questions. One needs to look to the usual custom and practice for guidance.

In general, attorney involvement in the preparation of expert reports is customary. Some aspects of attorney involvement are clearly appropriate. For example, for experts who have not previously prepared an expert report, it is wholly appropriate for an attorney to help the expert with formatting and organization, ensuring that the presentation is clear and logical and that it satisfies the requirements of the applicable rules. Assisting the expert with proofreading (identifying typographical errors) or checking citations is also clearly appropriate and common-place. Assisting the expert in understanding and properly using legal terminology (e.g., the defi-nitions of "a reasonable degree of medical certainly" or "a substantial contributing factor") is customary and appropriate. In addition, attorneys often take the lead in putting together the expert's list of materials considered.

With respect to more substantive matters, there is certainly no prohibition on an attorney having detailed discussions with an expert about substantive issues, including suggestions about how an expert's report can be strengthened. In fact, an attorney arguably would not be doing his or her duty if he or she did not try to ensure that the expert's report is as strong as possible. In federal court and states that follow the federal rules with respect to communications between experts and attorneys being privileged, such conversations would be outside the scope of appro-priate inquiry and would not be discoverable. In jurisdictions that do not treat such communi-cations as privileged, however, the expert would be required to disclose such conversations. In either event, as long as the expert ultimately takes ownership of all of the opinions in his or her report, such discussions are unlikely to detract meaningfully from the expert's credibility.

Regardless of whether the communication with the attorney is privileged or not, there is nothing unethical or inappropriate about an attorney suggesting that an expert consider add-ing a reasonable scientific opinion or argument to the expert's report; indeed, an expert should keep an open mind on such matters. An expert should not, however, allow himself or herself to be "talked into" including an opinion that the expert does not genuinely hold or that does not truly represent the expert's opinion. At the end of the day, the expert is the author of his or her report, and the report should only contain opinions that the expert is prepared to stand behind.

Daubert and the importance of methodology

In 1993, the US Supreme Court decided a seminal case, *Daubert v Merrell Dow Pharmaceuticals, Inc.*,[7] that addressed the admissibility of expert testimony in federal courts. One of the require-ments set forth in the Federal Rules of Evidence is that expert testimony be based on "scientific . . . knowledge."[8] The Supreme Court clarified that the term "scientific" in the rule "implies a grounding in the methods and procedures of science" and the term "'knowledge' connotes more than subjective belief or unsupported speculation." The court emphasized the importance of expert opinions being "derived by the scientific method."[9]

This landmark decision had the practical effect of requiring experts to follow an accepted sci-entific methodology in reaching expert opinions that will be offered in court. What it means as a practical matter, for an expert who is a clinician and is reviewing a case or preparing an expert report, is that the expert must use the same scientific approach in evaluating the issues in the litigation case as the expert uses in evaluating patients in his or her own clinical practice. It is important for experts to discuss with the attorney with whom they are working how to ensure that the expert's methodology will pass muster under *Daubert* or one of the many state stan-dards that have followed the *Daubert* model.

Methodologic challenges to an expert's opinion can be made on numerous possible grounds. One common basis for such motions is that the opinion lacks foundation (i.e., it lacks reliable medical or scientific evidentiary support). So, for example, in a case in which an expert testifying on behalf of plaintiffs opines that a plaintiff's cancer was caused by exposure to a certain chemical, such an opinion might be challenged if there is no reliable epidemiologic evidence supporting that the exposure caused that particular type of cancer or, alternatively, there is no reliable evidence that the exposure causes cancer at the plaintiff's level of exposure.

Another potential ground for exclusion is an expert's failure to consider and rule out alternative causes. Take, for example, a case involving a 55-year-old female plaintiff with a 35-pack-year history of cigarette smoking who developed follicular lymphoma. If an expert on behalf of the plaintiff opined that the plaintiff's follicular lymphoma was due to a chemical exposure and failed to consider the role of cigarette smoking, the expert's opinion might be challenged for failure to exclude other potential causes on the grounds that there are numerous studies demonstrating a statistically increased risk of follicular lymphoma in cigarette smokers, particularly in women, and there is even a specific translocation that is commonly found in these patients.[10]

The fact that a party challenges an expert's opinion, of course, does not mean that the expert's opinion will be excluded. Ultimately, the trial judge needs to decide whether the expert's methodology was reasonably reliable to support the expert's opinion.[11] It is important, however, for experts to ensure—at the time they are formulating their opinions—that their opinions have a reliable scientific foundation. Courts have limited tolerance for *ipse dixit* opinions—roughly translated as "it is so because I said so"—and require that expert opinions be well grounded in science, not just in the expert's say-so.[12]

Qualifications of experts

In litigation, there are two important considerations related to an expert's qualifications. The first is a legal inquiry as to whether the expert is sufficiently qualified for his or her testimony to be admissible. In other words, will the judge allow the expert to testify in the first place? The second and more practical concern is whether an expert's qualifications are strong enough to be convincing to the fact finder (usually the jury). In many instances, an expert may be able to satisfy the minimum requirements for admissibility but would be a poor choice as an expert witness at trial.

The rules of evidence that apply in federal courts and a great many state courts refer to "[a] witness who is qualified as an expert by knowledge, skill, experience, training, or education."[8] The operative word is "or," and numerous courts have held that the bar for the admissibility of expert testimony is relatively low; although, of course, an expert's lack of qualifications would always be fair game for cross-examination, and an unqualified expert is unlikely to be convincing to a jury.

Demonstrating these concepts are two court decisions reaching differing conclusions. In *Hartke v McKelway*, the plaintiff, over the defendant's objection, was permitted to introduce the testimony of a physician regarding the standard of care for performing laparoscopic cauterization of the fallopian tubes.[13] Although the expert had performed several hundred tubal ligations, she had never performed a laparoscopic cauterization, had never assisted in the performance of such surgery, and had observed such an operation only twice. The appellate court noted that laparoscopic cauterization was a new procedure that was significantly different from the tubal ligation procedure. The court held that "[h]er reading of literature and conferring with other physicians on the eve of trial did not qualify her" and she "should not have been allowed to testify about the standard of care for laparoscopic cauterization."[13] The court concluded that "to give an opinion on whether the defendant complied with the applicable standard of care, the witness must be familiar with that standard."[13]

On the contrary, in *Hedgecorth v United States,* the trial court considered whether two physicians—an ophthalmologist and an emergency medicine specialist—were qualified to give expert testimony regarding the standard of care for performing cardiac stress tests even though they were not cardiologists.[14] The court made a specific finding that both physicians "have demonstrated to this court that they are familiar with the appropriate standard of care with regard to stress tests. The fact that [these physicians] are not cardiologists does not render their testimony on stress testing inadmissible, but merely goes to the weight given it by . . . the trier of fact."[14]

Following are three practical points of guidance concerning expert qualifications:

Rule 1—Experts should stay in their comfort zone. Experts are most likely to be effective and convincing when they stick with what they know. Let's say, for example, that a prospective expert is a board-certified oncologist, but 95% of his or her practice over the past decade has been related to colon cancer, pancreatic cancer, and other cancers of the gastrointestinal tract. If the expert is asked to testify in a case involving breast cancer, he or she would almost certainly meet the minimum standard of admissibility by virtue of his or her training and board certification. Although the expert probably knows a great deal more about breast cancer than most other subspecialists in internal medicine, the fact that the diagnosis and treatment of breast cancer are not a regular part of the expert's practice would provide the opposing party with a reasonable basis for suggesting to the jury that his or her testimony should not be given great weight, particularly if the expert on the other side has extensive experience in that specific area. Ultimately, so long as the expert is forthright about his or her experience, it is up to the attorney who has retained the expert to evaluate and determine whether he or she would be a good expert at trial given the totality of the circumstances. An expert's credibility is likely to be greatest, however, when he or she stays in his or her comfort zone.

Rule 2—Experts should not readily concede to lack of expertise in a subject matter. A lot of confusion stems from the fact that the term *expert* has a distinctly different meaning in normal medical vernacular than in the context of legal proceedings. Many medical experts think of "experts" as those few people, usually in academia, who are on the cutting edge of new research frontiers. So, the instinct of many physicians is to say "no" when they are asked whether they are "an expert" in a certain field. Because the legal definition for expert testimony is broad, it is important, at deposition, for example, not to "give away" soundbites about lack of expertise because of a misunderstanding of the different ways these terms are used in the medical and legal arenas. Most oncologists, for example, are knowledgeable about chimeric antigen receptor (CAR)-T cell therapy; they know what it is, they know the circumstances in which it might be useful, and they understand the physiologic underpinnings. So, if an expert is an oncologist, he or she is probably an "expert" in CAR-T cell therapy within the legal meaning of the term regardless of whether his or her practice is focused on hematologic malignancies and regardless of whether the expert has actually been involved with using CAR-T cell therapy to treat one of his or her own patients.

Rule 3—Experts should not get defensive about "the small stuff." The vast majority of experts, no matter how impressive their credentials, have some small points that the opposing party will pick away at on cross-examination. Perhaps the expert did not pass his or her board certification exam on the first attempt or let his or her general board certification lapse, maintaining only more specialized certification. Perhaps the expert's medical license once lapsed because of a busy schedule and inattention. Perhaps the expert has never written an article or given a talk on the topic that is the subject of the litigation. Whatever it is, the expert should not be defensive about it and should answer questions honestly at deposition and trial, trusting that the attorney who has retained the expert would not have chosen him or her unless the attorney was confident that the expert was well qualified and would be convincing to a jury.

Depositions

In federal courts and in many state courts, after expert reports have been served, counsel for the opposing party has the right to take the deposition of the opposing side's testifying experts. The deposition is a formal proceeding that typically lasts several hours, with the expert's testimony being taken down by a court reporter and often memorialized on a videotape as well. Most commonly, expert depositions are taken in a law firm conference room. Although typically there is no judge in attendance, the testimony is taken under oath as if it were being given in court.

Detailed guidance on the deposition process and preparation for depositions is discussed in a separate chapter within this book. Nonetheless, a few important observations about expert depositions warrant brief discussion to help understand the role of the expert deposition in the litigation process overall.

By definition, the main purpose of an expert deposition is discovery. The deposition is the opposing counsel's opportunity to explore in greater detail the opinions offered in the expert's report and the bases for those opinions, in addition to exploring the expert's methodology in reviewing the case and reaching his or her opinions. Additionally, questions related to discovery of bias or interest are also considered fair game.

As a practical matter, attorneys use expert depositions for many purposes other than strictly discovery. Attorneys use depositions, for example, to obtain key concessions about facts that are not in dispute or about areas as to which the expert does not intend to testify at trial. Attorneys use expert depositions to try to lock down "sound bites" that might be useful on cross-examination (e.g., "You would agree that although you are trained in general oncology, you have no particular expertise in hematologic malignancies?"). The attorney with whom an expert is working should prepare the expert in advance for how to testify truthfully while at the same time avoiding "traps" caused by ambiguous, oversimplified, or conclusory questions. But make no mistake; the objective of the opposing attorney is to score points and to prepare for trial; it is *not* to embark on a quest to find the scientific truth about the facts of the underlying case.

Far too often, physicians go into expert depositions with the mistaken impression that they are embarking on an intellectual discourse, with the typical give-and-take that one might encounter at a grand rounds presentation in an academic setting with the objective ultimately being the search for scientific truth. Such physicians are sadly disappointed to learn that the primary objective of the opposing attorney is to win the case and that the search for scientific truth is way down the list of priorities, if there at all.

It is important to have reasonable expectations about one's own performance. Physicians who are unfamiliar with the litigation process and who are convinced in the correctness of their own opinions often expect that once the opposing attorney hears the expert's compelling explanation and sound scientific reasoning, that he or she will simply fold up shop. That almost never happens no matter how outstanding an expert's performance, so it is important for experts not to set too high a bar for themselves.

Finally, attorneys routinely use expert depositions to evaluate an expert's potential effectiveness as a trial witness. On occasion, attorneys will try to "push the expert's buttons" by asking about potentially sensitive subjects (e.g., a previous case in which the expert was a defendant in a medical malpractice case, a lapse in medical licensure, failing a board certification exam) to determine whether the expert will quickly become defensive, hostile, or aggressive when asked about such subjects. Remaining respectful, maintaining self-control, and "being the adult in the room" are always the best course of action, even if the examining attorney is being snide, sarcastic, mean-spirited, or abusive.

Most important characteristics of an excellent expert witness

Both at deposition and while testifying at trial, the three most important characteristics of an excellent expert witness are good communication skills, humility, and credibility.

Communication skills

Being a good communicator is the single most critical skill an expert can possess. Using words and terms that lay people can understand to get one's message across is essential. If it is necessary to use acronyms or complex medical terminology, an expert needs to take the time to define them and explain what the terms mean before using them. Experts should look at the jury as they are testifying to gauge whether they are getting through to the jury or talking over their heads, just as the experts would do when explaining something to a patient. Effective experts will make adjustments as necessary to make sure their message is getting through.

Humility

Humility is paramount; no matter how accomplished experts are or how many feathers they have in their cap, people in general, and juries in particular, are not enamored by experts who are impressed with themselves. Experts who are proverbial "legends in their own mind" are a huge turn off in the courtroom, as in life. That is not to say that an expert should not take pride in reviewing his or her professional accomplishments; indeed, highlighting one's key certifications or publications and showing the jury how one's knowledge and experience are particularly germane to the case at hand are always incredibly useful. But there is no room for boastfulness, and experts need to check their egos at the courtroom door if they hope to be effective.

Credibility (perception of honesty and integrity)

An expert's credibility is critical to being an effective expert. The jury needs to know they can trust the expert and that the expert is "telling it to them straight." Experts should not be afraid to look the jury in the eyes when giving their testimony.

In every case, there are always some points that are helpful to the other side. Making concessions that need to be made on cross-examination without requiring the opposing attorney to pull it out of the expert often enhances an expert's credibility. Similarly, maintaining the same demeanor on cross-examination as was displayed on direct examination goes a long way toward establishing credibility. By contrast, when an expert goes from pleasant and cordial on direct examination to combative and defensive on cross-examination, it signals that the expert may be serving as an advocate, not an impartial expert.

CONCLUSION

Experts are essential to the litigation process, and they play an important function in advancing the administration of justice by helping juries to understand complex scientific and medical facts and principles. Serving as an expert can be a rewarding professional experience assuming that the expert keeps many of these basic principles in mind.

References:

1. Fed R Civ P 26(b)(4).
2. Code of Medical Ethics Opinion 9.7.1. American Medical Association. https://www.ama-assn.org/delivering-care/ethics/medical-testimony. Accessed August 6, 2021.
3. Fed R Civ P 26(b)(4)(E).
4. Fed R Civ P 26(a)(2)(B).
5. See, for example, 231 Pa Code Rule 4003.5(a).
6. Fed R Civ P 26(a)(2)(B).
7. *Daubert v Merrell Dow Pharmaceuticals*, 509 US 579, 592 (1993).
8. Fed R Evid 702(a).
9. *Daubert v Merrell Dow Pharmaceuticals*, 509 US 590 (1993).
10. See, for example, Diver WR, Patel AV, Thun MJ, Teras LR, Gapstur SM. The association between cigarette smoking and non-Hodgkin lymphoid neoplasms in a large US cohort study. *Cancer Causes Control*. 2012;23(8):1231–1240; Liu Y, Hernandez AM, Shibata D, Cortopassi GA. BCL2 translocation frequency rises with age in humans. *Proc Natl Acad Sci U S A*. 1994;91(19):8910–8914; Morton LM, Hartge P, Holford TR, et al. Cigarette smoking and risk of non-Hodgkin lymphoma: a pooled analysis from the International Lymphoma Epidemiology Consortium (Interlymph). *Cancer Epidemiol Biomarkers Prev*. 2005;14(4):925–933.
11. See, for example, *Salem v United States*, 370 US 31, 35 (1962). ("Furthermore, the trial judge has broad discretion in the matter of the admission or exclusion of expert evidence, and his action is to be sustained unless manifestly erroneous.")
12. *Kumho Tire Co. v Carmichael*, 526 US 137 (1999). ("Nothing in either *Daubert* or the Federal Rules of Evidence requires a district court to admit opinion evidence that is connected to existing data only by the *ipse dixit* of the expert [i.e., only by the statement of the expert himself].")
13. *Hartke v McKelway*, 526 F Supp 97, 101 (DDC 1981); aff'd, 707 F2d 1544 (DC Cir), cert denied, 464 US 983 (1983).
14. *Hedgecorth v United States*, 618 F Supp 627, 631 (ED Mo 1985).

PART II

The Practice of Clinical Oncology

CHAPTER 6

Radiation Oncology

Terry J. Wall, JD, MD

INTRODUCTION

This chapter will cover the intersection of the practice of radiation oncology with the legal system by examining the epidemiology of medical malpractice risk, strategies to avoid malpractice risk, and advice to radiation oncologists who are sued. It will also provide examples of how the elements of a claim of negligence manifest in the specific context of radiotherapy practice. Radiation oncology risk in the business practice of medicine will also be briefly considered.

EPIDEMIOLOGY OF MALPRACTICE RISK IN RADIATION ONCOLOGY

Several strategies have been employed to create a picture of legal liability in the specialty, including surveys of members of the American Society for Radiation Oncology (ASTRO)[1] or of radiotherapy alumni groups.[2] These surveys have their limitations, as do reviews of cases reported in the legal literature, since only a minority of malpractice claims (around 8%)[3] ever make it to completed litigation and only a portion of those cases are reported in the legal literature. Proprietary "jury verdict" reporting services can provide supplemental information,[4] as can information from malpractice insurers, but there is no single pool of data for all malpractice claims against radiation oncologists. A survey of ASTRO members calculated an approximate annual cumulative risk of being sued to be on the order of 3%, making it likely that a practitioner will experience a claim at some point in their career.[1] A "claim" does not equate to an indemnity payment of damages, however, as only a small percentage of claims result in a payment. One recent study looked at the radiation oncology claims collected by a trade association of malpractice insurers that insure approximately 60% of the private practice market. A "claim" against a radiation oncologist resulted in a payment in 28% of cases in this database.[3] The average and median settlement values for the ten years of this study, ending in 2012, were $372,000 and $250,000, respectively. Radiation oncology settlements were 14% higher than the "all specialty" average, and claims were most common for radiation oncologists between the ages of 45 and 54 years.[3] The most common disease sites were breast, prostate, and lung cancers. Another study of this same database, but through a different period of time, found that solo practitioners were more commonly sued.[5] A study of yet another database, this one containing data from 30 academic institutions, found that head and neck, central nervous system, benign disease, and brachytherapy were the most common scenarios resulting in indemnity payments and that "technical skill, clinical judgment, and communication" were the top two contributing factors involved in a payment.[6]

STRATEGIES TO MINIMIZE MALPRACTICE RISK

The headwater of a malpractice case is a disgruntled patient; a bad outcome or even clear physician fault does not generate a court case without a patient making a "human" decision to sue. The source of that unhappiness may be fairly clear: wrong-sided treatment or improper dose delivery that creates harm, so-called "hard risks." But there are also "soft risks" that may lead an unhappy patient to use the legal system to "punish" their radiation oncologist in the absence of objective negligence. Both risks can be managed.

Moreover, both risks can be managed without impairing the patient or the health care system. In the only known study of the issue in radiation oncology, a survey of radiation oncologists in Italy[7] found that 75% admitted to practicing at least one of eight identified defensive strategies in the 12 months prior to the survey, including "ordering more tests than medically indicated" (39%), "suggesting an invasive procedure against professional judgment" (4%), or "prescribing more medications than medically indicated" (35%).[8] A primary driver was concern over the risk of litigation. In the United States, a 2006 study by the accounting firm PricewaterhouseCoopers estimated that "defensive medicine" increased US health care costs by 10%.[9] Fear of litigation *should* change behavior, but it should just change the correct behaviors.

Controlling the soft risks

Good documentation doesn't prevent lawsuits; good patient rapport does. (Good documentation certainly helps win lawsuits, though!) But the "best" lawsuit is not the one that you win; it's the one that is never filed. There is consensus among the defense bar that certain behaviors are wise, including avoiding ostentatious displays of wealth in the clinic, such as expensive jewelry and clothing. Insurers have noted that patients who complain about physician billing and collection policies are more likely to litigate.[10] Run to the problem. Address these patient concerns and encourage staff to report such patient concerns. In the clinic, taking a seat while visiting with a patient and listening without interruption as much as possible build rapport. Be sympathetic to patient feelings, and be empathetic to patient concerns.[11]

CASE LAW # 1

An example of what is hopefully the low-water mark in radiotherapy was an Arkansas case[12] where a patient, Meryln Jones, became quadriplegic following his course of radiation therapy. He made an appointment with his radiation oncologist who, the court noted, greeted him by saying, "Well, Merlyn, what did you do, come up here to make idle threats?" Merlyn, not surprisingly, did more than that.

Other unhelpful comments to patients by radiotherapists reported in different litigation include the following: "Let's face it, you are 72; if cancer did not get you, it would be your time to check out anyway."[13]

It is important to involve the family when a patient is having pronounced side effects or complications. Uninvolved family members are often felt to be fomenters of litigation.[10] If the radiation oncologist is late, it is important to apologize for the delay. Apologizing for a bad outcome is a more contentious strategy and is discussed in detail below.

Physician risk in the use of social media is usually more subtle than the case of the pediatric radiation oncologist and residency program director who committed the statutory offense of "knowingly accessed with intent to view" in the act of downloading files of dozens of images of child pornography to his work computer, including images of prepubescent children and images depicting sadistic and masochistic behavior. Imprisonment, fines, becoming a registered sex offender, and loss of a medical career followed.[14] In less egregious misadventures in social media, physicians have been disciplined for posting derogatory information about patients with sufficient detail that they were identifiable, thus violating the Health Insurance Portability and Accountability Act (HIPAA) privacy laws.[15] Even in the absence of a statutory violation, disgruntled patients may cruise a practitioner's social media sites looking for something they do not like about the practitioner to "trigger" their decision to file suit.[16] All physicians are well served to have written social media rules for their practices. They are well advised to keep professional and personal social media presences separate and to strictly limit access to their personal social media sites, if they choose to have any at all. The American Medical Association (AMA)'s Council on Ethical and Judicial Affairs has issued a profitable report entitled, "Professionalism in the Use of Social Media."[17]

There is a sarcastic saying among lawyers: "A good lawyer knows the law. A great lawyer knows the judge." In medicine, more presciently, the following applies: "A good doctor knows medicine. A great doctor knows their patients." Controlling the soft risks by good patient rapport and discretion in nonprofessional self-revelation is the best strategy to avoid frivolous lawsuits.

Controlling the hard risks

Real patient injury leads to real liability, as it should. The epidemiology of radiation oncology lawsuits already suggests some strategies for risk reduction. Solo practitioners should investigate some mechanism for chart rounds with other radiotherapists, possibly using some online resources. Heightened attention should be given to high-risk areas of practice, such as the treatment of benign disease and brachytherapy. Seriously consider referring patients who need procedures or treatments for which a practitioner is only marginally qualified or which they do not perform routinely. For example, a radiation oncologist who only treats one or two gynecologic brachytherapy cases a year (and considering that it is a disease site with documented improvement in patient outcome with greater physician experience)[18] may well conclude, on mature reflection, that the fees from doing the procedure are not likely worth the risk to either the radiation oncologist or the patient.

A systematic review of 34 cases reported in the legal literature looked at whether participation in the ASTRO Accreditation Program for Excellent (APEx) and the ASTRO/American Association of Physicists in Medicine (AAPM) Radiation Oncology Incident Learning System (RO-ILS) programs would have caught the errors that were ultimately litigated.[19] The review found that the "pillars" of the APEx program could potentially have flagged all cases and the RO-ILS system would have potentially alerted a radiation oncologist to impending risk in all but one case. Participation in both programs could reasonably be expected to reduce the risk of error and consequent malpractice suits, although prospective data are lacking.

The necessity of hypervigilance to correcting causes of near misses in a radiation oncologist's personal practice is obvious. More globally, the RO-ILS program reports on specialty-wide trends. A review of 2344 event reports in 2016,[19] for example, found that 44% of events were due to "problematic plan approved for treatment," "wrong shift instructions given to therapists," or "wrong shift performed on treatment." In the "problematic plan approved for treatment" category, the majority of cases (65%) related to physician error in contouring or dose pattern prescription (i.e., lack of clarity about the desired dose and fractionation schedule intended).[20] Specific recommendations are forthcoming from RO-ILS reporting (which is updated quarterly), such as, "Peer review of target definition before planning commences deserves more attention, especially for hypofractionated cases."[20] Institutional incident learning experiences, such as that at Johns Hopkins, affirms the RO-ILS basic concept that "events [fall] into relatively small group(s) of common categories, which suggest that targeted interventions to prevent future events is likely to be a successful approach."[21]

Special challenges in defending radiation oncology malpractice cases

Radiation oncologists are generally aware that the biological effects of radiation on human tissue are something of a mysterious "black box" to the public and even to other physicians. Fear of the effects of radiation has been documented to be a barrier to women accepting radiation as part of breast-conserving treatment.[22] One study documented that "when describing radioactivity, patients repeatedly recall and describe the same images: the explosion of a nuclear bomb or the destroyed reactor in Chernobyl are part of the standard repertoire of the interviews."[23] Judges and juries are members of the public and bring these notions to a malpractice trial. One striking example is a judge's completely credulous acceptance of a patient's testimony about her alleged "injury" from radiation therapy. The judge's decision reads, in relevant part: "patient's reaction to the radiation therapy . . . deteriorated to such an extent, for instance, that her skin burned 'so severely that I bandaged myself so that nobody would see the smoke come out of me.'"[24] The case was appealed to the state supreme court, where that court did not blink at the description of a smoking patient and reiterated that the patient's side effects were "dramatically calamitous." In *Prete v Rafla-Demetrious*,[25] the court seemingly accepted the plaintiff's claim that cranial radiation caused "peeling and breaking of the skin all over his body." The public perception of radiation will need to factor into a radiotherapist's calculus about whether to take a case to trial.

Sometimes the efforts of radiation oncologists to address the complexities of cancer care in overly simplistic language will come back to haunt them. In a case where a patient successfully litigated against a radiation oncologist for their failure to affirmatively recommend radiation for their prostate cancer (and whose documentation was scanty), the ruling court summarized the patient's testimony against the radiation oncologist as follows: "He told me that if those wild Indian cells had been going to cause me cancer, I would have been in pain a hell of a long time before."[26] Further, the court quoted the patient remembering that his radiation oncologist said, "We'll burn that prostate to a cinder; and that he thought that the treatment was unnecessary." The advisability of discussing complex medical issues in understandable terms does not commend the adoption of rustic colloquialisms.

Steps a radiation oncologist should take if sued

1. Have no conversation with the patient, a spouse, colleagues, or *anyone else* until the physician has consulted with the attorney that will be assigned by the malpractice carrier or insuring institution. These conversations, while perhaps reassuring to physician ego, may well be discoverable and used against physician interest. If the physician needs to talk to someone, the physician should consult a mental health practitioner; those conversations will generally be privileged and immune from discovery. If a physician is not satisfied with the attorney assigned by the insurer, the physician can request a change. In rare cases, a physician may need to seek separate counsel.

2. Notify the malpractice carrier as soon as the existence of a claim is known. Many hospital bylaws also require that physicians notify the medical staff office, and their employment contract may require notification of the employer.

3. Secure the radiation therapy record. The physician should make no alterations to the chart and allow no one else to make alterations to the chart; these will be discovered and are highly prejudicial to a physician's chance of success in litigation and may even result in assessment of additional damages.

CASE LAW # 2

In the Ohio case *Moskovitz v Mount Sinai Medical Center, Figge, et al.*,[27] it was determined that an orthopedic surgeon had altered his office notes to indicate that, rather than it being *his* recommendation that a nodule be monitored, it was *the patient* who declined workup. When the patient developed metastatic sarcoma and sued, the alterations were discovered when unaltered copies of the office notes that had been sent, *inter alia*, to the radiation oncology department were produced. A $1 million punitive damage was entered against the orthopedic physician for making the alterations, and the Ohio court stated: "An intentional alteration, falsification, or destruction of medical records by a doctor to avoid liability for his or her medical negligence, is sufficient to show actual malice, and punitive damages may be awarded whether or not the act of altering, falsifying or destroying records directly causes compensable harm." Malpractice policies will generally not cover punitive damages, so the risks of record alteration are huge. Make no addendums without advice of counsel, and clearly date any such "preapproved" addendums.

4. Physicians should become acquainted with the details of their medical malpractice policy: What are the limits in aggregate and per occurrence? Often insurance companies can settle without physician consent (within the policy limits), and physicians will be stuck with additional paperwork in the credentialing process for years as a result. If a physician refuses to settle and the ultimate judgment exceeds what the insurance company was initially able to settle for, they may be liable for the difference (the so-called "hammer clause"). If there is a settlement or a judgment, a report will go to the National Practitioner Data Bank, although physicians have the right to object to the wording of that report and seek modification. Are the costs of defense included in malpractice limits? If so, there will be less financial freeboard to absorb a judgment. Physicians should know whether their state has a guarantee fund and whether their insurer is an admitted carrier to that guarantee fund, which provides some protection if an insurer becomes insolvent. There is a distressing radiation oncology case where the radiation oncologist's insurance company was declared insolvent just as a suit was filed against him by a prostate patient.[28] Fortunately, the case was filed in Florida, which had a state guarantee fund for just such a contingency, and his former carrier, Philco, had been admitted to participate in the system, so his defense was eventually taken up by the Florida Insurance Guarantee Association. Otherwise, the radiation oncologist would have had no insurance.

5. Do not speak with opposing counsel. A very famous radiation oncologist and department chair in Massachusetts made the mistake of speaking with an attorney who was representing other physicians who were being sued by one of his patients.[29] He spoke with counsel opposing his patient's claim on the day before he was to be deposed with counsel for both parties present and did so without the patient's permission. She complained to the Board of Registration in Medicine who disciplined the radiation oncologist for "gross misconduct," although that determination was ultimately overturned on appeal. In cases where the physician is the defendant, anything they say may be admissible as an "admission of a party," so all communications from a defendant physician should be made through counsel.

6. Prepare for a long haul. A study performed by the RAND Corporation based on data provided by The Doctor's Company, the nation's largest physician-owned medical malpractice insurer, found that, on average, medical malpractice suits will occupy 50.7 months of physician time during their career.[30]

7. Should you apologize? Some 39 states and the District of Columbia have enacted so-called apology laws, most only applicable to medical malpractice cases, which are intended to "promote healing, understanding and dispute resolution"[31] by making physician apologies inadmissible in subsequent malpractice trials. The laws were passed in hopes of decreasing both litigation and the damage amounts awarded. A 2019 study, based on proprietary insurance data covering 90% of an unidentified medical specialty and reported in the *Stanford Law Review*,[31] found that, for nonsurgeons within this specialty (where some practitioners performed surgery and others did not), "apology laws increase the probability of facing a lawsuit and increase the average payment made to resolve a claim" and also increase the cost to insurers of defending a claim. They found that "on balance, apology laws increase rather than limit medical malpractice liability risk." The authors' theory is relevant to radiation oncology practice and posits that surgical misadventures would be more obvious to a patient, and thus an apology by a surgeon would not come as a surprise to a patient, who already knew that there was something to apologize for. However, in the case of a nonsurgeon, the patient might be more surprised by an apology, which could be a first signal that something had gone wrong. That such an apology

(involving, as it does, the disclosure of asymmetric information) might reverse the intended effect of an apology law is relevant to radiation oncology, since patients generally are not immediately aware of a radiation error. This is not to say that disclosure should not be made to a radiation oncology patient who has been subject to medical error but might suggest that the information not be initially shared in the form of an apology. The authors of the *Stanford Law Review* study state: "Our advice to physicians is simple: Do not apologize without specific training," such as that offered by the Agency for Healthcare Research and Quality in their Communications and Optimal Resolution (CANDOR) toolkit. They ultimately conclude: "Prior to the advent of the apology law 'movement' attorneys routinely advised their physician clients not to apologize. Though this advice has been criticized, our results suggest that the attorneys offering it were right all along."[31]

LEGAL LIABILITY IN THE CLINICAL PRACTICE OF RADIATION ONCOLOGY

To review some basic civics, it is recalled that there exists both civil and criminal liability. To be sent to prison, there has to be a violation of a criminal statute passed by a legislature (e.g., Congress passed a criminal statute regarding accessing child pornography with intent to view). Civil liability does not risk jail time. There are three sources of civil liability: acts of the legislature, the common law (created by courts), and administrative liability for violating regulations passed by bureaucrats under a grant of power to promulgate them issued by a legislature. This section will only cover civil liability in the clinical practice of radiation oncology.

Choice of cause of action

In general, the plaintiff (in our context, a patient) gets to choose the legal theory under which they express displeasure with a physician. Often, this is by using a recognized "cause of action" under the common law or a statute to receive monetary damages from the offending physician. However, the patient may choose, instead, to seek "revenge" through an administrative action. In this scenario, the patient will not receive monetary damages, but the physician's license to practice medicine may be at stake. For example, in a case filed in Montana,[32] a radiation oncologist undertook treatment of a patient with inflammatory breast cancer and received her permission to make marks on her breast at the time of simulation. In the court's words, "in addition to the marks directing radiation beams, [the radiation oncologist] drew a smiley face on the woman's breast by drawing two dime sized 'eyes' above the nipple of the breast and outlining the scar from the breast biopsy for the 'mouth.'" While the patient might have elected to sue for the civil cause of action called "battery" (an "unpermitted touching") and possibly receive monetary damages, she chose instead to file a complaint with the Montana Board of Medical Examiners, who entered into a stipulation with the radiation oncologist that included a report to the National Practitioner Data Bank. Subsequent filings with the Board indicate that the radiation oncologist in question was having difficulty finding employment after having been dismissed over this incident.

If a patient elects to pursue a civil cause of action, they may pursue any combination of different legal theories including, for example, negligence, battery, breach of contract, breach of warranty, misrepresentation, or fraud/deceit, depending on the facts of the case. Not all states recognize the same causes of action. For example, in some states, a patient can sue for negligent infliction of emotional distress, whereas other states simply do not recognize that cause of action and will summarily dismiss a suit brought on those grounds. What a plaintiff has to prove differs between different causes of action. For example, a claim of negligence requires a showing of damages, whereas a claim of battery does not. It is generally the patient's choice as to the legal theory—that is, the cause of action—under which they make their suit. In a case arising in North Carolina,[33] the patient alleged lack of informed consent. The radiation oncologist essentially responded that his informed consent was so poor as to be nonexistent and argued therefore that the suit should, as the law says, "sound" in battery and not negligence. Why would he make that argument? The statute of limitations for battery was one year and had passed, whereas the statute of limitations for informed consent was two years and had not passed. The argument (perhaps not surprisingly) was rejected by the court but illustrated the point. Most civil liability in radiation oncology has been imposed under the legal doctrine of negligence, which will be considered in greater detail.

Negligence in radiation oncology

A plaintiff must present a case that proves the basic elements of negligence, generally taken to be the existence of a duty, a breach of that duty, causation in fact, proximate causation, and damages. If they do not submit proof of all elements, the defendant can move for summary judgment, and if granted, the case is over. Two of the elements require expert testimony: the elements of breach and causation. There are various defenses available to a defendant, as well. This section will provide examples from the radiation oncology case law of the different elements of a cause of action for medical malpractice and the defenses to such a claim.

The practicing radiation oncologist who surveys reported cases in the legal literature would encounter a spectrum of professional practice ranging from the unbelievable to instances where medical judgments were puzzling. Other cases involve seemingly reasonable judgments that resulted in litigation or routine practice that generated frivolous lawsuits. The radiotherapy details of many cases are only available from descriptions made when a procedural issue is appealed and before final findings of fact are made at trial. However, taking the plaintiff's allegations at face value, there are cases, for example, where a radiation oncologist, who was performing a prostate implant, placed a perineal template straight from the autoclave onto the perineum, causing second- and third-degree burns.[34] Other seemingly outlandish cases include a 23-year-old patient with bulky Hodgkin disease who was treated via a mantle field to radiosurgical doses, resulting in transverse myelitis,[35] and a case where a patient with colon cancer was treated postoperatively with high-dose rate brachytherapy and external beam radiotherapy to doses of 90.5 Gy.[36] Puzzling judgments arguably include treating a patient for glioblastoma multiforme (GBM) without a tissue diagnosis where the lesion subsequently proved to be a meningioma (resulting in patient death).[37] Other such cases include using a mixed photon/neutron beam on a 49-year-old patient with early-stage prostate cancer (subsequent death)[38] and the use of protons on a desmoid tumor, alleged to have caused severe fibrosis and edema.[39]

The fairly common judgment to use bilateral, rather than ipsilateral, treatment for a tonsillar tumor resulted in a suit by a cured patient, who sued for xerostomia.[40] In another case, a patient was given lorazepam (Ativan) in radiation oncology before expansion of a MammoSite balloon, and was dismissed from the clinic to drive home without warnings about the effects of sedation, crashed into a tree, and successfully sued.[41]

Jurisdiction

Before a malpractice case can proceed, the court where the suit is brought has to have what is called "personal jurisdiction" over the physician or practice, and this requires a "sufficient nexus" between the jurisdiction and the potential defendants such that trying the case in the jurisdiction where the suit is filed does not "offend traditional notions of fair play and substantial justice."[42]

CASE LAW # 3

In *Advanced Rad Solutions v ICAD, Inc, Western Radiation Oncology and Western Radiation Oncology Medical Group,*[42] Advanced Rad Solutions (ARS), which was a Texas company, signed a contract with ICAD, Inc, a Delaware company that had their principle offices in New Hampshire. For some unknown reason, the contract specified that any dispute between the two companies would be governed by the laws of Massachusetts. Western Radiation Oncology was a California practice with absolutely no contact with Massachusetts. ARS attempted to force Western Radiation Oncology, who was not even a party to the contract between ARS and ICAD, to submit to litigation in Massachusetts, and the US District Court dismissed the suit against Western Radiation Oncology for lack of personal jurisdiction.

On the other hand, when a Minnesota resident brought suit in a Minnesota court against the North Dakota radiation oncologist who had treated him in North Dakota for metastatic cancer without a biopsy[43] but was later found not to have metastatic disease, the outcome was different. The radiation oncologist argued that the practice maintained minimal contact with Minnesota, did not pay Minnesota taxes, and was not registered to do business in Minnesota. However, the court noted that the radiation oncology practice had relationships with several Minnesota outreach clinics, "pursuant to which it treats patients in Minnesota," and also had an agreement to provide medical services for the state of Minnesota from which it had received "tens of thousands of dollars" and, as such, that there was sufficient nexus to warrant personal jurisdiction in Minnesota over the North Dakota radiation oncology practice. Decisions in these jurisdiction cases—and there are several dealing with radiation oncology—are all very case fact specific.

A related concept to jurisdiction is the concept of *forum non conveniens,* where a court may decline to accept jurisdiction because their venue would be too inconvenient for rational adjudication. For example, in *Patricia Vargas v General Electric Company,*[44] some 99 residents of Costa Rica sought to sue General Electric (GE) in Connecticut for wrongful death and injuries sustained by GE's alleged negligence in the calibration and maintenance of a cobalt machine at a hospital in Costa Rica. The court declined to accept jurisdiction because the facts would be more readily determined if the trial were held in Costa Rica.

If health care was delivered by the government, plaintiffs have a special problem. The law generally bars citizens' suits against the government under the theory that, in a democracy, citizens *are* the government and that "you cannot sue yourself." Congress has provided exceptions to this general rule through the Federal Tort Claims Act (FTCA), as amended by the Westfall Act.[45] So, in *Lackro v Kao*,[46] when a patient received a prostate implant at a Veterans Affairs hospital that he alleged inadequately treated the tumor and gave excessive doses to surrounding normal tissue, the radiation oncologist was able to get himself dismissed from the case because "the FTCA affords certain federal employees absolute immunity from state law tort claims."[46] If the statute applies, the United States has to be substituted as defendant if it is shown that the physician was a federal employee acting with the scope of their employment at the time of the alleged negligence.

Choice of law

Related to the question of jurisdiction is the question of which state's laws will be applied to a case. For example, in *Dasha v Adelman*,[47] a patient, who had lived and was treated in Maine but who had moved to Massachusetts, sued for brain damage he claimed resulted from radiation therapy that was occasioned by the negligent diagnosis rendered by a Massachusetts neuropathologist. The case was initially dismissed because the Maine statute of repose (a type of statute that limits the time in which a suit can be brought) had expired, but a Massachusetts appellate court determined that "Massachusetts had more significant relationships to the parties than did Maine and thus the Massachusetts three-year medical malpractice statute of limitations applied,"[47] and the case was allowed to proceed.

Existence of a duty

Usually, the existence of a duty arises from establishment of a doctor-patient relationship. In most jurisdictions, if there is no such relationship, no duties arise, and therefore, no negligence suit can proceed. Take, for example, the case of a breast patient who sued the chairman of a radiation oncology department over injuries she claimed from an interstitial boost administered for breast cancer.[48] The chair had specified the use of interstitial boosts within his department, reviewed charts of patients so treated, reported results of the technique in the literature, and so on. However, he never saw the patient during treatment, although he saw her once with other physicians when radiation necrosis developed at the implant site. The chair was dismissed from the case, with the court holding, in relevant part: "There are no facts which would warrant a conclusion that a consensual relationship between the plaintiff and the defendant (existed) at the time of the alleged negligent treatment."[48] Similarly, in the case discussed earlier where a radiation oncologist treated for a GBM without a tissue diagnosis and the lesion turned out to be a meningioma,[37] the patient also sued a neurosurgeon who the radiation oncologist talked to over the phone about the images. The neurosurgeon, who never saw the patient, had told the radiation oncologist that the lesion "looked like a GBM to him." The court stated, "in general it is stated that a *prima facie* case for medical malpractice requires that a doctor-patient relationship be established . . . That means that in most cases, the absence of the relationship does prevent the creation of a duty . . . [and] a finding of liability when there is no doctor patient relationship remains the exception and not the norm."[37] The neurosurgeon was dismissed from the case.

CASE LAW # 4

An interesting radiation oncology case that appears to be one of first impression is the Connecticut case of *Streifel v Bulkley*.[49] In this case, a radiation oncology *nurse* sued a radiation oncology *patient*, alleging that the patient had breached a duty of care owed toward the nurse. The patient, Mr. Bulkley, described by the court as having "a large body habitus," was in an exam room, supine. The court continues: "The defendant then attempted to transition from a supine to a seated position on the examining table. In attempting to change positions, he grabbed hold of the plaintiff, who was the registered nurse assisting him. As a result of the defendant's physical contact with her, the plaintiff suffered several physical injuries." The court ruled: "We conclude, as a matter of law, that the law does not impose a duty of care on a patient to avoid negligent conduct that causes harm to a medical care provider while the patient is receiving medical care from that provider."[49]

Changing the scope of duties that the law will automatically impose once the doctor-patient relationship is established

Practitioners need to be aware that they may inadvertently expand their liability by making promises to patients about outcomes or freedom from side effects that would give patients additional causes of action under contract law or under the laws of warranty and guarantee. Holding yourself out as having special expertise may also increase the number of legal theories that a plaintiff could employ to seek damages. Most states acknowledge something called a "therapeutic reassurance," but practitioners need to be sure their conduct does not shade into contract or guarantee liability.

Negligence defined

Generally stated, negligence is conduct that falls below a minimum standard, defined by the law, for the protection of others against reasonably foreseeable risks of harm. This is assessed by comparing the physician behavior complained against to how an idealized reasonable and prudent physician would behave, in employing the knowledge, skill, and care ordinarily possessed by members of the profession in good standing to avoid conduct "involving unreasonably great risk of causing foreseeable and recognizable harm." Law students spend a semester unpacking the meaning of that formulation, which is chock full of "words of art." It is sufficient for present purposes to note that it is the *law's theoretical construct of a reasonable and prudent physician* and not what is commonly done in radiation oncology practice that ultimately determines what behavior is acceptable. In what may be one of the most quoted sentences uttered by the US Supreme Court, "what is usually done may be evidence of what ought to be done, but what ought to be done is fixed by a standard of reasonable prudence, whether it usually is complied with or not."[50] Several broad parameters of duty can be parsed from the case law.

Duties that arise in the physician patient relationship

Employing the knowledge, skill, and care ordinarily possessed by members of the profession in good standing

CASE LAW # 5

In *Esfandiari v United States*,[26] a case referenced earlier where the radiation oncologist had apparently discussed burning a prostate "to cinders," the radiation oncologist testified that it was his understanding that the administration of radiation made no difference in the outcome of prostate cancer. The radiation oncologist's testimony, in relevant part was as follows: "My understanding then is as it is today; that there is no difference in the ultimate survival rate with or without radiation treatment. The value of radiation is to keep the urinary tract open. This was a man who had just required a transurethral resection of his prostate. The only benefit of giving him radiation would have been to preserve patency of the urinary tract. Treatment would not have prevented subsequent development of metastatic disease." The court said, in relevant part, that the radiation oncologist's failure to "affirmatively recommend radiation therapy . . . as well as [his] failure to insure follow up . . . violated the standard of care and was a proximate cause of injury."

The duty to attend the patient diligently Perhaps the most egregious example of failure to give diligent attendance was a low-dose rate gynecologic brachytherapy case, where a radiation oncologist received a telephone referral, never consulted in person with the patient before surgery, performed an implant, and then, apparently, forgot about the patient for days.[51] No follow-up was established, and the patient later developed a radiation-induced fistula. Another case involved a world-famous genitourinary radiation oncologist who prescribed flutamide (Eulexin) for a prostate cancer patient and never arranged liver function tests in follow-up.[52] The patient died of fulminant liver failure as a result, and a judgment of over $3.3 million was entered against the radiation oncologist, which was greater than the limits of his malpractice policy.

Conversely, there can be risk in overzealous care. In *Tranum v Hebert*,[53] a patient was referred to M.D. Anderson with the diagnosis of a malignant tumor of the posterior pharynx. His "outside" slides were requested for in-house review, but he was sent to dental oncology for evaluation prior to anticipated radiation therapy and multiple teeth were extracted. He was ultimately found not to have cancer and filed suit over the needless removal of the teeth. The physicians were ultimately dismissed, but it is a cautionary tale. Tests should not be ordered if they do not affect treatment, and if tests are ordered, results should be awaited to permit logical progression of workup.

Duty to inform the patient of the nature and extent of disease and the extent of hazards of treatment The existence of a legal requirement for informed consent stems from the principle that every adult of sound mind has the right to control their body; it is a right founded upon patient autonomy. It is interesting that the first state supreme court decision that highlighted this aspect of negligence law, *Natanson v Kline*,[54] was actually a radiation oncology case involving a radiation oncologist's failure to discuss potential risks of postmastectomy chest wall irradiation in a patient who suffered areas of necrosis. There are dozens of cases in the radiation oncology literature based on a lack of informed consent to treatment.

The imposition of a legal requirement that a patient gives informed consent to a medical procedure requires a practitioner to engage in *a communication process,* not to secure a signed form.[55] It is entirely possible to have a signed form and yet not have met the legal requirements of informed consent. Conversely, it is also entirely possible to have no signed document but to have successfully completed the legal requirements for obtaining consent. Outside of the research setting and a few other special areas, the only *federal* law requiring a *signed form* in ordinary clinical practice is for physicians participating in Medicare and Medicaid who are performing surgery.[55] That being said, it is obviously always wise to have documentation that the informed consent process took place in the event of litigation, but the point is that the law's emphasis is actually on the *process, not the form!* Sometimes, clinicians seem to focus on the form. Sometimes, there is good reason for that; for example, in some states, the presence of a signed form is taken as *prima facie* evidence of informed consent, and at least three states (Texas, Louisiana, and Hawaii)[55] have an approved inventory of consent forms that, if used by a practitioner, provide additional protection. Many of these forms are specific to radiation oncology practice. Incidentally, physicians who delegate the communications process to another member of the health care team do so at their peril (under the legal doctrine of *respondeat superior*).

What must be disclosed to "inform" a patient? States differ on whether the patient must be told what a reasonable and prudent *practitioner* would disclose or what a reasonable and prudent *patient* would want to know! A minority of jurisdictions even require disclosure of what *this particular patient* would want to know. Acknowledging, therefore, that there are state and federal variations on the theme, in general, a patient must be told the indications for the treatment (i.e., the diagnosis). They must have an explanation of the proposed treatment, a description of other options, and an explanation of the probable risks and benefits associated with the proposed treatment and the other options, as well as some description of the consequences of declining recommended treatment. Some states hold that a practitioner facing a patient who declines recommended treatment must obtain an "informed refusal" of care.

The issue of causation, to be considered in greater detail later in this chapter, is particularly troublesome in the informed consent context.

CASE LAW # 6

In *Ashe v Radiation Oncology Associates*,[56] the Supreme Court of Tennessee was confronted with a patient who became paraplegic from radiation myelitis following postoperative radiation for lung cancer. She received 200 cGy at midplane on 25 fractions. The question became: Is causation established by Ms. Ashe's testimony that, had she been warned of the risk of myelitis, that she would have declined treatment? Obviously, such a test of causation would hinge on her credibility, since it would inevitably be self-serving and influenced by hindsight and bitterness. Or, is the correct standard of causation what a reasonable and prudent patient in similar circumstances would have decided (the so-called objective standard)? Tennessee, like most jurisdictions, opted for the objective standard of causation, and the case has been influential.

Is there a duty to refer patients for nonconventional treatment? In an unusual California case, the parents of a child diagnosed with a rhabdoid brain tumor that partially encased the spinal cord sued under a breach of informed consent theory because they were not offered antineoplaston therapy, an "alternative medicine" not approved by the US Food and Drug Administration offered by a single physician in Texas,[54] whose interstate transportation of antineoplastons was banned at the time of the child's illness. In fact, the administration of antineoplastons was prohibited by statute in the state of California, where the child underwent chemotherapy and radiation, ultimately dying of radiation necrosis of the brain. *After six years of litigation*, a California appeals court determined that a physician's duty to disclose available forms of treatment did not extend to include treatments that were illegal to administer in the state.

Need for expert testimony on breach of the duty

This is one of two places in a malpractice trial that requires expert testimony, and failure to provide such testimony will promptly end the plaintiff's case. For example, in *Roman v Kim*,[57] Mr. Roman, a prostate cancer patient, had fiducials implanted by a urologist (performing the procedure for the first time) who was being advised during the procedure by Mr. Roman's female radiation oncologist. Although he later sued, in part, due to the pain involved, he apparently still felt frisky at the completion of the procedure. The court notes that after the urologist departed the procedure room "while lying prone, naked from the waist down, Roman asked her [the radiation oncologist] twice to kiss him on the cheek." The fiducials ultimately proved to have been implanted in the wrong place and needed to be reinserted at a second procedure. Made uncomfortable by the patient's advances and after he filed suit, the radiation oncologist "informed him she would no longer treat him." He sued her for abandonment (a corollary of the duty to attend diligently) but presented no expert testimony on what the radiation oncologist's follow-up duties were. On appeal of the dismissal of his claim for abandonment, the appellate court stated, "Roman's failure to provide an expert declaration on the issue of patient abandonment was fatal to his claim. Accordingly, we conclude the court did not err in granting" dismissal of the claim.

The testimony on breach of duty must be fairly specific; an expert must state that the conduct complained of fell below the *minimum* standard of care, not just that some different conduct was considered the standard of care. This is a subtle but important distinction that has been pivotal in several radiation oncology cases.

CASE LAW # 7

In *King v Bauer*,[58] a Texas case with a long procedural history and multiple appeals, Mrs. King underwent split-course thoracic radiation therapy postoperatively for a node-positive bronchioalveolar adenocarcinoma. Her first phase of treatment was 250 cGy, followed by 300 cGy for the rest of her treatment, to a total of 5398 cGy. Estimates of total cord dose, uncorrected for EQD2 (equivalent dose in 2-Gy fractions) biological effect, was 4650 cGy. She developed transverse myelitis. There was testimony at trial as to what the standard of care was, but as the first appellate division put it, "we find that there was no evidence for the jury to have found that Dr. Bauer fell below that standard. All of the medical experts agreed that 200 rads per dose was a common manner to fractionate when treating a patient with radiation. On the other hand, there was no testimony that 300 rad dosages, as such, fell below or violated the standard of care." Ultimately, Mrs. Bauer received no compensation.

There is, in some states, an exception to the requirement of expert testimony if the breach is obvious to a layman. For example, in *Nowacki v Community Medical Center, et al.*,[59] expert testimony was not required when radiation therapists did not assist a wheelchair-bound metastatic patient who fell while attempting to get on the treatment table.

Who can be an expert in a radiation oncology case?

States differ on the identity of who qualifies as an expert in a radiation oncology case. Some jurisdictions are fairly liberal, allowing the trier of fact to give appropriate weight to the witness's credibility if the witness is not a radiation oncologist.

CASE LAW # 8

In *Swope v Razzaq*,[60] a radiation oncologist was allowed to testify that a urologist breached the standard of care in a prostate implant, but the urologist was free to argue, in closing, that a urologist should have determined the standard of care. *Swope* was tried in a federal court, but the same decision, that a radiation oncologist could give expert testimony in the case of a urologist treating prostate cancer, was reached in a Pennsylvania case, *Gbur v Golio*.[61] Some states are more proscriptive; for example, Tennessee requires the expert physician to have practiced in Tennessee or a contiguous state within a year of the events claimed to be negligent. In *Stryczek v The Methodist Hospitals*,[62] it was held that a nurse could not act as an expert in a radiation oncology case.

Causation in fact

In general, jurisdictions adopt either a "but for" test of causation (i.e., the injury would not have been caused *but for* the actions of the defendant) or a test that holds that the defendant's actions were a "material and substantial factor" in causing the injury.

CASE LAW # 9

As an example of the former, consider *Conti v Lende*.[63] In this case, a four-year-old child was admitted, found to have a brain tumor, and underwent subtotal resection. The hospital pathologist rendered a diagnosis of malignant mixed glioma (which the plaintiffs contend was the correct diagnosis), whereas a consulting neuropathologist rendered a diagnosis of subependymal astrocytoma, which the plaintiffs claimed was erroneous. The hospital rules required consultation with the neuropathologist and regarded the in-house pathologist's role in brain tumor cases to consist of routine processing, giving only a guarded diagnosis and not a "discrete diagnosis," which was ultimately deferred to the neuropathologist. The radiation oncologist was sued under the allegation that he had "deviated from sound medical practice" by relying on the neuropathologist's diagnosis. However, all of the testimony at trial indicated that the radiation therapy would have been identical under either diagnosis. While the court did not explicitly rest its decision on causation grounds, the argument could clearly be made that the radiation to the child would not have occurred *but for* the neuropathologist's alleged negligence. In a similar fashion, the Supreme Court of Connecticut in *Cohen v Yale-New Haven Hospital*[64] upheld a finding that *but for* the radiation oncologist's failure to act on a radiologist's recommendation for a follow-up magnetic resonance imaging scan of a sarcoma patient, the patient could have subsequently avoided the side effects of brachytherapy when a recurrence was detected after a more prolonged follow-up interval.

Proximate causation

If causation is parsed between causation in fact and proximate causation, as it is in some jurisdictions, a rough approximation of the difference is that causation in fact is actual causation and proximate cause is policy causation, which attempts to draw a circle of reasonable liability around a chain of events that, theoretically, can extend retrograde to the Big Bang and extend forward infinitely in time, space, and consequence. Expert testimony is required to say that a plaintiff's injury was caused by the defendant's lack of due care. A breach of a duty that does not proximately cause injury is not actionable.

CASE LAW # 10

As an example, consider *Hamby v University of Kentucky Medical Center*.[65] This was a hyperthermia case where a patient had head and neck cancer that had progressed through multiple therapies and who then underwent a course of hyperthermia that led to the necrosis of her ear. The jury found that the radiation oncologist's behavior in using surface-mounted probes instead of interstitial probes fell below the minimal standard of care, but they also found that this negligence had not led to the injury of which the patient complained. The malpractice case was accordingly dismissed, and the dismissal was upheld on appeal.

Damages

In the absence of "willful, wanton, reckless" conduct, punitive damages are not generally available in a malpractice case. We have already noted an exception in some jurisdictions allowing punitive damages if the physician attempts to alter the records in cover-up. Usual damages that are allowed to plaintiffs in malpractice typically include costs of treatment, lost income, pain and suffering, and loss of consortium by their spouse. Noneconomic damages are limited in some states as a mechanism of tort reform.

Res ipsa loquitur ("the thing speaks for itself")

Sometimes, there are cases in which an injured plaintiff is unable to identify specific acts of negligence that led to their injury. In some states, a legal doctrine called *res ipsa loquitur* can be applied in a malpractice case. The effect of applying the doctrine varies by jurisdiction. In some, for example, it creates a permissible inference of negligence; in others, its application creates a rebuttal presumption of negligence that the defendant needs to counter. In still other jurisdictions, it is merely considered a rule of evidence.

CASE LAW # 11

The factual settings in which the doctrine is applied are sometimes strange, as in the case of *Pillars v R.J. Reynolds Tobacco Company*,[66] where the plaintiff found a human toe in his chewing tobacco. He could not identify any specific acts of negligence by Reynolds that led to this outcome and sought to get his case to a jury on a *res ipsa* theory. The Supreme Court of Mississippi allowed the case to go to the jury on those grounds and presumably delighted in the composition of this holding: "We can imagine no reason why, with ordinary care, human toes could not be left out of chewing tobacco, and if toes are found in chewing tobacco, it seems to us that somebody has been very careless."

For those jurisdictions that allow *res ipsa* in medical malpractice, the necessary elements may include the following: (1) the injury must be one that would not have occurred in the absence of negligence; (2) the agency or instrumentality causing the injury is in the sole control of the defendant; (3) there is no contributory negligence or assumption of the risk by the plaintiff; and (4) the true explanation of what happened is more accessible to the defendant than to the plaintiff. There are several relevant radiation oncology cases; for example, in the perineal burn case,[34] both a urologist and a radiation oncologist were involved in the case and the patient could not categorically state which cosurgeon had applied the 270°F metal template to his perineum. The Iowa Court of Appeals stated that the jury should have been given a *res ipsa* instruction, *inter alia*, because "burn injuries to patients do not occur in the ordinary course of events without negligence."[34] In the case involving the 23-year-old Hodgkin patient who was treated with a "stereotactic dose"[35] to a mantle field (plus additional fractions) who developed myelitis, the Supreme Court of Washington allowed the application of *res ipsa* and stated, "paralysis does not ordinarily result from radiation therapy unless the therapy has been negligently administered."

Defenses to negligence

The most common defense to a claim of medical malpractice is that the plaintiff did not provide evidence to satisfy all of the elements of the cause of action or did not provide expert testimony for those elements that require it or that the expert testimony did not say, precisely, what was necessary.

Judgment notwithstanding the verdict

In rare cases, a judge may reject a jury's findings if the judge feels that the verdict was against the substantial weight of evidence in the case. Discussion of one such case might be useful, as it may reasonably be interpreted as an example of juries reacting extremely negatively to any suggestion of a cover-up by a health care provider.

CASE LAW # 12

The central issue in *Scuzzaro v Loma Linda University Medical Center*[67] was the appropriateness of the staging of a moderately differentiated squamous cell carcinoma of the gingiva. At no time was there pathologic confirmation or unequivocal radiographic evidence of mandibular invasion. Ms. Scuzzaro claimed that, at most, she had a T2 lesion. She proceeded to surgery and had a mandibular resection. *The hospital lost the resected jawbone.* The patient's fibular free graft failed, a second flap failed, the donor site on her leg became infected, and she would ultimately have some 22 surgeries. Based on the assumption that the lost jaw showed tumor invasion, she underwent radiation therapy, resulting in xerostomia so severe that she required a feeding tube. The jury awarded over $1.6 million. The judge entered a judgment notwithstanding the verdict, and the dismissal of the case was upheld by the Fourth District California Court of Appeals.

Statutes of limitation

These statutes place a limit on how long after treatment a patient can file a suit. They are frequently invoked in radiation oncology cases, not surprisingly, because the deleterious effects of radiation often manifest quite some time after the completion of treatment and statutes for medical malpractice are typically only one to two years in duration. Operation of statutes of limitation, however, varies widely from state to state based on other factors. Some states have what is called the "continuing course of treatment" doctrine, which holds that the statute does not start to run until the course of treatment (often including follow-up care) has concluded. The duration of liability for radiation oncology is increased if a state has what is called a "discovery rule," which states that the statute does not begin running until the patient discovers, or with reasonable diligence would have discovered, the injury. Some states also add "and knows that it results" from the radiation therapy. States with the discovery rule may or may not have what is called a "statute of repose," which sets an absolute outer limit to when a suit can be brought, irrespective of when the patient discovered the injury. There is not much a radiation oncologist can do about how the statutes exist in the state of their practice, but there is a great deal that they can do to prevent depriving themselves of its benefit, not the least of which is to document when the patient knows of an injury and when the possibility that it was from radiation was made known to the patient. Radiation oncologists can potentially deprive themselves of the benefit of a statute of limitations if they engage in fraudulent concealment that can "toll" the operation of the statute.

Fraudulent concealment

As an example, sadly, of several such radiotherapy cases, return to the case of *Jones v Central Arkansas Radiation Therapy Institute*,[12] where the radiation oncologist greeted his newly quadriplegic patient with the greeting, "Well, Merlyn, what did you do, come up here to make idle threats?" The court continues its findings of facts, stating that the radiation oncologist "told appellant [Merlyn Jones] that he was not convinced that the radiation treatment had caused [the quadriplegia]. He told appellant that he would have to secure his files from the Veteran's Hospital and arrange another appointment. No appointment was arranged, however and after repeated calls, appellant was only able to arrange an appointment . . . after the statute of limitation had run." Further, the radiation oncologist "claimed that he could not obtain the necessary information from the Veteran's Hospital to make a diagnosis and informed appellant that he would need to undergo certain tests." The radiation oncologist then said that he would contact a neurosurgeon about Jones's condition before seeing him again. "Jones agreed but never heard from [the radiation oncologist] or his office again." The court concluded: "We believe the appellant's allegations present a factual issue as to fraudulent concealment. It may reasonably be inferred that [the radiation oncologist's] representation concerning his uncertainty was false and that his conduct thereafter was purposefully dilatory to cover up its fraudulent character and to prevent Jones from seeing another physician. But for the fraud, Meryln Jones could have discovered the alleged malpractice before the statute of limitation ran."[12] The operation of the statute of limitations was tolled, and the case was allowed to proceed.

LEGAL LIABILITY IN THE BUSINESS PRACTICE OF RADIATION ONCOLOGY

Restrictive covenants not to compete

Restrictive noncompete clauses are, unfortunately, common in radiation oncology contracts, with Association of Residents in Radiation Oncology (ARRO) surveys showing that up to 80% of new graduates are faced with such a clause in their initial employment contract.[68] Illegal in every US jurisdiction for lawyers, this author has elsewhere argued their ethical problems in the practice of medicine.[69] As discussed later in this chapter, they are often the anvil upon which the hammer of injustice is applied against radiation oncologists. They exist to protect business interests, not the interests of patients. Some states have outlawed them in the practice of medicine by court decision or statute. But in states where they are enforced, their breach represents a huge financial risk.

CASE LAW # 13

The case of *Weatherall Radiation Oncology v Caletri*[70] arose in Louisiana, a state with a "public policy against noncompetition agreements" where there was, nevertheless, statutory exceptions to that general policy. One statutory exception required the employer to carry on "a like business" in the area covered by the restrictive covenant for the covenant to be valid. When the radiation oncologist left the practice with which he had signed a restrictive covenant, and even though his former employer did not send another radiation oncologist to practice in the restricted area, the radiation oncologist lost the suit, and damages of $520,000 were upheld on appeal. Similarly, three radiation oncologists employed by the Iowa Clinic (through a contract containing a restrictive covenant) thought that they were entitled to go into business on their own when the clinic entered a joint venture with their competitors to buy a CyberKnife.[71] The clinic successful enforced the "liquidated damages" provision of the restrictive covenant in a judgment, upheld on appeal, costing the radiation oncologists over $800,000.

With large sums of money at stake, restrictive covenant litigation can be fierce to the point of being histrionic. For example, Florida has a statute, Section 542.336 of Florida Statutes, invalidating restrictive covenants when the entity seeking to enforce such a covenant "contracts with all physicians practicing in a given specialty in a given county." 21st Century Oncology sought vigorously to enforce a restrictive covenant in that precise situation,[72] and the language of the chief US district judge that decided against giving 21st Century Oncology a preliminary injunction is strikingly unusual in its language and is quoted to emphasize that these contract provisions should not be agreed too lightly, as employers take them seriously:

In February, 1954, the classic horror film *Creature from the Black Lagoon* was released. The plot is now a familiar trope, a prehistoric monster emerges from the fetid depths of a jungle swamp to terrorize a scientific expedition . . . As the real-world setting for the eponymous lagoon, the filmmakers chose Wakulla Springs, Florida—a state park located less than fifteen miles from this Court's courtroom in Tallahassee. Sixty-five years later, Plaintiff contends, another monster has emerged, this time in the heart of Tallahassee itself. The primordial pool in question is the Florida State Capitol and the role of the hadean hominid is played by section 542.336, Florida Statutes.

Medicare fraud and abuse, false claims, and violation of anti-kickback statutes

The ability of whistleblowers to file what is called a *qui tam* action wherein they may collect a variable percentage of an ultimate settlement has led to the majority of radiation oncology liability in matters relating to the legality of billing and business practices. Basically, the whistleblower (formally called "the relator") files a suit, under seal, in the name of the government. If the government decides to "intervene," that is, take up the case (which is often the first time the practice learns that the suit has been filed—and that can be years after the filing), the relator is eligible for a certain percentage of the settlement (15%–25%). If the government decides not to take over the case, the individual can still prosecute the case in the name of the government and is eligible for a higher percentage of any ultimate settlement (25%–30%). Relators in radiation oncology cases have been physicists, other radiation oncologists, therapists, and administrators. *In short, those who practice aggressive billing and business relationships find themselves "surrounded by assassins."* The stakes are significant.

CASE LAW # 14

In *US ex rel. Johnson-Prichardt v Rapid City Regional Hospital,*[73] the hospital allegedly gave the radiation oncologists a "sweetheart" lease arrangement where they paid $19,000 per year for space and services whose fair market value was $136,441. An administrator relator ultimately received 24% of the over $1.5 million settlement. In *United States ex rel. Barker v Columbus Regional Healthcare System,*[74] the US government intervened in some of Barker's allegations, which included, *inter alia,* fraud (IMRT billed but not performed), kickback schemes regarding patient referrals, and overvaluation of practice purchase, but not others. Columbus settled on all counts, and Barker, a cancer center administrator, received a total whistleblower reward of $5.337 million.

Some practical advice for avoiding liability in the business practice of radiation oncology

1. **Have your own lawyer.** A cautionary tale in this regard is *Jackson v Levine.*[76] In this case, a radiation oncologist owned a 10% interest in a practice valued at $26 million that was about to be sold. *Radiation oncologists in the group had executed restrictive covenants.* The radiation oncologist was summoned

CASE LAW # 15

In a fascinating and complex litigation, *US ex rel. Rahman v Colkitt, et al.*,[75] involving some 80 "shell" corporations and attempts to hide assets overseas, a radiation oncologist was the whistleblower. The government alleged some $12 million of fraudulent billing, and because fraud and abuse statutes allow for triple damages in some cases, this inflated the government's claim against the two principally involved radiation oncologists to $86 million. A complex settlement was ultimately reached, and the whistleblower received nearly $2 million as a result.

to a meeting with *the group's attorney.* Also present was the physician head of the group. The radiation oncologist was told to sign some documents or be fired. The group's lawyer informed her that he was looking after her interests as a partner and as an individual, that she would have until the close of the agreement to make changes in the agreement, that it was in her best financial interest to sign, that signing would not affect ownership in the practice, and that the attorney would secure a release from her noncompetition agreement. In fact, none of that was true, and as a result of signing the documents, the radiation oncologist received zero dollars and zero cents from the sale of the practice. After spending $84,000 in litigation costs against the attorney, the radiation oncologist received a judgment of $1.471 million (in part because this was a trial in a comparative negligence jurisdiction and her reward was reduced by the 25% that the court felt was her fault, essentially from naiveté). The moral here is to get *your own* lawyer.

2. **Read what you sign; it's important.** In the "smiley face" case discussed earlier, the radiation oncologist later challenged the stipulation that he had signed with the Montana Board of Medical Examiners, wherein he agreed that he had engaged in unprofessional behavior and consented to a National Practitioner Data Bank entry, both of which subsequently led to difficulty in his finding employment. The Supreme Court of Montana ruled that while it "is certainly understandable that [the radiation oncologist] experienced mental distress concerning his license, such distress does not amount to duress sufficient to negate this stipulation."[32]

CLINICAL VIGNETTE # 1

A patient was diagnosed with metastatic prostate cancer and received an initial course of radiation therapy for a hip metastasis. Seven months later, he developed slurred speech, disorientation, and unfocused vision. A computed tomography (CT) scan was read as showing a parenchymal metastasis to the brain of prostate cancer, and based on this CT scan, a radiation oncologist administered whole-brain radiation. The patient claims that side effects of radiation included hair loss, skin reaction, exhaustion, and weakness. Three months later, further imaging disclosed that the patient had experienced a stroke and did not have metastatic disease. He brought suit and provided expert testimony that radiation therapy for parenchymal metastasis of prostate cancer to the brain without tissue diagnosis fell below the minimum standard of care. A jury awarded $175,000, and the radiation oncologist appealed. What was the outcome of the appeal?

This is essentially the case of *Prete v Rafla-Demetrious*,[25] and the outcome was that, on appeal, the verdict was reversed and the case dismissed because the patient did not provide expert testimony that the radiation treatment was the proximate cause of the hair loss, skin reaction, and fatigue.

CONCLUSION

Liability in radiation oncology can arise from both poor patient rapport and technical lapses. Various "hard" and "soft" strategies can mitigate those risks. Attention to how legal theory applies to the clinical practice of radiation oncology can strengthen a practice's resilience to litigation and prevent it from being deprived of legitimate defenses. Billing practices represent a second major threat to a radiation oncology practice.

KEY POINTS:

- It is likely that most radiation oncologists will have a claim filed against them during their career and that, although chances of a payment ultimately being made are small, considerable time will be spent in dealing with the claim.
- Managing "soft risk" by concentrating on patient rapport and responding to concerns patients express about billing and payment could reasonably be expected to decrease the incidence of nuisance suits.
- "Hard risks" related to radiation planning, dose delivery, fractionation, and plan implementation can likely be reduced by participating in chart rounds and in ASTRO's APEx program and the ASTRO/AAPM RO-ILS system.
- If sued, a radiation oncologist must not alter the records or speak to anyone except the attorney assigned to them by their insurance carrier or in privileged communication with their personal mental health provider. Other actions to be taken in the event of a suit are reviewed in this chapter.
- If a patient has an adverse reaction to therapy, the radiation oncologist should carefully note when the patient was aware of the complication and when they were aware that it might be related to radiation therapy. The radiation oncologist should never commit fraudulent concealment of facts that a patient is entitled to know.
- Medical malpractice is governed by the law of negligence, and the application of the various elements of negligence to radiation oncology practice is reviewed.
- Restrictive covenants can prove problematic to practitioners.
- What practitioners sign is important. Practitioners should read and review documents with their own counsel.
- Those engaging in aggressive billing and business practices face considerable risk from whistleblowers filing qui tam actions.

References:

1. Wall TJ. Refresher course. Presented at the Annual Meeting of the American Society for Therapeutic Radiology and Oncology, Miami Beach, FL, October 8–11, 1995.
2. Sherman N, Rich T, Peter L. Professional liability in radiotherapy: experience of the Fletcher Society. *Int J Radiat Oncol Biol Phys.* 1991;20(3):563–566.
3. Marshall D, Tringale K, Connor M, et al. Nature of medical malpractice claims against radiation oncologists. *Int J Radiat Oncol Biol Phys.* 2017;98(1):21–30.
4. Thomson-Reuters. NexGen Westlaw Jury Verdicts. St Paul, MN: Thomson-Reuters.
5. Marshall D, Punglia RS, Fox D, et al. Medical malpractice claims in radiation oncology: a population-based study 1985–2012. *Int J Radiat Oncol Biol Phys.* 2015;93(2):241–250.
6. Royce T, Dwyer K, Yu-Moe CW, et al. Medical malpractice analysis in radiation oncology: a decade of results from a national comparative benchmarking system. *Int J Radiat Oncol Biol Phys.* 2019;103(4):801–808.
7. Ramella S, Mandoliti G, Trodella L, et al. The first survey on defensive medicine in radiation oncology. *Radiol Med.* 2015;120(5):421–429.
8. Pernet A, Mollo V, Bibault JE, Giraud P. Evaluation of patient's engagement in radiation therapy safety. *Cancer Radiother.* 2016;20(8):765–767.
9. The factors fueling rising healthcare costs. PricewaterhouseCoopers. 2006. https://www.pwc.com/il/he/publications/assets/4the_factors_fueling.pdf. Accessed August 7, 2021.
10. Reiboldt J. Seven steps to reduce your malpractice risk. *J Med Pract Manage.* 2004;19(6):324–328.
11. Spindler J. Reduce your malpractice risk: top 10 documenting mistakes to avoid. *J Mich Dent Assoc.* 2015;97(12):24–29.
12. *Jones v Central Arkansas Radiation Therapy Institute Inc, et al.,* 270 Ark 988 (1980).
13. *Jacobs v SUNY at Buffalo School of Medicine,* 2007 WL 1655652 (2002).
14. *US v Pelloski,* 31 FSupp3d 952 (2014).
15. Federation of State Medical Boards. Social media and electronic communications. April 28, 2019. https://www.fsmb.org/siteassets/advocacy/policies/social-media-and-electronic-communications.pdf. Accessed August 7, 2021.
16. Lagu T, Greyson S. Physician, monitor thyself: professionalism and accountability in the use of social media. *J Clin Ethics.* 2011;22(2):187–190.
17. Shore R, Halsey J, Shah K, et al. Report of the AMA Council on Ethical and Judicial Affairs: professionalism in the use of social media. *J Clin Ethics.* 2011;22(2):165–172.
18. Chargari C, Deutsch E, Blanchard P, et al. Brachytherapy: an overview for clinicians. *CA Cancer J Clin.* 2019;69(5):386–401.
19. Zaorsky N, Ricco AG, Churilla TM, et al. ASTRO APEx and Ro-ILS are applicable to medical malpractice in radiation oncology. *Future Oncol.* 2016;12(22):2643–2657.
20. Ezzell G, Chera B, Dicker A, et al. Common error pathways seen in the RO-ILS data that demonstrate opportunities for improving treatment safety. *Pract Radiat Oncol.* 2018;8(2):123–132.
21. Wright J, Parekh A, Rhieu BH, et al. Real-time management of incident learning report in a radiation oncology department. *Pract Radiat Oncol.* 2018;8(5):e337–e345.
22. Guidolin K, Lock M, Brackstone M. Patient-perceived barriers to radiation oncology for breast cancer. *Can J Surg.* 2017;61(20):141–143.
23. Freudenberg L, Beyer T. Subjective perception of radiation risk. *J Nucl Med.* 2011;52(Suppl 2):29S–35S.
24. *Lopez v Sawyer, et al.,* 62 NJ267 (1973) (and cases precedent, eg, 115 NJ Super 237, 279 A2d 116).
25. *Prete v Rafla-Demetrious,* 224 AD2d 674 (1996).
26. *Esfandiari v United States,* 810 F Supp 1 (1992).
27. *Moskovitz v Mount Sinai Medical Center, Figge, et al.,* 69 Ohio St3d 638 (1994).
28. *Halili v Radiation Oncology Consultants,* 820 So2d 415 (2002).

29. *Hellman v Board of Registration in Medicine*, 404 Mass 800, 537 NE2d 150 (1989).
30. Anderson R. Pending malpractice claims consume physicians' careers. The Doctor's Company. YouTube. https://www.youtube.com/watch?v=6io2h4Xgy0w. Accessed August 7, 2021.
31. McMichael B, Van Hor L, Viscuis W. "Sorry" is never enough: how state apology laws fail to reduce medical malpractice risk. *Stanford Law Rev*. 2019;71(2):341–409.
32. *Hughes v Pullman, et al.*, 306 Mont 420 (2001); *Hughes v Montana Board of Medical Examiners*, 318 Mont 181 (2003).
33. *Nelson v Patrick*, 58 NC App 546 (1982).
34. *Verwers v Rhoades*, 771 NW2d 651 (2008 WL 5233068).
35. *ZeBarth v Swedish Hospital Medical Center*, 81 Wash 2d l2, 499 P2d 1067 (1972).
36. *Daniels v Gamma West Brachytherapy*, 221 P3d 256 (2009).
37. *Scafide v Bazzone*, 962 So2d 585 (2007).
38. *Burek v Hart*, 779 NW2d 809 (2009 WL 3683313).
39. *Black v Delaney*, 91 Mass App Ct 1108 (2017).
40. *Natale v Riverview Cancer Care Medical Associates, et al.*, 68 AD3d 1574 (2009).
41. *Drew v Tenet St. Mary's*, 46 So3d 1165 (2010).
42. *Advanced Rad Solutions, LLC, v ICAD, Inc, Western Radiation Oncology and Western Radiation Oncology Medical Group*, WL 4461082 (2012).
43. *Breiland v Meritcare Health System, et al.*, WL 1782198 (2010).
44. *Patricia Vargas v General Electric Company*, WL 2196666 (2010).
45. 28 UDC SS 1346(b)(i).
46. *Lackro v Kao*, 748 FS2d 2145 (2010).
47. *Dasha v Adelman*, 45 Mass App Ct 418 (1998).
48. *Doherty v Hellman*, 547 NE2d 931 (1989).
49. *Streifel v Bulkley*, WL 7053742 (2017), *Streifel v Bulkley*, 195 Conn App 294 (2020).
50. *Texas & Pacific Ry v Behymer*, 189 US 468 (1903).
51. *Pegram v Sisco*, 406 FSupp 776 (1976).
52. *Rittenhouse v Hanks, et al.*, 777 A2d 1113 (2001).
53. *Tranum v Hebert*, 581 So2d 1023 (1991).
54. *Natanson v Kline*, 186 Kan 393, 350 P2d 1093 (1960), clarified on motion for rehearing, 187 Kan 186, 354 P2d 670 (1960).
55. Rozovsky F. *Consent to Treatment*. 5th ed. Philadelphia, PA: Wolters Kluwer; 2019.
56. *Ashe v Radiation Oncology Associates, et al.*, 9 SW3d 119 (2000).
57. *Roman v Kim*, WL 4594206 (2019).
58. *King v Bauer*, 767 SW2d 197 (1989).
59. *Nowacki v Community Medical Center, et al.*, 279 NJ Super 276 (1995).
60. *Swope v Razzaq*, 428 F3d 1152 (2005).
61. *Gbur v Golio*, 932 A2d 203 (2007).
62. *Stryczek v The Methodist Hospitals, Inc*, 604 NE2d 1186 (1998).
63. *Conti v Lende*, 194 AD2d 892 (1993).
64. *Cohen v Yale-New Haven Hospital*, 260 Conn 747 (2002).
65. *Hamby v University of Kentucky Medical Center*, 844 SW2d 431 (1993).
66. *Pillars v R.J. Reynolds Tobacco Co.*, 78 So 365 (1918).
67. *Scuzzaro v Loma Linda University Medical Center*, WL 22683416 (2003).
68. Wall TJ. Results of annual ARRO survey. ASTRO Annual Meeting 2019, Chicago, IL, September 15–18, 2019.
69. Wall T. Ethics in the legal and business practice of radiation oncology. *Int J Radiat Oncol Biol Phys*. 2017;99(2):265–268.
70. *Weatherall Radiation Oncology v Caletri*, WL 2061460 (2012).

71. *McGinnis v The Iowa Clinic*, 776 NW2d 110 (2009 WL 2424643).
72. *21st Century Oncology, Inc. v Moody, et al.*, 402 F Supp 3d 1351 (2019).
73. *US ex rel. Johnson-Pochardt v Rapid City Regional Hospital, et al.*, 252 F.S.2d 892 (2003).
74. *US ex rel. Barker v Columbus Regional Healthcare System*, WL 1241095 (2016), *US ex rel. Barker v Tidwell*, WL 3505554 (2015).
75. *US ex rel. Rahman v Colkitt, et al.*, 106 Fed Apps 804 (2004).
76. *Jackson v Levine*, 127 Nev 1154, 373 P3d 936 (2011).

CHAPTER 7

Head and Neck Surgery

Veling W. Tsai, MD, JD, FCLM

INTRODUCTION

Head and neck cancers account for a significant portion of annual incidence of cancers in the United States. Although not as prevalent as breast, lung, or colon cancer, head and neck malignancies represent over 10% of all cancers diagnosed each year, accounting for over 100,000 patients diagnosed with head and neck malignancies.[1] Despite the large numbers of newly diagnosed patients every year, the mortality rate from head and neck malignancies consistently hovers around 4% of total deaths from cancers in the United States.[2] This low mortality rate is due to the good response to treatment modalities for cancers originating in the head and neck. The traditional therapies of surgical resection, chemotherapy and radiation treatment, and the newer therapies of immunomodulation treatment, have all contributed to the increased survival rate of patients with head and neck cancer. However, patients still experience poor outcomes and surgical complications, which may result in alleged wrongdoing by health care professionals. This chapter will focus on the areas of head and neck malignancies with respect to the disease in particular anatomic locations and the resulting cause of the potential allegations of medical malpractice. This chapter will also discuss aspects of care of head and neck cancer patients that may minimize the potential risk of malpractice claims.

HEAD AND NECK MALIGNANCIES

The head and neck anatomy is composed of a complex system of cranial nerves, elaborate vasculatures, and an intricate group of muscles that provide the primary tool for human communication and allow for continued sustenance by processing the food eaten for later digestion. As a result, treatment of malignancies in the head and neck may result in mild to severe alterations of the most basic human functions. From extirpative resection of the face causing disfigurement to laryngectomies that decimate the ability to talk and glossectomies resulting in the loss of the ability to swallow, all patients will need pretreatment counseling and posttreatment rehabilitation. Knowledge of the various head and neck malignancies will better prepare the health care professional to diagnose, treat, and rehabilitate the patient.

Skin

Skin cancer is the most common malignancy in the United States, and a sizeable percentage arise in the head and neck area.[3] The most common types of skin cancer are nonmelanoma skin cancers and melanoma skin cancers. Nonmelanoma skin cancers comprise basal cell carcinoma and squamous cell carcinoma, with an incidence ratio of 3 to 1.[4] Although malignant melanoma accounts for only 5% of all skin cancers, it accounts for 75% of deaths from skin cancers.[2] Health care professionals who specialize in the head and neck area must be vigilant in monitoring for suspicious skin lesions, especially in population groups that are more susceptible to skin cancers, for example, patients with fair skin and light hair, patients with a history of sun exposure, and patients with a family history of skin malignancies. Because of the ease of examination of the skin in the head and neck area, lesions that are appreciated can be further evaluated and worked up to determine their malignancy potential. If patients with head and neck skin cancers are not identified and worked up by primary care physicians or head and neck specialists, there is a high risk for medical malpractice due to the ease of noting the lesions just by looking at the patient.

Salivary

Salivary neoplasms arise from minor or major salivary structures and account for 6% of all head and neck tumors, with the majority of neoplasms being benign.[5] The incidence of malignant salivary neoplasms in the United States is estimated to be about 1 in 100,000.[6] Due to the poor response of salivary malignancies to primary chemotherapy or radiation therapy, the treatment modality is mainly surgical resection, possibly followed by postoperative radiation. The major salivary glands include the parotid, submandibular, and sublingual glands. The parotid glands are located bilaterally in the preauricular area. The facial nerve that provides the innervation to facial muscles lies between the superficial and deep lobes of the parotid gland. The submandibular glands are located bilaterally anterior-inferior to the angle of the mandible. The hypoglossal nerve that innervates the tongue lies just deep in to the gland. Due to the location of the salivary structures in the head and neck, there is a high degree of concern for intraoperative cranial nerve injury, which can lead to loss of facial movement or oral dysphagia. As a result, preoperative counseling of the risks for the resection must be complete and comprehensive so that informed consent can be obtained.

Upper aerodigestive tract

Malignancies of the upper aerodigestive tract in the head and neck extend from the nasal cavity to the cervical esophagus and larynx. The most common type of malignancy of the upper aerodigestive tract is squamous cell carcinoma.[7] The risk factors for squamous cell carcinoma in the head and neck are tobacco use, marijuana use, alcohol use, exposure to human papillomavirus, and genetics.[8] With malignancies in the upper aerodigestive tract, patients will usually present with symptoms ranging from nasal congestion to hoarseness and dysphagia. Lesions of the aerodigestive tract are usually appreciated through a comprehensive physical exam, with focus on the area of the complaint. A thorough exam with appropriate workup will result in timely diagnosis. Moreover, treatment of malignancies in the upper aerodigestive tract has shifted from large and debilitating composite resections to organ-sparing modalities, with comparable results in response to chemotherapy and radiation treatment. These added modalities will require the health care professionals treating upper aerodigestive tract malignancies to be updated on the success of treatment as efficacy is difference for different subsites of the head and neck. For example, the five-year survival rate for nasopharyngeal carcinoma treated with radiation ranges from 60% to 80%, whereas a stage IV base of tongue malignancy treated with primary radiation has a five-year survival rate of 26%.[9,10] With surgical resection providing a greater chance of cure at certain anatomic locations, it is very important to detail the surgery with resulting sequelae so the patient is aware of the postoperative condition. To resect a large base of tongue cancer will likely require a total glossectomy via a mandibular split approach, with modified radical neck dissection, tracheostomy, and gastrostomy tube placement. In addition, the reconstruction of the defect will likely need a radial forearm free flap transfer and skin graft. When a choice is presented to the patient to choose either surgical resection or radiation therapy with adjuvant chemotherapy, health care professionals should not only delineate which therapeutic modality is "better" but also detail the associated risks and consequence associated with each treatment option. This might help alleviate the patient's fear regarding the cancer treatment and prevent future allegations by the patient that the risks and consequences of the treatment options were not disclosed.

Neck

Primary neck malignancies are rare. Most cases of cancer in the neck result from metastatic spread because the neck is rich with lymphatics and serve as a drainage basin for the upper aerodigestive tract. Lymphoma is the second most common malignancy of the head and neck, and 25% of extranodal lymphomas occur in the head and neck.[11] Thus, the type of malignancy will dictate the workup of neck masses regarding whether to search for the primary location or evaluate the extent of disease. The origin of the cancer will affect the prognosis and treatment choice of the patient; for example, the five-year survival rate for patients with metastatic carcinoma of the neck with an unknown primary tumor is different than that of patients with an upper aerodigestive tract carcinoma with metastatic disease to the neck.[12-14] Surgery of the neck may involve risk to several cranial nerves and injury to the great vessels. Patients will need to be advised of these potential risks, especially in light of the possible complications. For instance, a risk of neck dissection surgery is possible injury to the spinal accessory nerve. The spinal accessory nerve provides motor innervation to the trapezius muscle. If a golfer suffered an injury to the nerve during a neck dissection surgery, her golf swing would be permanently affected, which would definitely impact her golf career. This risk should be disclosed to all patients, but it is especially important to highlight this risk for patients who value the range of motion of their arms (e.g., athletes).

Endocrine

Endocrine cancers of the head and neck include thyroid and parathyroid malignancies. Thyroid and parathyroid cancers accounted for about 3% of newly diagnosed cancers in the United States in 2020.[15] The thyroid cancer rate has doubled over the past 20 years, whereas the mortality rate has remained stable during the same period.[15] This has led to speculation that the increase in incidence of thyroid cancer is due to the improvement in the ability to detect and diagnose the malignancy. Thyroid cancer is commonly a slow-growing cancer with a five-year survival rate of over 98%.[15] Advancements in technology have also reduced the number of thyroidectomy surgeries performed. Genetic analysis of thyroid cells can now quantify the risk of malignancy. Prior to genetic analysis, all patients with suspicious nodules underwent thyroid lobectomy for histologic evaluation, with confirmed cases undergoing completion thyroidectomy. With the ability to analyze genetic markers, testing can stratify the risk of malignancy, and physicians are better able to assess which patients actually need surgery. This detailed risk quantification has decreased the risk of complications, especially to the laryngeal nerve, by lowering the number of thyroid surgeries done for pathologic diagnosis. Injury to the superior and recurrent laryngeal nerves can result in devastating consequences to the quality of life of patients, especially if patients use their voice as an important aspect of their life. For example, the famous 20th-century opera singer Amelita Galli-Curci suffered a superior laryngeal nerve injury after thyroid surgery and was unable to recover her vocal range, and she subsequently retired from performing.[16] Thyroidectomy patients will need to be aware that hoarseness is a possible surgical sequela, but rehabilitation to improve the voice is possible, even if the injury is permanent. However, even with rehabilitation via therapies and procedures, the vocal quality will likely never return to normal.

ISSUES IN MALPRACTICE OF HEAD AND NECK MALIGNANCIES

Medical negligence and informed consent are the primary causes of action for patients with head and neck malignancies. Medical negligence cases can often be divided into missed or delayed diagnosis and treatment of perioperative complications.

Informed consent

The concept of informed consent is thoroughly detailed in Chapter 2, but this chapter will briefly discuss the importance of informed consent in treatment of the head and neck patient. The concept of informed consent was forged over 100 years ago, and the idea that patients should have control over the decisions of their body was defined in 1914 by Justice Cardozo: "Every human being of adult years and sound mind has a right to determine what shall be done with his own body; and a surgeon who performs an operation without his patient's consent commits an assault for which he is liable in damages."[17]

The informed consent principle has evolved over the years, but most jurisdictions have adopted the modern law version of the reasonable person standard—what a reasonable person, in the same or similar circumstance, would want to know in order to make an informed decision as to whether to have the recommended medical treatment.[18] The informed consent for the head and neck patient requires the health care provider to disclose the procedure to be performed, the result of the surgery with possible consequences, the common and dangerous risks of the surgery, the postoperative rehabilitation, and the possible permanent sequelae of the surgery. The surgeon will also need to offer the alternative therapies of chemotherapy and/or radiation therapy and the option of palliative care if no aggressive treatment is desired.

Unlike other surgeries of the body, the patient may not be fully aware of the complexities of the surgery and the resulting effects as compared to other parts of the body. For example, if a patient with sarcoma of the tibia was to undergo resection of the cancer that entailed the amputation of the leg, it is reasonable to assume that the patient would expect part of the leg to be removed and that they would need a prosthesis after surgery to be able to walk again. However, if a patient was diagnosed with a tonsil cancer extending to the base of tongue with invasion of the mandible, it is highly unlikely to expect the patient to be aware that the surgical resection would require a composite resection of the lateral pharynx with partial glossectomy, a partial mandibulectomy with ipsilateral neck dissection, a tracheostomy, and a gastrostomy tube placement. These numerous procedures would only be the extirpative portion of the treatment of the cancer. The reconstruction of the surgical defect would involve a fibula free flap with a split-thickness skin graft. The patient might be aware that the defect would need reconstruction but might not be aware of the need for tracheostomy or a gastrostomy tube. Thus, the discussion should focus on not only the oncologic resection but also the reconstruction and the postoperative recovery course. The tracheostomy is necessary to protect the airway during the perioperative period because the resection will involve the oral pharynx and cause swelling that may obstruct the airway. The tracheostomy is a temporary surgical airway to prevent airway obstruction and is usually removed about a week after surgery. During this period with a tracheostomy, the patient's speech will be impaired, and the patient should be aware of this temporary result. Additionally, resection of the base of the tongue may lead to dysphagia, and the gastrostomy tube is needed to allow alternative routes for enteral nutrition postoperatively. If the base of tongue resection crosses to the contralateral side, dysphagia may be permanent due to the lack of a functioning tongue to propel food bolus to the hypopharynx. After the resection, the reconstruction portion will likely require the transfer of a fibula free flap to allow bone replacement of the mandible that is resected. Resection of the mandible is necessary to ensure clear surgical margins, which is paramount in oncologic surgeries. A potential complication of the fibula flap transfer is the peroneal nerve palsy that will result in foot drop.

After surgery, there is also the possible need for postoperative radiation therapy, as pathology of the resected specimen may show high-risk findings (i.e., perineural or lymphovascular invasion of the carcinoma). Although surgical margins may be free of cancer, these high-risk pathologic findings in the specimen may warrant postoperative radiation therapy to increase local and regional control of the cancer, thereby reducing the risk of recurrence. Rehabilitation also needs to be clearly disclosed to the patient because speech and swallow therapy will be necessary to recover the swallow function.

The most common and most significant risks of the surgical procedure must be disclosed to the patient.[19] Additionally, the risk that is of particular importance to the patient must also be discussed. For example, if a patient is to undergo a parotidectomy for a salivary gland malignancy, the risk to the facial nerve is material and must be clearly expressed to the patient. If injury to the facial nerve in any of its branches to the areas of the face were to occur, facial expression would be compromised. Although the nerve injury may be temporary, this nerve deficit will have immediate impact on the patient's ability to nonverbally communicate. If the patient is an actor who relies on their appearance and ability to express themselves via facial expressions, this facial nerve impairment would significantly affect the patient's career, as the actor would not be able to work until the deficit resolves. The patient should also be aware that there is a risk, albeit low, of permanent facial nerve paralysis. This surgical risk will affect the patient's choice of treatment and is an important aspect of the informed consent principle.

Health care professionals often neglect the last component of an informed consent, which is to explain the choice of palliative care. Because the patient has autonomy over his or her body, all choices need to be disclosed to the cancer patient, and palliative care is an acceptable option. Some patients may decide that active treatment is not worth the end result and may choose end-of-life care. Health care professions may dismiss the choice of palliative care due to the appearance of "giving up." This avoidance to discuss palliative care as an alternative may be considered as lack of informed consent because a valid alternative to treatment was not offered to the patient.

CASE LAW # 1

Mrs. Allan was a 33-year-old woman with newly diagnosed right papillary thyroid cancer seen and treated by Dr. Kolb, an otolaryngologist at Fort Belvoir Community Hospital. Mrs. Allan was treated at the hospital as the spouse of an active military serviceman. Dr. Kolb and the endocrine consultants all recommended a total thyroidectomy due to diagnostic findings and the patient's risk factors, although the patient preferred a right hemithyroidectomy. The patient was consented with the knowledge of the risks of total thyroidectomy, including vocal cord paralysis resulting in need for tracheostomy and hypocalcemia from the possible injury to the parathyroid glands. The patient signed the consent for the total thyroidectomy and, knowing the risks, underwent the procedure. However, due to the extracapsular spread of the thyroid cancer, there was aggressive dissection of the right recurrent laryngeal nerve. Additionally, the contralateral recurrent laryngeal nerve was accidentally transected during the surgery. The patient's parathyroid glands were also accidentally removed and injured during the surgery, resulting in postoperative hypocalcemia. The patient underwent a tracheostomy after the thyroidectomy to secure a stable airway.

Mrs. Allan filed suit in federal court alleging that her doctor committed medical malpractice by falling below the standard of care in her treatment of thyroid cancer and failing to adequately inform her of the alternative treatments and procedures associated with her thyroid cancer, thereby failing to obtain her informed consent.

An interesting aspect of this case is the lack of adequate informed consent claim. It is accepted that patients have the right to be informed of the most common and the most dangerous risks that a reasonable person in the same or similar situation would want to know about the procedure. In addition to the risks of the procedure, the patient also needs to be advised of the alternatives to the proposed procedure. In this case, Mrs. Allan was informed of the possibility of the vocal cord damage and the need for possible tracheostomy if the bilateral recurrent laryngeal nerve were to be injured, and she did sign the consent forms before surgery, indicating that she wished to proceed with the surgery knowing the possible risks and complications. However, Mrs. Allan argued that she was not informed of the alterative procedures or treatments, namely, that she could have been offered a sub-total thyroidectomy, where residual thyroid tissue is left behind to minimize possible injury to the recurrent laryngeal nerve. The defense argued that the standard of care did not require the option of subtotal thyroidectomy to be offered to the patient in her condition. The various literature sources cited by the experts during trial concluded that when, comparing subtotal and total thyroidectomy for treatment of thyroid cancer, total thyroidectomy offers no statistically significant increased benefits in long-term survival rates in thyroid cancer; thus, the court sided with Mrs. Allan in deciding that subtotal thyroidectomy should have been offered as an alternative in the informed consent process. As a result, the court agreed that there was a lack of informed consent when Dr. Kolb failed to disclose and offer the alternative option of a subtotal thyroidectomy during the consent process of the total thyroidectomy.[20]

Missed or delayed diagnosis

The second major area in medical malpractice involving the head and neck patient is the issue of missed or delayed diagnosis. Although different legal standing is used, the cause of action in medical malpractice is the same and is the result of the lack of appropriate care and evaluation of the patient.[21] This appropriate care requires a complete history obtained from the patient, a thorough physical examination, an appropriate diagnostic workup, and the proper treatment and follow-up of the patient. These four elements, if properly and timely completed, can help avoid any missed diagnoses or delays in diagnosis.

The first element is the complete history taking and information gathering from the patient. As the great physician Dr. William Osler professed to his students, "Listen to your patient, he is telling you his diagnosis."[22] Health care professionals will need to gather the needed information to make the correct diagnosis. Additionally, clinicians also need to constantly maintain the current breadth of knowledge because medical knowledge is constantly advancing. For example, the link between human papillomavirus and squamous cell carcinoma in the upper aerodigestive tract was established in the last ten years, and this became an important risk factor for younger populations developing squamous cell carcinoma in the head and neck.[23] This risk factor changed the index of suspicion for younger patients who present with oral lesions or neck masses and have no history of tobacco or alcohol use. Previously, patients with a long history of smoking or alcohol use were at higher suspicion for head and neck cancers; thus, abnormal lesions were carefully worked up and followed, whereas younger patients without these risk factors were usually suspected of having an infectious etiology and treated with antibiotics and assurance. Clinicians with a current, up-to-date knowledge base are able to generate a more appropriate list of differential diagnoses and are less likely to miss suspicious lesions. In addition, gathering a complete history and eliciting pertinent information indirectly results in building rapport with the patient. This rapport is a critical element in the foundation of a strong doctor-patient relationship and, in turn, can decrease the risk of a medical malpractice claim.

The second element is to perform a thorough physical exam. In the head and neck patient, this will usually require endoscopic examination because some parts of the upper aerodigestive tract cannot be clearly examined by direct visual exam. Clear and detailed documentation in the patient's file is necessary to avoid future allegations that lesions were not appreciated on the physical exam. Due to advances in technology, the examination of the nasopharynx, hypopharynx, and larynx is now performed with endoscopes with photographic and video capabilities. What once was a description of the exam of the upper aerodigestive tract in the patient's chart is now a visual landscape that can be seen by the clinician, the patient, and even the future jury. Prior to the advent of the endoscope, the hypopharyngeal and laryngeal exam was done with an indirect mirror exam, and the only description was documented by the clinician who performed the exam. If there were questions regarding the accuracy of the exam, the only documentation was in the patient's chart and it was difficult to controvert the documentation. However, with photographic and video documentation, the legal examination is of the recorded video or photographic exam instead of the clinician's description in the patient's chart. Health care professionals need to be extremely careful to document all findings of the endoscopic exam so that the findings corroborate with the written and photographic findings for an accurate assessment of the anatomy.

The third element is the appropriate diagnostics workup with radiology and pathology. For patients with suspicious lesions of the head and neck, in addition to the history and physical exam, a short list of differential diagnoses should be generated. Imaging will likely consist of a combination of computed tomography scan, magnetic resonance imaging, positron emission tomography, and ultrasound exams to evaluate the location and extent of disease. Fine-needle aspiration or open biopsy of the lesion is necessary for a pathologic diagnosis. These modalities, when used appropriately, can lead to the diagnosis of the patient's condition. Using the appropriate imaging modality is also important to avoid unnecessary radiation or intravenous contrast exposure of the patient.

The last element is the appropriate treatment of the patient after diagnosis is confirmed. For the head and neck oncology patient, treatment may include surgery, chemotherapy, and/or radiation therapy. Except for early-stage disease, rarely are single treatment modalities sufficient for the treatment of head and neck cancers.[24] Multiple specialties are often involved in the care and treatment of head and neck cancer patients. Tumor boards, composed of head and neck surgeons, radiation therapists, and oncologists, are often convened to discuss the most appropriate treatment modalities for the particular patient. Moreover, tumor boards often also include prosthodontists and prosthetics specialists to discuss reconstruction and rehabilitation of the intraoperative defect. Tumor boards offer the patient comprehensive cancer care by gathering all the specialists that may participate in the care of the patient and providing continuity of care in the perioperative period.

The appropriate treatment modality is based on the treatment's evidence of success in treatment of head and neck cancers. With continued advances in chemotherapeutic drugs and the focused targeting of radiation treatments, the shift away from composite surgical resection to organ-sparing treatment has accelerated in the past ten years.[25] Currently, most squamous cell carcinoma surgical resections are performed as salvage surgery in patients who failed chemoradiation treatment or performed for recurrent disease that no long is eligible for further radiation treatment. Advances in treatment are constantly being updated in the literature, and the clinician is required to offer the best treatment modality to the patient to provide the best care. For example, in early-stage squamous cell cancer of the upper aerodigestive tract, five-year survival rates are equivalent for surgery versus radiation plus adjuvant chemotherapy.[23] Thus, what once was treated with a large resection, resulting in cosmetic and functional sequelae, is now treated with chemoradiation therapy that offers comparable local regional control with preservation of anatomy and function.

In contrast, salivary malignancies do not respond well to chemotherapy or radiation therapy. Hence, in a patient with a small adenoid cystic carcinoma of the parotid gland, the primary treatment would still be parotidectomy with facial nerve dissection, with possible selective neck dissection and possible postoperative radiation therapy if pathology showed perineural or lymphovascular spread.[26] Additionally, oncologic treatment options are being reevaluated for slow-growing papillary thyroid cancers. Previously, papillary thyroid cancers were treated with thyroidectomy followed by possible postoperative radioactive iodine treatment if high-risk factors were noted on pathology. Currently, the availability of advanced fine-needle aspiration has reduced the number of thyroidectomies performed for pathologic diagnosis. Furthermore, the ability to analyze genetic point mutations from the fine-needle aspirates has further helped stratify the risk of malignancy on previous indeterminate cytology samples, thus further reducing the need for thyroidectomies.[27] With new data on the behavior of papillary thyroid cancers, the American Thyroid Association has updated its recommendation on whether patients with well-differentiated thyroid cancers need to undergo partial or total thyroidectomies.[28] In addition, for certain patients, such as elderly patients or those with high morbidity, there is even evidence that these patients can be observed for papillary thyroid cancer due to its slow-growing character.

Because of the various types of pathology in head and neck oncology, health care professionals need to be aware of the latest treatment modalities and their associated success. This will enable an informed discussion with the patient regarding the treatment options. Patients can thus choose the option that is best after evaluation of the risks, benefits, side effects, and long-term sequalae of the treatment choice. Legal issues may arise if the clinician directs the patient toward a single option, especially if that option is surgery.

CASE LAW # 2

In 1991, Ms. Ivanjack, a 21-year-old woman, was seen by her primary care physician with complaints of unilateral right otalgia and right hearing loss. She was diagnosed with otitis media and treated with antibiotics. When she failed to improve after several weeks of antibiotics, she was referred to an otolaryngologist for further evaluation and treatment. Dr. Bond, an otolaryngologist who saw the patient a month later, confirmed the diagnosis of right otitis media because his examination of the ear showed effusion behind the tympanic membrane. Dr. Bond continued to treat Ms. Ivanjack for the next two months for the persistent ear infection and progressive ear and neck pain. The ear pain worsened and started to radiate to the throat and neck. Dr. Bond diagnosed tonsillitis and subsequently performed a tonsillectomy in hopes of resolving the patient's persistent and progressing pain. Over the two months of treatment, Dr. Bond did not evaluate the nasopharynx to evaluate for possible obstruction of the eustachian tube. The pain did not resolve with the tonsillectomy, and the patient was seen by another otolaryngologist who noted cervical lymphadenopathy; the resulting biopsy of the neck nodes showed metastatic nasopharyngeal carcinoma.

The nasopharyngeal carcinoma was diagnosed three months after the patients was first seen by the specialist, Dr. Bond. As a result of the delay, the patient was diagnosed with stage IV cancer. Ms. Ivanjack was treated with chemotherapy and radiation therapy, with no evidence of cancer six years after treatment completion. A malpractice lawsuit was filed due to the patient's persistent anxiety of recurrent disease. With late-stage cancer, there is a higher chance of recurrent disease. The patient argued that if she had been adequately evaluated and properly worked up with a nasal endoscopy when Dr. Bond initially saw and treated her, her cancer stage, with lack of cervical metastasis, would have been stage II. The defense presented experts who testified that the three-month delay made no significant difference in the patient's treatment outcome. The jury believed that, due to Dr. Bond's delay in diagnosis, the patient's recurrent disease rate was significantly worse for stage IV compared to stage II disease. The jury returned a verdict for Ms. Ivanjack in the amount of $2.2 million.[29]

Perioperative care and complications

The head and neck surgeon will need to provide the highest level intraoperative and postoperative care due to the complexity of the surgical procedure. Injury of the cranial nerves located in the head and neck can lead to temporary or permanent functional deficits. The hypoglossal nerve affects swallowing, the spinal accessory nerve controls the range of motion for the arm, the recurrent laryngeal branch of the vagus nerve controls speech and voice, and the facial nerve influences facial movement. Intraoperative attention to these vital structures must be paid. In addition, injury to the great vessels of the neck can lead to strokes and cerebral edema. Both intraoperative and postoperative care are directly related as inattentive care during a neck dissection can cause a chyle leak and, if noted intraoperatively, it can be ligated and treated. If the chyle duct injury is not recognized intraoperatively, then the leak can result in postoperative leak and possible fistula formation. Even if the chyle leak is missed intraoperatively, if it is discovered and treated appropriately postoperatively, then fistula formation and the associated increased hospital stay can be avoided.

In the perioperative period, the clinician is required not only to provide care and ameliorate complications that should happen but also to coordinate postoperative rehabilitations and treatments (i.e., referral to radiation therapy or speech and swallow therapy), when appropriate. The care does not end after the patient is discharged from the hospital but continues for at least five years for patients with cancer. After the perioperative period, when the wound has healed and the patient can resume daily activities, the surveillance period begins, because there is a risk the patient may develop recurrent disease. Posttreatment surveillance is an integral part of the care of the cancer patient and may require routine endoscopic surveillance and possible imaging modalities.

In addition to surveillance for recurrence, patients must also be assessed and followed for posttreatment side effects that can occur anytime from immediately after treatment to decades after treatment. For example, the most common sequela of radiation therapy is xerostomia, or dry mouth, and patients usually begin experiencing this symptom during, or immediately after, completion of the treatment course.[30,31] The xerostomia will usually improve but is unlikely to permanently resolve. Xerostomia can cause dysphagia, and patients will usually learn to cope with this discomfort. Additionally, a long-term risk of radiation therapy is the development of secondary malignancies (i.e., sarcomas), usually many years after treatment has been completed.[32] These long-term results and risks require the clinician to be astutely aware so that appropriate care and management can be provided.

MINIMIZING LEGAL LIABILITY IN THE CARE OF THE HEAD AND NECK CANCER PATIENT

Although the percentage of head and neck cancer patients is relatively low in comparison to other malignancies of the body, for the head and neck specialist, this population is a part of the daily medical practice. The first step in minimizing liability is ensuring that complaints are addressed and signs and symptoms are worked up appropriately, rather than dismissed or ignored. Although this is not a legal requirement, fostering the physician-patient relationship will decrease the risk of future malpractice claims. If the patient understands that the clinician is listening to and addressing their complaints and symptoms, then the patient will feel that appropriate care is being rendered. However, if the patient believes the clinician is dismissive of their concerns and symptoms, even if appropriate workup is done, the patient may not believe that appropriate care has been provided. Many medical malpractice lawsuits are filed so that patients can make their doctors listen to their grievances.

To provide care for this vulnerable group of patients in an ever-changing environment of advancing medical knowledge, combined with the ease of access to Internet knowledge, a clinician must be able to provide comprehensive knowledge and care. Patients will often present to the clinic having done Internet research on various diagnostic and treatment modalities from wide-ranging and diverse sources. Patients should be aware of the appropriate treatment options, and discussing the standards of treatment with patients, including the risks and benefits, ensures that awareness. The discussion of standard treatment modalities can avoid the pitfalls of falling below the standard of care. One need not be the foremost expert in treating head and neck cancers, but one needs to be aware of the standards for treatment of the various types of cancers.

The surgical care for the head and neck cancer patient is complex and can result in various morbidities. This is stressful and frightening to the patient. The clinician must exercise care during the perioperative care period to prevent complications and must be able to recognize complications early so the complications can be managed and treated without resulting in permanent sequelae. Mismanaging the early signs and symptoms of complications may lead to permanent damage and result in medical malpractice claims from the patient.

CLINICAL VIGNETTE # 1

A week before Thanksgiving, a 38-year-old Asian woman presents for evaluation of right hearing loss after being referred by her family physician. The patient states that she has had new onset of hearing loss in the right ear for the past three months. The symptom was originally isolated right aural fullness at the onset but now has progressed to hearing loss. The hearing loss is constant, and there is associated tinnitus and mild otalgia on the same side. According to the patient, the left ear is normal and asymptomatic. She denies otorrhea and headaches. She was previously treated with antibiotics and steroids, which improved the symptoms but did not resolve the problems. After completing the course of medications, the symptoms have progressively worsened.

Upon further questioning regarding her medical and social history, she states that she has a history of seasonal allergies that are worse in the winter, but otherwise, she is in good health without any chronic medical problems. She emigrated from Hong Kong ten years ago after attending graduate school in southern California. Her parents and siblings are in good health, except for well-controlled hypertension in her father. She has a history of social tobacco and alcohol use until her pregnancy ten years ago and has since not smoked or used alcohol. She has no known medical allergies and is no longer taking any prescription medication after completing the course of amoxicillin and prednisone.

A thorough review of systems reveals sneezing, rhinorrhea, and postnasal drip, which are worse in the morning. The patient also admits to occasional epistaxis from nose blowing and nasal congestion, both isolated to the right side.

Pertinent physical exam findings during the visit include right tympanic membrane with serous effusion. The nasal exam shows pale boggy mucosa with a right deviated septum with excoriated mucosa. There is no evidence of tonsil hypertrophy or palpable cervical lymphadenopathy.

The patient is treated with fluoroquinolones and both oral and nasal steroids and has a scheduled audiogram in one week. At the audiogram evaluation, the patient is noted to have a unilateral conductive hearing loss on the right with a 40-dB air-bone gap. The tympanogram on the right is flat (type B).

The patient is recommended to undergo a myringotomy with pressure equalization tube placement to resolve the otitis media and hearing loss. The patient agrees after consent discloses a small risk of a persistent tympanic membrane perforation after tube extrusion. After the tube is placed in the right tympanic membrane and the serous effusion is suctioned, the patient experiences immediate relief and resolution of the hearing loss.

A nasal endoscopy is also performed due to the patient's risk for nasopharyngeal malignancy. The endoscopy shows an exophytic mass in the right torus tubarius area. Biopsy of the mass shows non-keratinizing squamous cell carcinoma. Positron emission tomography and computed tomography fusion scans are done and show a hypermetabolic lesion in the right nasopharynx with bony erosion of the skull base; there are also numerous small hypermetabolic lesions noted in the right neck. No distant metastatic lesions are appreciated on the scans.

The patient is counseled on her new diagnosis. Although surgical intervention is not recommended for the treatment of nasopharyngeal carcinoma, the pathophysiology of the cancer and her particular risk factors are explained in detail to her. The treatment options and modalities are recommended, and the posttreatment surveillance plans are also discussed. The patient is then referred to radiation oncology and hematology-oncology specialists for chemoradiation treatment. The patient will be followed after treatment with routine nasal endoscopy for cancer surveillance and also with regular ear exams until the right tympanostomy tube is extruded.

This case illustrates the need for a complete and thorough medical history and physical exam to prevent a misdiagnosis or delay in diagnosis of the patient's nasopharyngeal carcinoma. A young healthy patient with a history of allergies and middle ear effusion may lead many clinicians to presume a straightforward diagnosis of otitis media.

Audiogram and tympanogram evaluation indeed showed a conductive hearing loss representing a middle ear condition of otitis media. The typical treatment of otitis media that fails medical intervention with steroids and decongestants is a pressure equalization tube. If the clinician only placed a tube in the ear to resolve the hearing loss, the malignancy would not have been found.

Understanding the pathophysiology of nasopharyngeal carcinoma will heighten a clinician's suspicion when encountering a unilateral conductive hearing loss. In addition, the carcinoma has a predilection for Southeast Asians due to genetics, dietary habits, and Epstein-Barr virus exposure. This understanding and awareness will lead to more specific questions during the patient's medical history interview.

Diagnostic biopsy and imaging are crucial to staging and determining treatment options for head and neck cancers. The pivotal nasal endoscopy in this case is the procedure that resulted in the biopsy that confirmed the diagnosis. Pathology and imaging will determine which interventions are more appropriate, ranging from surgery to radiation to chemotherapy, or any combination of the three. In this case, due to the presence of cervical metastasis and appearance of skull base erosion, chemotherapy would be recommended, whereas if the disease was localized to the nasopharynx, then chemotherapy might not be necessary as a treatment modality.

The persistence of symptoms after lack of response to treatment prescribed by the primary physician necessitates the otolaryngologist to expand the list of differential diagnosis. If the patient was treated with more medications without other diagnostic workup, then misdiagnosis and delay in care and treatment would have occurred. Similarly, the isolated procedure to resolve the middle ear effusion without nasal endoscopy would also have led to a misdiagnosis and delay in treatment. This is no secret; to prevent medical malpractice issues, a physician needs to be thorough and do what is appropriate for the patient.

CONCLUSION

Health care professionals who care for head and neck cancer patients should be compassionate, competent, and comprehensive. These qualities will allow the clinician to provide appropriate evaluation and treatment. In providing this specialized care, clinicians need to be aware of the appropriate workup required to ensure an accurate diagnosis. Once a diagnosis is confirmed, then the treatment modality chosen by the patient must be clearly and thoroughly discussed with the patient, including the potential risks, temporary and long-term sequelae, and various alternatives with comparable results. This truly informed consent will then be deemed adequate under any legal lens. Providing the appropriate perioperative care and postoperative surveillance is essential to ensure the success of the treatment. This vigilance in perioperative and postoperative care will minimize the possibility of devastating complications and is the minimum standard required of patient care. Accomplishing these goals will not only minimize the potential for legal entanglements but also is the foundation for building a solid patient-clinician relationship.

KEY POINTS:

- Head and neck malignancies represents about 10% of all cancers diagnosed each year.
- Head and neck malignancy survival rates are increasing due to new treatment modalities.
- Skin malignancies are the most common cancer in the United States.
- Salivary cancer resections involve a higher risk of intraoperative cranial nerve injury compared to other head and neck malignancies.
- Upper aerodigestive tract cancers have traditionally been associated with smoking and alcohol use, but now there is increased association with human papillomavirus exposure.

- Primary malignancies of the neck are rare. Instead, neck tumors more often indicate metastatic spread of a primary cancer.
- Thyroid malignancy incidence has increased over the past 20 years, but the survival rate has remained unchanged.
- Informed consent is determined by what a reasonable person, in the same or similar circumstance, would want to know regarding the risks, benefits, and alternatives of the medical treatment.
- Missed or delayed diagnosis can be avoided by taking a comprehensive medical history, performing a thorough physical exam, ordering the appropriate diagnostic tests, and providing timely and appropriate treatments.
- Postoperative care is a part of the medical treatment and requires the surgeon to provide monitoring and treatment, even after the procedure.

References:

1. Cancer facts and figures 2020. American Cancer Society. https://www.cancer.org/content/dam/cancer-org/research/cancer-facts-and-statistics/annual-cancer-facts-and-figures/2020/cancer-facts-and-figures-2020.pdf. Accessed July 28, 2020.
2. NPCR and SEER incidence—U.S. cancer statistics 2001–2016 public use database data standards and data dictionary. Centers for Disease Control and Prevention. https://www.cdc.gov/cancer/uscs/public-use/pdf/npcr-seer-public-use-database-data-dictionary-2001-2016-508.pdf. Accessed July 28, 2020.
3. Rogers HW, Weinstock MA, Feldman SR, et al. Incidence estimate of nonmelanoma skin cancer (keratinocyte carcinomas) in the U.S. population, 2012. *JAMA Dermatol*. 2015;151(10):1081–1086.
4. Cancer stat facts: melanoma of the skin. National Cancer Institute. https://seer.cancer.gov/statfacts/html/melan.html. Accessed July 28, 2020.
5. Stenner M, Klussmann JP. Current update on established and novel biomarkers in salivary gland carcinoma pathology and the molecular pathways involved. *Eur Arch Otorhinolaryngol*. 2009;266(3):333–341.
6. Pinkston JA, Cole P. Incidence rates of salivary gland tumors: results from a population-based study. *Otolaryngol Head Neck Surg*. 1999;120(6):834–840.
7. Sanderson RJ, Ironside JA. Squamous cell carcinomas of the head and neck. *BMJ*. 2002;325(7368):822–827.
8. Dhull AK, Atri R, Dhankhar R, et al. Major risk factors in head and neck cancer: a retrospective analysis of 12-year experiences. *World J Oncol*. 2018;9(3):80–84.
9. Mendenhall WM, Million RR, Cassisi NJ. Elective neck irradiation in squamous-cell carcinoma of the head and neck. *Head Neck Surg*. 1980;3(1):15–20.
10. Al-Sarraf M, LeBlanc M, Giri PG, et al. Chemoradiotherapy versus radiotherapy in patients with advanced nasopharyngeal cancer: phase III randomized Intergroup study 0099. *J Clin Oncol*. 1998;16(4):1310–1317.
11. Wulfrank D, Speelman T, Pauwels C, et al. Extranodal non-Hodgkin's lymphoma of the head and neck. *Radiother Oncol*. 1987;8:199–207.
12. Grau C, Johansen LV, Jakobsen J, et al. Cervical lymph node metastases from unknown primary tumours. Results from a national survey by the Danish Society for Head and Neck Oncology. *Radiother Oncol*. 2000;55(2):121–129.
13. Lou J, Wang S, Wang K, et al. Squamous cell carcinoma of cervical lymph nodes from an unknown primary site: the impact of neck dissection. *J Cancer Res Ther*. 2015;11(suppl 2):C161–C167.
14. Hoffman HT, Porter K, Karnell LH, et al. Laryngeal cancer in the United States: changes in demographics, patterns of care, and survival. *Laryngoscope*. 2006;116(9 Pt 2 Suppl 111):1–13.
15. Cancer stat facts: thyroid cancer. National Cancer Institute. https://seer.cancer.gov/statfacts/html/thyro.html. Accessed July 28, 2020.

16. Marchese-Ragona R, Restivo DA, Mylonakis I, et al. The superior laryngeal nerve injury of a famous soprano, Amelita Galli-Curci. *Acta Otorhinolaryngol Ital*. 2013;33(1):67–71.

17. *Schloendorff v Society of New York Hospital*, 105 NE 92 (NY 1914).

18. *Spence v Canterbury*, 409 US 1064, 93 S Ct 560, 34 L Ed 2d 518 (US 1972). See, for example, Cal Code Regs Tit 9 § 784.29; Wash Rev Code Ann § 7.70.050 (West); NY Pub Health Law § 2805-d (McKinney).

19. *Sard v Hardy*, 379 A2d 1014 (Md 1977); *Dunn v Yager*, 58 So 3d 1171 (Miss 2011); *Downs v Trias*, 49 A3d 180 (2012); *Scott v Bradford*, 606 P2d 554 (Okla 1979).

20. *Allan v United States*, 401 F Supp 3d 681 (2019).

21. See, for example, *Mann v United States*, 300 F Supp 3d 411 (ND NY 2018); In re Barker, 110 SW3d 486 (Tex App 2003); *Daniel v Jones*, 39 F Supp 2d 635 (ED Va 1999), aff'd sub nom *Daniel v Pearce*, 213 F3d 630 (4th Cir 2000).

22. Pitkin RM. Listen to the patient. *BMJ*. 1998;316(7139):1252.

23. D'Souza G, Dempsey A. The role of HPV in head and neck cancer and review of the HPV vaccine. *Prev Med*. 2011;53(Suppl 1):S5–S11.

24. Chitapanarux I, Traisathit P, Komolmalai N, et al. Ten-year outcome of different treatment modalities for squamous cell carcinoma of oral cavity. *Asian Pac J Cancer Prev*. 2017;18(7):1919–1924.

25. Cognetti DM, Weber RS, Lai SY. Head and neck cancer: an evolving treatment paradigm. *Cancer*. 2008;113(7 Suppl):1911–1932.

26. Reddy EK, Mansfield CM, Hartman GV, et al. Malignant salivary gland tumors: role of radiation therapy. *J Natl Med Assoc*. 1979;71(10):959–961.

27. Cerutti JM. Employing genetic markers to improve diagnosis of thyroid tumor fine needle biopsy. *Curr Genomics*. 2011;12(8):589–596.

28. Haugen BR, Alexander EK, Bible KC, et al. 2015 American Thyroid Association management guidelines for adult patients with thyroid nodules and differentiated thyroid cancer: The American Thyroid Association Guidelines Task Force on Thyroid Nodules and Differentiated Thyroid Cancer. *Thyroid*. 2016;26(1):1–133.

29. *Bond v Ivanjack*, 740 A2d 968 (1999).

30. Tolentino Ede S, Centurion BS, Ferreira LH, et al. Oral adverse effects of head and neck radiotherapy: literature review and suggestion of a clinical oral care guideline for irradiated patients. *J Appl Oral Sci*. 2011;19(5):448–454.

31. Yeh SA. Radiotherapy for head and neck cancer. *Semin Plast Surg*. 2010;24(2):127–136.

32. Singh GK, Yadav V, Singh P, et al. Radiation-induced malignancies making radiotherapy a "two-edged sword": a review of literature. *World J Oncol*. 2017;8(1):1–6.

CHAPTER 8

Medical and Pediatric Oncology

Randall Y. Chan, MD, Quynh La, JD, and Viney Hardit, MD, JD

INTRODUCTION

Despite the challenges and hazard of poor outcomes inherent to the practice of treating patients with cancer, oncologists enjoy an overall low risk of medical malpractice claims, and malpractice insurance costs for a medical oncologist are similar to those of a general internist.[1] In addition, payouts are comparatively rare.[2] Nonetheless, the practice of medicine in a high-stakes field such as medical and pediatric oncology will expose practitioners to risk; many of these risks are mitigatable.

CHEMOTHERAPY ERRORS

While the overall coordination of cancer care generally is assumed by the medical or pediatric oncologist, the legal responsibility of detection, diagnosis, staging, excision, and palliation of cancer is generally the burden of other specialties. Thus, the primary procedure of the oncologist is the prescribing of chemotherapeutic medications. As these medications are toxic by nature, this procedure is also the primary source of litigation risk to oncologists.

The vast majority of cancer patients treated with systemic therapy will receive chemotherapy. Chemotherapy drugs, in general, have narrow therapeutic windows, which is the difference between effective and toxic or lethal doses, in comparison to other commonly used medications.[3] Thus, medication errors involving chemotherapy are likely to cause harm.[4] Unfortunately, chemotherapy errors are common; for example, in an exploratory survey of oncology nurses, 63% reported an occurrence of a chemotherapy medication error.[5]

Chemotherapy errors often result from errors in dosing or route or insufficient supportive care. Dosing errors may occur due to incorrect measurement of the patient's body size or miscalculation of the resulting dose; certain medications, such as carboplatin, are of particular note due to the complexity of calculations as a result of factors such as targeting the area under the curve.[6] Route errors can be particularly lethal; a review of the pediatric literature described a series of reports of vincristine given via the intrathecal route with 100% lethality despite various attempts to remove or flush the drug from the space.[4] Supportive care for many medications involves hydration and/or diuresis, and some medications such as methotrexate require specific antidotes or protectants to be given to avoid toxicity.[7]

Malpractice as a legal concept in relationship to chemotherapy errors is relatively straightforward. The correct dosing and administration of chemotherapy medications are the standard of care; thus, errors in dosing and administration are both considered under the standard of care. Resolution of a malpractice claim thus depends primarily on who is at fault and whether harm was caused to the patient.

CASE LAW # 1

In 1995, Vincent Gargano was undergoing systemic chemotherapy as part of his therapy for testicular cancer.[8] His physician intended etoposide 197 mg and cisplatin 39.4 mg every 24 hours for five consecutive days from May 26 through May 30. The resident physician wrote orders for etoposide 39.4 mg and cisplatin 197 mg instead, and the patient received the incorrect dosages four times before a nurse caught the error on the morning of May 30.

Even with omission of the final dose, the patient received four times the intended cumulative dose of cisplatin. He experienced acute kidney injury and ultimately failure, electrolyte wasting, hearing loss, and severe bone marrow suppression. Ultimately, the overdose proved fatal within two weeks of the overdose. The family filed a lawsuit claiming wrongful death, noting as well that the patient would have had an excellent prognosis overall, with an overall survival rate of 95% for his tumor type and stage. The university settled out of court for $7.9 million.

CASE LAW # 2

Betsy A. Lehman was enrolled in a clinical trial for advanced-stage breast cancer in 1994.[9] She was to receive an autologous stem cell transplant, a technique in which myeloablative doses of chemotherapy are given, with a rescue using the patient's own cryopreserved hematopoietic stem cells. A fellow physician wrote for 6520 mg of cyclophosphamide daily for four days; the correct dose should have been 1630 mg daily for four days to a total dose of 6520 mg. The patient received the entire dose followed by the thawed stem cells. She died as she was being prepared for discharge home; an autopsy did not reveal the cause of death and also noted no evidence of cancer.

Two months after her death, during data review for the clinical trial, the error was uncovered. A second death that had occurred for the same reason (four times the dose of cyclophosphamide given) on the same protocol within two days of this case was discovered at the same review. Audits from the Massachusetts Department of Public Health as well as The Joint Commission for the Accreditation of Healthcare Organizations (since renamed to The Joint Commission) revealed numerous deficiencies, and an internal investigation resulted in numerous formal reprimands for the staff. The fellow physician who wrote the orders was stripped of his license to practice medicine in Massachusetts for three years. The medical center settled a wrongful death suit for an undisclosed amount that was reported by the *Boston Globe* to be in the multimillion dollar range.

Most, if not all, chemotherapy errors are considered preventable, although human error cannot be fully omitted. Numerous strategies have been employed; some of these are mandated by regulatory bodies.

Most revolve around the Swiss cheese model of error prevention.[10] Understanding that human error cannot fully be prevented, the model instead focuses on multiple checks and safety stops to reduce the chance for an error to actually reach the patient and cause harm. In the case of chemotherapy, once a physician orders the chemotherapy, the pharmacist checks dosing, timing, and volume of administration prior to preparation and dispensing of the medication. The nurse again checks dosing, timing, and volume prior to actual administration. This model does require a free sharing of information, including chemotherapy protocols and intended dosages and regimens.

Beyond the Swiss cheese model, error prevention methods commonly employed include extra formal training for the dosing of chemotherapy, the use of preprinted order forms, and computerized physician order entry (CPOE).[11] Extra training for chemotherapy is often obtained in advanced oncology training (fellowship). The use of preprinted order forms allows for simplified error checking via the Swiss cheese model; this method may be supplemented or even supplanted by CPOE methods that reduce error rates by alerting prescribers to unusually high doses and/or incorporating automatic calculations.[12]

It is worth noting that trainee status may afford some protection from liability, but ultimately, it is not complete protection. In Case Law No. 2, it was ultimately the fellow physician (i.e., subspecialist in training) who was found to be liable, rather than his attending physician supervisor. It should be assumed that any licensed practitioner can potentially be liable; thus, multiple persons may be potentially liable for any single harmful error.

CLINICAL VIGNETTE # 1

The patient is a 56-year-old woman who is undergoing doxorubicin, cyclophosphamide, and docetaxel chemotherapy for six cycles for a T1cN2M0 infiltrating ductal cancer of the left breast status post lumpectomy in the setting of breast conservation therapy. On her third cycle, she feels a burning sensation in her arm. Dr. Jones, her medical oncologist, brings her into clinic and notes extravasation for the doxorubicin. He checks the dose of the chemotherapy and realizes that, instead of 60 mg/m^2, the patient was given 600 mg/m^2 of doxorubicin. During the clinic encounter, the patient loses consciousness and is swiftly admitted to the inpatient intensive care unit.

One of the primary responsibilities of an oncologist is the appropriate prescribing of medically indicated chemotherapeutics for patients with malignant conditions. Because chemotherapeutic drugs are toxic by nature and typically have very narrow therapeutic windows, the prescribing of these medications is part of the standard of care for oncologists. This includes the correct dosing and administration of the medication. In the vignette, the individual who accidentally amplified the dose from 60 mg/m^2 to 600 mg/m^2 would likely be held liable for the error.

Whether that individual is the physician is indeterminate from the vignette. It is possible that the physician correctly dosed the medication but a pharmacy and/or nursing error was to blame for the incorrect administration of the medication. Ultimately, liability would be contingent upon who was responsible for the error (e.g., physician, pharmacist, nurse) and whether the patient actually suffered harm (which, in this case, the patient clearly did).

Had this error been a "near miss" where, although a medication error occurred, the patient suffered no adverse consequences as a result of the error, then resolution of the patient's malpractice claim would likely result in the recovery of minimal damages.

EVOLVING STANDARD OF CARE

More troubling than errors in the use of chemotherapy are systematic errors in knowledge or judgement. Human error in the use of chemotherapy will generally harm only the patient who is directly involved. In contrast, the consistent misapplication of oncologic knowledge and/or tools in the process of treatment planning exposes an oncologist to potential litigation from essentially every patient affected. Nowhere is this more apparent than in the case of an oncologist with outdated knowledge.

Cancer care is a constantly evolving field, requiring practicing oncologists to stay updated regarding the latest standard of care. Complicating this matter in pediatrics is that forward progress in the field is reliant primarily on large cooperative group trials with long follow-up, many of which do not publish results until many years after the study has been performed; it is not unusual to publish final results from a trial a decade after the research was initiated.[13]

Nonetheless, it should be recognized that progress can occur relatively quickly. For example, from the 1960s through the 2000s, each decade saw interval improvement in outcome for patients with pediatric acute lymphoblastic leukemia (ALL).[14] Pediatric ALL was almost uniformly fatal at the start of the 1960s, whereas long-term survival was achievable in nearly half of patients by the end of 1970s and is over 80% today.[15] Much of this success has been achieved through refined treatment strategies, such as single-drug regimens in the 1950s, combination chemotherapy in the 1960s, intrathecal chemotherapy in the 1970s, prolonged intensification in the 1980s, and so on.[14]

Other tumors saw similar progressive improvements; for example, Wilms tumor showed progressive improvement as surgery alone was augmented with external beam radiation in the 1940s, chemotherapy in the 1960s, and complex regimens stemming from cooperative group trials in the 1980s and onward.[16] Other tumors saw major shifts in therapy due to breakthroughs such as the use of retinoic acid derivatives to treat acute promyelocytic leukemia or the use of intraocular photoablation to treat retinoblastoma.[17,18]

As new large cooperative group trials are completed every five to ten years, the standard of care slowly shifts around the world regardless of resource availability.[19] Failing to maintain pace with the evolving standard of care puts one at risk for legal action due to the very real risk of suboptimal outcomes.

CASE LAW # 3

The pediatric oncology program at University of New Mexico Hospital (UNMH), under the direction of Dr. Marilyn Duncan, came under fire for the treatment of pediatric patients with cancer using outdated treatment regimens in 1998.[20] Two new physicians, who had recently joined the practice, had written a letter of concern to the department chair after having first contacted two outside experts regarding the therapy given. The memorandum named 217 patients who received outdated therapy for ALL over the course of 17 years. Dr. Duncan was a member of a cooperative trial group (the Pediatric Oncology Group) and thus presumably had full access to modern protocols, but she had not been using them.

The UNMH escalated the concern to the dean of the medical school, and after a full investigation, the university notified patients and at least two patient health insurance carriers in 1998. Dr. Duncan was placed on extended leave and eventually surrendered her license to practice medicine. Reportedly, UNMH has settled litigation with over 50 families of former patients, and two class action lawsuits have been initiated against UNMH.

Of note, during legal proceedings, it came to light that the UNMH pediatric oncology program had undergone a review by physicians at the Dana-Farber Cancer Institute in 1986 and was notified in 1987 that the program was using outdated protocols. It also came to light during legal proceedings that the university instructed staff to avoid giving details regarding who was the treating physician, which protocols were used, what problems may have arisen as a consequence of using old protocols, and how the problem was uncovered. The script read to families included the statement, "We do not know if that treatment was equally effective for your child."

Case Law No. 3 illustrates the pitfalls of systematically practicing below the standard of care. In legal terms, the standard of care is not necessarily the most optimal care nor the most cutting-edge care. Technically and practically, the standard of care is defined as what another competent (specialist) physician within the community would reasonably be expected to do. Medical oncology and pediatric oncology are rapidly evolving fields, as are most other fields of medicine. It would be expected that practicing physicians will have variations in their practice in regard to types of chemotherapy regimens, particularly in areas of oncology where no single accepted regimen or approach exists (e.g., cancers resistant to multiple frontline therapies).[21]

A breach in the standard of care only becomes medical malpractice when the substandard care results in harm to the patient. In the case of systematic substandard care (e.g., the application of outdated protocols), however, death from cancer could be considered a wrongful death and therefore grounds for a medical malpractice suit. Further, suitable guidelines do exist for the management of most de novo cancers and even relapsed cancers, via the National Comprehensive Cancer Network for adults, for example, or through the use of proven cooperative group or large institution protocols for children (e.g., from the Children's Oncology Group or St. Jude Children's Research Hospital, respectively). The UNMH case discussed earlier demonstrates that the courts will take such protocols into account, generally via an expert witness as proxy.

CLINICAL VIGNETTE # 2

A 12-year-old girl is diagnosed with acute promyelocytic leukemia (APL) after presenting with bruising and confusion. Aggressive systemic chemotherapy, including approximately 950 mg/m^2 (doxorubicin equivalent) of anthracycline agents, results in complete remission. Within three months of completion of therapy, the patient develops progressive exercise intolerance, difficulty breathing at rest, and edema (swelling) of both feet to mid-calf. She is diagnosed with early-onset cardiomyopathy, a rare but known complication of anthracyclines that is associated with high cumulative doses. She dies while awaiting a cardiac transplant, and an autopsy shows no evidence of cancer recurrence. Her family files suit for wrongful death.

The field of oncology is a constantly evolving specialty, and new developments in the standard of care occur rapidly. Oncologists are obligated to stay current on new developments and therapeutic options. Failing to maintain pace with the evolving standard of care puts one at risk of legal action due to the very real risk of suboptimal outcomes. The patient in this vignette was diagnosed with APL, which is highly curable.

In the past, this condition required very high doses of cardiotoxic anthracycline chemotherapeutic agents, such as doxorubicin. In recent years, however, the standard of care for APL has evolved to incorporate a newer therapy: all-trans retinoic acid (ATRA). The new standard of care still involves anthracycline therapy, but doses are now reduced by 50% or more, thus greatly reducing the risk of developing dilated cardiomyopathy later in life.

The patient in the vignette received a substantially higher cumulative anthracycline dose (950 mg/m^2) following an outdated therapeutic protocol than she would have received her physician adhered to more recent guidelines for the treatment of APL. The patient's death secondary to the development of early-onset cardiomyopathy is directly attributable to the substandard care received and would most likely be deemed medical malpractice.

PARENTAL RIGHT OF REFUSAL

In contrast to cancer in adults, cancer in children is often curable with standard-of-care therapy. In particular, the most common pediatric cancer, ALL with favorable characteristics, has cure rates well above 90%.[22] With a lack of definitive targeted therapy for most tumors, however, most cures will be achieved using a combination of surgery, systemic chemotherapy, and/or external beam radiotherapy. Thus, toxic events and late effects affect both survivability and quality of life significantly in both the short and long term.[23,24] Moreover, many pediatric cancers have intermediate or poor cure rates.[25]

Due to a combination of variable prognosis, concern for morbidity and/or mortality, medical mistrust, misinformation, religious beliefs, and/or other reasons, parents of children with cancer may choose to refuse potentially lifesaving therapy for their children.[26] In situations where treatment is likely futile, the treating physician may very well agree.[27] This may occur at initial diagnosis or later in the disease course (e.g., in response to overwhelming toxicity or disease progression). However, despite aspirations toward a shared decision-making process, situations will arise where the physician will determine that refusal of cancer therapy is not in the best interests of the child.

While in general the law gives the family unit a fair degree of autonomy, the courts have stated multiple times that medical teams are not under obligation to carry out the wishes of the parents if the child's health and well-being are clearly endangered. Whether the parents are legally permitted to refuse potentially lifesaving therapy is determined by the perceived threat of morbidity or mortality from withholding cancer therapy, as illustrated by the following cases.

CASE LAW # 4

In 1977, a 20-month-old child presented to a family physician for fever in Nebraska and was ultimately referred to Omaha University Medical Center for suspicion and later diagnosis of acute lymphocytic leukemia.[28] Systemic chemotherapy was given, and the patient was found to be in complete remission after one month. The parents transferred care to another physician in Massachusetts and stopped oral chemotherapy shortly after.

When the disease relapsed, the family admitted to stopping chemotherapy and refused all further care. Probate court issued temporary guardianship and returned the child to therapy. Treatment was continued by order of the superior court, noting "denial of the recommended medical treatment means certain death for the minor, whereas continuation of such treatment offers him substantial hope for life." His parents appealed to the Supreme Judicial Court of Massachusetts, which upheld the ruling.

CASE LAW # 5

A three-year-old child was brought to a medical center for evaluation of anorexia and frequent emesis. The parents noted to the court that they had brought their child for evaluation reluctantly due to their religious beliefs prohibiting medical therapy, but ultimately, they did so due to fear of litigation.[29] Initial radiographs were inconclusive, and observation was recommended; however, the parents left the hospital with the child against medical advice.

The child presented again after one week and was found to have a 15-cm mass in the abdomen, pathologically confirmed as a non-Hodgkin lymphoma. The family was given a prognosis of 40% survival with chemotherapy and 0% without; the family refused therapy and instead went to a Christian Science practitioner in accordance with their religious beliefs.

The Delaware Division of Child Protective Services (DCPS) successfully petitioned for temporary custody of the child from the family court. However, the court issued a stay allowing for immediate appeal to the Supreme Court of Delaware. The court reversed the decision of the lower court, stating that the potentially toxic therapy offered to give a 40% chance of survival was not clear and convincing evidence that separating the child from the parents was necessary to ensure the health and safety of the child.

As these cases illustrate, in situations where parental refusal of curative-intent therapy is not in line with medical advice, the state has the obligation to consider removing custody of the child from the parents. However, the state and its designated agency (e.g., child protective services) have the burden of proof to demonstrate the necessity of such a disruptive action.

Interestingly, in Case Law Nos. 4 and 5, most, if not all, practicing pediatric oncologists will recognize that almost any child with newly diagnosed non-Hodgkin lymphoma in 1995 would have a markedly better prognosis than a child with partially treated acute lymphocytic leukemia with relapse at seven months in 1978.[30,31] Therapy in the former case would also have been far less toxic. Nonetheless, the outcome of the courts granting custody and decision-making capacity to the state only in the latter (relapse) case clearly illustrates its role in interpreting the evidence presented.

While the presentation of evidence is a multifaceted process in which both plaintiff and defendant play a role, it is paramount that the treating physician presents known prognostic information and anticipated complications of therapy to the family and documents this information clearly. Documentation of this conversation, including the details conveyed, can be critical not only to families weighing difficult decisions but also, in some cases, to the state and the courts as they weigh the harms and benefits of revoking parental custody to allow cancer therapy. (A detailed discussion of informed consent and its application to the law can be found in Chapter 2.)

CLINICAL VIGNETTE # 3

A seven-year-old boy with neuroblastoma presents with recurrent stridor (an abnormal high-pitched sound during inhalation). His tumor had been previously treated with a partial resection and two courses of chemotherapy, and he had finished his therapy six months ago with anticipation of an excellent prognosis. Radiographic imaging of his chest confirms that his tumor has progressed, however. Due to its location, it is not amenable to complete resection.

The medical team recommends salvage chemotherapy, with the possibility of further treatments including surgery, external beam radiotherapy, hematopoietic stem cell transplantation, and immunotherapy. The family requests to terminate the therapeutic relationship instead, citing loss of trust in the treatment team. They disclose plans to go seek an alternative therapy in Mexico as the practitioner has promised 100% cure rates. The oncology team requests that child protective services file suit for custody.

Health care providers have a duty to educate patients and assist them in making informed decisions. This entails presenting all reasonable treatment options to patients, including relevant risks and benefits, and allowing patients and their families to make voluntary choices about potentially life-changing health care interventions. Although, in general, the law gives the family unit a fair degree of autonomy, courts have repeatedly held that medical teams are under no obligations to execute the wishes of the parents if a child's health and well-being are clearly endangered.

The patient in the vignette has relapsed neuroblastoma, which requires an intensive regimen of salvage chemotherapy, radiotherapy, immunotherapy, and stem cell transplantation. In addition to the risk imposed by the cancer itself, many patients undergoing such therapy will experience life-threatening and sometimes fatal complications.

Despite the claims of the practitioner the parents have consulted in Mexico, there is no known efficacious alternative therapy with any proven ability to cure neuroblastoma. Relapse therapy for unresectable tumors has a much lower rate of long-term cure, and unfortunately, the majority of patients will eventually die of their cancer. Nevertheless, therapy after relapse does have the ability to prolong life considerably, in many cases for years.

Whether the parents are legally permitted to refuse potentially lifesaving therapy is determined by the perceived threat of morbidity or mortality from withholding cancer therapy, which in this case appears to be substantial. Therefore, most courts would likely rule against the patient's parents.

CHILD'S RIGHT OF REFUSAL

One of the guiding principles in medical ethics is respect for patient autonomy.[33] This principle dictates that although health care providers have a duty to educate patients and assist them in making informed decisions, the provider does not possess the authority to make the decision for patients themselves.[34] Instead, all reasonable options should be presented with information regarding risks and benefits, allowing patients to make voluntary choices about potentially life-changing health care interventions.[35]

The responsibility to make treatment decisions for pediatric patients typically falls to the parents because most children lack the agency required to be truly autonomous agents, so long as the patient is not an emancipated minor (e.g., is married, is a member of the armed services, has received a declaration of emancipation from a court of law).[36] As children either willingly comply with the wishes of their parents with regard to therapeutic options or lack the capacity to make decisions in most circumstances, this distinction rarely presents itself as an ethical dilemma for most clinical encounters.

In general, it is advisable that the decision-making process involve soliciting the child's treatment preferences. However, situations may arise where patient and parental decisions diverge; in such situations, pediatricians may have an obligation to treat children over their objections.[33] Therefore, on a practical level, soliciting the child's concerns may allow for further discussion that ultimately results in a decision that can be supported by all stakeholders (child, parent, and physician). Furthermore, the obligation to treat a child against refusal to give assent is not absolute[37]; whether a child's preferences will be overridden by a court of law depends, among other things, on the child's capacity to reason and to fully grasp the consequences of his or her treatment decisions.

CASE LAW # 6

In 1991, a 15-year-old adolescent boy was found to have a tumor in the anterior mediastinum, which can be immediately life-threatening.[38,39] He was scheduled to undergo needle biopsy at Olean General Hospital in Olean, New York, as was the standard of care for this tumor. However, due to the patient's fear of needles, he refused to undergo the procedure against the wishes of his mother. Perceiving the situation as both critical and life-threatening without immediate intervention, the mother petitioned the court for an order requiring the respondent to submit to diagnostic surgery, under physical restraint if necessary.

The Family Court of Cattaraugus County granted an order authorizing the hospital to immediately admit, examine, and treat the 15-year-old patient using surgical intervention. The order also included direction for the minor patient to cooperate fully and for the sheriff's department to take all necessary steps to enforce the order.

Although the court noted that it was "reluctant to summarily and precipitately disregard the emphatic protests of the fifteen-year-old," it concluded that the court also "has a strong interest in protecting the health and welfare of a child within its jurisdiction." Since those who are 18 years of age or older may give consent for medical services, the court found that an implicit corollary of that is that those under 18 years of age may not give consent. In addition, by extension, those under 18 years of age may also not withhold consent.

Cases such as the one above are few and far between—more often seen are cases where the parents agree with and support the child's decision, such as in the case of Ernestine Gregory, where the Illinois Supreme Court ultimately upheld a 17-year-old's right to refuse lifesaving transfusion.[40] And while some state legislatures and courts have in recent years adopted laws conferring mature adolescents with legal authority to consent to medical treatment without parental involvement—colloquially referred to as "mature minor laws"—these laws often only apply to general medical treatment.[41] Application of this doctrine is questionable in cases involving more serious procedures.

It is useful to note that in this case of the 15-year-old boy, the court found that immediate medical attention was required after the mother and Department of Social Services demonstrated that time was of the essence with respect to medical treatment. While the parent and state likely have the burden of proof to demonstrate that "time is of the essence" with respect to medical treatment, the proof provided will ultimately be the documented provider's opinion.

CONCLUSION

The primary areas of substandard care that expose an oncologist to liability include chemotherapy errors and out-of-date care. Ultimately, errors related to the use of chemotherapy, whether in the prescribing or administering, are human errors and are either preventable or possibly preventable. Systems, such as CPOE with automated checking and/or multidisciplinary efforts to detect errors, can and should be used to avoid chemotherapy errors. Additionally, practitioners are expected to stay up to date in all aspects of care, particularly in situations where the overall survival of patients is improving over time; the consistent use of outdated knowledge and protocols will expose a practitioner to potentially numerous malpractice claims or even a class action lawsuit.

Patient autonomy is another complex medicolegal issue in oncology, particularly in regard to pediatric patients. The approach to informed consent changes markedly for the treatment of children, where the welfare of the child is considered over the autonomy of the family unit. Multiple decision options may be considered within the best interest of a child, however, and the court often relies on practitioner documentation and expert opinion to determine said best interest. Ultimately, due to the subjective nature of risk versus benefit analyses, cases have widely varied outcomes (often within a single case at the time of appeal or settlement).

A child's right of refusal is still relatively uncharted territory. The few cases that have arisen generally tend to side with the parents and state, particularly in oncology cases where procedures are seen as serious and time sensitive. The relevancy of mature minor laws is still uncertain as applied to pediatric oncology cases.

KEY POINTS:

- -

- Chemotherapy medications and regimens often have a narrow therapeutic window, resulting in a high risk of harm if errors are made. Systems exist to prevent errors from reaching the patient, and error-free care is considered the standard of care in medical and pediatric oncology. All oncologists should strongly consider employing one or more systems to prevent inevitable human errors from reaching the patient and causing harm.
- Oncologists must stay abreast of current management strategies to avoid systematic litigation risk. National guidelines and/or cooperative group protocols are available to reduce the risk of practicing outdated care. Conversely, ignoring the recommendations of colleagues or outside expert reviewers also exposes an oncologist to substantial risk.
- Children are considered incompetent wards of the state, and their health and outcome are considered over the autonomy of the person and family unit.
- Documented known prognostic information and risks of therapy are both considered as evidence in cases where a state agency (e.g., child protective services) sues for custody of a child in order to forcibly render therapy. It should not be assumed that a judge will find in favor of medical opinion by default.
- Respect for pediatric autonomy should involve soliciting children's preferences about treatment and acknowledging that their preferences matter, even though in certain situations the child's preferences may ultimately be overridden.
- Whether a child's preferences should be overridden in a particular case depends, among other things, on the child's capacity to reason and to fully grasp the consequences of their treatment decisions.
- In general, it is not required that there be an emergency or immediate danger to a child's life before a court may act, only a requirement that the child be within the jurisdiction of the court and appear to the court to be in need.

References:

1. Legant P. Oncologists and medical malpractice. *J Oncol Pract*. 2006;2:164–169.
2. Jena AB, Seabury S, Lakdawalla D, Chandra A. Malpractice risk according to physician specialty. *N Engl J Med*. 2011;365:629–636.
3. Canal P, Gamelin E, Vassal G, Robert J. Benefits of pharmacological knowledge in the design and monitoring of cancer chemotherapy. *Pathol Oncol Res*. 1998;4:171–178.
4. Trinkle R, Wu JK. Errors involving pediatric patients receiving chemotherapy: a literature review. *Med Pediatr Oncol*. 1996;26:344–351.
5. Schulmeister L. Chemotherapy medication errors: descriptions, severity, and contributing factors. *Oncol Nurs Forum*. 1999;26:1033–1042.
6. Liem RI, Higman MA, Chen AR, Arceci RJ. Misinterpretation of a Calvert-derived formula leading to carboplatin overdose in two children. *J Pediatr Hematol Oncol*. 2003;25:818–821.
7. Cohen IJ, Wolff JE. How long can folinic acid rescue be delayed after high-dose methotrexate without toxicity? *Pediatr Blood Cancer*. 2014;61:7–10.
8. Berens MJ. U. of C. to pay $7.9 million in death of cancer patient. *Chicago Tribune*. 1999. https://www.chicagotribune.com/news/ct-xpm-1999-10-08-9910080243-story.html. Accessed May 7, 2020.
9. Altman LK. Big doses of chemotherapy drug killed patient, hurt 2d. *The New York Times*. 1995. https://www.nytimes.com/1995/03/24/us/big-doses-of-chemotherapy-drug-killed-patient-hurt-2d.html. Accessed May 11, 2020.

10. Walsh KE, Kaushal R, Chessare JB. How to avoid paediatric medication errors: a user's guide to the literature. *Arch Dis Child*. 2005;90:698–702.
11. Cohen MR, Anderson RW, Attilio RM, Green L, Muller RJ, Pruemer JM. Preventing medication errors in cancer chemotherapy. *Am J Health Syst Pharm*. 1996;53:737–746.
12. Fortescue EB, Kaushal R, Landrigan CP, et al. Prioritizing strategies for preventing medication errors and adverse drug events in pediatric inpatients. *Pediatrics*. 2003;111:722–729.
13. Matloub Y, Lindemulder S, Gaynon PS, et al. Intrathecal triple therapy decreases central nervous system relapse but fails to improve event-free survival when compared with intrathecal methotrexate: results of the Children's Cancer Group (CCG) 1952 study for standard-risk acute lymphoblastic leukemia, reported by the Children's Oncology Group. *Blood*. 2006;108:1165–1173.
14. Gutierrez A, Silverman LB. Acute lymphoblastic leukemia. In: Orkin SH, Fisher DE, Ginsburg D, Look AT, Lux, SE, Nathan DG, eds. *Nathan and Oski's Hematology of Infancy and Childhood*. 8th ed. New York, NY: Saunders; 2015:1527–1554.
15. Hunger SP, Mullighan CG. Acute lymphoblastic leukemia in children. *N Engl J Med*. 2015;373:1541–1552.
16. Green DM. The evolution of treatment for Wilms tumor. *J Pediatr Surg*. 2013;48:14–19.
17. Huang ME, Ye YC, Chen SR, et al. Use of all-trans retinoic acid in the treatment of acute promyelocytic leukemia. *Blood*. 1988;72:567–572.
18. Shields JA, Shields CL, Parsons H, Giblin ME. The role of photocoagulation in the management of retinoblastoma. *Arch Ophthalmol*. 1990;108:205–208.
19. Marjerrison S, Antillon F, Fu L, et al. Outcome of children treated for relapsed acute lymphoblastic leukemia in Central America. *Cancer*. 2013;119:1277–1283.
20. *Cummings v Board of Regents of University of New Mexico*, 444, P 3d 1058 (2018).
21. Mangan JK, Luger SM. Salvage therapy for relapsed or refractory acute myeloid leukemia. *Ther Adv Hematol*. 2011;2:73–82.
22. Angiolillo A, Schore RJ, Kairalla J, et al. Excellent outcomes with reduced frequency of vincristine and dexamethasone pulses in children with National Cancer Institute (NCI) standard-risk B acute lymphoblastic leukemia (SR B-ALL): a report from Children's Oncology Group (COG) Study AALL0932. *Blood*. 2019;134:824.
23. Decoster G, Stein G, Holdener EE. Responses and toxic deaths in phase I clinical trials. *Ann Oncol Off J Eur Soc Med Oncol*. 1990;1:175–181.
24. Landier W, Bhatia S, Eshelman DA, et al. Development of risk-based guidelines for pediatric cancer survivors: the Children's Oncology Group long-term follow-up guidelines from the Children's Oncology Group Late Effects Committee and Nursing Discipline. *J Clin Oncol Off J Am Soc Clin Oncol*. 2004;22:4979–4990.
25. Johnson KJ, Cullen J, Barnholtz-Sloan JS, et al. Childhood brain tumor epidemiology: a brain tumor epidemiology consortium review. *Cancer Epidemiol Biomarkers Prev*. 2014;23:2716–2736.
26. Hord JD, Rehman W, Hannon P, Anderson-Shaw L, Schmidt ML. Do parents have the right to refuse standard treatment for their child with favorable-prognosis cancer? Ethical and legal concerns. *J Clin Oncol Off J Am Soc Clin Oncol*. 2006;24:5454–5456.
27. Nassin ML, Mueller EL, Ginder C, Kent PM. Family refusal of chemotherapy for pediatric cancer patients: a national survey of oncologists. *J Pediatr Hematol Oncol*. 2015;37:351–355.
28. *Custody of a Minor*, 379 NE 2d 1053 (Mass 1978).
29. *Newmark v Williams*, 588 A 2d 1108 (Del 1991).
30. Patte C, Auperin A, Gerrard M, et al. Results of the randomized international FAB/LMB96 trial for intermediate risk B-cell non-Hodgkin lymphoma in children and adolescents: it is possible to reduce treatment for the early responding patients. *Blood*. 2007;109:2773–2780.
31. Salzer WL, Devidas M, Carroll WL, et al. Long-term results of the Pediatric Oncology Group studies for childhood acute lymphoblastic leukemia 1984–2001: a report from the children's oncology group. *Leukemia*. 2010;24:355–370.
32. Caplan AL. Challenging teenagers' right to refuse treatment. *Virtual Mentor*. 2007;9:56–61.

33. Wasserman JA, Navin MC, Vercler CJ. Pediatric assent and treating children over objection. *Pediatrics*. 2019;144:e20190382.

34. Entwistle VA, Carter SM, Cribb A, McCaffery K. Supporting patient autonomy: the importance of clinician-patient relationships. *J Gen Intern Med*. 2010;25:741–745.

35. O'Connor AM, Bennett CL, Stacey D, et al. Decision aids for people facing health treatment or screening decisions. *Cochrane Database Syst Rev*. 2009;1:CD001431.

36. Katz AL, Webb SA, Committee on Bioethics. Informed consent in decision-making in pediatric practice. *Pediatrics*. 2016;138:e20161485.

37. San Martin N. Defiant transplant patient dies at home. *Sun Sentinel*. 1994;1A. https://www.sun-sentinel.com/news/fl-xpm-1994-08-21-9408210035-story.html. Accessed August 9, 2021.

38. *Matter of Thomas B*, 152, Misc 2d 96 (NY 1991).

39. *Matter of Thomas B*, 574, NYS 659 (NY 1991).

40. In Re EG, 133, Ill 2d 98 (Ill 1989). https://law.justia.com/cases/illinois/supreme-court/1989/66089-7.html. Accessed April 8, 2021.

41. Minor consent to medical treatment laws. National District Attorneys Association. https://ndaa.org/wp-content/uploads/Minor-Consent-to-Medical-Treatment-2.pdf. Accessed August 9, 2021.

CHAPTER 9

Anatomic and Clinical Pathology

Claire E. Murphy, MD, Richard Harlin Knierim, MD, Benjamin Pardue, JD, and
Timothy Craig Allen, MD, JD

INTRODUCTION

Pathology is the branch of medicine that specializes in the examination of samples of body tissue and fluids for diagnostic or forensic purposes, and pathologists are physicians who subspecialize in pathology. Pathology is divided into (1) anatomic pathology and (2) clinical pathology (also termed *laboratory medicine*). Major subdivisions of anatomic pathology are surgical pathology, cytopathology, and autopsy pathology. Clinical pathology includes clinical chemistry, hematology, microbiology, and transfusion medicine. Pathologists frequently subspecialize, and there are Accreditation Council for Graduate Medical Education (ACGME)–accredited fellowships in breast pathology, cytopathology, dermatopathology, gastrointestinal pathology, genitourinary pathology, gynecologic pathology, hematopathology, medical microbiology, molecular genetic pathology, neuropathology, pediatric pathology, renal pathology, forensic pathology, and clinical informatics.

Procedures for acquiring tissue specimens in anatomic pathology include fine-needle aspirations, biopsies, excisional biopsies, excisions, and resections. Needle core biopsies are often used for the initial workup of a mass. Fine-needle aspirations are frequently used for initial evaluation of easily accessible masses such as thyroid nodules. Clinical laboratory specimens include blood, urine, cerebrospinal fluid, pleural fluid, ascites, saliva, sputum, and cellular material from aspirations, swabs, and scrapes. Some of these specimens are also used in cytopathology. Many organs, tissues, and fluids are examined during autopsies.

The pathologist examines the tissue and renders a report containing an expert opinion regarding a diagnosis. The pathology report confirms that the specimen examined is from a clearly identified individual. The date of specimen collection is given. The time of specimen collection may be required; breast specimens have minimum and maximum times of formalin fixation for optimal prognostic and predictive studies. The pathologist or pathologist's assistant performs a gross examination of the tissue specimen, and the gross description in the report describes the physical nature of the biopsy, surgical specimen, or cytology specimen. A microscopic description, which may be present in the report, describes the slides containing the tissue examined under the microscope and reports any immunohistochemical stains or other special studies performed. The final diagnosis is the pathologist's final interpretation based on clinical information and all the features of gross and microscopic examination. A comment may be included in the report. It discusses differential diagnosis, certainty, or other clinically related comments. A comment would also state whether consultation and additional studies are pending.

DEFINING ERROR AND RISK IN PATHOLOGY

Patient testing performed in the clinical laboratory informs clinical decision making every day. Clinical decisions based on laboratory testing frequently lead to an invasive procedure, new or altered therapy, patient admission or discharge, radiologic workup, or a host of other activities that impact the patient's health, any of which potentially exposes the patient to increased risk of harm. Pathologists therefore are charged with the responsibility of maintaining consistently high quality and trustworthy laboratory practices, with the provision of accurate laboratory results. These results are important for patient care and patient safety.

Potential errors in the laboratory setting, whether in the clinical laboratory or anatomic pathology laboratory, are divided into three types: preanalytical, analytical (actually performing the test), and postanalytical. Many of the sources of error originate in the preanalytical phase, which includes the clinical patient assessment, test order entry, requisition completion, patient identification and labeling, specimen collection and submission, specimen transport and routing, and specimen receipt in the laboratory. One of the most problematic preanalytical phase issues is mislabeling of a patient specimen, with approximately 1 in 18 identification or mislabeling errors resulting in adverse events.[1] In an analysis of nearly 300 legal surgical pathology claims, 5% involved issues with specimen mix-up between patients.[1] In response, laboratories have restrictive specimen acceptance policies and procedures, electronic labeling and identification systems, and a cooperative culture between the laboratory and collection personnel. Transfusion medicine specimens require even stricter procedures due to the high risk of serious, even fatal transfusion-related complications.

The analytical phase encompasses the moment the patient specimen is received in the laboratory for testing until the result is communicated. Sources of error in the analytical phase include sample mix-ups, undetected failure in quality control leading to an unknown need for recalibration, procedures not being followed correctly, and instrument issues, among others. Recognizing the risk of analytical error, laboratories are routinely inspected by accreditation organizations to ensure quality laboratory practices encompassing all elements of laboratory testing. These accrediting organizations include the College of American Pathologists, the US Food and Drug Administration, The Joint Commission, and the Centers for Medicare and Medicaid Services (CMS) through the Clinical Laboratory Improvement Amendments (CLIA), among others.

Statistical errors may also occur in the analytical phase. For example, a random error is caused by variables that are relatively unknown that can affect a result positively or negatively. These types of unknown variables result in evenly distributed data around a mean. The standard deviation represents the error range in that data set. A systematic error can originate from the instrument, leading to positive or negative bias away from the "true" value. The pathologist looks at this type of data during method validation when considering a new test.

In surgical pathology, the preparation of a specimen for examination and diagnosis starts with the gross evaluation of a specimen. The pathologist selects portions of a larger specimen for submission for microscopic examination, or the pathologist may select the entirety of a smaller specimen for submission. These pieces of tissue submitted for processing are later represented on a glass slide. In this process, specimen mix-up or tissue contamination can occur; however, these can be minimized by the habitual use of clean workspaces, one-piece flow, specimen identification scanning, and other standardized processing methods.

The postanalytical phase encompasses the reporting phase. The sources of error in this phase may include a failure to report at all or in a timely manner, improper manual data entry, or failure to retrieve the result by the clinical team. In response to these risks, laboratories develop critical value lists that require documentation of receipt of a critical laboratory result that may require the patient to be immediately evaluated by the clinical care team. In surgical pathology, an incorrect diagnosis reported either on routine permanent processing or intraoperative or intraprocedural consultation (frozen section or rapid onsite evaluation) can lead to patient harm such as incorrect surgery or treatment modification.

Surgical pathology has undergone significant change in the postanalytical reporting phase over the years, with an emphasis on synoptic and standardized reporting. The analytical phase has also undergone significant change, with the evolution of secondary reviews of diagnoses, including consensus review.[2] Cognitive errors in diagnosis are the most challenging to overcome. These errors lead to false positives, false negatives, tumor grading errors, and/or misreading of margins or tumor type. Some specific biases include anchoring bias, blind spot bias, confirmation bias, and overconfidence. Development of a culture of safety, subspecialization of practice, external expert consultation, and second review procedures help minimize these issues. Fortunately, error rates in surgical pathology are relatively low. For example, in a review of almost 9000 cases in one surgical pathology department, the error rate was approximately 0.8%.[3] Ideally, however, this number should be even closer to zero. The use of Six Sigma (6σ), a data-driven improvement methodology typically used in manufacturing, assists laboratories to strive for near error-free operational performance. Ideally, a system would reduce errors down to 6σ, which would translate to a "defect-free product" 99.99966% of the time, allowing only 3.4 errors/defects per 1 million opportunities (DPMO). Laboratory error rates are estimated to be 3030 to 6098 DPMO, which translates to a level of quality on a sigma scale of approximately 4σ, which is average for any given industry.[4]

Not all sources of error translate into legal claims. In searches performed by various authors of jury verdicts and settlement cases, trends emerged. The most common error cited in litigation was the missed diagnosis of melanoma (false negative) on a skin biopsy.[5] Other common specimen types included breast biopsies, gynecologic specimens of various types (biopsies and Papanicolaou smears), lung biopsies, genitourinary system biopsies, and transfusion-acquired human immunodeficiency virus (HIV) infection.[5] There was a mix of false negatives, false positives, and delay in diagnosis.[5,6] Some causes of false-negative or false-positive diagnoses on biopsy are tissue artifacts, limited diagnostic material, and poor slide quality. Interestingly, a more recent search demonstrated a decrease in claims related to melanoma, Papanicolaou smear, and breast specimens, but melanoma remains the number 1 malpractice claim.[7]

Overall, pathologists face a lower lawsuit dismissal rate when compared with other specialties (36.5% vs. 61.5% for internists) and have the highest "resolved before a verdict" rate (49.6% vs. 33.3% for internists). The frequency at which claims progressed to a trial verdict is also relatively low across specialties but highest among pathologists (7.4% for pathologists vs. 2.0% for anesthesiologists).[8]

While second opinions are sought daily interdepartmentally by pathologists as a quality assurance tool, many large tertiary academic centers and small referral centers have adopted policies requiring an institutional review of the patient's completed pathology case prior to the patient being seen by the oncologist or oncologic surgeon. Major discrepancies typically result in a change of treatment for the patient, while minor discrepancies typically do not. In a study of head and neck–related pathology institutional reviews, major discrepancies occurred in 4% of cases. Dysplasia versus invasive squamous cell carcinoma was the most common specific type of discrepancy (35%). Of the major discrepant diagnoses, 60% involved a change from benign to malignant, one involved a change from malignant to benign, and 30% involved tumor classification.[9] In another study of a slide review service in gynecologic pathology, there was a 14% minor discrepancy rate and 2% major discrepancy rate among 720 cases.[10] In the cases of a major discrepancy, clinical implications included canceled or modified surgeries or changes in radiation or chemotherapy treatment. In a study of 535 needle biopsies of the prostate, 1.3% involved a change from malignant to benign, leading to canceled surgeries.[11] Unfortunately, despite its great value, second opinion review is typically not reimbursed by payers.

Specimen contamination–related errors are rare in pathology but do occur. This can happen at different phases of laboratory testing (preanalytical [collection], analytical [group slide staining], and postanalytical [patient report or slide mismatch]). Stainer baths are a known source of contaminating tissue fragments. Specific rates of these types of errors (and others) are difficult to determine because the documentation of error is variable between laboratories; however, as noted previously, laboratories' level of quality on a sigma (σ) scale is approximately 4σ, which is average for any given industry. Pathologists are acutely aware of specimen contamination and should interpret the findings within the clinical and histopathologic context. Treating physicians should communicate with the pathologist immediately if the diagnosis does not fit with the patient's clinical findings. Decreasing or eliminating cross-contamination from one specimen to another is an important aspect of quality within the specimen-processing component of the laboratory.[12] Molecular studies can help resolve this by determining if the contaminating tissue is truly from the patient; however, these studies are time consuming and expensive.

THE LOSS OF CHANCE DOCTRINE

As medical therapies continue to improve, patients experience better therapeutic responses and greater survival. Nowhere recently has this improvement been more remarkable than with cancer patients treated with molecular-based therapies. Lung cancer patients with tumors that have specific actionable molecular biomarkers have shown dramatic responses and increased survival times with what would have previously been quickly fatal lung tumors. Other nonneoplastic areas of medicine have also benefitted from improved treatments and survival recently, such as with the diagnosis and treatment of the various forms of amyloidosis, a previously difficult-to-diagnose and uniformly fatal condition. These laudable improvements have made filing successful malpractice lawsuits more difficult, especially in areas like these, with fast-changing diagnostics and therapeutics.

Traditional tort theory requires that, for a plaintiff to succeed in a medical malpractice lawsuit, a physician's actions must be proved to "more likely than not" have caused the injury.[13] As discussed in an article by Dyer, "If the plaintiff had a 51% chance of survival, and the misdiagnosis reduced that chance to zero, the estate is awarded full wrongful death damages, but if the patient had only a 49% chance of survival, and the misdiagnosis reduced it to zero, the plaintiff receives nothing. Thus, whenever the chance of survival is less than even, the 'all or nothing' rule gives a 'blanket release from liability for doctors and hospitals . . . regardless of how flagrant the negligence.'"[14] There has been a judicial inclination over the past quarter-century to adopt a looser, perhaps more just, approach, viewing the "prospect for surviving a serious medical condition as something of value, even if the possibility of recovery was less than even (i.e., less than a 50% chance) prior to the physician's allegedly tortuous conduct."[14,15] Under this doctrine, courts can accept any injury as the "loss of chance" for a patient's clinical improvement or prolonged survival and impose liability. The loss of chance doctrine allows the plaintiff the ability to recover a percentage of the total damages equal to the percent reduction in the patient's chance of survival. For example, if a patient would have had a five-year survival of 40% had the diagnosis been made accurately at the time of the alleged negligence but now has a five-year survival of 5% due to the alleged delay in diagnosis or misdiagnosis, then the patient will recover the difference, which, here, is 35% of the total damages awarded. The loss of chance doctrine has been considered as an alternative to traditional tort and adopted by about half of the states, whereas it has been explicitly rejected by others.

The loss of chance doctrine remains controversial. Adopting states have relaxed the causation standard, providing potential recovery of damages despite the plaintiff's inability to prove causation by a preponderance of the evidence, as is required under traditional tort theory. Here, expert testimony showing that the plaintiff was deprived of a substantial possibility of recovery or survival due to the physician's alleged negligence could suffice in allowing plaintiff recovery.[16] The doctrine is used to increase a plaintiff's success, particularly in situations where the patient is extremely ill or near death, with comorbidities that make it difficult or impossible to prove causation under traditional tort theory. Late-stage cancer patients and patients with amyloidosis, as mentioned earlier, may fit well into this situation. The ultimate success of the doctrine remains to be seen; proponents of the loss of chance doctrine cite its fairness, whereas critics denounce its expansion of liability and its holding physicians to a tort standard not held by any other group under negligence law.

THE FUTURE (MOLECULAR TESTING)

Molecular biomarker testing has progressed rapidly over the past several years from research to practice and from theory to reality, and it continues to develop rapidly, taking research concepts to the patient's bedside with extraordinary speed. As medical genomics and molecular pathology continue to mature, it is likely that medical error in this arena will garner plaintiff attorneys' attention.[17] Because genomic testing affects generations of relatives, not just the patient being tested, pathologists will likely be called upon to "balance the interests of physicians with single and multi-generational plaintiffs, while providing a realistic framework for courts to follow."[18] Undoubtably, improved physician education about molecular and genomic medicine, with the development of clear standards, will be required.[19]

Integral to the maturation of genomic medicine and molecular diagnostics and therapeutics will be the integration of artificial intelligence (AI) and digital pathology. AI is expected to reduce malpractice liability by improving diagnosis and therapy, thus reducing medical error and preventing unnecessary and ineffective treatments; however, there is a fear that it will instead increase liability risk by raising the standard of care by introducing measures a physician may or may not choose to use for patient diagnosis and therapy. Please note that the overview here is focused on pathology; see Chapter 21 for an in-depth discussion of AI. One potential solution might be the replacement of traditional medical malpractice theory with enterprise liability in these situations.[20] Enterprise liability removes the barrier of requiring the plaintiff prove negligence and spreads loss and victim compensation. Because AI will likely never be capable of guaranteeing every patient a good outcome, there will exist AI-related "unpreventable calculable harm," providing an opportunity for enterprise liability to successfully manage the risk of patient harm.[20]

The medicolegal issues related to digital pathology generally concern licensure and the provision of medical malpractice insurance for diagnoses rendered by the pathologist across state lines. Pathologists risk exposure to uninsured claims for interstate, digital pathology–based diagnoses that extend outside their typical coverage arena and also risk claims of practicing without a license if rendering an interstate diagnosis. Various solutions, including a mutual-recognition interstate compact, have been proposed.[21]

Direct-to-consumer molecular testing is also an area of future medicolegal concern. Without a treating physician ordering or a pathologist overseeing the molecular testing, consumers (not patients) must consider themselves whether tests being offered are useful or accurate. Tests must measure accurately, the result itself must be correct, and the test must, in fact, provide benefit to the consumer. Inaccurate test claims can cause psychological, economic, and indirect physical injury to the consumer.[22] Litigation has not yet begun in earnest based on claims of injurious direct-to-consumer molecular testing; however, given the fast pace of the development and offering of genetic and molecular tests directly to consumers, the vast amount of ongoing research in the area, the powerful consumer interest in these tests, and the great potential commercial profit involved, legal issues are certain to arise. Laboratory and pathologist liability in these cases remains to be determined.[23]

ILLUSTRATIVE EXAMPLES

Melanocytic lesions

Pigmented (melanocytic) and nonpigmented skin lesions are frequently biopsied or excised. Glass slides containing stained thin sections of biopsies may be examined with a microscope by dermatologists, general pathologists, and dermatopathologists. The diagnosis given will determine subsequent treatment. Wider and deeper excision margins are used for malignant melanomas than are used for other malignant tumors. Some of these lesions, initially called benign, are subsequently determined to be malignant melanomas. The differential diagnosis of malignant melanoma versus benign melanocytic nevus versus other benign and malignant disorders is usually straightforward but, at times, can be difficult.[24-28] In some malignant tumors, including a subset of malignant melanomas, malignant cells closely resemble benign cells. Claims for a false-positive diagnosis of melanoma are uncommon but have occurred. Missed opportunities due to false-negative diagnoses have been one of the most common reasons for professional liability (malpractice) claims that name a pathologist as a defendant.[29]

Nevoid melanoma is one type of melanoma associated with an occasional incorrect diagnosis. According to North et al., "Nevoid melanoma is a rare histologic subtype of vertical growth phase melanoma, which on low-power inspection may be (and often is) confused with a banal melanocytic nevus. It can be equally challenging to recognize clinically on patient skin examinations as well. Diagnosis depends on a high index of suspicion and careful attention to cytological detail including a thorough search for dermal mitotic activity. A practical or functional definition of nevoid melanoma is the 'diagnosis of a nevus which one later regrets.' Because nevoid melanoma is commonly misdiagnosed as a banal nevus, subsequent delay in appropriate treatment is common, with potentially devastating consequences."[26] Along the same lines, the differential diagnosis concerning a Spitz nevus, atypical Spitz nevus, and spitzoid malignant melanoma may be difficult. Some lesions in this spectrum are called melanocytic lesions (or neoplasms) of uncertain biologic behavior. Special studies, including immunohistochemistry, comparative genomic hybridization, and fluorescence in situ hybridization, have been used in attempts to separate benign and malignant melanocytic tumors with some success.[24,27] In addition, desmoplastic malignant melanomas are uncommon tumors that are sometimes extremely difficult to identify, especially with a small biopsy.[24-26] Lymphocytic infiltrates, which are common in these tumors, and features of scar may draw attention away from subtle scattered malignant cells. Immunohistochemistry studies may help establish the correct diagnosis.

Breast lesions

Breast cancer is the most frequently diagnosed cancer among women, and claims involving breast lesions and breast cancer diagnoses are among the most common claims brought against pathologists.[6,29] Breast biopsy–related claims are a close second to melanoma-related claims in frequency.[6] In a breast cancer malpractice litigation review over ten years (2005–2015), plaintiffs tended to be younger than the median age of women at the time of diagnosis, with multimillion-dollar payouts being common. While pathologists can be named in these lawsuits, typically radiologists are most commonly involved.[30] The systems-related processes leading to a breast cancer diagnosis can involve many physicians (pathologist, radiologist, surgeon, oncologist), which can lead to communication errors. Most cases allege negligence related to a delay in diagnosis, with a median delay of 17 (± 14) months.[29,30] Certain breast lesions such as atypical ductal hyperplasia and certain forms of ductal carcinoma in situ can have a certain amount of intraobserver variability, especially needle core biopsy specimens (up to 25% disagreement with an expert consensus panel), which can sometimes lead to differing management of patients clinically.[31] Assurance practices commonly used by breast pathologists include ordering additional immunohistochemistry tests (60% of pathologists surveyed), recommending additional surgical sampling (56%), requesting additional external or internal colleague reviews (84%), and choosing more severe diagnoses in borderline cases (15%).[32]

CASE LAW # 1

The plaintiff underwent a needle biopsy of her left breast mass. The pathologist reviewed the slides from the biopsy specimen and issued a diagnosis of "infiltrating ductal carcinoma grade 1." At the time of her diagnosis, the patient was pregnant. Three weeks later, she underwent a left breast radical mastectomy. Upon examination of the slides from the mastectomy specimen, the pathologist issued a diagnosis of "multifocal sclerosing adenosis and fibroadenomatoid changes," with no malignancy identified. The previous biopsy specimen was pulled from the archives and reviewed, and the pathologist realized that the initial diagnosis was an error. The plaintiff had undergone an unnecessary mastectomy for benign changes.[33]

Sclerosing adenosis is a complex lesion and is a well-known mimic of breast cancer, particularly with diagnoses made based on small core biopsies. Often, sclerosing adenosis can be a straightforward diagnosis; however, occasionally the lesion is complex, with fibrosis and obliterated glands present in infiltrative-appearing glandular structures. In addition, there may be a loss of myoepithelial cells (the presence of these cells is useful for proving the lesion is benign). In a small core biopsy, sclerosing adenosis can mimic invasive ductal carcinoma.[34] In the end, the trial court awarded the plaintiff damages, including $475,000 for physical pain, suffering, mental anguish, and loss of enjoyment of life ("general damages"). On appeal, the Louisiana state appellate court ruled that this award was not excessive.[33]

CLINICAL VIGNETTE # 1

A 52-year-old woman saw her family practice physician for a routine gynecologic and breast exam after her first mammogram. A small abnormal density with grouped coarse heterogeneous calcifications, BI-RADS (Breast Imaging–Reporting and Data System) category 4B, was identified on the mammogram. Therefore, the lesion was recommended for a stereotactic core needle biopsy. The core biopsy was interpreted by the pathologist as "focal atypical ductal hyperplasia, arising in a background of flat epithelial atypia, and associated calcifications. Fibrocystic changes were also seen." The treating physician reviewed the biopsy results with the patient and discussed the patient's options of surveillance and excisional biopsy. An excisional biopsy was recommended, and the patient was referred to a breast surgeon. The breast surgeon performed a large lumpectomy and placed it in formalin fixative, and the operating room staff transported the specimen to the surgical pathology laboratory on a Friday evening, without calling the on-call pathologist. On Monday morning, the lumpectomy was cut per protocol, showing a central mass. Slides from the breast specimen were delivered to the pathologist on Tuesday. Invasive intermediate-grade ductal carcinoma was identified. A sentinel lymph node biopsy was later performed and showed no malignancy. The estrogen receptor (ER), progesterone receptor (PR), and human epidermal growth factor receptor 2 (HER2) studies were negative. Due to the patient's triple-negative status, adjuvant chemotherapy including an anthracycline- and taxane-containing regimen was initiated. The patient suffered significant cardiac side effects and could not complete treatment. Two years later, a liver mass was biopsied and confirmed to be metastatic breast carcinoma that was ER positive, PR negative, and HER2 negative. Due to the ER positivity, the accuracy of the original hormone receptor status was questioned.

Had the original lumpectomy specimen been handled correctly, a false-negative report of the tumor's ER status could have been avoided. The patient could have received endocrine therapy and potentially avoided the cardiac toxicity from the regimen typically used for triple-negative breast cancers. Does she have a negligence claim?

The Defendant-practitioners fail to meet a reasonable standard of care when they fail to do what a reasonably prudent pathologist would have done in like or similar circumstances at the time of the care in question. While not determinative, and do not define the standard of care, expert witnesses whose testimony defines the standard of care may rely upon guidelines set out by professional organizations, such as the American Society of Cytopathology and the College of American Pathologists, to help explain to a jury the standard of care and whether it was met or breached.

To establish liability under medical malpractice, the plaintiff-patient must establish a breach of the standard of care and proximate causation. Missed opportunities due to false-negative diagnoses are among the most common ways of establishing proximate causation where a pathologist is a named defendant. Specifically, if a patient could have sought a more effective treatment "but for" the false-negative diagnosis, the patient may be able to establish causation through her missed opportunity.

Here, the physician appropriately referred the patient for surgical excision, as atypical ductal hyperplasia (ADH) is a borderline lesion, qualitatively or quantitatively not abnormal enough to be classified as carcinoma in situ. ADH diagnosed on tissue biopsy has a mean upgrade rate (finding something malignant subsequently in a much larger excision specimen) of 29% on surgical excision, as reported in a large literature review.[35]

The issue in this case is the probable false-negative ER result by immunohistochemistry. This false-negative result supported the diagnosis of a triple-negative breast cancer, leading to inappropriate therapy. To prevent this from occurring, the American Society of Clinical Oncology/College of American Pathologists issued ER and PR testing guidelines for breast cancer specimens. These guidelines provide recommendations on tissue handling, a scoring system with standardized interpretation, and optimal immunohistochemical staining performance. The guidelines state that the time (ischemic time) from tissue acquisition to fixation (in 10% neutral buffered formalin) should be as short as possible, which did not occur in this case. Also, the lumpectomy should be sliced at 5-mm intervals or at least bisected before fixation to allow for maximum fixative penetration in a shorter time interval which was not performed by the pathologist or the pathologist's staff. The central tumor was not adequately fixed in a short time frame, increasing the ischemic time before fixation. Samples should be fixed for 6 to 72 hours.[36] Had a false-negative result for ER been avoided, the patient could have received endocrine therapy and potentially not suffered the cardiac toxicity from the regimen she received for triple-negative breast cancers. That the patient could have pursued endocrine therapy likely constitutes a "missed opportunity," and therefore, proximate causation could likely be established. The American Society of Clinical Oncology/College of American Pathologists recommendations would not be determinative in establishing a reasonable standard of care. However, a jury would likely consider their recommendations as strong evidence that the pathologist should have minimized the time from tissue acquisition to fixation and sliced samples at 5-mm intervals before fixation to allow for maximum tissue penetration. Because the pathologist had not been informed of the lumpectomy's presence in the laboratory after hours on a Friday, the pathologist failed to appropriately slide and fix the patient's lumpectomy specimen. The pathologist was not notified of the lumpectomy specimen, and communication to the pathologist of the specimen's existence is a necessary precursor to the pathologist acting. Had the pathologist known that of the specimen's existence, the pathologist could have processed the specimen Friday evening so that the specimen would have been properly formalin-fixed for continued processing on Monday morning, best ensuring that the tissue's fixation would provide for accurate biomarker testing were a cancer found to be present. As that did not occur here, the hospital may find itself vicariously liable for the actions of its employees who breached the standard of care

As medicine becomes more molecular based, physicians should expect that other types of biopsies and surgical specimens will require special handling and timely attention so that appropriate fixation and sectioning of the specimen can occur. Strong communication between departments will be necessary going forward to ensure patients are fully served in this evolving molecular era.

CLINICAL VIGNETTE # 2

A woman was seen by her gynecologist for a routine exam. As part of that examination, a Pap test, a test for cervical dysplasia (premalignancy) and cervical malignancy, was performed. The pathologist interpreted the patient's specimen as "negative for any abnormalities." Clinically, this seemed congruent with the cervical exam. Three years later, the patient contacted her physician's office with complaints of left-sided abdominal pain. Workup with repeat sampling, including a repeat Pap test and cervical biopsy, confirmed the presence of invasive squamous cell carcinoma of the cervix. Despite chemotherapy, surgery, and radiation therapy, the patient died of metastatic cervical cancer shortly thereafter.

If upon review of the original Pap test abnormal cells are identified, is the pathologist liable for causing a delay in diagnosis and, ultimately, death? The currently recommended screening for high-risk human papillomavirus (HPV) DNA in addition to Pap tests (co-testing) will detect most significant lesions of the uterine cervix. There is also convincing evidence that the HPV vaccine is effective in preventing new and persistent infections of the genital tract with the two types of HPV most commonly associated with cervical cancer and its precursors.[37] Despite the decrease in cervical cancer incidence and mortality in the United States, the Pap test is an imperfect test, which in the pathology laboratory is usually based on slides initially screened by cytotechnologists. Approximately 50,000 to 100,000 cells are present on a slide and require screening, and the workload limit per the College of American Pathologists for cytotechnologists is 100 slides per day (80 in California).[38] Some quality assurance studies have shown failures with sensitivity, where the false-negative rates vary between 3% and 13%, and specificity, with false-positive rates of less than 5%.[39] Because of this inherent error rate, the finding of a false-negative smear alone is not, by itself, evidence of practice below the standard of care. Errors must be judged in the context of overall laboratory performance.[39]

A diagnosis of "atypical squamous cells of undetermined significance" is a poorly defined entity. Poor inter- and intraobserver reproducibility have been described. Disputed cases of atypical squamous cells or glandular cells of undetermined significance are not likely to be reasonable grounds for allegations of practice below the standard of care. Pap tests secondarily reviewed by an expert hired for possible litigation are optimally reviewed without the screener/evaluator knowing the patient's intent of litigation or current health status (e.g., development of carcinoma). Biased review does not accurately reflect screening in a normal working environment.[40–42]

In 1998, the American Society of Cytopathology and the College of American Pathologists published rescreening guidelines to ensure unbiased evaluation when Pap test findings are litigated. The guidelines' key recommendation is that the expert witness pathologist conduct a blinded review, a review in a manner similar to that performed at the time the Pap test was initially evaluated, without knowing the result or current clinical information in advance.[40–50] Essentially, expert witnesses are typically required to base their testimony on generally accepted procedures. When their testimony is novel (i.e., not a generally accepted scientific principle), they must show that the methodology used to come to their novel conclusion is based on generally accepted science.[42–49] This is important for pathologists considering evaluating Pap tests and providing expert witness testimony. Standards set out by professional organizations such as the American Society of Cytopathology and College of American Pathologists can inform a court as to whether the defendant met a reasonable standard of care.[40–50] However, such standards are not determinative; courts are hesitant to allow professional organizations to define their own standard of care out of a fear of an incentive to "race to the bottom." Expert witnesses should explain their methodology and reasoning as clearly as possible in their report in language that an educated layperson could reasonably understand. In this case, whether the physician met the standard of care will likely depend upon the severity of the dysplasia later identified on rereview, the frequency of the dysplastic cells in the Pap test specimen, and the presence or absence of any great degree of inflammation or other cells that obscure the dysplastic cells.

CONCLUSION

As a medical specialty, pathology presents many opportunities for malpractice liability. All laboratory tests have an error rate, and such errors present legal risks for both the laboratory and the pathologist. Additionally, many steps in the process provide an opportunity for a claim-producing error, including mislabeling, statistical errors, failure to timely report findings, improper manual data entry, and the failure to retrieve the results by a clinical team. Such claims may lead to costly payouts. Recent developments in the legal landscape, such as the loss of chance doctrine, complicate these risks.

KEY POINTS:

- Pathology is the branch of medicine that specializes in the examination of samples of body tissue and fluids for diagnostic or forensic purposes, and pathologists are the physicians who specialize in pathology. Pathologists frequently subspecialize, and there are several specific ACGME-accredited fellowships.
- Pathologists produce reports confirming the source, date, and physical nature of the tissue specimen. The final diagnosis is the final interpretation by the pathologist. An accompanying comment may include differential diagnoses and degree of uncertainty.
- Medicolegal issues in pathology often arise from errors including patient specimen mislabeling, statistical errors (both random and systematic), failure to timely report all findings, improper manual data entry, and failure to retrieve the results by the treating physician.
- Missed opportunities due to false-negative diagnoses, which can result in delay in diagnosis and delay in appropriate treatment, are a common cause of pathologist professional liability (malpractice) claims.
- Breast cancer misdiagnosis is a common type of malpractice claim against pathologists. Plaintiffs are typically younger than the median age of women diagnosed with breast cancer, and lawsuits may result in multimillion-dollar awards.

- False-negative Pap tests are also a basis for malpractice claims against pathologists and laboratories. While all laboratory tests have an error rate and a false-negative result does not conclusively demonstrate failure to practice standard care, pathologists are, as with other medical malpractice claims, held to a standard of care of a reasonably prudent physician with similar training performing under similar circumstances.
- Traditional tort theory requires that, for a plaintiff to succeed in a medical malpractice suit, a physician's actions must be proved to "more likely than not" have caused the injury. However, recent cases tried under the loss of chance doctrine have adopted a looser approach, viewing the prospect for surviving a serious medical condition as something of value, even if the possibility of recovery was less than even (i.e., less than a 50% chance) prior to the physician's allegedly tortuous conduct. About half of states impose liability for the loss of chance in a patient's clinical improvement or prolonged survival.
- As medical genomics and molecular pathology mature, pathologists will likely be called upon to balance the interests of physicians with single and multigenerational plaintiffs, while providing a realistic framework for courts to follow. It will be necessary to advance physician education about molecular and genomic medicine and develop clear standards to protect the interests of all parties who may be affected by testing.

References:

1. Valenstein PN, Raab SS, Walsh MK. Identification errors involving clinical laboratories: a College of American Pathologists Q-Probes study of patient and specimen identification errors at 120 institutions. *Arch Pathol Lab Med.* 2006;130(8):1106–1113.
2. Hollensead SC, Lockwood WB, Elin RJ. Errors in pathology and laboratory medicine: consequences and prevention. *J Surg Oncol.* 2004;88(3):161–181.
3. Renshaw AA, Gould EW. Measuring errors in surgical pathology in real-life practice: defining what does and does not matter. *Am J Clin Pathol.* 2007;127(1):144–152.
4. Carlson RO, Amirahmadi F, Hernandez JS. A primer on the cost of quality for improvement of laboratory and pathology specimen processes. *Am J Clin Pathol.* 2012;138(3):347–354.
5. Kornstein MJ, Byrne SP. The medicolegal aspect of error in pathology: a search of jury verdicts and settlements. *Arch Pathol Lab Med.* 2007;131(4):615–618.
6. Troxel DB. Medicolegal aspects of error in pathology. *Arch Pathol Lab Med.* 2006;130(5):617–619.
7. Troxel DB. Trends in pathology malpractice claims. *Am J Surg Pathol.* 2012;36(1):e1–5.
8. Jena AB, Chandra A, Lakdawalla D, Seabury S. Outcomes of medical malpractice litigation against US physicians. *Arch Intern Med.* 2012;172(11):892–894.
9. Mehrad M, Chernock RD, El-Mofty SK, Lewis JS Jr. Diagnostic discrepancies in mandatory slide review of extradepartmental head and neck cases: experience at a large academic center. *Arch Pathol Lab Med.* 2015;139(12):1539–1545.
10. Santoso JT, Coleman RL, Voet RL, Bernstein SG, Lifshitz S, Miller D. Pathology slide review in gynecologic oncology. *Obstet Gynecol.* 1998;91(5 Pt 1):730–734.
11. Epstein JI, Walsh PC, Sanfilippo F. Clinical and cost impact of second-opinion pathology. Review of prostate biopsies prior to radical prostatectomy. *Am J Surg Pathol.* 1996;20(7):851–857.
12. Platt E, Sommer P, McDonald L, Bennett A, Hunt J. Tissue floaters and contaminants in the histology laboratory. *Arch Pathol Lab Med.* 2009;133(6):973–978.
13. Leslie K, Bramley D, Shulman M, Kennedy E. Loss of chance in medical negligence. *Anaesth Intensive Care.* 2014;42(3):298–302.
14. Dyer C. Negligence through loss of chance. *Br Med J (Clin Res Ed).* 1986;293(6561):1560–1561.

15. Renehan JF. A new frontier: the loss of chance doctrine in medical malpractice cases. *Boston Bar J*. 2009;53:14–15.

16. Warzecha CM. The loss of chance doctrine in Arkansas and the door left open: revisiting *Holt ex rel. Holt v. Wagner*. 2010, 63 *Ark L Rev* 785, 803. https://heinonline.org/HOL/LandingPage?handle=hein.journals/arklr63&div=36. Accessed August 9, 2021.

17. Marchant GE, Lindor RA. Genomic malpractice: an emerging tide or gentle ripple? *Food Drug Law J*. 2018;73(1):1–37.

18. Lovell K. CRISPR/Cas-9 technologies: a call for a new form of tort. *San Diego Int Law J*. 2018;19:407.

19. Westbrook MJ. Transforming the physician's standard of care in the context of whole genome sequencing technologies: finding guidance in best practice standards. *St. Louis U J Health Law Policy*. 2015;9:111–148. https://core.ac.uk/reader/234183904. Accessed August 9, 2021.

20. Swanson A, Khan F. The legal challenge of incorporating artificial intelligence into medical practice. *J Health Life Sci*. 2012;6(1):90.

21. Allen TC. Digital pathology and federalism. *Arch Pathol Lab Med*. 2014;138(2):162–165.

22. Duranske S. This article will make you smarter! (Or, regulating health and wellness claims). *Am J Law Med*. 2017;43:7–8.

23. Allyse MA, Robinson DH, Ferber MJ, Sharp RR. Direct-to-consumer testing 2.0: emerging models of direct-to-consumer genetic testing. *Mayo Clin Proc*. 2018;93(1):113–120.

24. Busam KJ, Gerami P, Scolyer RA. *Pathology of Melanocytic Tumors*. New York, NY: Elsevier; 2019.

25. Hosler GA, Patterson JW. Desmoplastic/spindle-cell melanomas, minimal deviation melanoma, nevoid melanoma. In: Patterson JW, ed. *Weedon's Skin Pathology*. 4th ed. New York, NY: Elsevier Limited; 2016:837–901.e38.

26. North JP, Bastian BC, Lazar A. Minimal deviation melanoma, nevoid melanoma, spitzoid melanoma, desmoplastic and neurotropic melanomas. In: Calonje E, Brenn T, Lazar A, Billings S, eds. *McKee's Pathology of the Skin, with Clinical Correlations*. 5th ed. New York, NY: Elsevier Limited; 2020:1310–1362.e19.

27. Luzur B, Bastian BC, North JP, Calonje E. Spitz nevus, atypical Spitz nevus, intermediate tumors (dysplastic/atypical nevi), melanocytic tumors of uncertain malignant potential. In: Calonje E, Brenn T, Lazar A, Billings S, eds. *McKee's Pathology of the Skin, with Clinical Correlations*. 5th ed. New York, NY: Elsevier Limited; 2020: 1234–1309.e16

28. LeBoit PE. Fire your dermatopathologist! *Arch Dermatol*. 1999;135(2):137–138.

29. How common is breast cancer? American Cancer Society. January 2021. https://www.cancer.org/cancer/breast-cancer/about/how-common-is-breast-cancer.html. Accessed August 9, 2021.

30. Lee MV, Konstantinoff K, Gegios A, Miles K, Appleton C, Hui D. Breast cancer malpractice litigation: a 10-year analysis and update in trends. *Clin Imaging*. 2020;60(1):26–32.

31. Allison KH, Reisch LM, Carney PA, et al. Understanding diagnostic variability in breast pathology: lessons learned from an expert consensus review panel. *Histopathology*. 2014;65(2):240–251.

32. Reisch LM, Carney PA, Oster NV, et al. Medical malpractice concerns and defensive medicine: a nationwide survey of breast pathologists. *Am J Clin Pathol*. 2015;144(6):916–922.

33. *Monroe v State*, 2012–1683 (La App 1 Cir 2013)

34. Cui X, Wei S. Carcinoma in situ involving sclerosing adenosis: seeking the salient histological characteristics to prevent overdiagnosis. *Ann Clin Lab Sci*. 2017;47(5):529–534.

35. Schiaffino S, Calabrese M, Melani EF, et al. Upgrade rate of percutaneously diagnosed pure atypical ductal hyperplasia: systematic review and meta-analysis of 6458 lesions. *Radiology*. 2020;294(1):76–86.

36. Allison KH, Hammond MEH, Dowsett M, et al. Estrogen and progesterone receptor testing in breast cancer: ASCO/CAP guideline update. *J Clin Oncol*. 2020;38(12):1346–1366.

37. Collaço LM, Zardo L. Cytologic screening programs. In: Bibbo M, Wilbur DC, eds. *Comprehensive Cytopathology*. 4th ed. New York, NY: Elsevier Saunders; 2015:44–53.e2.

38. CLIA-related Federal Register and Code of Federal Regulation announcements, and the FDA's Clinical Laboratory Improvement Amendments (CLIA). Centers for Medicare and Medicaid Services. https://www.cms.gov/Regulations-and-Guidance/Legislation/CLIA/CLIA_Regulations_and_Federal_Register_Documents. Accessed March 16, 2021.

39. Davey DD. Quality and liability issues with the Papanicolaou smear: the problem of definition of errors and false-negative smears. *Arch Pathol Lab Med.* 1997;121(3):267–269.
40. Frable WJ. "Litigation cells" in the Papanicolaou smear: extramural review of smears by "experts." *Arch Pathol Lab Med.* 1997;121:292–295.
41. McCoy DR. Defending the pap smear: a proactive approach to the litigation in gynecologic cytology. *Am J Clin Pathol.* 2000;114(Suppl):S52–S58.
42. Adoption of guidelines for review of pap smears in the context of potential litigation. September 1996; amended January 1997. California Society of Pathologists. www.calpath.org. Accessed August 9, 2021.
43. DeMay RM. Should we abandon pap smear testing? *Am J Clin Pathol.* 2000;114(Suppl):S48–S51.
44. Steigman CK, Vernick JP. The Pap smear: a victim of its own success? *Med Lab Obs.* 2002;34:8–14.
45. Skoumal SM, Maygarden SJ. Malpractice in gynecologic cytology: a need for expert witness guidelines. *Mod Pathol.* 1997;10:267–269.
46. Frable WJ. Guidelines for experts reviewing Papanicolaou smear litigation cases. *Arch Pathol Lab Med.* 1997;121:331–334.
47. Wood TP. A consensus on Pap smear review. *CAP Today.* 1998;12:12.
48. Freckelton I. Gynaecological cytopathology and the search for perfection: civil liability and regulatory ramifications. *J Law Med.* 2003;11:185–200.
49. Ducatman BS, Ducatman AM. How expert are the experts? Implications for proficiency testing in cervicovaginal cytology. *Arch Pathol Lab Med.* 2005;129:604–605.
50. Austin RM. Results of blinded rescreening of Papanicolaou smears versus biased retrospective review. *Arch Pathol Lab Med.* 1997;121(3):311.

CHAPTER 10

Emergency Medicine

Mary J. Wall, MD, JD, FCLM, FAALM, DABR

INTRODUCTION

Emergency medicine liability for oncology had been minimal in past decades, but this is changing. The intersection of oncology and emergency medicine liability has widened in recent years. In order to understand this, it is necessary to explore the history of emergency medicine and recent changes in American health care delivery.

Ancient roots

The history of emergency medicine is both long and short. Emergency medicine has its deepest roots in ancient Greece. Around 400 BC, Hippocrates realized the importance of rapid removal of projectiles from soldiers during battle. As such, the origins of emergency medicine lie in the military.

Military origins of emergency medicine

In more modern times, emergency medicine found its early progress in the 19th-century French army, specifically during the Napoleonic wars. One of Napoleon's chief military surgeons, Dominique Jean Larrey (1766–1842), can be considered the grandfather of emergency medicine. Larrey analyzed Napoleon's military tactics and the resultant changes in military combat injuries. Compared to the 17th and 18th centuries, tactical changes resulted in more widely scattered battlefield casualties.

The biggest military tactical change in the 19th century was the use of wheeled, quickly moving artillery as opposed to prior lines of slower-moving infantry, thus resulting in the scattered wounded. Larrey developed a system of carriage evacuation for battlefield casualties, labeled "flying ambulances," to ensure more rapid treatment of the wounded. Further building on that efficiency, Larrey also developed a system to categorize battlefield injuries based on the level of need for care. In essence, Larrey introduced the first emergency medicine triage system, which replaced the prior loose system based on military rank (or nationality in the case of multinational forces).[1]

In the United States, emergency evacuation and treatment were introduced during the Civil War by Dr. Jonathan Letterman in 1862. Letterman instituted forward first aid stations, which served to reduce mortality. He was instrumental in establishing the US Army Medical Corps.

Previously, military medical care was delivered by a division of the Army Quartermasters.[2] In 1864, the US Congress established forward line treatment, evacuation, and triage for the entire US Army, the earliest codification of what evolved into modern American emergency medicine.[2] Emergency medicine principles primarily remained within the military until the mid-20th century, including the introduction of early physician extenders, the military medics.

Civilian emergency medicine

Prior to the 1960s and 1970s, no emergency medicine specialty existed in the United States. Civilian emergency medical care was delivered by general practice physicians and surgeons. The first emergency medicine "group" was started in 1961 at Alexandria Hospital in Alexandria, Virginia, by five doctors: James DeWitt Mills, Chalmers A. Loughbridge, William Weaver, John McDade, and Steven Bender. The group provided 24-hour medical coverage, and this model became known as the "Alexandria Plan," thus ushering in a template for the structure of the modern civilian emergency department (ED).[3]

In 1968, the American College of Emergency Physicians was founded, and the late 1960s and early 1970s saw discussion at the American Medical Association regarding the establishment of emergency medicine as a US board-recognized medical specialty. In 1970, the first emergency medicine residency started at the University of Cincinnati, and in 1971, the University of Southern California established the first US medical school department of emergency medicine.[4] In 2018, emergency medicine residents represented 5.47% of total active medical residents in the United States.[5]

The evolution of emergency medicine as a specialty has been influenced by changes in patient demographics, payor mix, and medical care delivery patterns paired with decreasing numbers of primary care physicians. All of these factors tie into increased liability for emergency medicine and increased numbers of patients with oncologic conditions accessing the ED, resulting in increased emergency medicine liability for patients with oncologic conditions.

EMERGENCY DEPARTMENT UTILIZATION

Currently, EDs provide almost 50% of total medical visits in the United States each year. In 2017, 137 million ED visits occurred in the United States; 40 million were injury related, whereas almost 100 million were related to medical conditions. These numbers represent 43.3 visits per 100 population.

Currently, 37% of ED noninjury visits involve general family practice issues, 33.6% involve emergent medical problems, and 23.5% pertain to non–primary care specialty problems such as joint pain and general orthopedics, rash and other dermatologic conditions, and vision dysfunction. Included in the above are patients with known and heretofore undiagnosed oncologic conditions.

A discussion of US ED utilization is incomplete without analysis of the changing medical care delivery factors in the past few decades. The severe shortage of primary care physicians is a significant driver of this situation. Due to the high debt load faced by many US medical school graduates, many choose more lucrative specialties, as family practice, internal medicine, and pediatrics are typically lower-paid medical specialties compared to orthopedics, specialty surgery, ophthalmology, dermatology, and plastic surgery.[6]

Another driver of ED utilization is payor mix. Currently, in the United States, federal and state governments are the primary payers for most patients in most states. Medicare and Medicaid do not restrict ED usage. Private insurers often use reimbursement rules that encourage the patient to use non-ED resources for nonaccident occurrences.

Emergency medical treatment and labor act

An unintended factor driving up ED utilization over the past couple of decades was the passage of the Emergency Medical Treatment and Labor Act (EMTALA) by Congress in 1986. EMTALA was part of the Congressional Omnibus Budget Reconciliation Act (COBRA).[7]

EMTALA was passed in response to a practice commonly referred to as "dumping" patients. Some hospitals, upon discovering that a patient was uninsured, would transfer patients to neighboring hospitals or tertiary care facilities without properly assessing the patient's condition or need for emergent care prior to transferring or transporting the patient, leading to risk that the patient would worsen or decompensate during transfer. Sometimes, the receiving facility was unaware of the transfer, the patient's condition, or the acuity of the patient's condition. In some cities, the initial hospital would even place the patient into a public conveyance such as a cab and send them off to another unknowing recipient facility.[8]

EMTALA requires hospital EDs that accept payments from Medicare to provide an appropriate medical screening examination (MSE) to anyone seeking treatment for a medical condition, regardless of citizenship, legal status, or ability to pay. The law specifically prohibits delays in assessment or treatment in order to ascertain the patient's ability to pay.[8] Participating hospitals may not transfer or discharge patients needing emergency treatment except with the patient's informed consent, upon stabilization of the patient, or when the patient's condition requires transfer to a health care facility better equipped to administer needed treatment to the patient.[8]

EMTALA applies to "participating hospitals." The statute defines participating hospitals as those that accept payment from the Department of Health and Human Services, Centers for Medicare and Medicaid Services (CMS) under the Medicare program.[8] Because there are very few hospitals that do not participate in Medicare, the law applies to nearly all hospitals.[8] The combined payments of Medicare and Medicaid, $602 billion in 2004, or roughly 44% of all medical expenditures in the United States, make not participating in EMTALA impractical for nearly all hospitals.[9] In addition, EMTALA's provisions apply to all patients, not just to Medicare patients.[8] The penalty for an EMTALA violation might involve exclusion of the hospital or provider from CMS participation, meaning all Medicare and Medicaid patients, a devastating financial penalty that most, if not all, facilities and providers cannot survive financially.

The cost of emergency care required by EMTALA is not directly covered by the federal government, as it extends to patients not covered by the Medicare and Medicaid programs, so it has been characterized as an unfunded mandate.[8] Uncompensated care represents 6% of total hospital costs. Fully 12.6% of EDs in the United States closed between 1991 and 2011.[10]

Because EMTALA is unclear in its definition of what constitutes emergency care and stabilization, EMTALA has "opened the floodgates" and has resulted in the ED serving as the primary US point of service for health care.[11] EMTALA provisions are widely known among the public. Many people understand that they likely will not incur any out-of-pocket costs for accessing most of their medical care via the ED, thus raising utilization rates. From 1993 to 2003, the US population grew 12%, while ED visits increased by 26%.[12]

Nonemergent patient utilization of the ED for routine medical care usurps skilled care from patients with more emergent or complex conditions, including oncology problems. This diversion of intense resources can result in decreased, truncated, or rushed care for patients with known or undisclosed oncologic disease. Additionally, EMTALA extends to on-call physicians, creating an uncompensated burden on them, including oncologists.

Emergency liability

Approximately 3.8 per 100,00 ED visits result in a malpractice claim. Most claims involve patient in the 18 to 64 age range; 74.1% of claims are attributable to cancer, vascular events including cardiac, and infections.[13]

The following is a breakdown of elements of care as factors involved in ED liability claims[8]:

- Documentation/notes, 6%
- History and physical, 11%
- Ongoing monitoring, 30%
- Diagnostic tests/imaging, 65%
- Performance of tests, 5%
- Test interpretation, 22%
- Transmittal to ED, 7%
- Consultation management, 26%
- Discharge plan, 43%
- Follow-up after diagnosis, 9%
- Patient compliance, 5%

The major general factors underlying emergency medical liability include time limitations during patient encounters, unpredictable patient workflows, discontinuity of care, handoffs, and problems with follow-up.

Approximately 47% of emergency medicine claims involve failure to diagnose a condition, with 39% related to missed diagnosis, 41% involving inadequate analysis or workup or premature discharge, and 24% related to poor or inadequate medical management.[14]

ED encounters are measured and judged by a number of standards. One of the most important of these standards is patient waiting times and turnaround times or length of visit. A common benchmark for non–emergency medical services visits is a waiting time of 30 minutes or less before having an initial evaluation by a health care professional, usually the triage nurse. Although this is not a Health Care Finance Administration rule, some states, such as West Virginia and New Jersey, have codified this standard of the 30-minute emergency consultation into state regulations.[15]

Another standard is returning visits for the same condition. Sometimes these benchmarks are included in the emergency physician's annual performance review. This time pressure can result in an incomplete patient assessment, which raises the risk of medical error and subsequent risk of a malpractice claim.

Workflow

Due to increased and high patient utilization of the ED, the patient load, and therefore the workflow, may be unpredictable. This is markedly accentuated during mass trauma or casualty events, such as a multiple-vehicle crash on a highway, explosion, or mass shooting. Additionally, the specialty and nature of emergency medicine place high demands on the individual physician's physical, intellectual, and emotional reserves. As a result, burnout is a prevalent condition among emergency medicine physicians, with the average time in specialty of ten years.[16]

These intermittent patient surges can disrupt routine workflows and result in an overwhelming amount of information and analysis for the ED physician to handle, raising the chance that a medical error is made. Data analysis has revealed that the percentage of medical errors increases with increased patient workload.[17]

This workflow disruption can involve multiple point sources including lab, imaging, nursing, medications, transport, disposition, and even housekeeping. For example, unclean or contaminated workspaces or patient areas raise the risk of infection, sometimes exponentially. Infection risk is especially dangerous for oncology patients, particularly those undergoing active oncology treatment.

Handoffs and communication

Much has been written in recent years about discontinuity of care and handoffs. Handoffs occur when a patient's treatment or care is not completed before the treating doctor or nurse finishes their work shift, transferring the patient to another's care. This handoff period is risky and can result in diagnostic, treatment, medication, and therapeutic errors, among others. Handoffs require a report of the patient's condition, the current progress of the workup, proposed treatment plan, if developed, and probable disposition of the patient. The rate of some type of communication error occurring during an emergency care handoff has been calculated at 18 per 100 patient transfers.[18]

If an ED is busy, chaos may ensue. The handoff report on a patient might be incomplete or brief or may have gaps in important clinical information. Communication surrounding the handoff may be ambiguous, difficult to follow, or perfunctory. Approximately 30% of ED malpractice claims are related to failures in communication. Communication problems were a contributing factor in 7149 cases (30%) of 23,000 medical malpractice claims filed between 2009 and 2013, according to a report published by research/analysis firm CRICO Strategies.[19]

Handoffs have increased in recent years, particularly at teaching hospitals, necessitated by the limitation in the number of hours an intern, medical student, or resident is permitted to work due to guidelines or regulations.[20]

The military has developed a system to minimize the risk of miscommunication during hand-offs, represented by the acronym SPAR—Situation, Problem/Background, Action, Reports—renamed from the SBAR system developed for nuclear submarines.[21]

Follow-up care

Follow-up issues are myriad in today's ED environment. In past decades, teaching hospitals with residency programs staffed free or low-cost clinics for lower-income or uninsured patients. As the federal government has reduced Medicare reimbursement to residency programs, these clinics have mostly disappeared, leaving the emergency physician in the risky situation of having to complete workups on patients while in the ED rather than referring them for clinic follow-up, leading to more costly, lengthy, and complex visits. Follow-up care is particularly essential for patients with discovered or suspected cancers secondary to ED visits who do not meet the criteria for hospital admission.[22]

THEORIES OF LIABILITY

It is well established that the elements of a malpractice claim include the following: a duty due to the patient-plaintiff; a breach of that duty by the treating physician or health care provider or health care worker; a proximate cause; that the breach resulted in the harm claimed by the plaintiff, commonly referred to as causation; and that the patient suffered an actual injury.

Primary liability

Primary liability pertains to the individual relationship between the treating physician, in this case the ED physician, and the patient presenting for treatment with little question as to the duty owed to the patient by the physician; relationship is established once the patient presents to the ED and is seen by the physician. The usual elements of duty, breach of duty, proximate cause, and injury are straightforward elements.

Negligence liability

A medical corporation is responsible when it fails to protect patients presenting for care under its sphere of control from harm. In the past, the hospital was held to an innkeeper standard in that they provided a facility in which the physician treated the patient. The hospital has been the primary organization for civilian emergency medical care in the 20th and 21st centuries. Along these lines, the hospital traditionally was responsible for the safety of its physical facilities and equipment as well as its employees, such as nurses, technicians, and so on. In prior times, the hospital was deemed harmless for any breaches of care committed by physicians.[23]

Corporate negligence theory has replaced that "innkeeper model" with the view that a hospital owes the patient a separate and independent duty to protect them from harm.[24] The duty includes a number of responsibilities: to provide sufficient global monitoring of the quality of patient care services[25] and to perform standard of care in maintaining the facility and providing medical instruments and equipment.[26]

Currently, while hospitals might contract with an emergency medicine physician group to provide services, many directly employ emergency medicine specialists as employees. The hospital has a responsibility to oversee adequate credentialling of physicians and to regularly monitor their performance, whether they are independently contracted or employed physicians.

A primary justification for hospital corporate negligence responsibility is the custody over the patient. Therefore, this principle may extend to a managed care organization or closed insurance plan, which may have liability for inadequate scrutiny of or selection processes for participating physician panels, particularly if the entity fails to exercise reasonable care in the credentialling or selection process (see *Harrell v total Care, Inc.*).[27] This is pertinent where a managed care organization has its own hospitals or an exclusive contract with a hospital or health care system to provide emergency care.

CASE LAW # 1

In *Darling v Charleston Community Memorial Hospital*, the patient, who broke his leg while playing in a college football game, was awarded $150,000 by a jury after his leg was amputated because of the attending doctor's negligence. The court rejected the historical view of a hospital's limited duty.[28] The first and most widely followed corporate negligence case, the court recognized the hospital's obligation to oversee the quality of patient care services.[29]

Vicarious liability

Yet another liability theory is the doctrine of *respondeat superior* or vicarious liability, which holds a health care facility liable for the negligent acts of an employee arising in the course of his or her employment. In 1965, the courts began to extend liability to hospitals on some theory other than the doctrine of *respondeat superior*.[30]

Up until that time, liability turned on the character of the physician-hospital relationship, that is, whether the physician was an independent contractor or an employee. More recently, courts have held a hospital vicariously liable, under certain conditions, for the negligence of a physician who was an independent contractor.[31]

Vicarious liability decisions hold, for example, that a health care facility or organization that carelessly credentials or retains an independent contractor physician may be directly liable for injuries resulting from the negligence of the physician independent contractor.[32] Further, a health care facility may be vicariously liable for the negligence of an independent contractor performing care outside of the delineated scope of practice or nondelegable duties. In recent years, such vicarious liability has also been found under the doctrine of ostensible agency.[33]

As a theory of liability for care decisions based on cost, the doctrine of *respondeat superior* might subject a third-party payer to liability if a physician were employed by the managed care product endorsed or contracted for by the third-party payer and the health care provider made negligent decisions based on utilization review or financial risk shifting.[23]

With more frequency, courts are applying theories of vicarious liability to third-party payers. This is true where the managed care product limits a patient's choice of providers to those who have contracted to provide care to its beneficiaries.[34] Many insurance cost containment care products, such as preferred provider organizations, do not directly employ physicians.[35]

Additionally, many injury-producing decisions fall within a hazy area in which medical decision making, though motivated by considerations other than the patient's best interests, such as financial or performance benchmarks, may lie within the appropriate standard of care. Under such situations, third-party payers would not be liable for resulting injuries. Furthermore, cost control measures move more health care professional performance from the clearly negligent arena into the nonnegligent (or judgment) arena, resulting in compensation for fewer injured patients. Therefore, as Randall writes, "the doctrine of respondeat superior would not be effective in spreading the cost of cost containment injuries to all responsible parties."[23]

Present-day hospitals regularly employ on a salary basis a large staff of physicians, nurses, and graduate medical education employees (e.g., residents), as well as ancillary services providers and administrators. Certainly, people who avail themselves of the ED expect that the hospital will attempt to adequately treat them, not that its nurses or other employees will act on their own responsibility.[36] Health care facility corporate negligence does not turn on the relationship between the physician and the health care organization. A primary justification for the corporate negligence doctrine is the hospital's custody of the patient.[29]

Although a managed care product does not have custody, the duty to protect from harm may nevertheless arise from the process of vetting physicians, physician extenders, or ancillary health care staff for the insurance managed care product. This is particularly true when the managed care product structure serves to severely restrict a patient's choice of provider. Thus, a managed care product should be liable for failing to properly review, vet, and utilize primary source verification of the credentials and expertise of provider panel applicants.[37] Court decisions have discussed the extension of the corporate negligence doctrine to independent practice association model managed care products.

CASE LAW # 2

In *Harrell v Total Health Care, Inc.*, the plaintiff brought an action against a health service corporation alleging damages resulting from alleged malpractice. The trial court entered summary judgment for the health service corporation.[27] The Missouri Supreme Court held that (1) a former statute that exempted health service corporations from some forms of liability for injuries to patients applied to a patient's action that alleged that the corporation was negligent in its selection of the surgeon who treated the patient and (2) the statute was not unconstitutional.

Ostensible agency

Ostensible agency liability is vicarious liability under which a hospital can be held liable for a provider's negligence, as the patient, in presenting to a health care facility, has a reasonable expectation that the care provided is adequate. The liability extends to the hospital when it appears to the patient that the provider is either employed by the health care organization or facility or is under facility or health care entity control. The view here is that the patient might have reasonably relied on the perceived quality of care based on the appearance that the physician was under the control of the entity.[38]

In order to find a hospital liable for the negligent acts of an independent physician with staff privileges, courts have generally required the following: (1) the plaintiff must show that the hospital or its agent acted in a way that would lead a reasonable person to conclude that the negligent physician was operating as an agent under the hospital's authority; (2) where the acts of the agent create the appearance of authority, the plaintiff must prove that the hospital had knowledge of the authority and acceded to the agent; and (3) the plaintiff must have acted in reliance on the ostensible agency relationship.[39]

Courts analyzing this doctrine have usually accepted the ostensible agency doctrine on two bases. First, the courts recognize that the changing role of the health care facility, including advertising, creates a reasonable assumption that patients will look to the institution and not to the individual physician for care.[40] Second, the courts say that ostensible agency liability should attach when the hospital holds out. A "holding out" occurs "when the hospital acts or omits to act in some way which leads the patient to a reasonable belief he is being treated by the hospital by one of its employees."[41]

Will the ostensible agency doctrine be extended to third-party payers? If applicable, will the doctrine be an effective tool to promote safety, to protect the physician-patient relationship, and to minimize access problems? The managed care product market is changing radically and expanding rapidly. This rapid change and expansion, coupled with an increase in the number of inexperienced people who develop and manage managed care products increases the probability that ostensible agency will extend to third party payers.[42]

SPECIALTY-SPECIFIC EMERGENCY MEDICINE LIABILITY

Diagnostic radiology liability

Nearly half of all radiology malpractice claims involve patients treated in the ED, according to a new study published in the *Journal of the American College of Radiology*. "Diagnostic errors are the primary source of liability risk in radiology," wrote Jeffrey D. Robinson, MD, MBA, department of radiology at the University of Washington in Seattle, and colleagues. "Radiologists are in the midrange of subspecialists with respect to both the frequency of claims and the cost of settlements."[43]

The high percentage of imaging claims arising from the ED might be because studies are distributed to a large variety of specialists, the researchers wrote, or because "the pace and coverage hours demanded by emergency radiology can lead to an increase in diagnostic errors."[43]

An important part of diagnostic radiology liability associated with the ED is missed diagnosis. Multiplanar imaging studies consisting of hundreds, even thousands, of images raise the chance that a small incidental detail might be overlooked. However, the small overlooked incidental detail, if not flagged for surveillance, might be the first sign of a developing malignancy. Lack of follow-up could lead to delay in diagnosis, with the malignancy discovered at a later stage, decreasing the patient's chance for a successful treatment.

Additionally, the emergency physician who fails to completely read the details in the imaging report might miss an important detail signaling the beginnings of a malignancy. This miss might result in delayed discovery of cancer and shared liability between the radiologist and the emergency physician. To prevent this, the careful radiologist will have a well-developed impression, including delineation of incidental findings and follow-up recommendations, incorporating best practice guidelines developed by the American College of Radiology.[44]

Oncology-specific emergency medicine liability

As previously noted, 47% of emergency medicine malpractice claims involve failure to diagnose a condition. Of these conditions, cancer is the most prevalent, at 30% of cases, with 18% involving cardiovascular conditions, 17% complicated medical conditions, 7% gastrointestinal, and 2% neurologic, with some overlap. The top cancers involved in emergency medicine delayed or missed diagnosis are breast (16% of total medical missed diagnoses), lung (14%), colorectal (10%), uterine or ovarian (7%), and skin (6%).[45]

Breast cancer

Missed diagnosis of breast cancer in the ED is more common due to the realities of the usual workflow in discovering breast cancer. Most breast conditions are worked up in the outpatient setting, with the diagnostic radiologist, primary care physician, OB/GYN physician, or surgeon as the initial access of care point. A patient accessing care for an acute or chronic breast condition through the ED is more likely to have low income, be a minority, and have multiple comorbidities that can mask the cancer.

A patient coming in with an obvious ulcerating or grossly palpable breast mass is unlikely to have a missed diagnosis. More problematic are younger women who present with breast pain, a vague lump, or redness and swelling. These symptoms may be related to a benign limited condition such as abscess, mastitis, or a medication side effect, such as breast pain related to lipid-lowering medication. However, these patients may be harboring breast cancer. Redness might be related to inflammatory or invasive breast cancer, not mastitis. Itchiness could be related to breast cancer, breast parenchyma or skin lymphoma, or rare cases of ductal carcinoma in situ or minimal Paget's disease of the breast.

Complicating the situation is that most insurance, including Medicare and Medicaid, does not reimburse for breast imaging in the emergency setting unless it is the primary diagnosis for the

ED admission. In addition, skilled dedicated breast imaging is usually not available in late evenings and not at all during the night, when these patients are more likely to present. Ultrasound is an assessment option but represents incomplete breast workup, with mammography the gold standard due to its ability to detect calcifications often associated with breast cancers, especially in situ or minimally invasive breast carcinomas. On-call ultrasound technologists rarely possess specialized training in breast scanning. Indeed, almost 40% of all breast ultrasound studies performed in the ED are deemed of nondiagnostic or poor quality by Mammography Quality and Standards Act–certified radiologists.

Breast diagnostic and care follow-up after the patient leaves the ED is fraught with risk. The emergency medicine physician is dependent on the patient following up afterward with a breast care department or specialist, and ensuring a follow-up appointment time after business hours can be almost impossible. The prudent health care facility will have a safety net built-in, such as a follow-up workflow to contact the patient the next day or an after-hours centralized scheduling protocol.

Another risk for the emergency physician regarding missed breast cancer diagnosis involves the electronic medical record (EMR) and best practices alerts. With some health care organizations, best practice alerts or screening reminders pop up on the screen alerting the emergency physician to missing patient screening studies, or absence of such, for example, mammograms and stool fecal tests or colonoscopy. It remains to be seen how these best practice screening reminders will affect liability for a missed cancer diagnosis for the emergency physician. Due to easily tracked audit trails embedded within the patient EMR, audit trail systems are capable of tracking whether an alert popped up and was ignored or not acted upon, with the patient developing cancer.

Lung cancer

Lung cancer, particularly small-cell carcinoma, might be difficult to diagnose from a single ED visit. Cough and shortness of breath are common presenting patient complaints in the ED. Concurrent pneumonia can hide a lung mass on chest radiographs and computed tomography (CT). Follow-up evaluation of presumed pneumonia is important. Additionally, it is imperative that a smoking history be obtained on every ED patient, especially in those with respiratory complaints. The person obtaining the history should also ask if there is any smoking history, ever. Patients who quit smoking long ago might reply in the negative. Pack-year history is also pertinent. Smoking raises the risk for development of most cancers.

Colon cancer

Asymptotic colon cancers can be easily missed in an ED setting. It is important to ask whether the patient has family history, is a smoker, has gastrointestinal symptoms, or has had a colonoscopy or a lab colon screening study, or to peruse the EMR for this information. Colon cancers are sometimes detected on CT chest exams, evidenced by hepatic lesions, deformities in the colon flexures, or abdominal adenopathy.

CASE LAW # 3

In *Sevanen v Houston NIU Medical Center*,[46] the patient Joseph Nicholson presented to a Houston hospital ED with complaints of sore throat, fever, and blood in his stool on November 13, 2016. The patient was discharged to home from the ED after treatment. Mr. Nicholson's condition rapidly deteriorated, and he died five days later, on November 18, 2016.

An autopsy revealed that the patient died of complications of acute myelogenous leukemia, namely, respiratory failure and cardiac arrest. The patient's EMR revealed that no blood work was ordered during his ED stay. Given his bloody stools, a complete blood count should have been ordered, which would have discovered an abnormal panel and the blood abnormality. Fever would have dictated ordering bloodwork.

Sore throat is a common ED complaint. Most times, it is a limited condition, with complete recovery, usually due to cold, sinus condition, or virus. However, it may be related to gastroesophageal reflux or possibly an esophageal abnormality, such as tonsillar abscess, lymphoma, oral cancer, or leukemia. In this instance, the physician had a duty of care to the patient to adequately develop a differential diagnosis and adequately investigate based on the differential.

CASE LAW # 4

A single 47-year-old woman with one daughter visited a hospital ED in October 2006, complaining of a persistent cough. The physician treating her was a radiologist who ordered a chest x-ray to rule out pneumonia. After examination, the physician ruled out pneumonia, interpreting the chest x-ray as normal. The physician diagnosed the patient with an upper respiratory tract infection, prescribed antibiotics, and discharged her from the hospital.[47]

Thirteen months later, the patient returned to the same hospital after her symptoms worsened. At this second visit, a different physician ordered a CT scan, which revealed signs of advanced stages of lung cancer. The patient's health declined quickly. Within seven months of the new diagnosis, the cancer had spread to her liver, spine, kidney, and pubic bone, and the patient ultimately succumbed to the advanced cancer in August 2008.

The patient's surviving daughter brought suit against the radiologist and the hospital. She claimed that the physician failed to identify a nodule in the initial chest x-ray, and she said that this mistake constituted negligence. The plaintiff presented the 2006 x-ray as evidence, and medical experts during trial clearly identified a 1.5-cm nodule in the upper right lung of the patient. By 2007, this nodule grew to about 2.5 or 3 cm, and the later x-rays revealed several additional nodules that were not present in the first x-ray.

The radiologist attempted to pass some of the blame to the patient herself by stating that he was not provided with the patient's full medical history. The patient was a smoker of 30 years, and her mother died of lung cancer, so the radiologist argued that without this vital information, his diagnosis could not have been completed correctly. Another attempted defense focused on causation. The defendants alleged that the patient's cancer was incurable at the time the radiologist became involved. The jury agreed with the plaintiff, found the radiologist and hospital liable, and awarded $16.7 million in damages, with the case hinging on deviation from standard of care.

CLINICAL VIGNETTE # 1

A 71-year-old patient with personal history of a low-grade colon carcinoma presented to the ED for a sinus infection. The ED physician, while perusing the EMR, noted via a best practice pop-up EMR alert that the patient had no recent screening mammography and counseled the patient to get a screening mammography, placing an order in her chart.

The patient followed up with her screening mammography, which showed an asymmetrical area that was worked up diagnostically and likely benign, with six-month follow-up including ultrasound recommended. At the six-month follow-up appointment, the breast appeared unchanged, but the axilla was scanned with ultrasound, demonstrating an irregular mass. Upon biopsy of the axillary mass, pathology was not consistent with breast cancer; instead, primary axillary squamous carcinoma was the favored diagnosis. This case points out the physician responsibility to act upon EMR best practice alerts.

CONCLUSION

In summary, medical liability attached to the ED setting has rapidly increased in recent decades, fueled by physician shortages, especially in primary care, difficulties in accessing outpatient care, systematic delivery changes, and EMTALA. The major liability risk in emergency medical care related to oncology is missed or delayed diagnosis of cancers. This liability extends beyond the ED physicians to include diagnostic radiologists, among others.

KEY POINTS:

- ED utilization has sharply increased in the past two decades.
- EMTALA has significantly contributed to ED utilization, particularly for nonemergent conditions.
- Most health care encounters in the United States currently occur in an ED setting.
- Changing physician service relationships with hospital EDs have changed over the past several decades.
- With changing physician service and employment relationships, the hospital liability for ED physician care has changed.
- Increased physician extender utilization has affected hospital liability for ED visits.
- Managed care liability regarding ED encounters is a fluid situation.
- Given ED utilization for non-emergent care, the ED physician must be vigilant to ensure follow up care when necessary.
- The ED healthcare provider must be alert to the EMR best practice alerts if available.

References:

1. Gabriel RA. *Between Flesh and Steel: A History of Military Medicine from the Middle Ages to the War in Afghanistan.* Dulles, VA: Potomac Books; 2013:145.
2. Early military medicine. US Army Medical Department, Office of Medical History. May 15, 2009. https://history .amedd.army.mil/booksdocs/HistoryofUSArmyMSC/chapter1.html. Accessed August 11, 2021.
3. Zink BJ. Commemoration of the Alexandria Plan at 50 years. August 1, 2011. https://www.acepnow.com/article/ commemoration-alexandria-plan-50-years/. Accessed August 11, 2021.
4. Zink BJ. *Anyone, Anything, Anytime: A History of Emergency Medicine.* Philadelphia, PA: Mosby Elsevier; 2006:30–32.
5. Report on residents, 2017-2018. Association of American Medical Colleges. https://www.aamc.org/system/files/ reports/1/report-residents-executive-summary-2018.pdf. Accessed August 12, 2021.
6. Sivey P, Scott A, Joyce C, Humphreys J. Junior doctors' preferences for specialty choice. *J Health Econ.* 2012;31(6):813–823.
7. 42 USC § 1395dd 1867.
8. Zibulewsky J. The Emergency Medical Treatment and Active Labor Act (EMTALA): what it is and what it means for physicians. *Proc (Bayl Univ Med Cent).* 2001;14(4):339–346.
9. Emergency Medical Treatment and Active Labor Act. Wikipedia. https://en.wikipedia.org/wiki/Emergency_ Medical_Treatment_and_Active_Labor_Act. Accessed August 11, 2021.
10. Dollinger T. America's unraveling safety net: EMTALA's effect on emergency departments, problems and solutions. *Marq L Rev.* 2015;98:1759–1802.
11. Ansell DA, Schiff RL. Patient dumping. Status, implications, and policy recommendations. *JAMA.* 1987; 257(11):1500–1502.
12. Institute of Medicine. *Hospital-Based Emergency Care: At the Breaking Point.* Washington, DC: The National Academic Press; 2007:XV.
13. Sams J. Research shows misdiagnosis leading cause of malpractice claims. *Claim J.* https://www.claimsjournal .com/news/national/2019/07/24/292140.htm. Accessed August 12, 2021.
14. CRICO annual benchmarking report, malpractice risks in emergency medicine. CRICO Strategies. crico_ benchmarking_emergency_medicine.pdf. Accessed August 12, 2021.
15. Glauser J. Screening examinations, stabilization, and the law. *Emerg Med News.* 2000:22.

16. Moore JD. Burnout: emergency medicine hit hardest. *MedPage Today*, November 29, 2015. https://www.medpagetoday.com/medpagetodayat10/burnout/54916. Accessed August 12, 2021.

17. Weissman JS, Rothschild JM, Bendavid E, et al. Hospital workload and adverse events. *Med Care*. 2007;45(5):448–455.

18. Fordyce J, Blank FS, Pekow P, et al. Errors in a busy emergency department. *Ann Emerg Med*. 2003;42(3):324–333.

19. Budryk Z. Healthcare miscommunication cost $1.7B—and nearly 2,000 lives. FierceHealthcare. February 1, 2016. https://www.fiercehealthcare.com/healthcare/healthcare-miscommunication-cost-1-7b-and-nearly-2-000-lives. Accessed August 12, 2021.

20. Wagner MJ, Wolf S, Promes S, et al. Duty hours in emergency medicine: balancing patient safety, resident wellness, and the resident training experience: a consensus response to the 2008 Institute of Medicine resident duty hours recommendations. *Acad Emerg Med*. 2010;17(9):1004–1011.

21. Stewart K, Hand K. SBAR, communication, and patient safety: an integrated literature review. UTC Honors Theses, 2016. https://scholar.utc.edu/cgi/viewcontent.cgi?article=1070&context=honors-theses. Accessed August 12, 2021.

22. Kyriacou DN, Handel D, Stein AC, Nelson RR. Brief report: factors affecting outpatient follow-up compliance of emergency department patients. *J Gen Intern Med*. 2005;10:938–942.

23. Randall VR. Traditional theories of liability, managed care, utilization review, and financial risk shifting: compensating patients for health care cost containment injuries. *U Puget Sound L Rev*. 1993;17:1.

24. *Rhoda v Aroostook General Hospital*, 226 A2d 530 (Me 1967) (holding that the nonliability rule of charitable immunity extends to shelter a hospital corporate charity from liability for its own corporate negligent acts, including the selection, training, and supervision or control of its personnel or employees).

25. *Fridena v Evans*, 622 P2d 463 (Ariz 1980) (finding that a hospital's duty includes an obligation to take reasonable steps to monitor and review the treatment being received by a patient); *Poor Sisters of St. Francis Seraph of the Perpetual Adoration, Inc. v Catron*, 435 NE2d 305 (Ind Ct App 1982) (holding that a hospital can be held liable for negligence when a nurse or other hospital employee follows a doctor's orders despite knowledge that the doctor's orders are not in accordance with normal medical practice); to properly probe, review, ascertain, and databank query the credentials and expertise of medical staff applicants before granting privileges: *Jackson v Power*, 743 P2d 1376 (Ak 1987) (finding a duty by a hospital to ensure that physicians granted hospital privileges are competent and to supervise medical treatment provided by members of its medical staff); *Insinga v LaBella*, 543 So 2d 209 (Fla 1989) (holding hospital liable for its negligent decision to grant staff privileges); *Joiner v Mitchell County Hospital Authority*, 186 SE2d 307 (Ga Ct App 1971) (finding that a hospital may be held liable for negligent selection of new staff physicians, but not when it selects authorized physicians in good standing), aff'd, 189 SE2d 412 (Ga 1972); *Copithorne v Framingham Union Hospital*, 520 NE2d 139 (Mass 1988) (holding hospital liable for the failure to withdraw staff privileges when it has received notice of the misconduct of a staff physician); *Blanton v Moses H. Cone Memorial Hospital, Inc.*, 354 SE2d 455 (NC 1987) (holding that a hospital owes duty of care to its patients to ascertain that a doctor is qualified to perform an operation before granting him the privilege to do so); *Corleto v Shore Memorial Hospital*, 350 A2d 534 (NJ Super Ct Law Div 1975) (holding a hospital liable for negligent selection and retention of a staff physician when the physician's incompetence was obvious); *Johnson v Misericordia Community Hospital*, 301 NW2d 156 (Wis 1981) (holding hospital liable when it failed to exercise reasonable care to determine whether physician was qualified to receive privileges); to protect patients from malpractice by members of its medical staff when, through customary care, it should have known that malpractice was likely: *Cordero v Shore Memorial Hospital*, 350 A2d 534 (NJ Super Ct Law Div 1975) (holding a hospital liable for negligent selection and retention of a staff physician when the physician's incompetence was obvious).

26. *Emory University v Porter*, 103 Ga App 752, 120 SE2d 668 (Ga Ct App 1961) (holding that a hospital could be held negligent for failing to furnish adequate equipment); *Hamil v Bashline*, 485 A2d 1204 (Pa 1982) (holding that a hospital is under a duty to adequately procure and maintain equipment); to use care in selecting and supervising medical personnel: Dee JH. Note, torts: corporate negligence: Wisconsin hospital held to owe a duty to its patients to select qualified physicians. *Marq L Rev*. 1981;65:139–156.

27. *Harrell v Total Health Care, Inc.*, 781 SW 2d 58 (Mo 1989).

28. *Darling v Charleston Community Memorial Hospital*, 33 Ill2d 326, 211 NE2d 253, 255, 257 (Ill 1965).

29. Hall RE. Hospital committee proceedings and reports: their legal status. *Am H Law Med*. 1975;2:245–282 (describing the premise of corporate negligence as being that the hospital, by virtue of its custody of the patient, owes a duty to exercise care in the construction, maintenance, and operation of the hospital).

30. *Schloendorff v Society of N.Y. Hospitals*, 211 NY 125 (NY Ct App 1914) (see, "The true ground for the [hospital's] exemption from liability is that the relation between a hospital and its physicians is not that of a master and servant. The hospital does not undertake to act through them but merely to procure them to act upon their own responsibility.")

31. See, for example, *Arthur v St. Peters Hospital*, 405 A2d 443 (NJ Super Ct Law Div 1979); *Capan v Divine Providence Hospital*, 430 A2d 647 (Pa Super Ct 1980); *Brownsville Medical Center v Garcia*, 704 SW2d 68 (Tx Ct App 1985); and *Adamski v Tacoma General Hospital*, 20 Wash App 98, 579 P2d 970 (1978). But see *Johnson v St. Bernard Hospital*, 399 NE2d 198 (Ill App Ct 1979) and *Reynolds v Swigert*, 697 P2d 504 at 55 (NM Ct App 1984).

32. *Albain v Flower Hospital*, 553 NE2d 1038, 1044 (Ohio 1990).

33. *Darling v Charleston Community Memorial Hospital*, 211 NE2d 253, 257 (Ill 1965); *Arthur v St. Peters Hospital*, 405 A2d 446 (NJ Super Ct Law Div 1979); *Albain v Flower Hospital*, 553 NE2d 1044 (Ohio 1990); *Capan v Divine Providence Hospital*, 430 A2d 643-649 (Pa Super Ct 1980); *Adamski v Tacoma General Hospital*, 20 Wash App at 111, 579 P2d at 977 (1978).

34. *Schleier v Kaiser Foundation Health Plan, Inc.*, 876 F2d 174, 177-178 (DC Cir 1989) (holding a health maintenance organization [HMO] vicariously liable for the negligence of a consulting physician); *Sloan v Metro. Health Council, Inc.*, 516 NE2d 1104, 1109 (Ind Ct App 1987) (holding that HMOs can be liable for the conduct of employee physicians under the doctrine of respondeat superior). But see *Williams v Good Health Plus, Inc.*, 743 SW2d 373 (Tex Ct App 1987) (holding an HMO not liable for physicians found to be independent contractors).

35. *Mitts v H.I.P.*, 478 NYS2d 910, 911 (App Div 1984) (rejecting the theory of *respondeat superior* and finding in favor of a staff model HMO in a medical malpractice suit on the grounds that the HMO "does not treat or render medical service or care to anyone"). But compare to *Schleier v Kaiser Foundation Health Plan, Inc.*, 876 F2d at 174 (DC Cir 1989) (holding an HMO responsible for the acts and omissions of a consulting physician who had no contractual relationship to the HMO).

36. *Bing v Thunig*, 143 NE2d 3, 8, 38 (NY 1957).

37. *Benedict v Saint Luke's Hospital*, 365 NW2d 499, 504-05 (ND 1985) (holding that the hospital will not be liable for negligent selection where the physician exercised the care and the skill ordinarily possessed by other emergency room physicians, and for failing to protect its insured from malpractice by provider panel members when it knew or should have known, through current standards of care, that such malpractice was likely); *Jackson v Power*, 743 P2d 1376 (Ak 1987) (finding a duty by a hospital to ensure that physicians granted hospital privileges are competent and to supervise medical treatment provided by members of its medical staff); *Insinga v LaBella*, 543 So 2d 209 (Fla 1989) (holding hospital liable for its negligent decision to grant staff privileges).

38. Weiner EP. Managed health care: HMO corporate liability, independent contractors, and the ostensible agency doctrine. *J Corp L*. 1990;15:535–538.

39. See generally *Grewe v Mt. Clemens General Hospital*, 273 NW2d 429, 433-434 (Mich 1978); *Albain v Flower Hospital*, 553 NE2d 1038, 1048-1049 (Ohio 1990); *Capan v Divine Providence Hospital*, 430 A2d 647, 648 (Pa Super Ct 1980) (citing Restatement [Second] of Torts S 429 [1965]); *Brownsville Medical Center v Garcia*, 704 SW2d 68, 74 (Tex Ct App 1985).

40. See *Grewe v Mt. Clemens General Hospital*, 273 NW2d 433 (Mich 1978).

41. *Adamski v Tacoma General Hospital*, 20 Wash App 98, 115, 579 P2d 970, 979 (1978) (the physician as its employee); see also *Howard v Park*, 195 NW2d 39, 40 (Mich Ct App 1972); *Capan v Divine Providence Hospital*, 430 A.2d at 649 (Pa Super Ct 1980); *Adamski v Tacoma General Hospital*, 20 Wash App at 115, 579 P2d at 978–979; see also *Brown v Moore*, 247 F2d 711, 719-720 (3d Cir 1957) (applying liability under *respondeat superior* when a holding out occurs).

42. See, generally, Stern J. Health maintenance organizations: development, growth and expansion. Whittier L Rev. 1986;8:377 (presenting a panel discussion of the reasons behind the surge of HMOs in California). The courts have heard several cases under the doctrine of ostensible agency. The leading cases are *Boyd v Albert Einstein Medical Center*, 547 A2d 1229 (Pa Super Ct 1988) and *Williams v Good Health Plus, Inc.*, 743 SW2d 373 (Tex Ct App 1987).

43. Robinson JD, Hippe DS, Deconde RP, Zecervic M, Mehta N. Emergency radiology: an underappreciated source of liability. *J Am Coll Radiol*. 2020;17(1 Pt A):42–45.

44. Berland LL, Silverman SG, Gore M, et al. Managing incidental findings on abdominal CT: white paper of the ACR Incidental Findings Committee. *J Am Coll Radiol*. 2010;7(10):754–773.

45. Ruoff G, Hoffman J, Yu W. Medical malpractice in America: 10 year assessments with insight. CRICO 2018 CBS Benchmarks. www.rmfstrategies.com.

46. *Sevanen v Houston NIU Medical Center, Iftikar Ahmet, PA, Bhushkan Kukkal, et al.*, Harris County District Court 71625 (Tex 2016).

47. Suffolk County Superior Court, MA. Case No. SUCV2010-00558. June 18, 2014. https://www.reliasmedia.com/articles/21632-family-members-awarded-16-7-million-after-radiologist-missed-evidence-of-lung-cancer. Accessed August 12, 2021.

CHAPTER 11

Radiology

Hamid R. Latifi, MD, JD, MA, FCLM, Taylor G. Maloney, MD, and Rebekah J. Maloney, JD*

INTRODUCTION

In 1999, the Institute of Medicine (IOM) reported that medical care was responsible for up to 98,000 deaths per year in the United States.[1] In 2016, Johns Hopkins University researchers estimated that medical errors account for more than 250,000 deaths per year in the United States, resulting in medical error representing the third most common cause of death in the United States.[2] The practice of defensive medicine to minimize failure to diagnose disease in a patient has led to increasing volumes of diagnostic tests ordered by physicians across a range of medical specialties.[3]

Radiology is an integral part of all oncology practices. Imaging of oncology patients constitutes a major portion of the studies performed at most hospital radiology departments.[4] Advanced imaging using high-resolution sonography, multidetector computed tomography (CT), 3-T magnetic resonance imaging (MRI), positron emission tomography (PET)–CT, and PET-MRI has increased the sensitivity and specificity of diagnosing, staging, restaging, and treatment monitoring of cancer patients. At the same time, the exponential growth in the number of images submitted for interpretation of each study contributes to a greater workload for the radiologists, only to be compounded by complexity of cases and greater demand for more detailed measurements required for patients enrolled in clinical trials evaluating the efficacy of novel systemic therapies. Screening examinations (e.g., mammography, low-dose CT scanning for lung cancer, coronary artery calcium scoring) have created new challenges for radiologists, and one can speculate that diagnostic errors on screening examinations will comprise an increasing liability for radiologists.[5]

Radiologists compose approximately 4% of physicians in the United States, but they rank sixth in the number of malpractice lawsuits naming physicians as defendants.[6] The likelihood of a radiologist being named as a defendant in at least one malpractice lawsuit by 60 years of age is 50%.[7] Diagnostic errors are an unfortunate, but inevitable, part of any radiology practice, and the most common reason for malpractice lawsuits against radiologists.[8] Another major contributor to malpractice litigation against radiologists is communication errors.[9] The technical advancements that have led to improved image quality combined with a greater volume of imaging over the past few decades also have resulted in detection of more incidental abnormalities ("incidentalomas") on routine or follow-up imaging of nononcology and oncology patients.

Reporting incidentalomas and assessing their clinical significance is challenging and has been a subject of a large volume of research and publications on the topic. Fortunately, incidentalomas have a less than 1% chance of representing a lethal cancer.[10]

The individual topics pertaining to medical malpractice liability against radiologists in general, and oncology imagers in particular, will be examined and discussed in more detail in the following sections of this chapter.

RADIOLOGY LIABILITIES

Diagnostic errors

In a review of malpractice cases in the United States from 2008 to 2012, radiology was the eighth most likely responsible service implicated in a medical malpractice lawsuit.[11] Approximately 44% of claims in that study pertained to diagnosis of cancer.[11] The most common missed diagnosis is breast cancer, with lung cancer being a frequent, but less common, missed diagnosis.[12] Up to 75% of all medical malpractice lawsuits against radiologists allege negligence related to errors in diagnosis.[8] Most radiologic errors occur in plain radiographs, followed by CT and MRI.[13] In a landmark study in 1949, Garland[14] showed that experienced radiologists missed 33% of positive chest radiographs and disagreed with themselves 20% of the time. The overall error rate in daily clinical radiology practice averages 3.5% to 4% of cases.[15] With approximately one billion worldwide radiologic studies performed annually, a 4% error rate would result in approximately 40 million interpretive errors per year.[16] This error rate has been confirmed by more recent studies and across imaging modalities. For instance, Muhm et al[17] reported their findings from the Mayo Lung Project in 1983, showing that in their lung cancer screening population, 90% of lung cancers were visible on serial chest radiographs in retrospect, some for as long as two years and one for 4.5 years. Based on their study results, they state that "failure to detect a small pulmonary nodule on a single examination should not constitute negligence or be the basis for malpractice litigation."[17] Austin et al[18] reported that 31% of overlooked lung cancers on CT scans in their study were greater than 2 cm. In a limited study looking at 14 patients with known lung cancer missed on CT scans, an experienced thoracic radiologist who knew there was a missed lung cancer overlooked 57% of lesions greater than 1 cm.[19] In 2010, Abujudeh et al[20] reported that there was 26% interobserver variability and 32% intraobserver variability in interpretation of abdominal CT scans. Discordant CT interpretations have been reported in 31% to 37% of cases, with 19% resulting in a change in radiologic cancer staging.[4] In 1993, Harvey et al[21] reported that breast cancer could be seen in retrospect in 75% of mammograms that were initially read as normal. Other studies have shown a mammographic "miss rate" ranging from 15% to 63%.[15]

As surmised from these studies, diagnostic errors in radiology are prevalent and unavoidable, although many strategies have been proposed to minimize them. In general, radiologists are sued because of observer errors, interpretation errors, communication errors, or failure to suggest an appropriate follow-up procedure.[22] Observer errors include recognition error (i.e., perceptual error), decision-making error (i.e., cognitive error), and satisfaction of search error.[22]

Perceptual errors account for 60% to 80% of radiologic errors, with the majority of the remaining errors attributed to cognitive errors.[15,23] In simple terms, perceptual error means a radiologist does not see the abnormality on the radiologic study, whereas a cognitive error means that the radiologist identifies the abnormality but attributes it to a benign etiology instead of cancer or somehow underestimates the significance of the finding, such that it causes a delay in diagnosis or treatment of the patient.[15] Satisfaction of search error means that a finding is missed because of failure to continue searching for additional abnormalities after the first abnormality is detected on a radiologic examination.[16]

From a practical point of view, errors in the practice of oncology imaging are different from other radiologic diagnostic errors that occur in the setting of outpatient nononcology practice or the emergency department. The difference mainly lies in the frequent and close follow-up of oncology patients and strict guidelines for clinical and imaging surveillance. For instance, a diagnostic error leading to a missed diagnosis of incidental lung cancer in a patient presenting to an emergency department after trauma is more likely to lead to an adverse outcome because of lack of follow-up from the acute clinical setting. However, an overlooked benign or malignant lesion in a breast cancer patient who is getting surveillance CT scans of the chest, abdomen, and pelvis every three to six months is more likely to be discovered on a follow-up CT, PET-CT, or other imaging study. Nevertheless, the implications of diagnostic errors in oncology patients can have grave consequences, including exclusion or withdrawal from a clinical trial, cessation of therapy, or erroneous change in treatment strategy.

Communication errors

Radiology reports are the work products of radiologists presented to the referring clinicians and patients as the products of the radiologists' labor. Unfortunately, 15% of clinicians admit that they do not read radiologic reports,[10] and only 38% of referring physicians read the radiology reports in full regardless of the length.[24] Effective communication requires more than generating a radiology report to be sent to the referring clinician.[10] Communication errors are the third most common malpractice allegation against radiologists.[25] In a study of malpractice cases from 2004 to 2008, communication failures played a role in 4% of cases.[26] In another study of malpractice claims from 2008 to 2012, however, communication failures were less common than previously thought, with 1.3% of claims involving communication failures as the primary allegation and communication errors representing an additional 4.6% of claims as a contributory factor to a diagnostic-related allegation.[11] Regardless of the actual numerical contribution of communication errors to malpractice claim cases, such errors are of great import and may lead to catastrophic outcomes. Failure to communicate critical or important unexpected results has been a cause of many malpractice claims against radiologists, with rising malpractice awards.[26]

The American College of Radiology (ACR) started publishing practice standards in 1990, including standards for communication of radiologic studies, which were subsequently renamed guidelines, parameters, and now *practice parameters and technical standards*. The most recent ACR Practice Parameters for Communication of Diagnostic Imaging Findings (referred to hereafter as ACR Parameters) state—and at least some courts, including the Iowa Supreme Court and Arizona appellate court have supported the statement—that "Practice Parameters and Technical Standards are not intended, nor should they be used, to establish a legal standard of care."[27] Nevertheless, plaintiffs' attorneys continue to argue that the ACR Parameters represent the standard of care in the radiology community. Although not intended as a legal standard of care, following the ACR Parameters pertaining to communication certainly is a reasonable starting point to ensure proper and timely patient care, as well as minimize liability. The ACR Parameters state that the duty of effective communication does not solely lie with the radiologist and that the ordering health care provider "shares in the responsibility for obtaining results of imaging studies he or she has ordered."[27]

In addition to routine communication of results by the usual channels, there are certain situations that warrant nonroutine communication. Situations that warrant nonroutine communication include urgent findings (e.g., tension pneumothorax, ruptured aneurysm), important unexpected findings (e.g., lung cancer detected on a preoperative clearance chest radiograph for an orthopedic procedure), and discrepancy between the preliminary and final reports. The most effective methods of nonroutine communication include in-person or telephonic contact, thus allowing free exchange of information and minimizing the risk of errors in conveying a crucial or important nonemergent finding. Regardless of the method of nonroutine communication, as the old adage of "if it isn't documented, it wasn't done" implies, documenting the direct nonroutine communication in the radiology report is crucial for risk management. In addition to direct person-to-person communication, there are also several commercial programs that are available on the market that may be used to relay nonroutine communications to the referring physicians and document the communication in the report. In cases of self-referred patients (e.g., mammography, whole-body or cardiac CT screening), the interpreting radiologist establishes a doctor-patient relationship and thus a duty to communicate the results directly to the patient and arrange for appropriate follow-up.[27]

Another potential liability arises in radiology residency training programs or private practice settings where a preliminary report is generated by a different individual than the one who reviews and finalizes the interpretation. It behooves the attending radiologist who makes the final interpretation to directly communicate with the appropriate health care provider any discrepancies between the preliminary and final reports, as it is inevitable that patient treatment decisions already have been made based on the preliminary interpretation and changes may be necessary to optimize patient management when there is a discrepancy in the reported diagnostic findings.

A newer challenge to effective communication has arisen from the Health Insurance Portability and Accountability Act (HIPAA), which states that patients have a right to access their personal health information, resulting in an increasing number of patients accessing and reading their radiology reports. This should serve as a reminder to the radiology community to continually strive to improve the quality of radiology reports, which are a reflection of the expertise, personality, and effort of the interpreting radiologist. Radiologists are encouraged to make every effort to avoid ambiguous medical jargon, proofread their reports, and certainly avoid the use of derogatory or judgmental terms to describe the patient or patient attributes.

Incidental findings

An incidental finding in diagnostic radiology is a mass or lesion that is found during an imaging examination, such as CT, MRI, ^{18}F-fluorodeoxyglucose PET, sonography, or other imaging, ordered for an unrelated reason. These incidental findings are often called "incidentalomas" as the suffix "-oma" denotes a tumor. Incidental findings are never anticipated but are frequently encountered in the field of radiology, particularly with the increasing rate of imaging procedures. A prudent radiologist will describe these findings and assist the referring provider by providing a recommendation for their surveillance or further workup. This section is not intended to detail all incidental findings that may be encountered in the vast field of radiology. However, the goal of this section is to discuss and provide examples of commonly encountered incidental findings, particularly those related to oncology.

Historically, many of these incidental findings, which often prove benign, were unnecessarily biopsied or treated; this strategy can bring unnecessary costs, risk, and anxiety to patients. The ACR has formed an Incidental Findings Committee composed of radiologists and consulting physicians who formulate general recommendations for managing incidental findings. These general "recommendations" or "guidance" are published by the ACR as a series of white papers. Although the white papers meet policy standards of the ACR, they neither represent official ACR policy nor meet any specific or formal national standard, and thus, they are not referred to as "guidelines." White papers should not be used to form the legal standard of care in any situation.[28]

Common oncology-related incidental findings include intracranial lesions (e.g., pituitary gland lesions and meningiomas), thoracic lesions (e.g., pulmonary nodules or masses), abdominal lesions (e.g., liver, adrenal, or renal lesions), and osseous lesions (e.g., metastases or multiple myeloma).

Incidental thoracic lesions

Pulmonary nodules are rounded lesions in the lungs that measure less than 3 cm. When the pulmonary lesions measure greater than or equal to 3 cm in size, they are characterized as masses, rather than nodules. The differential diagnosis for pulmonary nodules is broad and depends on their character and location. Malignant etiologies for pulmonary nodules include primary lung cancer, metastases, and lymphoma. Benign etiologies for pulmonary nodules include pulmonary hamartomas and pulmonary chondromas. Inflammatory etiologies for pulmonary nodules include granuloma, abscess, and rheumatoid nodule. Artifacts, such as buttons or nipple shadow on chest radiographs, can be mistaken for pulmonary nodules. The Fleischner Society publishes recommendations for pulmonary nodules incidentally detected on CT scans. However, it is important to note that these recommendations do not apply to lung cancer screening, patients with a prior cancer, immunosuppressed patients, or those who are not yet 35 years old.[29]

Incidental asymptomatic mediastinal lymph nodes with a short axis measurement less than 1.5 cm often require no further workup. If mediastinal lymph nodes have a short axis measurement greater than or equal to 1.5 cm with an explainable disease, then further management depends on the specific disease. However, if there is no explainable disease, then clinical consultation, PET-CT, and/or three to six month follow-up chest CT can be considered.[30]

Incidental abdominal lesions

Renal masses can be broadly classified into cystic or solid types. In 1986, a CT-based classification system known as the Bosniak classification was developed to characterize cystic renal masses.[31] The Bosniak classification has been modified over the years, and there are now five classes into which radiologists classify cystic renal lesions; classes I, II, IIF, III, and IV. The "F" in class IIF is to denote that it should be followed up on a subsequent examination. The lower the Bosniak class, the lower is the risk of malignancy. A proposed update to the Bosniak classification was published in 2019, which described the concordant MRI findings for each Bosniak class.[32]

Incidental renal masses identified on a noncontrast CT scan are often difficult or impossible to fully characterize. If the renal mass has abnormal margins, has a density above water density (0-20 Hounsfield units), or contains septations, thick walls, or soft tissue nodularity, then it would require a renal-mass protocol CT or MRI to fully characterize the lesion. The management recommendations for incidental solid renal masses largely depend on the size of the mass, with solid lesions greater than 3 cm that do not contain fat probably representing renal cell carcinoma and warranting surgery.[28] If the renal lesion contains fat, it likely represents a benign angiomyolipoma.

Incidental liver and adrenal gland lesions may represent benign etiologies, such as hepatic cysts or adrenal adenomas, or raise concern for metastases, particularly in the oncology patient population. The imaging characteristics of these lesions, as well as the clinical context for each patient, can help guide management or the need to pursue further diagnostic imaging, biopsy, or surveillance imaging.

Incidental osseous lesions

When a CT is performed, a common step in the radiologist search pattern is to evaluate the bones on bone windows. Bone windows modify the appearance of the image to highlight the bones and allow the radiologist to better evaluate and characterize osseous structures or lesions within them. Aggressive-appearing bone lesions are often more permeative, have periosteal reaction, and may cause cortical destruction. Metastatic bone lesions can be lytic, sclerotic, or mixed lytic and sclerotic. It is necessary to consider the clinical history when differentiating a metastatic bone lesion from infection or other process such as lymphoma, as each of these can have a permeative appearance. A common benign incidental lesion in the spine is a hemangioma, which has a characteristic "corduroy" appearance of uniform trabecular hypertrophy on sagittal views. In contrast, in Paget disease of the bone, the coarsened trabeculae are not uniform, and there may be cortical thickening, which is not seen in benign hemangiomata. Paget disease of the bone can occur in any bone, and similar to metastatic disease, it can appear lytic, sclerotic, or mixed lytic and sclerotic. It is not always possible by CT to differentiate Paget disease in the pelvis from another commonly sclerotic process such as metastatic prostate carcinoma. When an incidental bone lesion is encountered on CT, its margins, appearance, and correlation with plain radiographs as well as clinical history can aid in diagnosis and often prevent biopsy.

Incidental pituitary lesions

The two most common culprits responsible for incidental pituitary lesions are Rathke cleft cysts and pituitary adenomas. Rathke cleft cysts are small simple cysts located in the sella turcica with no enhancing solid component. When incidental Rathke cleft cysts are less than 5 mm in size in asymptomatic patients age 18 or older without potential pituitary pathology, no further follow-up imaging is needed.[33] Pituitary adenomas are tumors that arise from the pituitary gland and can be further classified into pituitary microadenomas when they are less than 10 mm in size or pituitary macroadenomas when they measure greater than or equal to 10 mm. Pituitary adenomas can cause hormonal imbalances or enlarge and compress surrounding structures, potentially leading to hypopituitarism or visual field deficits. Pituitary macroadenomas that compress or invade surrounding structures warrant endocrine or neurosurgical referral.

Screening examinations

The ultimate goals of screening examinations are to detect disease earlier, when it is still curable or treatable, and to prevent mortality from that specific disease. Some common screening examinations include mammography to detect breast cancer, low-dose CT to detect lung cancer, sonography to detect abdominal aortic aneurysms, and CT colonography to detect colorectal cancer.

Lung cancer is the leading cause of cancer death among both men and women. A large trial known as the National Lung Screening Trial conducted in the United States enrolled 53,454 patients at high risk for lung cancer. Patients at high risk smoked at least one pack per day for 30 years and were current smokers or quit smoking within the past 15 years. These patients were randomly assigned to receive either three annual low-dose CT screening examinations or three annual posteroanterior chest radiographs. The results in the low-dose CT group showed a reduction in mortality from lung cancer of 20% and an all-cause reduction in mortality of 6.7%.[34] A low-dose CT is most often performed with a lower current, which is measured in milliamperes (mAs). The lungs are less dense than many other structures in the body, and therefore, the necessary current to image them is less. This lowers the radiation dose to the patient. Regardless, radiation exposure to the patient poses a small risk to the patient, and it is necessary to weigh the potential benefit from the examination versus the risk from radiation.

Breast cancer is the second most common cancer diagnosis after skin cancer, and the second leading cause of cancer death in women after lung cancer. The mortality rate from breast cancer decreased by 36% from 1989 to 2012 after the implementation of screening mammography.[35] Radiographic advances have led to the implementation of digital breast tomosynthesis, which has increased the breast cancer detection rate, reduced false-positive results, and reduced the patient recall rate.

The gold standard in detecting colorectal cancer (CRC) is optical colonoscopy. However, colonoscopy can have potential complications, which include bowel perforation and gastrointestinal hemorrhage. CT colonography is an alternative option for CRC screening. A downside is that CT colonography exposes patients to radiation, whereas optical colonoscopy does not. If a polyp or abnormality is found on CT colonography, it would then require a colonoscopy in order to further evaluate it. Each of these examinations require a colon-cleansing preparation, and no screening examination is 100% sensitive in detecting colon polyps.

Whole-body CT screening is exactly as the name implies. It does not meet any standard for an effective screening procedure, and there are no professional medical societies that endorse whole-body CT screening for asymptomatic patients. Whole-body CT could potentially do more harm than good for patients by exposing them to unnecessary radiation, overdiagnosis, and needless financial cost. Further, the review of imaging from such full-body CT creates greater opportunity for the discovery of incidental findings, which could lead to an invasive procedure (e.g., biopsy), subjecting the patient to even more risk. A role of the US Food and Drug Administration (FDA) is to assure the safety and effectiveness of medical devices, such as CT systems. The FDA specifically prohibits CT system manufacturers from promoting the use of CT in whole-body screening of asymptomatic people.[36]

LEGAL CASE EXAMPLES

Because the majority of radiology is centered on diagnostics, it is not surprising that errors in diagnosis account for most of the lawsuits initiated against radiologists. The case examples below illustrate common fact patterns in litigation against radiologists, based on misdiagnosis or failure to diagnose cancer. As you read them, try to identify any legal rules or concepts used in each case. Following the case examples is a clinical vignette that describes the fact scenario of a hypothetical patient, and you will be asked to apply the same rules and concepts to determine the likely outcome in the event such hypothetical patient files a lawsuit.

CASE LAW # 1

At age 36, Lynda Carrozza underwent a baseline screening mammogram, the results of which were reviewed and interpreted by Roy Greenbaum, MD. Dr. Greenbaum's report identified a cluster of calcifications in the right breast but concluded that it was benign, stating that it "[did] not have a particularly suspicious appearance to it."[37] Two years later, Ms. Carrozza went in for her routine checkup and underwent another screening mammogram, the films from which were reviewed and interpreted by a different radiologist, Kathryn Evers, MD. Dr. Evers compared the films with the prior results, noting no change and concluding that the calcifications were benign. Approximately 15 months later, Ms. Carrozza noticed a lump in her right armpit and a mass in her right breast.

Needle biopsy results ultimately confirmed that the mass in her right breast was a carcinoma. Following an aggressive treatment plan, which included chemoradiotherapy and a radical mastectomy, Ms. Carrozza filed a malpractice complaint alleging negligence on the part of Dr. Greenbaum, Dr. Evers, and their respective practices and hospitals.[37]

Over the course of a seven-day jury trial, Ms. Carrozza presented evidence and offered the testimony of two experts regarding breach of the standard of care and causation, respectively. The expert testifying with respect to breach stated that Dr. Greenbaum and Dr. Evers "fell below the standard of care" for failing to order biopsies based on certain features of the clustered calcifications.[37] The expert testifying as to causation provided his professional opinion regarding Ms. Carrozza's chances of survival and severity of treatment required to treat the carcinoma on the date of diagnosis versus the initial screening. Each testimony served to bolster Ms. Carrozza's allegation that the misinterpretation of her mammograms was a breach of the standard of care, which led to a delay in diagnosis, ultimately resulting in an aggressive course of treatment and reduced life expectancy. The jury found that Ms. Carrozza presented sufficient expert testimony to prove negligence and causation and entered a verdict in her favor in the amount of $4 million, apportioning 50% of the liability to each of Dr. Greenbaum and Dr. Evers.[37]

CASE LAW # 2

Jaye Donnelly received an MRI of her left shoulder after she presented to her primary care physician, Surykant Parikh, MD, with complaints of pain in her upper left extremity.[38] The resulting study was reviewed and interpreted by Albert Zilkha, MD, who identified a "partial thickness tear of the infraspinatus tendon; subacromial-subdeltoid-subcoracoid bursitis; joint effusion with fluid extending to the biceps tendon sheath; a hypertrophic acromioclavicular joint; and muscle atrophy."[38] The orthopedic surgeon, John Saugy, MD, also reviewed the MRI results and diagnosed Ms. Donnelley's ailment as shoulder impingement syndrome and rotator cuff pain.[39] However, approximately seven years later, Ms. Donnelly filed a malpractice claim against Dr. Parikh, Dr. Saugy, and Dr. Zilkha for, among other things, failure to timely diagnose her lung cancer. With respect to Dr. Zilkha's missed diagnosis, the court granted his motion for summary judgment and dismissal of the complaint.[39] Although Dr. Zilkha failed to establish that he did not have a duty to discover a mass allegedly visible on the films he interpreted, he was successful in demonstrating adherence to the radiologic standard of care.[39] This was accomplished partly with the assistance of expert witness testimony, in which the expert noted that Dr. Zilkha's role was to interpret an MRI study that the record clearly indicated was for a left shoulder, and not a comprehensive screening to independently diagnose Ms. Donnelly's medical conditions.[38] Further, the court stated that Dr. Zilkha's "submissions demonstrated that . . . the plaintiff's tumor would present on an MRI as 'a mass in the apex of the lung,'" and none of the films he interpreted showed the apex of the lung.[39]

CLINICAL VIGNETTE # 1

Thomas, a 54-year-old man, presented to the emergency department with complaints of acute onset of severe right-sided flank pain, radiating to the groin. His only past medical history was hypertension. His workup included urinalysis, blood tests, and CT renal stone protocol, performed without oral or intravenous contrast. His blood tests did not reveal any abnormality, but his urinalysis showed microscopic hematuria. His noncontrast CT scan showed a 3 mm obstructing stone in the distal right ureter, explaining his symptoms. Thomas was provided the appropriate care for his renal colic and told to follow up with a urologist if he did not spontaneously pass his stone. Approximately eight months later, he presented with weight loss, anorexia, and back pain. Repeat CT scan, this time with oral and intravenous contrast, showed a 5 cm mass in the tail of the pancreas within the left upper quadrant. There was also evidence of metastatic disease to the liver. In retrospect, a 2 cm mass was present in the tail of the pancreas on his renal stone CT eight months earlier but was not appreciated by the radiologist because the examination was done without intravenous contrast material, which made the small tumor much less conspicuous. Furthermore, there was likely a component of satisfaction of search at work because of the findings of the obstructing renal stone contralateral to the tumor.

Was the radiologist who interpreted the first CT scan negligent for breaching the standard of care, and does Thomas have a valid malpractice claim against the radiologist for "missing" his pancreatic cancer, resulting in delayed diagnosis and treatment, with reduced chance of survival?

Rules and application of the law

If Thomas files a lawsuit and it goes to trial, we can assume that one of his claims would be negligent failure by the radiologist to detect his pancreatic cancer at the time of the initial CT scan. His success will depend on his ability to prove the elements of such tort claim by a preponderance of the evidence (i.e., >50% probability). As previously discussed in Chapter 1, the four elements of a malpractice claim are duty, breach, causation, and damage.

Rules related to the elements of a malpractice claim

In order to prevail against a defendant-physician, the plaintiff-patient must prove that (1) the physician owed a duty to the patient; (2) the physician breached that duty; (3) the breach was the proximate cause of, or a substantial factor in, producing the harm the patient suffered; and (4) the damage suffered was the direct result of the harm.[40]

The element of duty is established by the existence of a doctor-patient relationship.[41] Although diagnostic radiologists generally do not meet the subjects of the scans they interpret, given narrow exceptions, a doctor-patient relationship is formed nonetheless. This element, while not the most frequent source of contention in malpractice suits, can come into play for diagnostic radiologists in the context of radiologists reading under contract for a third party.

Breach of a physician's duty to the patient occurs if the physician deviates from the applicable standard of care.[41] The standard of care for a specialist is the degree of skill, care, and learning ordinarily possessed by fellow physicians in that particular specialty area, which is a higher standard than that imposed on general practitioners.[42] Thus, when evaluating radiologic misdiagnosis, the standard of care is what a diagnostic radiologist exercising due care and skill would have done under the identical factual circumstances.[41]

Causation is established by demonstrating a causal relationship between the physician's breach of the applicable standard of care and the injury suffered by the patient. Specifically, the plaintiff must prove proximate cause.[43] Two factors determine proximate cause: (1) causation in fact and (2) foreseeability.[43] In the realm of cancer misdiagnosis, the driving factor is causation in fact. That is because, generally, the type of injury for which the patient is at risk if cancer goes misdiagnosed or undiagnosed is readily foreseeable and not often disputed.[43] Thus, in this context, proximate cause is typically established by proving causation in fact, meaning the injury is more likely than not the result of the physician's negligence.[43] Commonly known as the "but for" test, in determining proximate cause, courts usually ask whether an injury would have occurred but for the negligent act. However, injury in a cancer misdiagnosis could be the advancement of the cancer, which is caused not only by the failure to discover it but also by the cancer's very existence.[43] Therefore, in cases alleging radiologic misdiagnosis of cancer, a plaintiff need only show that the negligence was a "substantial factor" in bringing about the injury.[43] Historically, this standard has been met if the condition was discoverable when the radiologist reviewed the scan at issue.[43,44]

Damage is established if the patient sustains injury or loss as a result of a physician's breach of the standard of care.[41] In determining damage, the harm that proper diagnosis and treatment would have prevented must be distinguished from the harm that the cancer would have caused if allowed to run its natural course.[43]

Application of the rules

Given the facts of the vignette, a malpractice lawsuit initiated by Thomas against his radiologist would likely turn on the elements of breach and causation. The analysis of the elements of duty and damage is relatively more straightforward. The radiologist clearly undertook a professional obligation with respect to Thomas's diagnosis by agreeing to interpret the medical record and noncontrast CT and produce a report with his findings, thereby evidencing a doctor-patient relationship. Given the potential for rapid spread in pancreatic cancer, the harm Thomas suffered is likely to include reduced life expectancy as a result of the radiologist's failure to diagnose his cancer, particularly if the cancer metastasizing in the interim means he is no longer a candidate for distal pancreatectomy.

To determine the existence or nonexistence of breach of the standard of care by the radiologist, the court must first define the applicable standard of care, and consider what a diagnostic radiologist exercising due care and skill would have done with respect to Thomas's scan. When considering the elements of causation, the fact that the mass was technically detectable in the noncontrast CT, even if less conspicuous, does not weigh in the radiologist's favor. As in Case Law No. 1, Thomas can assert that the failure to diagnose his pancreatic cancer at the time of the initial scan was a substantial factor in his reduced life expectancy. However, as in Case Law No. 2, the radiologist can wield the defense of compliance with the applicable standard of care to shield himself from liability. From a practical perspective, he will likely be able to show, through expert testimony and/or other evidence, that a diagnostic radiologist exercising due care and skill would have made the same call without the benefit of contrast. He might opt to rely on the perceptual error and satisfaction of search error as reasons for "missing" the tumor diagnosis.

In sum, based on the facts of the clinical vignette and the applicable standard of care, the radiologist likely has a viable defense to a malpractice claim on the theory that he upheld the standard of care in his review and interpretation of the noncontrast CT. However, it is critical to keep in mind that malpractice is a creature of state law and cases are ultimately decided by juries. Thus, if the case goes to trial, it is ultimately up to the judgment of 12 individuals based on their interpretation of evidence presented by both the plaintiff and the defendant. This makes the results of malpractice cases somewhat unpredictable, since no two juries are the same and no single jury's decision is binding on another case.

CONCLUSION

Radiologists play a major role in screening, diagnosing, staging, restaging, and treatment monitoring of cancer patients. The fundamental obligation of a diagnostic radiologist is to carefully and skillfully make diagnoses. What goes into each diagnosis is the precise identification of abnormalities, clear interpretation of the findings, and effective communication of results with the ordering providers. When a radiologist misdiagnoses or fails to diagnose a cancer, compliance with that fundamental obligation may be questioned in the form of a malpractice claim. However, it is important to keep in mind that radiologists are not called upon to be infallible, but instead to perform consistently with the accepted standard of care while making diagnoses.

KEY POINTS:

- Radiology is an integral part of oncology practice and plays a crucial role in diagnosis, staging, restaging, and treatment monitoring of cancer patients.
- Diagnostic errors are the most common cause of medical malpractice claims against radiologists, with breast cancer and lung cancer being the two most common missed diagnoses giving rise to malpractice claims against radiologists.
- Communication errors represent a much smaller primary cause, but nevertheless an important cause, of malpractice claims against radiologists. These types of errors are readily preventable, and thus, radiologist should make every effort to minimize failures in communication of their findings to the referring clinicians and patients.
- Screening examinations are performed for the specific purpose of detecting a malignancy in its early stages, in the hope of prolonging patient survival. Therefore, diagnostic errors on screening examinations are an important cause of malpractice claims against radiologists.
- Incidental findings on imaging examinations have become more frequent with technologic advances leading to greater image quality. Reporting these findings and recommending the appropriate follow-up are dilemmas for the radiologist, causes of uncertainty and frustration for the referring physicians, and sources of anxiety for the patient.
- In a diagnostic radiology malpractice action for failure to accurately and properly interpret submitted radiologic films, a plaintiff must prove all four elements of negligence by a preponderance of the trial evidence.

- Medical malpractice law is highly complex due to a constantly evolving landscape and the volatility of juries. The success of a defendant radiologist in a malpractice claim depends on the deployment of skilled legal counsel and substantial and competent expert testimony regarding the applicable standard of care and whether the radiologist breached it.

*The above-listed co-authors of this chapter (collectively, the "Co-Authors") have contributed to this publication solely in their personal capacities. All views and opinions expressed herein are the Co-Authors' own, do not reflect the positions of their respective employers or affiliates, including but not limited to Latifi Law, PLLC, Avicenna Consulting, PLLC, Sidley Austin LLP, Baylor University Medical Center, and their respective affiliates (collectively, the "Employer Entities"), and should not be interpreted as legal or medical advice. You should not act or rely upon this information without seeking advice from a lawyer or physician, in each case licensed in your own jurisdiction, as applicable. Neither the Co-Authors nor any of the Employer Entities are responsible for any errors or omissions in the content of this publication or for any damages arising from the use of this publication or any information provided herein, in whole or in part, in any format, under any circumstances.

References:

1. Institute of Medicine Committee on Quality of Health Care in America, Kohn LT, Corrigan JM, Donaldson MS, eds. *To Err is Human: Building a Safer Health System*. Washington, DC: National Academies Press; 2000. Copyright 2000 by the National Academy of Sciences. All rights reserved.; 2000.
2. Makary MA, Daniel M. Medical error-the third leading cause of death in the US. *BMJ*. 2016;353:i2139.
3. Berlin L. Medical errors, malpractice, and defensive medicine: an ill-fated triad. *Diagnosis (Berl)*. 2017;4(3):133-139.
4. Siewert B, Sosna J, McNamara A, Raptopoulos V, Kruskal JB. Missed lesions at abdominal oncologic CT: lessons learned from quality assurance. *Radiographics*. 2008;28(3):623-638.
5. Berlin L. Liability of performing CT screening for coronary artery disease and lung cancer. *AJR Am J Roentgenol*. 2002;179(4):837-842.
6. Srinivasa Babu A, Brooks ML. The malpractice liability of radiology reports: minimizing the risk. *Radiographics*. 2015;35(2):547-554.
7. Baker SR, Whang JS, Luk L, Clarkin KS, Castro A 3rd, Patel R. The demography of medical malpractice suits against radiologists. *Radiology*. 2013;266(2):539-547.
8. Berlin L. Radiologic errors and malpractice: a blurry distinction. *AJR Am J Roentgenol*. 2007;189(3):517-522.
9. Siegal D, Stratchko LM, DeRoo C. The role of radiology in diagnostic error: a medical malpractice claims review. *Diagnosis (Berl)*. 2017;4(3):125-131.
10. Berlin L. Contemporary risk management for radiologists. *Radiographics*. 2018;38(6):1717-1728.
11. Harvey HB, Tomov E, Babayan A, et al. Radiology malpractice claims in the United States from 2008 to 2012: characteristics and implications. *J Am Coll Radiol*. 2016;13(2):124-130.
12. Whang JS, Baker SR, Patel R, Luk L, Castro A 3rd. The causes of medical malpractice suits against radiologists in the United States. *Radiology*. 2013;266(2):548-554.
13. Brady AP. Error and discrepancy in radiology: inevitable or avoidable? *Insights Imaging*. 2017;8(1):171-182.
14. Garland LH. On the scientific evaluation of diagnostic procedures. *Radiology*. 1949;52(3):309-328.
15. Berlin L. Radiologic errors: past, present and future. *Diagnosis (Berl)*. 2014;1(1):79-84.
16. Bruno MA, Walker EA, Abujudeh HH. Understanding and confronting our mistakes: the epidemiology of error in radiology and strategies for error reduction. *Radiographics*. 2015;35(6):1668-1676.
17. Muhm JR, Miller WE, Fontana RS, Sanderson DR, Uhlenhopp MA. Lung cancer detected during a screening program using four-month chest radiographs. *Radiology*. 1983;148(3):609-615.

18. Austin JH, Romney BM, Goldsmith LS. Missed bronchogenic carcinoma: radiographic findings in 27 patients with a potentially resectable lesion evident in retrospect. *Radiology.* 1992;182(1):115-122.

19. White CS, Romney BM, Mason AC, Austin JH, Miller BH, Protopapas Z. Primary carcinoma of the lung overlooked at CT: analysis of findings in 14 patients. *Radiology.* 1996;199(1):109-115.

20. Abujudeh HH, Boland GW, Kaewlai R, et al. Abdominal and pelvic computed tomography (CT) interpretation: discrepancy rates among experienced radiologists. *Eur Radiol.* 2010;20(8):1952-1957.

21. Harvey JA, Fajardo LL, Innis CA. Previous mammograms in patients with impalpable breast carcinoma: retrospective vs blinded interpretation. 1993 ARRS President's Award. *AJR Am J Roentgenol.* 1993;161(6):1167-1172.

22. Pinto A, Brunese L. Spectrum of diagnostic errors in radiology. *World J Radiol.* 2010;2(10):377-383.

23. Busardò FP, Frati P, Santurro A, Zaami S, Fineschi V. Errors and malpractice lawsuits in radiology: what the radiologist needs to know. *Radiol Med.* 2015;120(9):779-784.

24. Clinger NJ, Hunter TB, Hillman BJ. Radiology reporting: attitudes of referring physicians. *Radiology.* 1988;169(3):825-826.

25. Waite S, Scott JM, Drexler I, et al. Communication errors in radiology: pitfalls and how to avoid them. *Clin Imaging.* 2018;51:266-272.

26. Gale BD, Bissett-Siegel DP, Davidson SJ, Juran DC. Failure to notify reportable test results: significance in medical malpractice. *J Am Coll Radiol.* 2011;8(11):776-779.

27. ACR practice parameter for communication of diagnostic imaging findings. American College of Radiology (ACR). https://www.acr.org/-/media/ACR/Files/Practice-Parameters/CommunicationDiag.pdf. Published 2014. Accessed July 25, 2020.

28. Berland LL, Silverman SG, Gore RM, et al. Managing incidental findings on abdominal CT: white paper of the ACR incidental findings committee. *J Am Coll Radiol.* 2010;7(10):754-773.

29. MacMahon H, Naidich DP, Goo JM, et al. Guidelines for management of incidental pulmonary nodules detected on CT images: from the Fleischner Society 2017. *Radiology.* 2017;284(1):228-243.

30. Munden RF, Carter BW, Chiles C, et al. Managing incidental findings on thoracic CT: mediastinal and cardiovascular findings. A white paper of the ACR Incidental Findings Committee. *J Am Coll Radiol.* 2018;15(8):1087-1096.

31. Bosniak MA. The current radiological approach to renal cysts. *Radiology.* 1986;158(1):1-10.

32. Silverman SG, Pedrosa I, Ellis JH, et al. Bosniak Classification of Cystic Renal Masses, Version 2019: an update proposal and needs assessment. *Radiology.* 2019;292(2):475-488.

33. Hoang JK, Hoffman AR, González RG, et al. Management of incidental pituitary findings on CT, MRI, and (18)F-fluorodeoxyglucose PET: a white paper of the ACR Incidental Findings Committee. *J Am Coll Radiol.* 2018;15(7):966-972.

34. Aberle DR, Adams AM, Berg CD, et al. Reduced lung-cancer mortality with low-dose computed tomographic screening. *N Engl J Med.* 2011;365(5):395-409.

35. Siegel RL, Miller KD, Jemal A. Cancer statistics, 2017. *CA Cancer J Clin.* 2017;67(1):7-30.

36. Full-body CT scans: what you need to know. US Food and Drug Administration website. https://www.fda.gov/radiation-emitting-products/medical-x-ray-imaging/full-body-ct-scans-what-you-need-know. Published 2017. Updated 12/5/2017. Accessed July 25, 2020.

37. *Carrozza v Greenbaum*, 866 A2d 369, 374-376, 391-393 (Pa Super 2004), aff'd on other grounds 916 A2d 553 (Pa 2007).

38. Order of the Supreme Court, Suffolk County (Jeffrey Arlen Spinner, J.), dated August 19, 2014.

39. *Donnelly v Parikh*, 150 AD3d 820, 821, 823-824 (NY 2017).

40. *Carrozza v Greenbaum*, 866 A2d 369, 379 (Pa Super 2004); *Loudin v Radiology & Imaging Servs., Inc.*, 2011-Ohio-1817, ¶ 13, 128 Ohio St 3d 555, 559, 948 NE2d 944, 949; *Holbrook v. United Hospital Medical Center*, 248 AD2d 358, 669 NYS2d 631 (2d Dep't 1998); *Armbruster v Edgar*, 731 P2d 757, 759-760 (Colo App 1986).

41. Diagnostic Radiology Malpractice Litigation, 75 Am Jur Trials 55 (originally published in 2000).

42. 61 Am Jur 2d, Physicians and Surgeons § 226.

43. 45 Causes of Action 2d 205 (originally published in 2010).

44. *Peterson v Ocean Radiology Associates, P.C.*, 109 Conn App 275, 951 A2d 606 (2008).

CHAPTER 12

Genetic Testing

Michelle L. McGowan, PhD, Kristen Fishler, MS, CGC, David Edul Dryburgh, JD, and Kenji Saito, MD, JD, FACOEM

INTRODUCTION

Both germline and somatic mutations contribute to tumor pathogenesis. The integration of genetic and genomic sequencing into cancer care has unveiled the presence of unique mutations that characterize tumors based on their molecular origins.[1] In some cases, specific molecularly targeted therapies may be incorporated into a personalized treatment plan based on the presence of a particular mutation biomarker.[2-5]

Germline variants

Germline variants are inherited and are present in all cells in the body. Health care providers may recommend genetic testing for germline mutations associated with a hereditary cancer syndrome based on a patient's family history of cancer, if they are diagnosed with particular types of cancer, and/or if they are diagnosed at an early age. Patients may also learn about familial germline mutations associated with cancer syndromes if someone in their family has received clinical genetic testing (gene panel, exome, genome) for a pediatric presentation of a rare genetic condition. People may also learn about germline mutations through direct-to-consumer (no interface with an ordering physician) or direct-to-provider testing (interface with a physician contracted with the lab).[6,7]

If a patient is found to carry a germline mutation associated with a hereditary cancer syndrome, these findings have implications for the patient and their family. First-degree relatives may have up to a 50% chance of having the same mutation, even if they do not present with cancer. Each mutation may confer risk for many different types of cancers, many of which have specific high-risk screening and management guidelines. With confirmation of a germline variant, risk management plans are tailored to patients beyond standard public health guidance regarding commencing cancer risk screening on the basis of one's age or sex or moderating health behaviors such as increasing exercise or quitting smoking.[8]

Somatic mutations

Somatic mutations are acquired in individual cells throughout a person's lifetime and make up the majority of mutations identified in tumor samples. In the context of molecular tumor testing for patients with a cancer diagnosis, somatic mutations are confined to tumor tissue. These mutations may be identified through tumor sequencing, which may or may not include a comparison to the germline (see Clinical Vignette No. 1). While both germline and somatic mutations may inform treatment and management options, there are no hereditary implications of purely somatic mutations. However, germline mutations may provide predictive information to an individual and their family about hereditary disease risk. If a mutation originally identified from a tumor sample is confirmed in the germline, the patient and their family may have a higher risk for cancer recurrence, additional cancers, or other diseases.[9-11] Currently, the National Comprehensive Cancer Network (NCCN) criteria recommend germline testing through a Clinical Laboratory Improvement Amendments (CLIA)–approved lab for any genes for which a patient meets criteria based on clinical and/or family history, because tumor sequencing is not designed to pick up germline variants and the interpretation may be misleading due to tumor testing's focus on treatment decision making (e.g., a variant of uncertain significance in tumor sequencing may be pathogenic in the germline).[12]

CLINICAL VIGNETTE # 1

When she was 45 years old, RL detected a palpable mass in her left breast. Her doctor detected suspicious masses in her left breast and ancillary lymph nodes. The pathology report from a core needle biopsy revealed grade 2, triple-negative, poorly differentiated invasive ductile carcinoma. RL's left ancillary lymph node showed metastatic adenocarcinoma with metastatic workup negative for distant disease. She tested negative for *BRCA* mutations. Following six cycles of chemotherapy, left partial mastectomy, and left sentinel and axillary lymph node dissection, pathology showed no invasive carcinoma in the breast and lymph nodes. She then received radiation. Twenty months after her initial diagnosis, RL had a recurrence in the skin overlying the left breast and regional nodes with similar pathology. She received an additional four cycles of chemotherapy and left mastectomy and right prophylactic mastectomy. Five months later, a clinical exam revealed a recurrence in the chest wall. She started chemotherapy but within five months had increasing neuropathy.

Following hyperthermia radiation for the chest wall recurrence now in remission, RL met with her oncologist, who recommended tumor sequencing to assess possible treatment and clinical trial options. A sample of the patient's tumor was sent to a commercial laboratory for sequencing and analysis. A multidisciplinary genomic tumor board met to discuss the results of tumor-only sequencing to make recommendations to the ordering oncologist, such as referring the patient to genetics for suspected germline variants, clinical trials, US Food and Drug Administration–approved on-label therapies, androgen receptor testing, and repeat human epidermal growth factor receptor 2 (HER2) testing. RL's tumor sequencing report listed a *FANCC* mutation, which is associated with autosomal recessive Fanconi anemia and autosomal dominant predisposition to breast and pancreatic cancer, although data on the cancer risk association are preliminary. The laboratory-generated tumor sequencing report recommended germline testing for this mutation in the "right clinical context." The tumor board debated what kind of recommendation to make on the basis of this mutation and the verbiage in the report. Tumor board members acknowledged that they had little knowledge of the relevance of this result in relation to the patient's family history. They were reluctant to refer the patient to genetics because, in their view, the *FANCC* gene was not directly related to hereditary breast or ovarian cancer syndrome. Ultimately, the tumor board decided against referring the patient to genetics for further evaluation of the *FANCC* variant reported in tumor-only sequencing. Although a legal duty to refer patients to genetics has not been established, professional societies have issued guidance weighted toward referring, and this issue may continue to surface as genomic testing is further incorporated into cancer care.

Genomic testing

In 2013, the American College of Medical Genetics and Genomics (ACMG) issued recommendations for reporting secondary or incidental findings from clinical genome and exome sequencing, including findings of mutations associated with increased cancer risks, indicating that "incidental variants should be reported for the normal sample of a tumor-normal sequenced dyad."[13] This statement raised logistical and ethical challenges regarding how commercial laboratories would incorporate additional interpretation, how health care providers would discuss the possible outcomes of the test during pretest counseling and results during posttest counseling, and whether it would change whether patients elect to undergo clinical genomic testing if secondary results could be returned. The American Society of Clinical Oncology states that incidental findings from all cancer genetic testing, including germline mutations identified through tumor sequencing, should be disclosed to patients.[14] However, physicians are not required to evaluate each mutation identified through somatic tumor sequencing to assess the mutation's potential of also being present in the germline. Therefore, it is possible that incidental findings in the germline may be overlooked by ordering physicians.

People may also learn about familial cancer variants in a pediatric setting, with increasing adoption of clinical genetic panels and exome and genome testing.[15] In this setting, parents of the proband have the opportunity to opt in or opt out of having secondary findings analyzed by the laboratory. Labs may provide additional options of reporting secondary findings for the proband only. If secondary findings are listed on the proband's report, the provider could be obligated to return them to the parents (see Case Law No. 4 and Case Law No. 5). However, a parent's choice to have secondary findings listed on the report is optional, given that their implications are usually secondary to the pediatric proband's care management in childhood. This decision is balanced with the potential of these variants to inform management and screening for cancer and other conditions in adulthood.

LIABILITY ISSUES

Introduction

Genetic tests and the implications of genetic test results have changed as more is learned about the human genome. While genetic and genomic testing has increasingly been integrated into cancer care, little professional society guidance exists on which genetic or genomic tests are most appropriate to order to address particular clinical scenarios. Decisions about which tests to order typically fall to physicians and genetic counselors, who may face challenges regarding the appropriateness or sufficiency of genetic testing.[16]

Ethical considerations that arise in the context of cancer genetic testing include how to ensure the adequacy of informed consent to undergo testing and the fair distribution of costs associated with cancer genetic testing and downstream care. Liability issues that have arisen as genetic testing has proliferated in cancer care include physicians' duties to warn and recontact patients and their families and whether commercial laboratories can patent a gene and privatize cancer genomic tests and data.

Pretest education and counseling

Professional societies have cautioned against predictive genetic testing in pediatric populations, except in cases when results can affect medical management in childhood.[17] Thus, most cancer genetic testing is offered in adult populations. According to NCCN guidelines, pretest counseling includes composing a three-generation family history, risk assessment based on family and personal history, discussion about the possible outcomes of testing, and education about inheritance patterns, penetrance, variable expressivity, and genetic heterogeneity. NCCN recognizes that genetic counselors, medical geneticists, oncologists, surgeons, oncology nurses, or other health professionals with experience in cancer genetics may be involved in the pre- and posttest counseling of patients. Ensuring the adequacy of informed consent is paramount, but the more complex genetic and genomic testing in oncology makes ensuring adequacy of informed consent increasingly difficult. In particular, the increasing size of genetic testing panels and the discovery of genes and genetic variants with uncertain management indications complicate the pretest education and counseling that underpin informed consent. Clinical germline and tumor sequencing has the potential to provide results related to one's personal risk of developing cancer or the genetic makeup of a tumor one already has. Genetics professional society guidelines for pretest education and counseling for genetic testing recommend including education about the purpose of the test; why the test is recommended; what it can and cannot reveal about the patient; the benefits, risks, and alternatives to undergoing testing; the potential impact of the results on one's own health, health care, and family members; whether there will be insurance coverage and costs that the patient will incur for the test; and to whom the results can be disclosed.[18,19] With genomic tests such as whole-genome and whole-exome sequencing that may return secondary findings that reveal increased cancer risk, it is important for patients to understand that these results may be returned even if they were not the reason for ordering testing. Particularly given what is known about patients' and families' concerns about the potential impact of genetic test results on employment and insurability,[20] it is important for health care providers to disclose the protections that the Genetic Information Nondiscrimination Act (see Clinical Vignette No. 2 and Case Law No. 1) provides for patients against discrimination in employment and health insurance on the basis of genetic test results and the gaps in this legislation in terms of discrimination potential in other forms, such as in long-term care insurance or for patients who are employed in a company with less than 15 people. Once a patient provides consent and the test results are available, posttest genetic counseling is pertinent for patients with positive results; this counseling should explain the implications for the patient's physical, emotional, and psychosocial health; recommended procedures and surveillance; benefits, risks, and alternatives to pursuing additional testing or care; and potential implications for family members.

CLINICAL VIGNETTE # 2

Physicians at an academic medical center are increasingly ordering clinical exome sequencing for pediatric patients with undiagnosed conditions. These tests may also include samples from biological parents to assist in the interpretation of variants present in the proband. The academic medical center implemented a policy that parents need to provide written informed consent for their DNA to be analyzed and permission for their child's exome to be sequenced. The consent document indicates that, in addition to the possibility of learning the genetic basis for their child's undiagnosed condition, they may also learn about secondary findings, including genes associated with increased risk of developing cancer or cardiac conditions. Physicians report to the director of the personalized medicine program at the academic medical center that parents express reluctance to consent to whole-exome sequencing because they are concerned about where genetic information about their child—or about themselves—could end up. Would the institution be obligated to place genomic test results in their child's or in their own electronic health record? If asked, would the parents be obligated to report these results to their health insurance provider or employer wellness programs? Parents are worried that they or their child might risk losing their insurance or their employment based on genetic diagnostic or risk information revealed by whole-exome sequencing that ends up in their electronic health record. How should physicians and the academic medical center administration respond to this concern?

Relevant federal law

Congress enacted the Genetic Information Nondiscrimination Act (GINA) in 2008,[21] but its prohibition against genetic discrimination in health insurance applied only to asymptomatic individuals. It was not until the implementation of the Patient Protection and Affordable Care Act that Congress prohibited all health-based discrimination in health insurance.[22] This universally applicable nondiscrimination law provides comprehensive protections and avoids coverage gaps that characterize genetic nondiscrimination laws. The Health Insurance Portability and

Accountability Act, initially enacted in 1996, prohibited exclusion from employer-sponsored group health plans on the basis of genetic conditions, but its protection was limited by its failure to prohibit differential rates. Other laws, such as the Americans with Disabilities Act, also provide some protection to those who are severely affected by genetic disorders.[23]

CASE LAW # 1

In *Ortiz v City of San Antonio Fire Department*, the Court of Appeals found that GINA prohibits an employer from discriminating or taking adverse actions against an employee "because of genetic information with respect to the employee."[24] GINA also makes it unlawful for an employer to request, require, or purchase genetic information with respect to an employee or a family member of the employee with some exceptions. In this case, the plaintiff argued that the department's mandatory wellness program was a form of discrimination and retaliation in violation of Title VII and GINA. Genetic information means information about the genetic tests of an individual or family member and information about a manifestation of disease or disorder in such individual or family members. Genetic test means an analysis of human DNA, RNA, chromosomes, proteins, or metabolites that detect genotypes, mutations, or chromosomal changes. The Court of Appeals concluded that there is a difference between genetic information and medical information and that the wellness program did not violate GINA by requiring the employee to participate in its mandatory wellness program. There is no evidence that the wellness program requested, required, or purchased his genetic information or discriminated against the plaintiff because of it.

Costs and accessibility of testing

The fair distribution of benefits and burdens of the integration of genomics into cancer care remains fraught. Academic medical centers and patients with private insurance were the earliest users and beneficiaries of cancer genetic testing, with the availability of a variety of genetic tests in community health care settings and public insurance coverage for cancer genetic tests lagging behind.[25] This raises the potential for uneven access to and benefits from the shift toward precision approaches to cancer care and may generate skewed knowledge about cancer genomics based on the demographic characteristics of participants in cancer clinical trials and population genetic studies that do not represent the population as a whole.[26]

Accessibility and ownership of cancer genetic variant reference data

As germline testing for mutations in the *BRCA1* and *BRCA2* genes associated with hereditary breast and ovarian cancer syndromes became available, commercial laboratories compiled patient samples to evaluate mutations in these genes. In part due to its efforts to patent processes to evaluate these mutations (see Case Law No. 2), Myriad Genetics became an industry leader in offering clinic genetic testing for *BRCA1* and *BRCA2* despite criticisms that, as a private company, it could not be an unbiased source of hereditary cancer genetic risk information.[27] This afforded Myriad Genetics the opportunity to amass samples from a significant market share of genetic tests, building a trove of data to categorize variants in cancer genes as pathogenic, likely pathogenic, of uncertain significance, or nonpathogenic. From a liability perspective, this has raised questions about (1) how to manage variant reclassifications and (2) the rightful ownership of cancer genetic risk information. Advocates have raised particular concerns about how racial and ethnic minority patients who have undergone *BRCA1* and *BRCA2* testing have been more likely to receive results indicating that they have a variant of uncertain significance due to limited knowledge of how variants more common in this population affect cancer risk, which diminishes the potential utility of predictive genetic testing in these populations.

With regard to ownership of cancer genetic information, patient organizations have fiercely advocated for the public release of cancer variant information held by commercial laboratories, arguing that there should be no proprietary value on their personal genetic information. They argue that making cancer risk information publicly available would enable researchers to more quickly translate cancer genetic findings into clinical trials and care, benefiting past patients who contributed their genetic information to these databases and future patients who face increased risk of developing cancer due to genetic variants associated with hereditary cancers.

CASE LAW # 2

The US Patent Office had accepted patents on isolated DNA sequences as a composition of matter, for example, *BRCA1* and *BRCA2* genes. Myriad Genetics had discovered the precise location and sequence of these two human genes, mutations of which can substantially increase the risks of breast and ovarian cancer. Myriad obtained a number of patents based on its discovery. In *Association for Molecular Pathology v Myriad Genetics, Inc.*, the Supreme Court of the United States needed to resolve whether a naturally occurring segment of DNA is patent eligible under 35 USC § 101 by virtue of its isolation from the rest of the human genome. The court also addressed the patent eligibility of synthetically created DNA known as complementary DNA (cDNA), which contains the same protein-coding information found in a segment of natural DNA but omits portions within the DNA segment that do not code for proteins. The court found that merely isolating genes that are found in nature does not make them patentable because "nature, natural phenomena, and abstract ideas are not patentable; they are the basic tools of scientific and technological work that lie beyond the domain of patent protection."[28] Furthermore, the court held, "a naturally occurring DNA segment is a product of nature and not patent eligible merely because it has been isolated, but cDNA is patent eligible because it is not naturally occurring."[28]

Return of reclassified results

As more is learned about the human genome, variants may be reclassified as pathogenic, likely pathogenic, of uncertain significance, or benign. While most variants of uncertain significance get reclassified as benign, some may be reclassified as likely pathogenic or pathogenic. While legal liabilities regarding the management of variants that are reclassified remain unclear,[29,30] health care providers face ethical dilemmas as to whether and how to notify patients if their genetic variants have been reclassified, particularly if they have been reclassified as pathogenic or likely pathogenic (see Clinical Vignette No. 3). Health care providers have raised questions about their legal liabilities in disclosing reclassified results, particularly if the patient who underwent cancer genetic testing is no longer living. Specifically, they have queried whether there is a duty to notify patients or family members of patients who have passed away if their cancer risk has changed as a result of variant reclassification. Current ACMG guidance on duties to recontact patients rest on the ethical principle of beneficence, urging reasonable effort to recontact when results may benefit patients' health or care management.[29] At the same time, ACMG distributes responsibility for checking on variant reclassification among genetic testing laboratories, health care providers, and their families, as clarity is lacking as to who ought to ensure communication of variant reclassifications.[29]

Health care providers have also raised questions about their legal obligations with regard to sharing cancer genetic risk results with people other than the patient. Do health care providers have a duty to warn patients' family members that they are at increased risk of developing cancer during their lifetimes, even if the patient does not want to disclose the results? The bioethics literature suggests that physicians' ethical obligations do not extend beyond returning results to their patients but that they should encourage their patients to share relevant cancer genetic risk with family members who could be affected. However, ethical obligations and legal liabilities are not always in alignment with one another, and it is possible that family members could claim withholding relevant risk information could result in harms to their health and well-being (see Case Law No. 4 and Case Law No. 5).

CLINICAL VIGNETTE # 3

A 47-year-old woman presented to her primary care physician for a breast lump. Workup included a mammogram, which showed a lesion at 1 o'clock in the left breast. Biopsy revealed infiltrating ductal carcinoma. She told her doctor that her grandmother and aunt also had breast cancer at an early age. The patient was a single mother to two daughters in their mid-20s. As part of her oncologic evaluation, she was referred for genetic counseling to determine whether there was a genetic driver of her cancer, especially given the age of onset and family history.

The genetic counselor ordered a gene panel, which identified a variant of uncertain significance in *CHEK2*. The genetic counselor informed the patient that this result may be associated with the cause for her cancer but that more information about this variant is needed. The genetic counselor discussed that, over time, this variant has been reclassified as benign, likely pathogenic, and pathogenic.

The patient received extensive cancer treatment but, unfortunately, died a few months after receiving genetic counseling. Six months later, the genetic testing lab reached out to the genetic counselor to let them know that the patient's variant had been reclassified as a likely pathogenic result. The genetic counselor and team felt obligated to return this result to the patient's next of kin, given that she had living children and siblings who all had a 50% chance of also having the variant. However, the only contact information remaining for her was that of an ex-husband. Following a consultation between legal counsel and the genetics team, institutional legal counsel approved the genetics team's request to contact the patient's ex-husband to attempt to get in touch with either her siblings or her children (without disclosing specific information about the variant to him). The genetic counselor was able to contact one of the patient's children, who was glad that there was an explanation for her diagnosis and actions that she, her siblings, and other relatives could take to be proactive in their care. This team made the decision to return this result. However, are all health care professionals obligated to contact next of kin? If so, under what circumstances? What if the lab had not reached out to the physician? Whose responsibility is it to check in on reclassification? Is it the patient's and/or their family's responsibility or that of the provider?

Duty to warn case law

CASE LAW # 3

In *Tarasoff v Regents of the University of California*, a woman was killed by her stalker after he had confided his intention of killing her to his therapist.[31] The court concluded that a physician or therapist has a duty to warn if (1) he or she has a special relationship with either the person who may cause the harm or the potential victim, (2) the person at risk is identifiable, and (3) the harm is foreseeable and serious. This definition is now commonly used in legal settings in cases involving a physician's duty to warn and was called upon in two suits regarding physicians' duty to inform families of inherited cancer risks.

CASE LAW # 4

In *Pate v Threlkel*, a woman received treatment for medullary thyroid carcinoma, which can be associated with an autosomal dominant condition called multiple endocrine neoplasia.[32] Three years later, her adult daughter was diagnosed with the same type of cancer and filed a complaint against the doctor who had treated her mother, arguing that if she had known earlier about the genetic risk of medullary thyroid cancer, she could have taken preventive action and her condition would have been avoided or detected at an earlier and curable stage. The prevailing standard of care at that time was that if there is a duty that is obviously for the benefit of certain identified third parties and the physician knows of the existence of those third parties, then the physician's duty runs to those third parties. When translated to the facts of this case, it was found that the physician owes a duty of care to the children of a patient to warn the patient of the genetically transferable nature of the condition for which the physician is treating the patient. Consequently, the court agreed with the daughter's argument that the physician had a duty to warn of the risk to his patient's children. However, the court concluded that this duty was satisfied by warning the patient about the risk to her relatives, including her daughters. Overall, *Pate v Threlkel* concluded that the physician had a duty to warn his patient that his patient's daughter was at risk of developing a lethal disease known to be genetically transferable, even though the physician was not in privity with the daughter. However, the court also held that the physician could discharge his duty to warn by telling his patient, the daughter's mother, of the risk and that the physician had no duty to personally warn the daughter.

CASE LAW # 5

In *Safer v Estate of Pack*, a woman was diagnosed with colorectal cancer due to familial adenomatous polyposis, an autosomal dominant condition predisposing to colorectal cancer.[33] She filed a complaint against the estate of Dr. Pack, the deceased physician who treated her father for the same condition 26 years earlier, alleging a violation of the physician's duty to warn her of her own health risks. She argued that if she had known about her risk of having this condition, her cancer could have been detected at an early and curable stage through regular surveillance. In a decision that differed from that of the *Pate v Threlkel* court, the *Safer v Estate of Pack* court found that the physician's duty to warn may not be satisfied in all cases by informing the patient of the risk to his relatives. The court pointed out that the exception to the *Pate* case would be somewhere along the lines of protecting the public health, where the trial court acknowledged that contagious or infectious diseases, which may be easily spread between persons, warrant public health protection. However, the trial court believed genetic diseases to be threats that are already present in an individual, do not spread between individuals, and, thus, do not rise to the public health level of contagious or infectious diseases. On appeal, the court asserted that, as a matter of law, the same duty that exists to warn of the risk of infectious diseases should require a warning for genetic risks. Consequently, the physician must take reasonable steps to guarantee that immediate family members are warned, and the duty to warn extends to family members in the case of hereditary conditions.

CONCLUSION

The integration of genetic testing into cancer care has been rapid, expansive, and uneven. As health care providers incorporate germline, somatic, and genomic testing modalities into their practices, familiarizing themselves with the purpose, benefits, limitations, and alternatives to testing is paramount to protect patients' autonomy, promote beneficence, and ensure just distribution of the benefits and burdens of precision medicine. Legal doctrine pertaining to clinical genetic testing is evolving; thus, health care providers should consult with institutional legal counsel when questions around their duties and obligations with regard to ordering tests and interpreting, returning, and managing genetic test results arise.

KEY POINTS:

- Patients who meet criteria for germline genetic testing based on personal and/or family history should be offered clinical testing through a CLIA-approved lab, regardless of tumor sequencing results.
- Families may become aware of germline cancer variants through exome/genome sequencing in a pediatric proband being evaluated for a rare disease. This testing is not comprehensive cancer testing and may exclude genes most relevant to other family members' care. Therefore, additional cancer genetic counseling and/or genetic testing may be indicated.
- Protection of patients' privacy is paramount, particularly when genetic and genomic test results may reveal sensitive information about the patient's health or risk of developing cancer in their lifetime. However, under some circumstances, there may be a legal and professional duty to inform people other than the proband about a genetic testing result or reclassification, including, for example, next of kin and first-degree relatives.
- GINA protects patients' genetic diagnostic and risk information from being used by health insurers and employers to discriminate against them. It is important for health care professionals and patients to understand the limitations of this legislation, particularly in that it does not protect against long-term care insurance discrimination and small employers do not have the same obligations as larger employers. Other federal law may provide additional nondiscrimination protections related to individuals' genetic information.

References:

1. Everett JN, Gustafson SL, Raymond VM. Traditional roles in a non-traditional setting: genetic counseling in precision oncology. *J Genet Couns.* 2014;23(4):655–660.
2. Meric-Bernstam F, Farhangfar C, Mendelsohn J, Mills GB. Building a personalized medicine infrastructure at a major cancer center. *J Clin Oncol.* 2013;31(15):1849–1857.
3. Meric-Bernstam F, Mills GB. Overcoming implementation challenges of personalized cancer therapy. *Nat Rev Clin Oncol.* 2012;9(9):542–548.
4. Schilsky RL. Personalized medicine in oncology: the future is now. *Nat Rev Drug Discov.* May 2010;9(5):363–366.
5. Johnson DB, Dahlman KH, Knol J, et al. Enabling a genetically informed approach to cancer medicine: a retrospective evaluation of the impact of comprehensive tumor profiling using a targeted next-generation sequencing panel. *Oncologist.* 2014;19(6):616–622.

6. McGowan ML, Fishman JR. Using lessons learned from BRCA testing and marketing: what lies ahead for whole genome scanning services. *Am J Bioeth*. 2008;8(6):18–20.
7. McGowan ML, Fishman JR, Settersten RA Jr, Lambrix MA, Juengst ET. Gatekeepers or intermediaries? The role of clinicians in commercial genomic testing. *PLoS One*. 2014;9:e108484.
8. Meagher K, McGowan ML, Settersten R, Fishman J, Juengst E. Precisely where are we going? Charting the new terrain of precision prevention. *Annu Rev Genomics Hum Genet*. 2017;18:369–387.
9. Schrader KA, Cheng DT, Joseph V, et al. Germline variants in targeted tumor sequencing using matched normal DNA. *JAMA Oncol*. 2016;2(1):104–111.
10. Meric-Bernstam F, Brusco L, Daniels M, et al. Incidental germline variants in 1000 advanced cancers on a prospective somatic genomic profiling protocol. *Ann Oncol*. 2016;27(5):795–800.
11. Catenacci DV, Amico AL, Nielsen SM, et al. Tumor genome analysis includes germline genome: are we ready for surprises? *Int J Cancer*. 2015;136(7):1559–1567.
12. Genetic/familial high-risk assessment: breast, ovarian, and pancreatic. National Comprehensive Cancer Network. https://www.nccn.org/professionals/physician_gls/pdf/genetics_bop.pdf. Accessed March 29, 2021.
13. Green RC, Berg JS, Grody WW, et al. ACMG recommendations for reporting of incidental findings in clinical exome and genome sequencing. *Genet Med*. 2013;15(7):565–574.
14. Robson ME, Bradbury AR, Arun B, et al. American Society of Clinical Oncology policy statement update: genetic and genomic testing for cancer susceptibility. *J Clin Oncol*. 2015;33(31):3660–3667.
15. Hart MR, Biesecker BB, Blout CL, et al. Secondary findings from clinical genomic sequencing: prevalence, patient perspectives, family history assessment, and health-care costs from a multisite study. *Genet Med*. 2019;21:1100–1110.
16. Marchant G, Barnes M, Evans JP, LeRoy B, Wolf SM. From genetics to genomics: facing the liability implications in clinical care. *J Law Med Ethics*. 2020;48(1):11–43.
17. Botkin JR, Belmont JW, Berg JS, et al. Points to consider: ethical, legal, and psychosocial implications of genetic testing in children and adolescents. *Am J Hum Genet*. 2015;97(1):6–21.
18. Ayuso C, Millán JM, Mancheno M, Dal-Ré R. Informed consent for whole-genome sequencing studies in the clinical setting. Proposed recommendations on essential content and process. *Eur J Hum Genet*. 2013;21(10):1054–1059.
19. ACMG Board of Directors. Points to consider for informed consent for genome/exome sequencing. *Genet Med*. 2013;15(19):748–749.
20. McGowan ML, Glinka A, Highland J, Asaad G, Sharp R. Genetics patients' perspectives on clinical genomic testing. *Per Med*. 2013;10(4):339–347.
21. Genetic Information Nondiscrimination Act, Pub L No 110–233 (2008).
22. Patient Protection and Affordable Care Act, Pub L No 111–148 111th Congress (2010).
23. Clayton EW. Why the Americans with Disabilities Act matters for genetics. *JAMA*. 2014;313:2225–2226.
24. *Ortiz v City of San Antonio Fire Department*, 15–50341 (5th Cir 2015).
25. McGowan ML, Settersten RA Jr, Juengst ET, Fishman JR. Integrating genomics into clinical oncology: ethical and social challenges from proponents of personalized medicine. *Urol Oncol*. 2014;32(2):187–192.
26. Popejoy AB, Fullerton SM. Genomics is failing on diversity. *Nature*. 2016;538(7624):161–164.
27. Matloff E, Caplan A. Direct to confusion: lessons learned from marketing BRCA testing. *Am J Bioeth*. 2008;8(6):5–8.
28. *Association for Molecular Pathology v Myriad Genetics, Inc.*, 569 US 576 (2013).
29. David KL, Best RG, Brenman LM, et al. Patient re-contact after revision of genomic test results: points to consider—a statement of the American College of Medical Genetics and Genomics (ACMG). *Genet Med*. 2019;21(4):769–771.
30. Roberts JL, Foulkes AL. Genetic duties. *William & Mary L Rev*. 2020;62(1):143–212.
31. *Tarasoff v Regents of the University of California*, 17 Cal 3d 425 (Cal 1976).
32. *Pate v Threlkel*, 661 So2d 278 (Florida 1995).
33. *Safer v Estate of Pack*, 677 A2d 1188 (NJ Super Ct App Div 1996).

CHAPTER 13

Prescribing Drugs and Services

Mudit Kakar, PhD, JD

INTRODUCTION

The practice of oncology requires compliance with a gamut of laws (rules and regulations) relating to prescription and administration of drugs and treatment regimens. Given that the practice of medicine is highly regulated, it is not a surprise that there are laws that may impinge on a physician's decision making when prescribing a drug or a treatment regimen. These laws, although seemingly burdensome to the everyday practice of oncology, are critical to what is in the best medical interest of patients and the overall health care system. These laws are meant to protect patients against undue influence of money in management of a disease or a condition while imparting the best medical treatment. This chapter provides a summary of four different laws, rules, and regulations—namely, the Anti Kickback Statute, the Physician Self-Referral law, the Right to Try Act, and Off-label Drug Use—that directly affect the act of prescribing a drug or a treatment regimen for a patient or making a referral regarding the same.

ANTI-KICKBACK STATUTE

The Anti-Kickback Statute, commonly referred to as *AKS*, is a criminal statute that makes it illegal to solicit or receive remuneration in return for prescribing a drug or a service or making a referral regarding the same to a patient, where payment of such drug or service is covered by a federal health care program.[1] The objective of *AKS* is to prevent undue influence of money or other favors on a physician's or other health care practitioner's ability to make sound clinical decisions that are in the best interest of a patient. Another objective of *AKS* is to prevent fraud and exploitation of federal health care programs by precluding claims for medically redundant or unnecessary services. Under the *AKS*, not only are some of the obvious acts, for example, bribes, prohibited, but even seemingly innocuous conduct, such as sponsored business dinners, paid speaking arrangements, or contributions to a physician's favorite charity, is considered illegal if it meets all other elements of an *AKS* violation. Since *AKS* is a criminal statute, an action under the *AKS* must be brought by the government.

Elements of AKS

The *AKS* is implicated when a physician or an entity:

- knowingly and willfully
- solicits, receives, offers, or pays any remuneration

- to induce or as an award for, referrals for or orders of, drugs or services
- paid for, fully or partially, by a federal health care program.

Knowingly and willfully

Although it may appear that the requirement that a physician "knowingly and willfully" acted in violation of the AKS must mean that the physician knew that the AKS prohibited receiving renumeration in exchange for referrals, yet intended to break the law; that is not the case. Actual knowledge of the AKS or the specific intent to violate the AKS is not required to show that a violation of AKS has occurred.[2] The government is only required to prove that the defendant willfully committed an act that violated the AKS.[3] As long as a physician or an entity provides services covered by a federal health care plan, they are presumed to have knowledge of the AKS.

Remuneration

Remuneration includes anything of value, received directly or indirectly, overtly or covertly, in cash or in kind.[1] Remuneration means payment or compensation.[4] The AKS's prohibition on remuneration is broad: physicians may not accept any payment in exchange for referrals. The law does not limit remuneration by the type or source of the payment.[5] Therefore, remuneration can include anything of value, tangible or intangible.[6]

Referral

The AKS criminalizes remuneration for referrals for "the furnishing or arranging for the furnishing of any item or service."[1] Therefore, according to the statute, the referred items or services need not have been provided, as long as they were arranged for, ordered, or recommended.[7] This makes sense because one of the objectives of the AKS is to address the potential for unnecessary drain on the federal health care system.[8] In the context of AKS, remuneration includes sums for which no actual service was performed in addition to those for which some professional time was expended.[9]

Practitioners must be cognizant of the remuneration-referral relationship to avoid AKS violation because AKS covers a variety of business relationships where the main purpose of a business arrangement may not be a kickback in exchange of a referral. What is commonly referred to as the *One Purpose Rule* states that a violation of the AKS requires only that "one purpose of the payment" be to induce referrals, even if that is not the primary purpose of the business relationship between the parties or the payments were also intended to compensate for legitimate professional services.[10]

Federal health care program

The final prong of AKS includes that the item or service referred by a physician be covered through a federal health care program. The statute defines federal health care program as "any plan or program that provides health benefits, whether directly, through insurance, or otherwise, which is funded directly, in whole or in part, by the United States Government"[11] or any state health care program, as defined in 42 USC § 1302a-7(h).

AKS safe harbors

The AKS includes exceptions and safe harbors that describe various remunerations and business practices that are protected from prosecution under the AKS *if* the parties to a business arrangement meet the specific criteria for such arrangement, as described in the corresponding safe harbor provision of the *AKS*.[12] These business practices may include arrangements such as investment interests, space rental lease, equipment rental lease, personal services and management contracts, sale of practice, referral services, warranties, practitioner recruitment, investment in group practices, ambulatory surgical centers, referral arrangements for specialty services, and electronic prescribing items and services. The safe harbor regulations, in their entirety, are codified in 42 CFR § 1001.952, which can be accessed online (http://federal.elaws.us/cfr/title42.part1001.section1001.952).

The Office of Inspector General (OIG), Department of Health and Human Services, is tasked with making rules regarding various safe harbor provisions of the *AKS*.[13]

OIG advisory opinions

The OIG issues advisory opinions (AOs) about the application of *AKS*, including its exceptions and safe harbor provisions, to a requesting party's existing or proposed business arrangement.[14] Practitioners are encouraged to review OIG's AOs or seek an AO if one relevant to a practitioner's situation is not available prior to entering into a business arrangement with an entity to make sure that the arrangement is not prohibited by the *AKS*. OIG provides advice through its AOs on application of the *AKS* in specific factual situations. The AOs are binding and may be legally relied upon on the party requesting it.

PHYSICIAN SELF-REFERRAL LAW (STARK LAW)

The Physician Self-Referral Law, commonly known as the *Stark law*, prohibits a physician from making a referral of designated health services (DHSs) payable by Medicare or Medicaid to a DHS provider if the physician or an immediate family member of the physician has a financial relationship with the DHS provider.[15] On the receiving end, the DHS provider may not bill Medicare, Medicaid, an individual, a third-party payor, or any other entity for DHSs provided under a prohibited referral.[16]

Elements of *Stark law*

The *Stark law* is implicated when a physician or an entity:
- refers a patient to an entity
- for furnishing of DHSs paid for by Medicare or Medicaid
- when the physician or an immediate family member of such a physician
- has a financial relationship with such entity.

Referral
Referral includes a request by a physician for an item or service, including the request by a physician for a consultation with another physician (and any test or procedure ordered by or to be performed by [or under the supervision of] that other physician).[17] This also includes a request for or an establishment of a plan of care by a physician that includes the provision of a DHS.[18] Notably, a request by a radiologist for diagnostic radiology services and a request by a radiation oncologist for radiation therapy, when such services are furnished by (or under the supervision of)

such radiologist or radiation oncologist pursuant to a consultation requested by another physician, *do not* constitute referrals.[19]

Designated health services

DHSs include clinical laboratory services; physical therapy services; occupational therapy services; radiology services, including magnetic resonance imaging, computed tomography scans, and ultrasound services; radiation therapy services and supplies; durable medical equipment and supplies; parenteral and enteral nutrients, equipment, and supplies; prosthetics, orthotics, and prosthetic devices and supplies; home health services; outpatient prescription drugs; inpatient and outpatient hospital services; and outpatient speech-language pathology services.[20] The DHSs are defined in federal regulations in detail.[21] A quick reference, however, is available from the Centers for Medicare and Medicaid Services (CMS), which maintains and annually updates lists that identify all items and services included within certain DHS categories.[22]

Immediate family member

For the purpose of the *Stark law*, an immediate family member is a husband or wife; birth or adoptive parent; child or sibling; stepparent, stepchild, stepbrother, or stepsister; father-in-law, mother-in-law, son-in-law, daughter-in-law, brother-in-law, or sister-in-law; grandparent or grandchild; or spouse of grandparent or grandchild.[21]

Financial relationship

A financial relationship under the *Stark law* is defined as an ownership or investment interest in an entity or a compensation arrangement with an entity.[23] Further, for the purpose of the *Stark law*, an ownership or investment interest in an entity may be through equity, debt, or other means and includes an interest in an entity that holds an ownership or investment interest in any entity providing the DHS.[24] A compensation arrangement includes any arrangement involving any remuneration between a physician and a DHS provider entity, where, just like in the *AKS* a remuneration is any payment or benefit, which may be direct or indirect, overt or covert, in cash or in kind.[25] The *Stark law* however, does not consider certain compensation arrangement as remuneration for the purposes of this law.[26]

Practitioners must be aware that a determination of a financial relationship between a physician and a DHS provider entity applies to a physician or an immediate family member of such a physician alike.[27]

Exceptions in *Stark Law*

The *Stark law* regulations include a wide range of exceptions that apply to financial relationships between a physician and a DHS provider entity. These exceptions include the following:

- General exceptions to both ownership and compensation arrangement prohibitions[28]
- General exceptions related only to ownership or investment prohibition for ownership in publicly traded securities and mutual funds[29]
- Exceptions relating only to ownership or investment prohibition[30]
- Exceptions relating to certain compensation arrangements[31]

Each *Stark* exception includes its own requirements. As a general rule, however, these exceptions require the compensation arrangement to be:

1. set at fair market value and not take into account the volume or value of referrals or business generated;
2. memorialized in writing, signed by the parties and specifying all the services and compensation provided under the arrangement; and
3. in compliance with state and federal law, including the *AKS*.[32]

CMS advisory opinions

Given that the nature of financial relationships can vary widely, practitioners are encouraged to seek guidance from CMS when referring patients to a DHS provider entity with which the physician or an immediate family member of such physician has a financial relationship. CMS issues certain written AOs that provide guidance on whether or not such referrals are allowed.[33] These AOs provide a binding opinion regarding the application of the *Stark law* to specific factual situations. CMS also operates a physician self-referral call center where physicians can direct their inquiries related to the *Stark law*.[34]

RIGHT TO TRY ACT

The Right to Try Act of 2017 provides patients who have been diagnosed with a life-threatening disease or condition and who have exhausted approved treatment options and who are unable to participate in a clinical trial involving an investigational drug a means to access the investigational drug without US Food and Drug Administration (FDA) approval.[35] This law is particularly relevant to oncology considering the life-threatening nature of cancer and the extent of research emphasis on finding novel therapies for oncology indications.[36]

A benefit of the Right to Try Act is that it exempts physicians from liability when prescribing drugs and treatments under this act unless they engage in reckless or willful misconduct, are grossly negligent, or commit an intentional tort.[37] Yet, physicians must be mindful of the regulatory requirements when prescribing a treatment under the Right to Try Act given the limited data available for such treatments.

Eligible patients

To access a treatment not yet approved by the FDA under the Right to Try Act, a patient must meet all of the following requirements:

- Patient must have a **life-threatening** disease or condition. For the purposes of the Right to Try Act, a life-threatening diseases or condition is one where the likelihood of death is high unless the course of the disease is interrupted, including diseases with potentially fatal outcomes, where the end point of a clinical trial analysis is survival.[38]
- Patient must have **exhausted approved treatment options** and must be **unable to participate in a clinical trial** for the investigational drug the patient is seeking.[39] Practitioners must note that *this requirement must be certified by a physician* who is in a good standing with the physician's licensing organization or

board and who will *not be compensated* directly by the sponsor or the manufacturer of the investigational drug for the certification.[39]
- Patient or their legally authorized representative must have provided written informed consent regarding the proposed treatment.

Eligible investigational drug

An investigational drug that may be prescribed for treatment under the Right to Try Act must
meet the following criteria:

- It must have completed a phase I clinical trial.
- It must not have been approved or licensed by the FDA for any use.
- It must be subject of either:
  - a New Drug Application (NDA) or Biologics License Application (BLA) submitted with the FDA, *or*
  - an active Investigational New Drug (IND) application filed with the FDA with clinical trials underway to
    form the primary basis of a claim of effectiveness in support of an NDA or a BLA to be filed with the FDA.
- It must be under active development or production and must not have been discontinued by the manufacturer or placed on a clinical hold.[40]

OFF-LABEL DRUG USE

Off-label drug use allows physicians to prescribe FDA-approved drugs for unapproved uses.[41] An
example would be when a chemotherapy is approved by the FDA to treat one type of cancer, but
a physician decides to use it to treat a different type of cancer. Off-label use is not per se illegal,[42]
rather it is quite common in oncology.[43-46] However, it must be carried out with caution and
based on experience, research, and sound medical judgment.

Since, by definition, an off-label drug use is not approved by the FDA, indiscriminate off-label
drug use without sufficient clinical and scientific basis may not meet the relevant "standard of
care" and give rise to medical negligence liability against a physician (see Chapter 1). Another
thing to keep in mind when prescribing a drug or treatment for an off-label use is informed
consent (see Chapter 2). Although there may not be a legal duty to inform patients of a drug's
regulatory status, to avoid liability for any unwanted effects and as a matter of good practice,
physicians should obtain an informed consent from a patient when prescribing a drug for its
off-label use.[47,48]

CASE LAW # 1

The government, through US attorneys, brought a case against senior administrators—Edward
Novak and Clarence Nagelvoort—of Sacred Heart Hospital in Chicago, Illinois, for offering
and paying kickbacks to physicians in return for patient referrals in violation of the *AKS*, as well as

conspiracy to commit fraud.[49] The government alleged, and eventually proved, that Sacred Heart Hospital paid kickbacks to physicians by concealing them as payments under various types of contractual agreements, namely, (1) direct personal services contracts; (2) teaching contracts; (3) lease agreements for the use of office space; and (4) agreements to provide physicians with the services of other medical professionals (e.g., physician's assistants). Novak was charged with 27 substantive counts of violating the *AKS*, and Nagelvoort was charged with ten such counts. After a seven-week trial, the jury found both Novak and Nagelvoort guilty of the conspiracy count and all but one of the substantive counts with which they were charged.

On appeal, Novak and Nagelvoort argued that the contractual agreements the hospital had with the physicians—personal services contracts, teaching agreements, and the leases—met various elements of the safe harbor provisions of the *AKS*. The court noted, generally, the safe harbors exempt written agreements for space rental and personal services if the terms are for less than a year; the compensation is consistent with fair market values; and the services or space is reasonably necessary to accomplish the business goals of the contracting entity. These safe harbors, however, do not protect any payment that "takes into account the value or volume of any referrals" for services to be paid for under a federal health care program.

The appeals court concluded that the jury correctly found a violation of the *AKS* because the evidence provided by the government showed that the various contractual agreements made by the hospital did not fall under the safe harbor provisions of the *AKS*. For instance, regarding direct personal services contracts, even though two physicians signed contracts with the hospital to spend a certain number of hours per month developing a cancer screening program at the hospital and providing education on palliative and hospice services, respectively, those physicians never performed the actual work or services outlined in the contract, yet they got paid for these services. The evidence showed that it was the physicians' understanding that they were not actually required to perform the work outlined and, instead, were required only to bring patients to Sacred Heart. Therefore, the jury correctly concluded that the agreements took into account the physicians' potential referrals, thereby placing them outside the safe harbor.

As to the teaching contracts, the appeal court noted that the evidence showed that attending physicians were already teaching residents as part of their normal duties before the creation of separate teaching contracts and no additional duties were created that would have justified the additional payments made under the contracts. Instead, it was one physician's understanding that the physician was being compensated for bringing surgical cases to the hospital. While certain other physicians testified that they did not perform all of the corresponding duties but were paid pursuant to the teaching contracts.

Regarding the lease agreement with a physician, the evidence showed that the arrangement was a quid pro quo, where the hospital leased an outside medical center in exchange for getting referrals from the medical center.

The appeal court affirmed all criminal convictions of the district court against Novak and Nagelvoort.

CASE LAW # 2

Tri-County, a Pennsylvania corporation, identifies as being in the "equipment leasing" business and provides computed tomography (CT) scan services.[50] Tyrone Hospital is a not-for-profit organization that provides inpatient and ancillary hospital services to residents of Blair County, Pennsylvania, and to residents of neighboring counties. The plaintiffs, former employees of Tyrone Hospital, brought a claim against the defendant Ashcroft, physician defendants, and Tri-County for making prohibited self-referrals, in violation of the Stark law.

Defendant Ashcroft and the physician defendants maintained significant ownership interests in Tri-County as shareholders. Defendant Ashcroft also served as the chief financial officer at Tyrone Hospital for a period. The plaintiffs claimed that the defendants participated in a patient referral scheme to generate revenue for Tyrone Hospital and Tri-County. Essentially, the defendants referred patients to Tyrone Hospital for inpatient services and other DHSs, and, in return, Tyrone Hospital maintained a business arrangement with Tri-County and its shareholders.

The record in the case showed that the physician defendants were shareholders in Tri-County. Indeed, one of the shareholders also served as the chairman of the radiology department at Tyrone Hospital, maintaining an exclusive contract to provide radiology services. Tri-County provided CT scanning services and leased office space on the property of Tyrone Hospital for that purpose. Tyrone Hospital arranged for at least some of its inpatients to receive CT scans at Tri-County. Tyrone Hospital paid Tri-County for those scans. The court found that there was a "financial relationship" between the physician defendants and Tyrone Hospital because the physician defendants were shareholders in Tri-County and there was an unbroken chain of persons or entities linking Tri-County to Tyrone Hospital. To elaborate on the chain:

1. Tyrone Hospital paid Dr. DiGiacobbe—both an employee of Tyrone Hospital and a shareholder in Tri-County—for CT scans performed at Tri-County.
2. Tri-County representatives deposited these payments in a Tri-County business account.
3. Tri-County representatives distributed these payments to Tri-County shareholders, which included the physician defendants.

The court also found that evidence showed that the physician defendants received aggregate compensation that varied with, or otherwise took into account, the volume of referrals to Tyrone Hospital. Because Tyrone Hospital arranged for some of its inpatients to receive CT scans at Tri-County, the number of patients the physician defendants referred to Tyrone Hospital would affect the number of scans performed at Tri-County. Thus, the "aggregate compensation" between Tyrone Hospital and Tri-County varied based on the volume of referrals that the physician defendants made to Tyrone Hospital.

Finally, the court also found that the defendants did not meet Stark law exceptions. The court granted summary judgment in favor of the plaintiffs on the issue of violation of the Stark law.

CLINICAL VIGNETTE # 1

Dr. Jones is a medical oncologist who works at Life Clinic, Inc., an outpatient cancer clinic, and has hospital privileges at St. Smith Cancer Hospital. She has a contract with St. Smith where she supervises care of cancer patients requiring long-term care. As per her contract with the hospital, Dr. Jones's compensation from the hospital is based on professional services she personally performs or supervises at the hospital. Additionally, the hospital also provides certain benefits, for example, paying for Dr. Jones's medical liability insurance. Dr. Jones's son is a pharmacist and owns a retail pharmacy, Life Pharmacy, LLC, which is located in the same building as the Life Clinic. Dr. Jones does not have any ownership interest in Life Pharmacy, nor is she affiliated with Life Pharmacy in any professional capacity. Both Dr. Jones and her son are shareholders in Your Recovery Center, LLC, a rehabilitation center providing physical therapy services and occupational therapy services.

Dr. Jones routinely refers patients from Life Clinic to St. Smith Cancer Hospital for long-term care services. She personally supervises the treatment and care of such patients at St. Smith. Dr. Jones also refers her patients to Life Pharmacy for filling prescriptions because Life Pharmacy is located in the same building as Life Clinic and stocks all medications that Dr. Jones prescribes. Dr. Jones refers her patients at St. Smith Cancer Hospital and Life Clinic to Your Recovery Center for rehabilitation services. St. Smith Cancer Hospital routinely bills inpatient services to federal health care programs, such as Medicare.

Dr. Jones's professional situation and her working relationship with various entities, although they may sound all too common and innocuous, may involve a violation of the Stark law and the *AKS*. The analysis below explains how these laws may be implicated in Dr. Jones's various interactions.

The Stark law prohibits a physician from making a *referral* to an entity, such as a hospital, with which the physician has a *financial relationship* for furnishing *DHSs*. If the physician makes such a referral, the hospital may not submit a bill for reimbursement to Medicare.[27]

The *AKS* makes it a criminal offense to knowingly and willfully solicit, receive, offer, or pay any *remuneration* to *induce* or *reward*, among other things, *referrals for*, or *orders of*, items or services reimbursable by a *federal health care program*.[51] When remuneration is paid purposefully to induce or reward referrals of items or services payable by a federal health care program, the *AKS* is violated.

ST. SMITH HOSPITAL

Inpatient and outpatient hospital services are considered DHSs under the law.[20] A referral includes the request by a physician for an item or service.[17] A referral, however, does not include "any designated health service personally performed or provided by the referring physician."[21] Therefore, every time Dr. Jones refers a patient from Life Clinic to St. Smith Hospital for an inpatient service, such as long-term treatment and care, where she personally supervises the long-term treatment and care of such patient at the hospital, Dr. Jones is not making a referral for a DHS under the Stark law. However, there is a catch. There is a referral under the Stark law when St. Smith bills a "facility fee" (also known as a "facility component" or "technical component") in connection with Dr. Jones's personal supervision of long-term treatment and care of her patients at the hospital.

To find for a violation of the Stark law, it is also required to show that Dr. Jones has a financial relationship with the hospital. A financial relationship constitutes a prohibited indirect compensation arrangement if (1) there is an unbroken chain of any number of persons or entities that have a financial relationship between them; (2) the referring physician receives aggregate compensation that varies with, or takes into account, the volume or value of referrals or other business generated by the referring physician for the entity providing the DHSs; and (3) the entity has knowledge that the compensation so varies.[52] Here, Dr. Jones's compensation from the hospital is based on professional services she personally performs or supervises at the hospital and also includes certain benefits, such as paying for her medical liability insurance. As explained earlier, Dr. Jones makes referrals under the Stark law. Here, referrals consist of the "facility component" of the inpatient services that Dr. Jones personally provides to or supervises for her patients and the resulting facility fee billed by the hospital based upon that component. Therefore, the more patients Dr. Jones refers to St. Smith Cancer Hospital for long-term care and treatment, the more facility fees are billed and collected by the hospital, and the more compensation Dr. Jones receives from the hospital in the form of compensation proportional to the personally performed services. Therefore, there is a violation of the Stark law.

The analysis, however, is not so simple and straightforward because the Stark law includes a number of exceptions. For instance, the statute does not bar indirect compensation arrangements where (1) the referring physician is compensated at fair market value for services and items actually provided, (2) the compensation arrangement is not determined in any manner that takes into account the volume or value of referrals, (3) the compensation arrangement is commercially reasonable, and (4) the compensation arrangement does not run afoul of any other federal or state law.[53] In the case of Dr. Jones, if the hospital does not bill a "facility fee" in connection with the professional services Dr. Jones provides or supervises at St. Smith and bills such fee separate from and irrespective of the volume or value of professional services provided by Dr. Jones to her patients at the hospital, then there may not be a violation of the Stark law. This may be the case even though Dr. Jones refers patients from Life Clinic to St. Smith for inpatient services and her compensation from St. Smith is based on the professional services she provides to or supervises for those patients directly. However, for Dr. Jones and the hospital to be in compliance of the Stark law, it is also necessary that her compensation from St. Smith be at a fair market value (i.e., Are the benefits she is getting from the hospital in addition to her compensation based on the services she provides? Do those take her aggregate compensation above the fair market value?) and be commercially reasonable; in addition, it must also not violate any other state or federal laws (e.g., *AKS*).

Dr. Jones's compensation arrangement and referrals to St. Smith Cancer Hospital may also implicate a violation of the *AKS*. Although liability under the *AKS* ultimately turns on *willfulness*, it is possible to identify arrangements or practices that may present a significant potential for abuse.

For analyzing Dr. Jones's arrangement with St. Smith under the *AKS*, the following two inquiries are useful[54]:

- Does St. Smith Cancer Hospital have a remunerative relationship with Dr. Jones, who is in a position to generate federal health care program business for St. Smith directly or indirectly? The answer here is yes. Dr. Jones's compensation from St. Smith is based on the personal professional services she provides at the hospital, which include such services to patients she refers from the outpatient clinic, Life Clinic, to the hospital.
- With respect to Dr. Jones's financial relationship with St. Smith, could one purpose of the remuneration be to induce or reward the referral payable in whole or in part by a federal health care program? The answer here is maybe. Under the AKS, neither a legitimate business purpose for the arrangement nor a fair market value payment will legitimize a payment if there is also an illegal purpose (i.e., inducing federal health care program business). If, for instance, St. Smith Cancer Hospital offered Dr. Jones additional benefits (thereby increasing her aggregate compensation) as an inducement to refer more patients from Life Clinic to St. Smith, such an arrangement would violate the *AKS*.

In short, a simple innocuous-appearing compensation arrangement between a physician and a hospital may implicate a violation of both the *AKS* and the Stark law.

LIFE PHARMACY, LLC

Dr. Jones's referrals to Life Pharmacy for filling of prescription may be found in violation of the Stark law. First, outpatient prescription drugs are considered a DHS.[21] Second, Dr. Jones's son has a financial relationship (shareholder) with the pharmacy, even though Dr. Jones does not have any financial relationship with the pharmacy.[21] Although patients are free to fill prescriptions at any pharmacy, referring patients to Life Pharmacy by offering discounts or by any other means may constitute a violation of the Stark law.

YOUR RECOVERY CENTER, LLC

Dr. Jones's referrals to Your Recover Center, either from St. Smith Hospital or Life Clinic, may violate the Stark law. First, rehabilitation services, such as physical therapy services and occupational therapy services, are considered DHSs. Second, Dr. Jones has a direct financial relationship with Your Recover Center; she is a shareholder in the company.

Dr. Jones's referrals to Your Recovery Center for rehabilitation of her patients may also be a violation of the *AKS*. One purpose of the *AKS* is to protect patients from inappropriate medical referrals or recommendations by health care professional who may be unduly influenced by financial incentives. The opportunity for a referring physician to earn a profit, including through an investment in an entity for which she generates business, could constitute illegal remuneration under the *AKS*. The *AKS* is violated if even one purpose of the remuneration is to induce such referrals. Because Dr. Jones is in a position to generate substantial business for Your Recovery Center and is an investor/shareholder in Your Recovery Center, her relationship with the center will be considered questionable under the *AKS*. This is because her financial interest as a shareholder in Your Recovery Center may induce her to refer patients to Your Recovery Center for physical therapy or occupational therapy that is not medically necessary.

CONCLUSION

The different laws and statutes discussed in this chapter, although they may seem burdensome, are enacted for good reason: to allow health care workers to do what is in the best intertest of a patient. Unfortunately, the laws are complex and necessitate that a health care worker be vigilant of legal aspects of practice of oncology, in addition to treatment and management of a disease or a condition. The resources discussed in this chapter are a good starting point when entering in a business or employment relationship to make sure no laws are broken inadvertently. When in doubt, seek legal counsel.

KEY POINTS:

- The AKS makes it illegal to knowingly and willfully solicit or receive remuneration in return of prescribing drugs or services (or making a referral) that are paid for by a federal health care program.
- Actual knowledge or intent to violate the AKS is not required to show that a violation of the AKS has occurred.
- A health care worker providing services that are covered by a federal health care program is presumed to have the knowledge of the AKS and must comply with it.
- Remuneration has a broad scope and includes anything of value, received directly or indirectly, overtly or covertly, in cash or in kind (e.g., free meals, paid speaking positions, memberships to clubs).
- A referral made in exchange of remuneration is sufficient for finding a violation of the AKS even if the referred services are not actually provided.
- An AKS violation is found if one purpose of a remuneration is to induce referrals, even if the primary purpose of a business relationship is to compensate for a legitimate professional service.
- A federal health care program for the purpose of AKS violation may include state health care programs.
- The OIG and its AOs provide guidance on business relationships that may implicate an AKS violation. When in doubt, review the OIG's AOs or seek an AO specific to your situation.
- The Physician Self-Referral Law (Stark law) prohibits a physician from referring a patient to an entity in which the physician or an immediate family member of the physician has a financial interest for fulfillment of a DHS.
- Referral under the Stark law includes any request by a physician for an item or service but excludes a DHS personally performed or provided by the referring physician.
- A DHS provider entity may not bill Medicare, Medicaid, an individual, a third-party payor, or any other entity for the DHS provided under a prohibited referral.
- DHSs range from clinical laboratory services to outpatient prescription drugs. The CMS maintains and annually updates lists that identify all items and services included within DHSs.
- Financial interest for the purpose of the Stark law includes ownership or investment interest or a compensation arrangement.
- The CMS provides tools and AOs on which referrals may (or may not) violate the Stark law.
- Both the AKS and the Stark law include a range of exceptions (safe harbors) to allow for legitimate professional interests.
- The Right to Try Act exempts physicians from liability unless they engage in reckless or willful misconduct, are grossly negligent, or commit an intentional tort.
- Off-label drug use does not exempt physicians from standard of care and informed consent requirements.

References:

1. 42 USC § 1320a-7b(b)(1)(A).
2. 42 USC § 1320a-7b(h).
3. *United States v St. Junius*, 739 F3d 193, 210 (5th Cir 2013).
4. Garner B. *Black's Law Dictionary*, 9th ed. McLean, VA: West Group; 2009:1409.
5. *United States v Goldman*, 607 F App'x 171, *4 (3d Cir 2015); *United States v Vernon*, 723 F3d 1234, 1253 (11th Cir 2013).
6. *Hanlester Network, et al, v Shalala*, 51 F3d 1390, 1401-1402 (9th Cir 1995).
7. *United States v Hong*, 938 F3d 1040, 1049 (9th Cir 2019).
8. *United States v Kats*, 871 F.2d 105, 109 (9th Cir 1989).
9. *United States v Greber*, 760 F2d 68, 71 (3d Cir 1985).
10. *United States v Kats*, 871 F2d 105, 108 (9th Cir 1989).
11. 42 USC § 1320a-7b(f).
12. 42 CFR § 1001.952.
13. Safe harbor regulations. Office of Inspector General, US Department of Health and Human Services. https://oig.hhs.gov/compliance/safe-harbor-regulations/index.asp. Accessed August 12, 2021.
14. Advisory opinions. Office of Inspector General, US Department of Health and Human Services. https://oig.hhs.gov/compliance/advisory-opinions/index.asp. Accessed August 12, 2021.
15. 42 USC § 1395nn(a)(1)(A).
16. 42 USC § 1395nn(a)(1)(B).
17. 42 USC § 1395nn(h)(5)(A).
18. 42 USC § 1395nn(h)(5)(B).
19. 42 USC § 1395nn(h)(5)(C).
20. 42 USC § 1395nn(h)(6).
21. 42 CFR § 411.351.
22. Code list for certain designated health services (DHS). Centers for Medicare and Medicaid Services. https://www.cms.gov/Medicare/Fraud-and-Abuse/PhysicianSelfReferral/List_of_Codes. Accessed August 12, 2021.
23. 42 USC § 1395nn(a)(2)(A).
24. 42 USC § 1395nn(a)(2)(A)(B).
25. 42 USC § 1395nn(h)(1)(B).
26. 42 USC § 1395nn(h)(1)(C).
27. 42 USC § 1395nn(a)(1).
28. 42 USC § 1395nn(b).
29. 42 USC § 1395nn(c).
30. 42 USC § 1395nn(d).
31. 42 USC § 1395nn(e).
32. 42 CFR § 411.357(p) (indirect compensation arrangement); 42 CFR § 411.357(a)-(b) (rental of office space and equipment); 42 CFR § 411.357(d) (personal service arrangements); 42 CFR § 411.357(e) (physician recruitment).
33. Advisory opinions (AOs). Centers for Medicare and Medicaid Services. https://www.cms.gov/Medicare/Fraud-and-Abuse/PhysicianSelfReferral/advisory_opinions. Accessed August 12, 2021.
34. Call center. Centers for Medicare and Medicaid Services. https://www.cms.gov/Medicare/Fraud-and-Abuse/PhysicianSelfReferral/Call-Center.
35. 21 USC § 360bbb-0a. Accessed August 12, 2021.
36. Lynch HF, Sarpatwari A, Vonderheide RH, Zettler PJ. Right to try requests and oncologists' gatekeeping obligations. *J Clin Oncol*. 2020;38(2)111–114.
37. Pub L 115-176, §2(b), May 30, 2018, 132 Stat 1374.
38. 21 USC § 360bbb-0a(a)(1)(A); 21 CFR § 312.81(a).
39. 21 USC § 360bbb-0a(a)(1)(B).
40. 21 USC § 360bbb-0a(a)(2).

41. *United States v Evers*, 643 F2d 1043 (5th Cir 1981).
42. *Buckman Co. v Plaintiffs' Legal Committee*, 531 US 341 (2001).
43. McCafferty J, Grover K, Li L, et al. A systematic analysis of off-label drug use in real-world data (RWD) across more than 145,000 cancer patients. *J Clin Oncol*. 2019;37(15 suppl):e18031.
44. Saiyed MM, Ong PS, Chew L. Off-label drug use in oncology: a systematic review of literature. *J Clin Pharm Ther*. 2017;42(3):251–258.
45. Conti RM, Bernstein AC, Villaflor VM, Schilsky RL, Rosenthal MB, Bach PB. Prevalence of off-label use and spending in 2010 among patent-protected chemotherapies in a population-based cohort of medical oncologists. *J Clin Oncol*. 2013;31(9):1134–1139.
46. Lim M, Shulman DS, Roberts H, et al. Off-label prescribing of targeted anticancer therapy at a large pediatric cancer center. *Cancer Med*. 2020;9(18):6658–6666.
47. Mithani Z. Informed consent for off-label use of prescription medications. *Virtual Mentor*. 2012;14(7):576–581.
48. Meadows WA, Hollowell BD. "Off-label" drug use: an FDA regulatory term, not a negative implication of its medical use. *Int J Impot Res*. 2008;20(2):135–144.
49. *United States v Nagelvoort*, 856 F3d 1117 (7th Cir 2017).
50. *United States ex rel. Bartlett v Ashcroft*, 39 F Supp 3d 656 (WD Pa 2014).
51. 42 USC § 1320a-7b(b)(1)-(2).
52. 42 CFR § 411.354 (c)(2).
53. 42 CFR § 411.357(p).
54. Office of Inspector General. OIG supplemental compliance program guidance for hospitals. *Fed Reg*. 2005;70: 4858, 4864.

CHAPTER 14

Primary Care Provider's Responsibility in Cancer Care

Santos Ruiz-Cordero, MD, JD, FCLM, Deni Malavé-Huertas, MD, and Johnson Wong, DO

INTRODUCTION

Family physicians are the medical practitioners who are specially trained to provide health care to all individuals regardless of age, sex, or type of health problem. They provide primary and continued care for the whole family in their communities. They tend to physical, psychological, and social problems as well as coordinate comprehensive health care with other specialties as needed. They are also known as a family physicians or generalists in different countries.[1]

According to the National Cancer Institute's Dictionary of Cancer Terms, a primary care doctor is one who manages a person's health over time. A primary care doctor is capable of providing a wide range of care, including prevention and treatment. This can include discussion of treatment options for cancer and referral of patients to specialists.[2]

Family medicine is the medical specialty concerned with providing comprehensive care to individuals and families, integrating biomedical, behavioral, and social sciences. It is an academic medical discipline that includes comprehensive systems of health care, education, and research.[2]

Current patient care has evolved greatly. With constant changes in the provision of medical services and medical care and the increase in intermediaries, the primary care of the patient does not fall solely on doctors (allopathic or osteopathic doctors). The term *provider* is now applied to individuals providing such care and, hence, its use in the chapter's title. These denominated "mid-level providers" are now partly responsible for providing primary care. Changes in the practice of medicine have also contributed to the increase in participation of mid-level providers in the system. Among these changes are the prominent part of paying intermediaries of health service, the increase in shortages in certain geographical areas of primary care physicians, and changes in delivery of medical care. The mid-level practitioner has been more and more present, out of necessity in some cases and for economic considerations in others, taking a prominent or principal role in the delivery of primary care to patients in our society. These mid-level practitioners include nurse practitioners (certified advanced registered nurse practitioners [ARNP-C]) and physician assistants (PAs). Depending on jurisdiction, these health care professionals have more or less autonomy when it comes to providing primary medical care, either supervised or unsupervised. As a result, they can be solely responsible for the primary care of patients. In this chapter, we will outline how this provider-patient relationship evolves into a professional responsibility of the physician/provider from a legal point of view. We will try to focus on the responsibility of the physician, from the point of view of a traditional and increasingly less frequent service delivery model that is directed by physicians. We will use the word *provider* except when discussing *vicarious responsibility* and the *agent model*, where the mid-level practitioners (ARNP or PA) are employees of a physician or medical group.

We will mainly focus on situations in which the primary physician is exposed to legal medical liability scenarios related to different types of cancer prevention or diagnosis.

There are several important notions to keep in mind about a primary care physician or practice. First, we need to keep in mind that the primary care provider is the initial contact for an ill patient. This occurs by tradition or as mandated by medical insurance companies' protocols and requirements. Primary care providers will then determine whether to manage the patient themselves or refer the patient to another specialist. Health insurance companies can drive this by either persuasive or incentivizing measures. For example, health maintenance organization (HMO) plans will require the patient to be referred by the primary care provider in order to receive evaluation and management by other specialists. In other instances, the medical insurance company will allow unlimited evaluations by primary physicians without the need for a deductible (co-payment) but require such additional expenses for evaluation by other specialists. This all leads to patient screening by a primary care physician before evaluation by other specialists.

Primary care practices are regulated and thoroughly scrutinized. Providers are evaluated and rated by multiple different algorithms and metrics. Some examples include the Healthcare Effectiveness Data and Information Set (HEDIS) score, the Consumer Assessment of Health Care Providers and Systems (CAHPS), and the Medicare Reimbursement Adjustment (MRA). The Centers for Medicare and Medicaid Services (CMS) contracted with the National Committee for Quality Assurance (NCQA) to develop strategies to oversee the quality of care given by a Special Needs Plan (SNPs). These same criteria have been adopted by other health care intermediaries such as Medicare Advantage and commercial insurance plans. As a result, if a physician wants to remain competitive in today's primary care environment, the physician must maintain acceptable scores (>4 on a base of 0–5). These measures were created to fulfill a commendable goal and provide better health care to the patient. Often, these regulations defeat their own purpose. Examples of these measurements include patient wait times in the provider's office, use of high-risk medications, after-hospital follow-up visits, and others. This is the most common system used in the managed care model of primary care system. Managed care is a health care delivery system organized to manage cost, utilization, and quality. Medicaid managed care provides for the delivery of Medicaid health benefits and additional services through contracted arrangements between state Medicaid agencies and managed care organizations (MCOs) that accept a set per-member-per-month (capitation) payment for these services.[3] Complying with the measures described can be time consuming and can inadvertently negatively affect patient care. A provider can be torn between spending time meeting metrics versus spending time providing patient care. This is common in larger, high-patient-volume practices.

Finally, consider that medical insurance companies discourage spending by primary care providers on their patients. A primary care provider receives a rating based on utilization of resources. The more the insurance company spends on referrals and tests, the lower the rating is for that physician.

LIABILITY OF THE FAMILY CARE PHYSICIAN

There are two important terms that we need to remember related to cancer: detection and diagnosis. Even when highly suspected cancer signs or symptoms, injuries, or "syndromes" are found, the definitive diagnosis of cancer requires histopathologic studies. It is rarely the responsibility of the primary care professional to perform such histopathologic studies. Detection, on the other hand, can be achieved in two different ways by a primary care provider. The first relies on screenings, which are based on recommendations by different organizations (also known as guidelines). These guidelines consider a patient's personal and family history, triggering testing accordingly. The second way relies on clinical suspicion based on the patient's symptomatology or clinical findings. Some cancers do not present symptomatology until very advanced stages, and others present nonspecific symptoms. Often, symptoms are subtle and difficult to identify by both doctors and patients. Both modes of detection can increase utilization of resources and can create backlash for providers. Also, keep in mind that screening tests are not diagnostic and require diagnostic tests or procedures to confirm diagnosis.

In the following section, some of the general recommendations and/or guidelines for primary health providers and how these can create medicolegal liability situations are discussed. The most common guidelines and recommendations for primary health providers given by the American Cancer Society are covered. It is important to mention that failure to diagnose cancer is the most common malpractice claim brought against internists and family practitioners, and failure to diagnose breast cancer is the most common of these claims.[4]

CANCER SCREENING AND EARLY DETECTION

Breast cancer

Breast cancer is the most common cancer in women and the second leading cause of cancer death.[5] The physician should offer patients the option to begin annual mammography screening for breast cancer after 40 years of age, with thorough discussion of associated risks and benefits. Women aged 45 to 54 years old should be offered mammography annually. Women aged 55 and older may opt to receive mammograms every one to two years.

Regular mammograms or cancer screenings should continue as long as a woman is in good health or has a life expectancy of ten years or more.

The imaging tool recommendation can vary depending on medical, genetic, and family history, as well as other factors, and can include mammogram, magnetic resonance imaging (MRI), and/or ultrasound.

Colon cancer

Colon cancer is the third most common cancer in men and the second most common cancer in women and the third leading cause of death from cancer in both sexes. For patients with average risk of colon cancer, it is recommended by the American Cancer Society to start screening at age 45. Recommendations include either sensitive tests that detect signs of cancer in the patient's stools (stool-based test) or visual tests (colonoscopy). The stool-based test is a screening test, whereas a colonoscopy is both a screening and diagnostic test.

Patients in good health should continue to undergo testing until age 75. Between the ages of 76 and 85 years, the decision should be made on a case-by-case basis with the physician or provider, based on the patient's preferences, patient's health condition, and results of previous studies. After age 85, the consensus is that routine testing is not recommended.

It is important to remember that any positive test that is not visual should be followed by visual test (colonoscopy).

Cervical cancer

The screening for cervical cancer should begin at 21 years. Between the ages of 21 and 29 years, female patients should have cervical cytology (Papanicolaou [Pap] smear) done every three years. The human papillomavirus (HPV) test should not be used in this age group unless it is necessary based on an abnormal Pap result.

Between the ages of 30 and 65, patients can have either cervical cytology (Pap smear) with HPV every five years or cervical cytology every three years. Women over the age of 65 who have had normal results over the past ten years should not be routinely evaluated for cervical cancer.

Patients who have had results with pre-carcinogenic findings are recommended to continue routine testing for 20 years, even if this time period extends past the patient age of 65 years.

Patients who have had a total hysterectomy (uterus and cervix removed) for reasons that are unrelated to cervical cancer or who do not have a history of cervical cancer or precarcinogenic lesions do not require further screening.

Women who have received HPV vaccines are advised to continue their testing according to their age group.

Endometrial cancer

Endometrial cancer is the third most common cancer in women and the sixth leading cause of cancer death. Women who have undergone menopause and experience vaginal bleeding should be screened for endometrial cancer with ultrasound and/or hysteroscopy with biopsy. Patients with medical problems, such as endometrial hyperplasia, should consider undergoing endometrial biopsies annually.

Lung cancer

Lung cancer is the second most common cancer in men and women and the leading cause of cancer mortality in both sexes. It is recommended that patients between the ages of 55 and 74 years who are in good health, who are smokers or have stopped smoking within the past 15 years, and who have at least a 30-pack-year smoking history are recommended to have a low-dose computed tomography (CT) scan performed annually. Pack-year is a way to measure the amount a person has smoked over a long period of time. It is calculated by multiplying the number of packs of cigarettes smoked per day by the number of years the person has smoked. For example, one pack-year is equal to smoking one pack per day for one year or two packs per day for half a year, and so on.[6]

Prostate cancer

Prostate cancer is the most common cancer diagnosed in males. Currently, studies have failed to demonstrate whether the potential benefit of testing outweighs the harm of testing and treatment for prostate cancer. That said, the primary care provider should discuss with the patient the risks and benefits of performing the tests before ordering them. If agreed upon, testing can start at age 50 years.

In African American patients with a family history of a father or brother with prostate cancer before age 65, it is recommended that tests begin at age 45 once the patient understands the risks, benefits, and alternatives.

If testing is done, it is recommended to perform prostate-specific antigen (PSA) measurement, with or without a digital rectal examination (DRE). However, there is no clear benefit to performing DRE.

CLINICAL VIGNETTE # 1

Dr. Bettercare is a solo primary care provider with a busy private practice. A 67-year-old male patient presents to Dr. Bettercare's practice as a new patient. He has a history of hypertension and high cholesterol and a body mass index (BMI) of 31. His social history includes tobacco use of 1 pack per day for 35 years. Based on his history, Dr. Bettercare ordered blood tests and a chest x-ray. The chest x-ray reported emphysematous changes and a nodule located in the right superior lobe, measuring 0.7 cm, and a low-dose CT scan to better characterize the nodule was recommended. Dr. Bettercare did not order the CT because the nodule was less than 1 cm and decided to reassess the patient at the next appointment. The next appointment was scheduled for six months later, but Dr. Bettercare had an emergency, and the patient's visit was postponed for another three months. On the next visit, Dr. Bettercare recommended repeating the chest x-ray, which reported the nodule as measuring 0.9 cm and recommended a chest CT. The report from the CT scan indicated that the nodule actually measured 1.1 cm and recommended a biopsy.

The radiologist called Dr. Bettercare's office, but Dr. Bettercare was not available, so the radiologist left a message indicated that he wanted to discuss the findings with Dr. Bettercare. The receptionist lost the message inadvertently. About two weeks before the patient's follow-up appointment, he became ill with a cold, had an episode of hemoptysis, and called Dr. Bettercare's office. At this point, Dr. Bettercare became aware of the CT report and decided to order a new CT and to follow up with the patient in two weeks. At the follow-up, the patient was not feeling any better and had experienced a ten-lb weight loss. The CT scan was done the day before the visit, and on that same afternoon, the radiologist called Dr. Bettercare to tell him personally that the CT scan showed a mass that was now 2.1 cm and a new adjacent lesion of 1.2 cm. A subsequent biopsy confirmed lung cancer with metastasis to the liver. The patient underwent treatment, but unfortunately, he died four months later. The patient's family sued Dr. Bettercare, the staff members who did not give Dr. Bettercare the results of the CT scan on time, and the radiologist for medical negligence. The family was awarded $4 million in financial compensation for the patient's negligent/wrongful death attributed only to Dr. Bettercare.

An analysis of the reasons why Dr. Bettercare is responsible for the patient's death can include that the patient was a victim of a delay in treatment because of the failure to diagnose cancer at an early stage. This is a direct result of Dr. Bettercare's failure to follow standards of care. Such standards are provided by several organizations, such as the American Cancer Society. The guidelines recommend "that patients between the ages of 55 and 74 who are in good health and who are smokers or have stopped smoking with in the past 15 years and who have a history of at least 30 years of smoking with one pack per year are to have low dose CT scan performed annually." Not following these recommendations is a negligent act on the part of Dr. Bettercare and one that makes him liable. Staff members who were sued are not responsible in this situation because their acts were not intentional or criminal, and the lack of supervision and diligence of these employees is the responsibility of Dr. Bettercare as their employer agent, under the doctrine of *respondeat superior*. This is a legal doctrine, most commonly used in court, that holds an employer legally responsible for the wrongful acts of an employee or agent if such acts occur within the scope of the employment or agency. Typically, when *respondeat superior* is invoked, a plaintiff will look to hold both the employer and the employee liable. As such, a court will generally look to the doctrine of joint and several liability when assigning damages.[8]

In this case, based solely on the patient's smoking history, Dr. Bettercare should have ordered a low-dose CT scan as recommended by guidelines. If not on the first occasion, he should have definitely done it on the second visit. Similarly important, he should have made sure to track the results and/or develop a system in his office through which all communications from other doctors would be delivered to him urgently and that ensured that no results would be filed in a patient's chart without them being previously evaluated by the doctor or a qualified medical provider, even if the results are within normal limits.

CLINICAL VIGNETTE # 2

Ms. Susisue is a 47-year-old female patient of Dr. Munzinger, who is a general practitioner. The patient has a history of common colds, one episode of a sexually transmitted disease (STD), and a prior history of HPV. At her routine follow-up appointment, the patient complained to Dr. Munzinger about having some occasional postcoital bleeding and some vaginal discomfort. Dr. Munzinger decided to order a urinalysis, other tests for STDs, and a Pap smear. All results were negative, except the Pap smear, which reported "vaginal epithelial cells present with minimal contamination of red blood cells in the background. Moderate numbers of squamous epithelial cells admixed with a mixed cellular infiltrate composed mostly of neutrophils and rare macrophages and lymphocytes." Dr. Munzinger told the patient that her labs came back normal and that she has mild inflammation, which was the reason for the discomfort and bleeding. Several months later, the patient experienced the same symptoms. She returned for evaluation, and Dr. Munzinger stated that since her symptoms are similar and she has had no change in her health status, she does not need to worry. The patient asked about a referral to a gynecologist, but Dr. Munzinger told her it was not necessary. She continued complaining of the same symptoms intermittently for another two years, but her complaints were dismissed by Dr. Munzinger as inflammation. The symptoms did not improve, and the patient developed new symptoms of weight loss, dyspnea, and increased postcoital bleeding. She decided to seek a second opinion and paid out of pocket for a gynecologic evaluation. The gynecologist performed a Pap smear and a biopsy, which demonstrated cervical cancer. A positron emission tomography (PET) scan showed metastases to the lungs, and International Federation of Gynecology and Obstetrics stage IVB cervical cancer was confirmed. The patient sued Dr. Munzinger for medical malpractice alleging that she was not diagnosed on time and Dr. Munzinger failed to refer her to a gynecologist.

Primary care providers need to understand the scope of their practice and need to be vigilant in all the areas in which they are practicing. A primary care provider who manages a woman's health needs to be proficient in cervical cytology collection and result interpretation. In this case, Dr. Munzinger needed to be suspicions of cervical cancer since the patient had a prior history of HPV. HPV is one of the most common risk factors for cervical cancer. In addition, the patient was in the age range when cervical cancer is mostly commonly diagnosed. Finally, Dr. Munzinger should have recognized the inadequacy of sample collection with the reported vaginal cells but no cervical cells identified in the sample. This should have prompted repeat cervical cytology. Furthermore, if a patient's gynecologic symptoms persist even in the presence of a normal Pap smear (this was not the case), the primary care provider should refer the patient for further evaluation by a gynecologist. At that time, a gynecologist would have recognized the inadequate cervical sample and repeated the Pap smear. In this situation, Dr. Munzinger was negligent.

CONCLUSION

Our recommendation is always to practice evidence-based medicine. Regardless of the possible medical insurance penalties for the use of resources, it is better to order testing or treatment based on medical recommendations or guidelines. A delay in diagnosis or failure to diagnose cancer can lead to suffering, permanent damage, or death. It is also important to remember that in certain jurisdictions, in cases where it is proven that no treatment or diagnostic test was ordered for a patient and that the decision to omit the test or treatment was based on a financial interest of the provider, a case of ordinary negligence may change to gross negligence ("what is a 1. A lack of slight diligence or care. 2. A conscious, voluntary act or omission in reckless disregard of a legal duty and the consequences to another to another party, who may typically recover exemplary damages. Also termed reckless negligence; wanton negligence; willful negligence; willful and wanton negligence; hazardous negligence; *magna neglegentia*"[9]) or culpable negligence ("negligent conduct that while not intentional, involves a disregard of the consequences likely to result from one's actions . . . 'Culpable negligence,' while variously defined, has been held incapable of exact definition; it means something more than negligence . . . The word 'culpable' is sometimes used in the sense of 'blamable,' and it has been regarded as expressing the thought of a breach of a duty of the commission of a fault, but culpable negligence has been held to amount to more than blameworthy conduct . . . It does not involve the element of intent . . . On the other hand, it has been said to be intentional conduct which the actor may not intend to be harmful but which an ordinary and reasonably prudent man would recognize as involving a strong probability of injury to others"[10]). In addition, a criminal indictment will be added to civil proceedings that may result in financial loss for the medical provider and in the loss of his or her freedom.

The primary care provider needs to be aware of the patient's health conditions and any other medical manifestations of disease and cancers that may occur. In the vast majority of cases in primary health, providers are responsible for detecting or not detecting (which is the biggest problem of liability) cancer, either by incidental findings or by identification through labs or physical examination. The physician should always be up to date on new scientific findings related to cancer and other health care conditions to either educate or treat the patient. Not only should the different types of cancer be evaluated and looked for using routine prevention screenings but those screening tests should be followed and interpreted as discussed. In addition, there are other types of cancer that should be considered and for which patients should be evaluated, even if they are not part of prevention guidelines. Examples of these are skin melanoma, non-Hodgkin lymphoma, kidney cancer, bladder cancer, uterine cancer, thyroid cancer, pancreatic cancer, leukemias, and others less frequent pathologies.[6] If a provider does not have the necessary continuity in medical education and does not have those diagnoses in mind when evaluating symptomatology and test results, the provider may miss the diagnosis until such a time that the provider may have incurred medical negligence and responsibility. Thus, providers need to be aware of a patient's risk factors for certain cancers, such as cigarette smoking for lung cancer, alcohol consumption for head and neck cancer, chemical exposures for certain cancers, and so on.

In recent years, the media has often reported on the link between cancer and frequently used products, such as herbicides (discussed in other chapters of this book), and drugs, such as ranitidine, which have been recalled or withdrawn from the market. As mentioned previously, the primary care physician is usually the one who first educates the patient and hears a patient's concerns about this information in the media. Primary care physicians need to be informed and up to date regarding what is being published in the media and its relation to health care.

KEY POINTS[11]:

- -

- Always document in patient's medical chart all the important details of tests and referrals, when they were discussed with the patient, and the plan of care.
- Explain to the patient when a test is of great importance and the risks of doing or not doing it. For example, "Mr. X, it is really important to do your chest CT scan because your history of significant long-term smoking and your symptoms put you at higher risk of having lung cancer."
- Follow up on the tests and results. It is impossible to remember every order for every patient. Be sure that you review your prior notes to refresh your mind and be sure you have all the tests you ordered.
- If there is any abnormal test result, be sure that you communicate the result to your patient and document the communication in the chart with the time and date. If you are not able to communicate with your patient by phone, send a certified letter to the patient's last known address, save a copy in the chart, and record when it was sent.
- If you discussed your patient case with a specialist, document that on the patient chart with the time, date, specialist name, and a brief summary of what was discussed.
- *Never alter records!*
- Take all patient complaints seriously and avoid the perception that you know the patient well and the patient is not experiencing what they say they are experiencing.
- Always perform a thorough physical examination with emphasis on the patient's actual complaint.
- Be sure to review the patient's prior medical, social, and family history. Patients may not be predisposed to certain types of conditions, such as cancer, by age, race, sex, or family history but might be predisposed by social history.
- When you have doubts about a test result or image reading, repeat the test or call the performing specialist (radiologist or other specialist).
- If you have a doubt about the diagnosis, the response to treatment is not as expected, or the condition is beyond your scope of practice, refer the patient to the proper specialist.
- Order tests, referrals, or services based on a patient's needs and not on the insurance company's preferences, patient or family request, or any other reason.
- Always tell the truth to the patient and practice evidence-based medicine. You can be cost-effective and comply with all the measures required by insurance companies and CMS and still practice good, honest, and safe medicine. Patient health and well-being are what is important.

References:

1. Kidd M, Haq C, De Maeseneer J, et al. *The Contribution of Family Medicine to Improving Health System: A Guidebook from the World Organization of Family Doctors.* New York, NY: Taylor & Francis; 2020.
2. Primary care doctor. National Cancer Institute. https://www.cancer.gov/publications/dictionaries/cancer-terms/def/primary-care-doctor. Accessed August 13, 2021.
3. Managed care. Centers for Medicare and Medicaid Services. https://www.medicaid.gov/medicaid/managed-care/index.html. Accessed August 14, 2021.

4. American College of Legal Medicine. *The Medical Malpractice Survival Handbook.* Philadelphia, PA: Mosby Elsevier; 2007:299–310.

5. Siegel RL, Miller KD, Jemal A. Cancer statistics, 2019. *CA Cancer J Clin.* 2019;69:7–34.

6. Estimated new cancer cases and deaths for 2020. Table 1.1. National Cancer Institute. https://seer.cancer.gov/archive/csr/1975_2017/results_merged/sect_01_overview.pdf. Accessed August 14, 2021.

7. Pack year. National Cancer Institute. cancer.gov/publications/dictionaries/cancer-terms/def/pack-year. Accessed August 14, 2021.

8. *Respondeat superior.* Legal Information Institute. law.cornell.edu/wex/respondeat_superior. Accessed August 14, 2021.

9. Garner BA. *Black's Law Dictionary.* 9th ed. Cleveland, OH: West Publishing; 2009.

10. 65 CJS Negligence § 1 (13) (1996).

11. Hawkins KA. Family practice and internal medicine. In: American College of Legal Medicine, ed. *The Medical Malpractice Survival Handbook.* Philadelphia, PA: Mosby Elsevier; 2007:299–310.

CHAPTER 15

Dental/Oral Surgery

Jenny L. Wong, DMD, MD, Thanh T. Ton, DDS, MS, MPH,
Bruce H. Seidberg, DDS, MScD, JD, DABE, FCLM, FACD, and Becky Bye, DDS, JD, FCLM

INTRODUCTION

Head and neck cancers are a significant public health concern. The United States alone reports approximately 46,000 new head and neck cancers each year, with an estimated 10,000 deaths from these cancers.[1] From a medicolegal perspective, delayed or missed diagnosis of oral malignant diseases, particularly the highly metastatic oral squamous cell carcinomas, can result in sizable damages claims. This is due to the impact of oral cancer on the cost of medical care, pain and suffering, possible disfigurement, lost income, impact on the quality of life, and possible loss of life.[2] Plaintiffs' recovery for dental malpractice lawsuits based on oral cancer can range from $1.03 million to $3.5 million, with failure to perform a biopsy or failure to refer being common allegations in dental negligence litigation.[2,3]

Long-term oral complications can arise in cancer survivors, such as osteonecrosis of the jaw, which includes medication-related osteonecrosis of the jaw (MRONJ) and osteoradionecrosis (ORN).[2] Osteonecrosis is a severe complication associated with cancer treatments, including radiation and cancer medication. Osteonecrosis is defined as the death of bone cells and structure due to decreased blood flow and can present in dentistry when the jawbone is exposed.[4,5] Most osteonecrosis cases occur after invasive dental procedures, such as tooth extractions. Osteonecrosis is a leading cause of potential morbidity and mortality in surviving cancer patients, and its complications are commonly involved in dental malpractice litigation.[2,5]

This highlights the need for health care practitioners to recognize and identify head and neck premalignant and malignant diseases through continuous training and education, in order to prevent and manage cancer growth and potential complications resulting from head and neck cancer therapy. It is essential to develop appropriate approaches to achieve a more definitive oral cancer diagnosis and to create strategies to prevent osteonecrosis in cancer survivors. Where there is an uncommon or unusual presentation of a disease or complication, dental and other health care providers should consult with other dental specialists or refer to medical providers who have additional training and experience.

COMMON LEGAL ISSUES RELATED TO HEAD AND NECK CANCER DIAGNOSIS

Delayed diagnosis of oral squamous cell carcinoma and head and neck cancers

Head and neck cancers are often at an advanced stage when initially diagnosed. Either patient delay or professional delay can cause such a delay in diagnosis.[6] Patient delay in diagnosis refers to the period between the onset of the patient's symptoms and the patient receiving an initial professional evaluation.[7,8] The delay by the dental professional is defined as the time between the dentist's first consultation with the patient and the date of the histopathologic diagnosis, including if and when no treatment or inappropriate treatment has occurred.[9,10] The greater the delay in diagnosis and later the onset of treatment, the more advanced is the stage of cancer, necessitating more aggressive therapy and resulting in a poorer prognosis.[11,12] Therefore, delays in diagnosis are the leading cause of why most patients are in the advanced stages (III and IV) when their diagnoses are finally made.

Oral squamous cell carcinoma

More than 90% of head and neck cancers are oral squamous cell carcinomas (OSCCs).[12,13] OSCC is a type of cancer that occurs between the vermilion border of the lips and the junction of the hard and soft palates or the posterior one-third of the tongue.[14] In the United States, OSCC affects approximately 34,000 people each year and composes 3% of cancers in men and 2% in women.[14] OSCC generally occurs in people over the age of 50 and in those who smoke and consume alcohol.[12,14,15] The combination of tobacco and alcohol use poses a 15-fold increased risk of oral cancer for users compared to nonusers.[16] Squamous cell carcinoma of the tongue may result from any chronic irritation, such as dental decay, overuse of mouthwash, chewing tobacco, or the use of betel quid.[14] Squamous cell carcinomas of the vermillion border of the lips are related to sun exposure.[14] OSCC is also linked to the human papillomavirus (HPV), but not to the same extent as compared to oropharyngeal cancer.[17] Future studies are needed to investigate the mechanisms of how HPV infection causes HPV-positive OSCCs and whether the HPV vaccine helps prevent OSCCs.[17]

Treatment for OSCC includes surgery, radiation, chemotherapy, or a combination of thereof.[14,18] Despite advances in cancer diagnosis and treatment, the overall five-year survival rate for OSCC remains the lowest among head and neck malignancies.[19] The clinical stage (tumor-node-metastasis [TNM] stage) at diagnosis influences the survival and prognosis of oral cancer patients. Sixty to 65% of patients present in TNM stages III and IV at the time of OSCC diagnosis.[20,21] Diagnosis delays of more than one month were reported to contribute to the diagnosis of advanced stages of the disease.[22–24] Patients with localized disease have a greater than 80% five-year survival rate compared to a five-year survival rate of less than 30% in patients with advanced disease.[25,26] In advanced oral cancers, reconstructive surgery may be required.[18]

Clinical signs and symptoms

OSCC can arise anywhere in the oral cavity, including the lips, tongue, upper and lower gingiva, oral floor, palate, and buccal mucosa.[27,28] Early, curable lesions are rarely symptomatic. In its early stages, OSCC can go unnoticed, and patients may have little to no discomfort.[2] OSCC can start initially as a painless lesion but may develop into a burning sensation or pain when it becomes more advanced, invading the deeper muscles and jawbone.[6,27] Pain and other symptoms, such as numbness, hoarseness, or dysphagia, are not frequently present unless the patient has advanced disease.[29,30] OSCC can negatively affect patients' chewing, swallowing, speech, and dental aesthetics, worsening their quality of life.[28] Therefore, OSCC requires early detection, which can be accomplished by routine oral screenings and a comprehensive record of any signs and symptoms at each dental exam visit.

Intraoral exam

A visual and tactile intraoral examination is essential for detection of OSCC and other cancers. The usual presentation of OSCC is an ulcer with fissuring or raised exophytic margins.[27] OSCC may present as a lump or as a nonhealing extraction site.[27,31] OSCC may also present as precancerous lesions in the oral cavity, such as red lesions (erythroplakia), white lesions (leukoplakia), or mixed white and red lesions.[27] High-risk sites are the ventral part of the tongue and floor of the mouth.[29,31] OSCC should be considered when any of these features persist for more than two weeks.

Extraoral exam

A thorough extraoral exam is important to identify abnormalities. OSCC tends to cause cervical lymph node metastasis because the lymphatic vessels in the oral cavity are rich and comprise numerous anastomoses.[32] Lymph nodes should be palpated to determine if there is lymphadenopathy. Invasive OCSS can present as a cervical lymph node enlargement, characterized by hardness or fixation.[27] Lymph nodes should be assessed by location, size, and texture and by whether they are tender or nontender or mobile or fixed.[29] Trismus and facial asymmetry may indicate infiltration of muscle and other adjacent structures.[29]

Misdiagnosis

OSCC may be misdiagnosed on clinical examination as reactive or inflammatory lesions such as frictional keratosis (e.g., bite trauma, benign alveolar ridge keratosis), traumatic ulcerations, contact desquamation, and lichen planus.[33] As such, any lesion of unclear etiology that has not responded to treatment or intervention or resolved in two weeks should elicit suspicion and be promptly biopsied. If a dental practitioner is not comfortable performing a biopsy or is unsure of the best area to sample, a referral to an oral medicine specialist, oral pathologist, or oral surgeon may be helpful.[31,33]

Diagnostic tests

The gold standard for oral cancer diagnosis remains incisional biopsy of the tissue from the suspicious tumor and histopathologic examination.[34] In half of the legal cases involving head and neck cancers, biopsies were allegedly indicated but not performed.[2] Diagnostic imaging evaluation of either computed tomography (CT) or magnetic resonance imaging (MRI) is necessary to assess the extent of local and regional tumor spread, the depth of invasion, and the degree of lymphadenopathy.[34] CT is superior in detecting early bone invasion and lymph node metastasis. MRI is still preferred for assessing the extent of soft tissue involvement and providing a three-dimensional display of the tumor.[34] One or both of these tests may be necessary since each can provide different information concerning the extent of the malignancy.

CASE LAW # 1

In *Leone v Bauman*,[35] a jury awarded the plaintiff $2.1 million for facial disfigurement that resulted from his long-term dentist's failure to diagnose OSCC. The monetary recovery Leone received was later reduced to approximately $1.4 million because he had a preexisting cancerous condition, which must be considered in assessing damages attributed to the defendant in this case and all medical malpractice cases.

Leone, a man in his 50s, went to see Dr. Bauman for a toothache. Dr. Bauman testified that he performed cancer screenings during Leone's May 2014 and April 2015 examinations but did not observe any signs of OSCC. By July 2015, Leone felt a lump in his mouth. In August 2015, he went to see Dr. Bauman again and was referred to an oral surgeon. Leone subsequently underwent a biopsy, which showed that he had stage IV OSCC. The oral surgeon removed half of Leone's face to identify and remove the cancerous lesion. The surgeon then had to use bone and soft tissue from Leone's lower leg to reconstruct his jaw.

During the trial, testimony by the oral surgeon who removed the cancer and by an expert dentist and oral pathologist suggested that the disease was diagnosable at the time of Leone's May 2014 dental visit with Dr. Bauman. The experts testified that had the cancerous lesion been detected earlier, Leone would not have had to undergo surgery, chemotherapy, and radiation. According to the plaintiff's attorney, the cancer and surgery permanently altered Leone's life. In addition to his disfigurement, Leone had trouble eating, drinking, and swallowing.

The jury determined that Dr. Bauman failed to meet the standard of care because he did not perform a proper cancer screening that would have led to the discovery of OSCC. Although Dr. Bauman claimed that he performed a ten-minute cancer screening exam, his records did not indicate it. A routine cancer screening usually takes one to two minutes, during which a patient's mouth and soft tissue are examined for redness and/or raised areas, which are indicative of a cancerous lesion. Additionally, a dentist should palpate the patient's intraoral and extraoral lymph nodes to see if there is any lymphadenopathy. Dr. Bauman also claimed that when he performed a cancer screening exam, he was more concerned with white lesions rather than red lesions. However, the expert dentist contended that 90% of red lesions and 10% of white lesions are, in fact, cancerous.

CASE LAW # 2

In *Hopton v Silvertson*,[36] the plaintiff sued her dentist, periodontist, and oral surgeon for failure to diagnose OSCC. Hopton's oral cancer went undiagnosed for more than one year, resulting in the need for her to have extensive excision, revision, and reconstructive surgeries of her lower jaw.

The plaintiff also underwent chemotherapy, radiation, hyperbaric therapy, skin grafts, and bone grafts. She had eight major surgeries and 21 minor surgeries. The Michigan jury awarded Hopton $15 million for misdiagnosis by Dr. Vallerand, the oral surgeon, for his failure to order a timely biopsy. The recovery amount was later reduced to $500,000 based on Michigan's medical malpractice cap and pursuant to an agreement with the defendant. The periodontist, Dr. Silvertson, paid $25,000 due to a prior agreement between the parties. The plaintiff's dentist, Dr. Maly, settled before the trial for an undisclosed amount.

In August 2005, Hopton, who was about 60 years of age, went to her dentist for an unexplained pain to her lower right jaw. She was examined by Dr. Maly, but no diagnosis was made. In February 2006, three of the plaintiff's lower anterior teeth became loose, and her dentist referred her to a periodontist. The periodontist made a diagnosis of an acute periodontal abscess and recommended extraction of the three teeth and placement of a bridge. At that time, the periodontist observed a white lesion, which he diagnosed as an aspirin burn but was likely a leukoplakia-type precancerous lesion. The lesion went away. In May 2006, a new lesion 10 to 15 cm from the site of the first one was discovered by the periodontist.

Hopton was then referred to an oral surgeon for an evaluation and biopsy. The oral surgeon made a differential diagnosis of a traumatic injury caused by the temporary bridge. Although oral cancer was also a differential diagnosis, the oral surgeon did not recommend or order a biopsy, and no follow-up appointments were scheduled. Hopton subsequently returned to the oral surgeon on November 27, 2006, because she developed a large lesion in her mouth that was causing her pain. The oral surgeon then diagnosed her oral cancer, with a biopsy confirming that Hopton had stage IV OSCC, which statistically has a 30% five-year survival rate.

COMMON LEGAL ISSUES RELATED TO OSTEONECROSIS OF THE JAWS

Oncologic therapy can cause numerous, lifelong complications and morbidity for both current cancer patients and survivors. Where these long-term complications intersect with dentistry and litigation, based on the most recent dental and legal literature, is osteonecrosis of the jaws.[2] Dental and other health care providers should be familiar with two specific types of osteonecrosis: ORN and MRONJ.

Background of ORN and MRONJ

ORN of the maxilla or the mandible occurs when prior radiation therapy, typically exceeding 5000 cGy cumulatively,[37] causes portions of these bones to be more susceptible to potential death, along with the overlying soft tissue; this may occur either spontaneously or following invasive trauma, infection, or injury. Direct radiation exposure is known to cause permanent changes in osseous structure and physiology by means of hypocellularity, hypovascularity, and relative hypoxia, creating a lifelong milieu of potentially inadequate metabolic and healing capabilities of the radiated bone.[37,38] The incidence of ORN following radiation treatment to the oral cavity is approximately 6%.[39]

MRONJ is an uncommon yet dreaded outcome of cancer therapy combined with a patient's dental factors. Awareness of MRONJ within the dental profession has drastically increased within the past two decades as long-term use of antiresorptive medications, by some patients starting these drugs in the 1990s, unveiled this adverse effect, which was first published in 2002.[40] North American dental schools have incorporated varying amounts MRONJ-related content in their curricula to educate new generations of dentists and dental specialists, and MRONJ is a common topic presented at numerous dental continuing education courses in Canada and the United States.

MRONJ is associated with two main categories of systemic, antiresorptive medications.[41] The first category is the bisphosphonates, which act by inhibiting osteoclastic activity within bone and serve to reduce osseous turnover and remodeling. This prevents bone density loss and fracture, especially in metastatic cancer and in patients with preexisting or concomitant bone density loss. Bisphosphonates can be administered orally or intravenously. The second category is represented by denosumab, which is a human monoclonal antibody that inhibits bone resorption by cellular deregulation of osteoclasts.[41] Denosumab demonstrated a slightly higher incidence of MRONJ when compared to bisphosphonate therapy.[41,42] When evaluating intravenous versus oral bisphosphonate therapy, the risk for developing MRONJ is markedly higher in patients given monthly intravenous bisphosphonates than those given a regimen of oral bisphosphonates.[43,44] Also, longer duration of either intravenous or oral bisphosphonate treatment is correlated with an increase in MRONJ incidence.[45] Antiangiogenic medications have also been implicated in MRONJ development. These agents impede blood vessel growth and are combined with other chemotherapy agents to hinder tumor progression in specific forms of cancer.[46] The rates of MRONJ incidence vary by medication and with length of time of administration.[44]

Patient susceptibility to ORN and MRONJ is multifactorial. The patient's age[47] and preexisting chronic diseases, especially uncontrolled diabetes,[42] can increase the risk of osteonecrosis. The use of systemic glucocorticoids as a factor in MRONJ development is controversial.[44] Tobacco smoking is a known risk factor for ORN[48] and may contribute to MRONJ susceptibility.[42] When bone repair is hindered by antiresorptive medications and especially if tissue vascularization is impaired by antiangiogenic agents concurrently, typically benign, intraoral insults such as microtrauma, infection, and invasive dental treatment can initiate osteonecrosis. Common forms of microtrauma include poorly fitting dentures, recurrent injury to bony exostoses, and heavy occlusion.[43,44] Chronic periodontitis, abscessed teeth, and dental caries are examples of typical intraoral infections.

Clinical considerations for potential ORN and MRONJ patients

The frequency of comprehensive general dentistry visits should be established between dental providers and each patient on an individual basis. As recommended by the 2019 MRONJ international clinical practice guidelines, routine general dentistry visits are recommended at six-month intervals for patients on antiresorptive medications.[42] These visits are important for everyone of all age groups, especially all current and former cancer patients, to screen for and detect these forms of infection and microtrauma and early signs and symptoms of MRONJ and to initiate prompt treatment to prevent the need for more invasive therapy. Invasive dental treatment occurs when there is surgical or inadvertent manipulation of the gingiva or oral mucosa, such as periodontal therapy, dental extractions, alveoloplasty, implant placement, or iatrogenic trauma during dental treatment.[44,46]

To officially diagnose either ORN or MRONJ, dental providers assess if patients meet key historical and clinical criteria. The definition of ORN is exposed, previously irradiated bone, present for at least three months, without the simultaneous presence of active malignancy.[49] Established by the American Association of Oral and Maxillofacial Surgeons (AAOMS), the diagnosis of MRONJ requires fulfillment of three criteria: (1) prior or current therapy with antiresorptive or antiangiogenic medications; (2) denuded or necrosed bone, or palpable bone through either an intraoral or extraoral fistula, which has been present for more than eight weeks; and (3) lack of metastatic disease or radiation exposure to the maxilla or mandible.[50] Despite different means of causing bone death, the clinical signs of MRONJ and ORN are similar.[37] The most common presentation of either MRONJ or ORN to a dental provider is an area of exposed, necrotic bone detected on clinical exam.[51,52] This area of exposed bone may not be symptomatic. However, when the surrounding soft tissue becomes inflamed or infected, the patient may experience soreness, swelling, and purulent drainage. Patients may develop these same symptoms, in addition to tissue ulceration, redness, tooth mobility, jaw pain, and even bone enlargement, prior to the development of exposed bone.[53] During healing of invasive dental treatment in susceptible patients, these same signs can occur also as MRONJ or ORN is developing postoperatively.

The morbidity seen with either MRONJ or ORN can include chronic bone and soft tissue infection, leading to unsightly fistulae, disfigurement, and pathologic fractures of the jaw bones, along with poor nutrition and reduced quality of life as a result of pain and discomfort. According to Khan et al., "There are no universally accepted treatment protocols for ONJ. In the absence of a defined treatment algorithm for ONJ, there is a generally accepted approach of palliation of symptoms and controlling associated infection."[46] Treatment modalities frequently used in combination include antiseptic mouth rinses, systemic antibiotic therapy, and surgical debridement.[43,49]

The predictability and success of osteonecrosis therapy can be as varied as dental practitioners' approaches in management.[54] In severe cases of osteonecrosis, surgical resection of either maxillary or mandibular bone may be indicated, along with vascular reconstruction efforts to restore bone and soft tissue at the resected area.[37] Hyperbaric oxygen therapy is prescribed on a per-case basis in the prevention and/or treatment of ORN, despite conflicting evidence in the literature.[48] Pharmacologic therapies such as pentoxifylline with tocopherol have shown promising results in studies, especially in ORN management, along with teriparatide in MRONJ management.[49,55,56] However, they have not been adopted into standard protocols for osteonecrosis treatment as additional clinical studies are necessary.[37,49]

Medicolegal considerations for dental providers treating ORN and MRONJ patients

ORN and MRONJ can significantly affect the quality of a patient's life. Several patients have pursued litigation against members of their health care team, particularly their physicians and dental providers, and even pharmacologic corporations, frequently seeking compensatory damages. In 2015, Epstein et al.[2] published a comprehensive report that reviewed medicolegal litigation outcomes in head and neck cancer cases. This review of malpractice cases involving the development of ORN or MRONJ, with dental providers named as defendants, demonstrated three main areas of wrongdoing: inadequate case preparation, negligent treatment, and insufficient informed consent. While the defendants prevailed in 8 of the 41 reviewed cases at the time of publication, 26 cases had resulted in verdicts and settlements awarded, with the average recovery value being $1,033,500.11.[2]

Inadequate case preparation occurs when a dental provider fails to obtain adequate information regarding the patient's medical history and current clinical status prior to treating the patient, especially before invasive procedures, such as surgeries and dental extractions. In assessing for the risk of osteonecrosis development, dental providers need to obtain thorough, comprehensive patient medical and medication histories. A detailed assessment of all prior and concurrent medical conditions and background risk factors, such as tobacco use in the patient's social history, should be obtained. Dosages, administration routes, and duration of all medications, especially antiresorptive, antiangiogenic, and immunomodulating medications, and all forms of past, current, or anticipated chemotherapy should be recorded. Any prior history of head and neck radiation should be investigated, and a review of previous surgery and dental/oral surgery, with dates of surgeries and assessment of any adverse outcomes from those surgeries, is critical to obtain.

Negligent treatment places the patient in direct harm when a dental provider performs invasive procedures without appropriately following standard-of-care protocols, guidelines, or precautions and thus fails to reduce the risk of known complications. For instance, a patient had dental extractions performed following radiation therapy, without the dental provider taking any precautions prior to treatment, in June 1985. The patient then developed ORN and pursued litigation, resulting in a settlement of $1,001,308 in 1989. ORN developed in another patient who had numerous teeth extracted in 1985, despite their dental provider being aware of the patient's extensive head and neck radiation history. This case went to trial in March 1994, with a settlement awarded of $2,960,000.[2]

The concept of insufficient informed consent can solely apply to the at-fault dental provider, or it can include liability extended to both the dental provider and the patient's medical team, especially in cases of MRONJ development. When a dental provider fails to discuss the risks of osteonecrosis with proposed invasive treatment when there are known, clear risk factors in the patient's history and when omission of exploring alternative, less invasive treatment options with the patient occurs, the informed consent process is incomplete. In 1996, a patient was awarded $1,454,319 after the patient developed ORN from a dental provider's failure to inform of the risk of necrosis, in addition to not providing information about other treatment options. Inadequate informed consent can occur with negligent treatment in some cases as well. In May

1992, a patient was not referred for hyperbaric oxygen therapy despite a known prior history of head and neck radiation; the patient subsequently developed ORN from dental extractions. The patient was awarded $1,018,000.[2]

Shared liability beyond the dental provider

In response to the growing number of legal proceedings associated with MRONJ internationally in the early 2000s, Lo Russo et al.[57,58] published two papers in 2013 and 2014 that examined the legal liability of both the prescribing physician and the dental provider in MRONJ cases, referred to as bisphosphonate-related osteonecrosis of the jaws (BRONJ) in these publications. The predominant theme in these papers is the shared responsibility among three parties: the prescribing physician and the oral health provider share in the duties of informing, diagnosing, managing, or referring at all stages of antiresorptive drug therapy for MRONJ development and risk assessment, and the patient is obligated to be compliant with therapy and required medical and dental follow-up visits. Current, international guidelines in the management of MRONJ also echo this concept.[42]

Lo Russo et al.[57,58] emphasize that liability in cases of MRONJ does not only squarely sit on the shoulders of dental providers. Medical providers face legal responsibilities throughout the course of an antiresorptive therapy regimen they prescribe. They should have current knowledge of these medications and the latest best practices in prescribing such agents. At the time of initial prescription of MRONJ-related medications, physicians need to inform patients of not only the benefits but also the risks of antiresorptive therapy, including MRONJ, and they should assess for possible medical and dental risk factors that can contribute to MRONJ development, such as poor oral health. Patients should be encouraged to undergo initial screening with a dental provider prior to starting antiresorptive therapy, and they should inform the dental provider of the anticipated new drug regimen. Initial prescription discussion, led by the medical provider, should also focus on educating the patient on the importance of compliance with all medical and dental appointments and awareness of the early symptoms and signs of MRONJ. These items should be captured in a written informed consent form, signed by both the patient and the physician, prior to the start of drug therapy.[57,58]

When assessing liability in ORN, there is a paucity of current literature that directly analyzes the roles of dental providers and radiation oncologists in medicolegal cases. Dental providers have a clear responsibility in preventing or mitigating risk of ORN in cancer patients in planning for and performing treatment. However, when considering patient management basics in radiation oncology, the radiation oncology team (including reception, nursing, and social work staff) should be developing rapport and actively counseling patients about their disease, radiation therapy, and possible adverse effects of radiation.[59] According to Wang,[59] the informed consent process for head and neck radiation should include discussion of ORN of the mandible, delayed wound healing, and fistulae development prior to radiation therapy. Radiation oncologists need to adhere to standard-of-care protocols and evidence-based radiation dosages to effectively treat tumors, while being mindful of the adverse effects of radiation therapy and risks of excessive dosing. Adverse events due to excessive radiation account for 11% of litigation cases against radiation oncologists.[60] Considering that the risk of ORN drastically climbs with the cumulative dose of radiation, the informed consent process for head and neck radiation targeting the jaws[37] should include ORN to be prudent.

During antiresorptive treatment, the patient and the physician are mutually obligated to work together to complete therapy and to monitor for adverse outcomes. Medication compliance, compliance with all medical appointments, and alerting the physician of any suspected adverse effects of therapy are the responsibilities of the patient. The physician should be reassessing for changes in overall health and MRONJ risk factors at each patient visit, in addition to inquiring about compliance and findings at recent dental visits, including the results of routine MRONJ screenings. Epstein et al.[2] encourage oncologists to foster and build "close working relationship with informed and experienced dental providers" when preventing and managing acute and chronic oral complications from cancer therapy.

Dental providers face several responsibilities and challenges in working with MRONJ-susceptible patients. Along with their medical colleagues, oral health providers should have knowledge of current scientific literature related to MRONJ, relevant to their scope of practice. Ideally, the dental provider should have training and experience in working with these high-risk patients as well. For optimal patient care, dental providers with such expertise and experience should be incorporated into multidisciplinary oncology teams.[2] Dental providers are encouraged to refer to colleagues with greater expertise when appropriate.[42]

Three documented cases illustrate the importance of both the medical and dental providers' roles in thoroughly educating patients about MRONJ risk and reducing a patient's risk of developing MRONJ with similar fact patterns.

CASE LAW # 3

In January 2005, a patient with metastatic breast cancer was being treated with intravenous bisphosphonates and proceeded with multiple dental extractions. She developed extensive MRONJ. Following trial in November 2012, the jury awarded the plaintiff $10.45 million, which included punitive exemplary damages and personal injury allocations for past pain and suffering and future pain and suffering.[2]

CASE LAW # 4

The case of *Streimer v Biondo* illustrates a situation where a plaintiff can allege fault with both an oncologist prescribing intravenous bisphosphonate therapy and an oral surgeon in causing MRONJ. In this case, the plaintiff suffered from metastatic breast cancer and was treated by her oncologist, Dr. Grace. This treatment included intravenous bisphosphonates with some side effects in the form of osteomas in her oral cavity around September 2004.

In February 2005, the plaintiff started seeing Dr. Biondo, an oral surgeon, for removal of her osteoma-like growths. The plaintiff failed to mention her prior discussions with Dr. Grace that these could be due to bisphosphonate treatment. Her oral surgery treatment caused permanent and widespread bone exposure.

In the plaintiff's lawsuit, she alleged, among other things, that Dr. Biondo lacked proper informed consent to do the surgery and Dr. Grace was negligent in not preventing the surgery.

The plaintiff alleged that both practitioners should have been aware that the bisphosphonate treatment would be a contraindication to the surgery. Plaintiff's counsel argued that, in late 2004 and 2005, Novartis issued "dear doctor" letters to physicians and dental providers regarding the link between intravenous bisphosphonate therapy, invasive dental treatment, and osteonecrosis of the jaws. Note that this case followed shortly after the publications regarding the risks of bisphosphonates with invasive dental procedures, and thus, both providers were aware of the contraindications.

Dr. Grace, the oncologist, argued that he did not receive this "dear doctor" letter and was not liable for the procedures of another provider. Dr. Biondo, the oral surgeon, argued that the knowledge regarding bisphosphonates and dental procedures was not widespread.

The plaintiff sought damages for past and future pain and suffering and demanded a total of $340,000 before trial. A New York jury returned a defense verdict after a seven-day trial.[61] Note that this case took place at the time when or shortly after the link between bisphosphonates and MRONJ was established; the outcome may be far different today.

Cases against pharmaceutical companies

Large pharmaceutical companies who produce antiresorptive agents have also been implicated and embroiled in patient-driven litigation. Corporations such as Merck & Co, Inc. (manufacturer of Fosamax), Novartis Pharmaceuticals Corp (manufacturer of Zometa), Teva Pharmaceuticals USA, Inc. (manufacturer of alendronate), and Amgen, Inc. (manufacturer of Prolia) have faced product liability suits alleging these medications cause MRONJ, with some proceeding to trials and resulting in large payouts.

In 2010, the US District Court for the Southern District of New York held a retrial of the "first Fosamax multidistrict litigation case."[62] In this bellwether case, the jury awarded $8 million in compensatory damages, with the verdict against Merck & Co, Inc.[62] However, later in 2010, the $8 million verdict was deemed "excessive" by a New York federal judge overseeing this case *sua sponte*. The judge then remitted the verdict to $1.5 million unless the plaintiff desired a new trial on damages alone.[63]

In another case, Novartis Pharmaceuticals Corp paid $10.45 million in liability to a woman who developed MRONJ while being treated with Zometa, decided by a New York federal jury in 2012. The plaintiff's claims against Novartis included "strict liability, negligent manufacture, negligent failure to warn and breach of express and implied warranty."[64]

Some suits have been ruled in favor of the defendant corporations. For instance, between 2005 and 2013, Merck won five of seven MRONJ cases tried to verdict.[65] However, large class action settlements have been awarded as well. Also in late 2013, Merck & Co, Inc., agreed to a $27.7 million payout in 2013 to settle approximately 1200 plaintiffs' claims of product liability, which alleged that Fosamax caused MRONJ.[65]

CLINICAL VIGNETTE # 1

Mr. Carr was a 64-year-old White male with a history of tonsillar squamous cell carcinoma five years prior to initial clinical presentation. The cancer was treated with surgery, radiation therapy, and chemotherapy. Two years later, he developed ORN of the left posterior mandible and was subsequently treated with hyperbaric oxygen therapy. However, Mr. Carr continued to have discomfort in the left lower jaw for three years. He was faced with the decision to proceed with surgical resection and reconstruction of the left mandible. He sought a second opinion in search of other treatment alternatives, which lead to an initial consultation at an academic center. This second consultation found no evidence of ORN and determined that his discomfort was likely related to neuropathy (Figure 15-1).

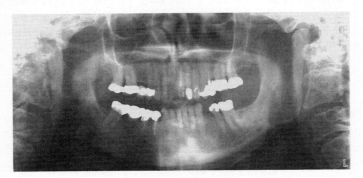

Figure 15-1. First pantomograph taken at an academic center during initial consultation. No overt radiographic findings of ORN at the left mandible.

A palliative, monitoring approach was deemed more appropriate than an aggressive, immediate surgical course. For three years, Mr. Carr was compliant with all follow-up, general dentistry, and hygiene treatment. The left mandibular site, previously with ORN, remained asymptomatic.

Unfortunately, at age 67 years, Mr. Carr developed a new, aggressive site of ORN of the right posterior mandible, below his fixed partial denture, with denuded bone and localized infection (Figure 15-2).

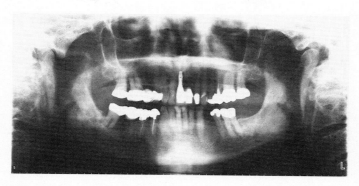

Figure 15-2. New ORN site detected on pantomograph affecting the alveolar bone of the posterior right mandible.

This lesion was palliatively managed for five years while it slowly grew and festered. Finally, the patient desired to proceed with surgical resection and reconstruction. The patient made this decision despite numerous professional and academic opinions to only extract the carious lower right tooth in the vicinity of the ORN lesion and not to proceed with surgery.

After further deliberation, Mr. Carr settled on having the carious tooth extracted in a private office. He then suffered postextraction infection with no wound healing and significant exacerbation of the existing ORN lesion, both requiring long-term antibiotics. To make matters worse, the private office that performed the high-risk extraction did not provide close follow-up for the patient, and the patient returned to the original academic center for management and care of the right mandible. Ultimately, seven months after the catastrophic extraction, Mr. Carr, at age 73 years, underwent a right hemi-mandibulectomy with a free fibular bone and tissue graft transfer to reconstruct his right mandible (Figure 15-3). Currently, he is still experiencing postoperative complications and is in the process of determining how to restore his teeth, speaking proficiency, and eating ability in the months to years ahead.

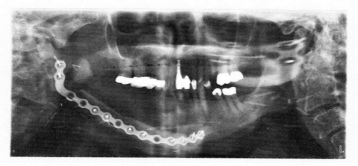

Figure 15-3. Post-operative pantomograph following resection and reconstruction of the right mandible to treat the infected, worsening ORN lesion.

Was the dentist negligent in extracting the carious tooth without additional preoperative and post-operative measures to manage Mr. Carr's ORN?

This case presents several unique variables for a case of negligence regarding ORN. As with all tort actions against health care providers, the patient must prove that the dentist's negligence caused his injuries; in this case, the injury was the right hemi-mandibulectomy and the damages were the pain and suffering related to restoring his teeth, speaking, and eating. Also note that Mr. Carr is 73 years old, and according to most mortality estimates, his remaining life span is a matter of years, not decades.

Before Mr. Carr chose to get his tooth extracted by the dentist, he appeared to make the decision to get the ORN resection but later changed his mind due to other professional opinions. He complied with these opinions by going to a dentist for the extraction. It seems that the dentist failed to provide proper informed consent about the procedure; the dentist also failed to engage in preventative measures, such as asking for medical clearance from his treating physicians, referring the matter to an oral surgeon, or performing the procedure in a hospital setting. Additionally, the dentist did not request hyperbaric treatment or other assessments to prevent this poor outcome and failed to provide thorough follow-up care.

Based on the facts and prior, similar cases, Mr. Carr has a good chance of some success if he chooses to pursue a case against his dentist, although he will still have to overcome challenges, such as the fact that he was planning this ORN surgery previously. If the case settled or a jury found in his favor, his damages for pain and suffering may be limited due to his limited life span.

The prevention of osteonecrosis

The prevention of osteonecrosis is the key consideration in dentistry when determining optimal clinical treatment for a cancer patient. Prior to a patient beginning any course of antiresorptive or radiation therapy, the dental provider must perform a comprehensive examination, initiate treatment and/or removal of unrestorable teeth, and engage in prophylactic efforts to prevent future invasive therapy.[42,66] During radiation or antiresorptive therapy, the dental provider should determine the least invasive means to complete treatment, such as avoiding tooth extractions, endosteal implant placement, and surgery to the gingiva and jaw bones.[37,42,49] For instance, in ORN prevention, avoidance of any surgical treatment in maxillary and/or mandibular regions with direct, prior exposure to high-dose radiation therapy is critical.[66] All invasive treatment in patients with a history of intravenous bisphosphonate use, current intravenous bisphosphonate use, or extensive oral bisphosphonate history with concurrent high-risk medications (antiangiogenic agents and corticosteroids) should be precluded to reduce MRONJ development.[49] Alternative treatments including endodontic therapy and strategic timing of invasive treatment in coordination with the medical team and current therapeutic guidelines should be considered in osteonecrosis-susceptible patient.[42,49]

For ORN, preoperative hyperbaric oxygen therapy (HBO) remains controversial because published studies have shown both reduced postoperative rates of ORN and unchanged or even increased rates of ORN development in irradiated patients. Perioperative and therapeutic HBO should be considered on a per-case basis.[48] However, current publications and prior litigation cases suggest that HBO should be considered and discussed with high-risk patients for preoperative optimization when weighing the potential morbidity of ORN.[2,48] Studies analyzing drug holidays for oncology patients on antiresorptive therapy have also generated mixed results in determining whether temporary perioperative drug cessation reduces MRONJ risk. While some publications recommend considering stopping antiresorptive therapy on a per-case basis,[46] there is a paucity of evidence in refuting or supporting these brief drug holidays in active cancer patients.[42]

Because cancer therapy is known to cause acute and chronic adverse effects, which include ORN and MRONJ, there have been international and national efforts to establish guidelines for preventing and managing oral complications. The Multinational Association of Supportive Care in Cancer (MASCC), the International Society for Oral Oncology (ISOO), and the American Society of Clinical Oncology (ASCO) jointly produced international practice guidelines for the management of MRONJ in 2019.[42] The National Institute of Dental and Craniofacial Research, a branch of the US Department of Health and Human Services' National Institutes of Health (NIH), maintains online reference guides for both oncologists and dental providers in the management of oral health care in oncology patients.[66,67]

CONCLUSION

The treatment of oncology patients requires consistent, accurate, and complete documentation during every step and interaction.[2,58,59] As emphasized by both Epstein et al.[2] and Lo Russo et al.,[58] acquiring all pertinent information, maintaining clear records of communication with both the patient and the medical team, documenting patient discussion and education, thoroughly assessing risk versus benefit in all treatment alternatives, and ensuring completeness of all records are vital in mitigating legal liability for the dental provider.

The intersection of oncology, dentistry, and litigation frequently centers on a missed or delayed diagnosis of OSCC and osteonecrosis of the jaws. These issues drastically impact patients' lives, especially their quality of life. The oncology team, the dental provider, and the patient have specific responsibilities and obligations in communicating about, monitoring, and managing dental-related issues and avoiding preventable adverse oral health outcomes. When there is breakdown in this network, litigation, with potential large payouts, may be pursued.

KEY POINTS:

- OSCC is the most common head and neck cancer.
- Failure to diagnose, failure to refer for diagnosis, and misdiagnosis of OSCC are common factors in dental malpractice litigation.

- The greater the delay in diagnosis of OSCC and the later the onset of treatment, the more advanced is the stage of the cancer, necessitating more aggressive therapy and resulting in a poorer prognosis.
- OSCC can initially be asymptomatic and progress to become symptomatic.
- Precancerous oral lesions can present as oral erythroplakia, leukoplakia, or a mixed lesion.
- An oral screening exam by a dentist is the standard of care.
- Biopsy remains the gold standard for oral cancer diagnosis.
- A multidisciplinary team approach, with the inclusion of knowledgeable and experienced dental providers, is vital to optimal prevention and management of oral complications, especially osteonecrosis of the jaws, in cancer treatment.
- Prior to any dental treatment, a thorough patient workup, which includes obtaining the patient's history of medical conditions, medications, substance use, prior/current/future cancer therapy information, known adverse events related to cancer therapy, and a thorough clinical exam with radiographs, should be performed and documented by the dental provider. Documented communication with the patient's oncology team to obtain or clarify necessary information prior to dental treatment is essential.
- Dental providers need to consider and discuss alternatives to invasive surgical treatment with the patient when treatment planning and evaluating ORN or MRONJ risk.
- If invasive dental treatment is necessary, a thorough informed consent process about the risk of osteonecrosis should occur, along with documentation of perioperative measures considered and taken to prevent osteonecrosis.
- Complete and accurate patient chart documentation is critical in abating liability if ORN or MRONJ development leads to medicolegal proceedings.
- The prevention of ORN or MRONJ is dependent on the triad of the medical provider/oncology team, the dental provider, and the patient. The medical provider and dental provider are responsible for maintaining current knowledge of respective care guidelines, patient education, patient health optimization, and monitoring and treating the patient's condition. The patient is responsible for complying with treatment, attending all medical and dental appointments, alerting providers to adverse effects and new symptoms, and maintaining healthy lifestyle choices. Open, ongoing communication connecting all three parties is ideal.

References:

1. USCS data visualizations. Centers for Disease Control and Prevention. https://gis.cdc.gov/grasp/USCS/DataViz.html. Accessed April 23, 2021.
2. Epstein JB, Kish RV, Hallajian L, Sciubba J. Head and neck, oral, and oropharyngeal cancer: a review of medicolegal cases. *Oral Surg Oral Med Oral Pathol Oral Radiol*. 2015;119:177–786.
3. Lydiatt DD. Cancer of the oral cavity and medical malpractice. *Laryngoscope*. 2002;112:816–819.
4. Osteonecrosis. American College of Rheumatology. https://www.rheumatology.org/I-Am-A/Patient-Caregiver/Diseases-Conditions/Osteonecrosis. Accessed April 23, 2021.
5. Osteoporosis medications and medication-related osteonecrosis of the jaw. American Dental Association. https://www.ada.org/en/member-center/oral-health-topics/osteoporosis-medications. Accessed April 23, 2021.
6. Gao W, Guo C-B. Factors related to delay in diagnosis of oral squamous cell carcinoma. *J Oral Maxillofac Surg Off J Am Assoc Oral Maxillofac Surg*. 2009;67:1015–1020.
7. Hackett TP, Cassem NH, Raker JW. Patient delay in cancer. *N Engl J Med*. 1973;289:14–20.

8. Mackillop WJ, Bates JH, O'Sullivan B, Withers HR. The effect of delay in treatment on local control by radiotherapy. *Int J Radiat Oncol Biol Phys*. 1996;34:243–250.

9. Carvalho AL, Pintos J, Schlecht NF, et al. Predictive factors for diagnosis of advanced-stage squamous cell carcinoma of the head and neck. *Arch Otolaryngol Head Neck Surg*. 2002;128:313–318.

10. Guggenheimer J, Verbin RS, Johnson JT, Horkowitz CA, Myers EN. Factors delaying the diagnosis of oral and oropharyngeal carcinomas. *Cancer*. 1989;64:932–935.

11. Felippu AWD, Freire EC, Silva R de A, Guimarães AV, Dedivitis RA. Impact of delay in the diagnosis and treatment of head and neck cancer. *Braz J Otorhinolaryngol*. 2016;82:140–143.

12. Grafton-Clarke C, Chen KW, Wilcock J. Diagnosis and referral delays in primary care for oral squamous cell cancer: a systematic review. *Br J Gen Pract J R Coll Gen Pract*. 2019;69:e112–e126.

13. What are oral cavity and oropharyngeal cancers? American Cancer Society. https://www.cancer.org/cancer/oral-cavity-and-oropharyngeal-cancer/about/what-is-oral-cavity-cancer.html. Accessed April 23, 2021.

14. Oral squamous cell carcinoma: ear, nose, and throat disorders [Internet]. Merck Manuals Professional Edition. https://www.merckmanuals.com/professional/ear,-nose,-and-throat-disorders/tumors-of-the-head-and-neck/oral-squamous-cell-carcinoma. Accessed April 23, 2021.

15. Head and neck cancers. Centers for Disease Control and Prevention. https://www.cdc.gov/cancer/headneck/index.htm. Accessed April 23, 2021.

16. Ogden GR. Alcohol and oral cancer. *Alcohol Fayettev N*. 2005;35:169–173.

17. Jiang S, Dong Y. Human papillomavirus and oral squamous cell carcinoma: a review of HPV-positive oral squamous cell carcinoma and possible strategies for future. *Curr Probl Cancer*. 2017;41:323–327.

18. Oral cavity cancer. American Head and Neck Society. https://www.ahns.info/resources/education/patient_education/oralcavity/. Accessed April 23, 2021.

19. Kim JW, Park Y, Roh J-L, et al. Prognostic value of glucosylceramide synthase and P-glycoprotein expression in oral cavity cancer. *Int J Clin Oncol*. 2016;21:883–889.

20. De Vicente JC, Recio OR, Pendás SL, López-Arranz JS. Oral squamous cell carcinoma of the mandibular region: a survival study. *Head Neck*. 2001;23:536–543.

21. Scott SE, Grunfeld EA, Main J, McGurk M. Patient delay in oral cancer: a qualitative study of patients' experiences. *Psychooncology*. 2006;15:474–485.

22. Allison P, Locker D, Feine JS. The role of diagnostic delays in the prognosis of oral cancer: a review of the literature. *Oral Oncol*. 1998;34:161–170.

23. Mackillop WJ, Zhou Y, Quirt CF. A comparison of delays in the treatment of cancer with radiation in Canada and the United States. *Int J Radiat Oncol Biol Phys*. 1995;32:531–539.

24. Fortin A, Bairati I, Albert M, Moore L, Allard J, Couture C. Effect of treatment delay on outcome of patients with early-stage head-and-neck carcinoma receiving radical radiotherapy. *Int J Radiat Oncol Biol Phys*. 2002;52:929–936.

25. Ragin CCR, Modugno F, Gollin SM. The epidemiology and risk factors of head and neck cancer: a focus on human papillomavirus. *J Dent Res*. 2007;86:104–114.

26. Oral cancer 5-year survival rates by race, gender, and stage of diagnosis. National Institute of Dental and Craniofacial Research. https://www.nidcr.nih.gov/research/data-statistics/oral-cancer/survival-rates. Accessed April 23, 2021.

27. Markopoulos AK. Current aspects on oral squamous cell carcinoma. *Open Dent J*. 2012;6:126–130.

28. Sasahira T, Kirita T. Hallmarks of cancer-related newly prognostic factors of oral squamous cell carcinoma. *Int J Mol Sci*. 2018;19:2413.

29. Chi AC, Day TA, Neville BW. Oral cavity and oropharyngeal squamous cell carcinoma: an update. *CA Cancer J Clin*. 2015;65:401–421.

30. Dolan RW, Vaughan CW, Fuleihan N. Symptoms in early head and neck cancer: an inadequate indicator. *Otolaryngol Head Neck Surg*. 1998;119:463–467.

31. Woo S-B, Grammer RL, Lerman MA. Keratosis of unknown significance and leukoplakia: a preliminary study. *Oral Surg Oral Med Oral Pathol Oral Radiol*. 2014;118:713–724.

32. González-García R, Naval-Gías L, Rodríguez-Campo FJ, Sastre-Pérez J, Muñoz-Guerra MF, Gil-Díez Usandizaga JL. Contralateral lymph neck node metastasis of squamous cell carcinoma of the oral cavity: a retrospective analytic study in 315 patients. *J Oral Maxillofac Surg.* 2008;66:1390–1398.

33. Warnakulasuriya S, Johnson NW, van der Waal I. Nomenclature and classification of potentially malignant disorders of the oral mucosa. *J Oral Pathol Med.* 2007;36:575–580.

34. Carreras-Torras C, Gay-Escoda C. Techniques for early diagnosis of oral squamous cell carcinoma: systematic review. *Med Oral Patol Oral Cirugia Bucal.* 2015;20:e305–e315.

35. *Anthony Leone v Lawrence Bauman, D.D.S.,* Vol 2019, Jury Verdicts LEXIS, 2019, p. 98968.

36. *Herta Hopton v John F. Silvertson, D.D.S.; Smith, Silvertson & Zahn PLLC; Periodontal Specialists Group; Waren Vallerand D.D.S., M.D, and the Center for Oral & Facial Surgery,* Vol 2009, Jury Verdicts LEXIS, 2009, p. 416137.

37. Bagheri SC. Head and neck pathology. In: *Clinical Review of Oral and Maxillofacial Surgery.* 2nd ed. Philadelphia, PA: Mosby; 2014:187–222.

38. Marx RE. Osteoradionecrosis: a new concept of its pathophysiology. *J Oral Maxillofac Surg.* 1983;41:283–288.

39. Gupta V, Kann BH. Oral cavity. In: Chao KSC, Perez CA, Wang TJC, eds. *Radiation Oncology: Managment Decisions.* 4th ed. Philadelphia, PA: Lippincott Williams & Wilkins; 2019:275–290.

40. Edwards BJ, Gounder M, McKoy JM, et al. Pharmacovigilance and reporting oversight in US FDA fast-track process: bisphosphonates and osteonecrosis of the jaw. *Lancet Oncol.* 2008;9:1166–1172.

41. Berenson JR, Stopeck AT. Risks of therapy with bone antiresorptive agents in patients with advanced malignancy. In: Post TW, ed. UpToDate. Waltham, MA: UpToDate; 2019. https://www.uptodate.com/contents/risks-of-therapy-with-bone-antiresorptive-agents-in-patients-with-advanced-malignancy?source=history_widget. Accessed July 19, 2020.

42. Yarom N, Shapiro CL, Peterson DE, et al. Medication-related osteonecrosis of the jaw: MASCC/ISOO/ASCO clinical practice guideline. *J Clin Oncol.* 2019;37:2270–2290.

43. Bagheri SC. Pharmacology. In: *Clinical Review of Oral and Maxillofacial Surgery.* 2nd ed. Philadelphia, PA: Mosby; 2014:29–64.

44. Berenson JR, Stopeck AT. Medication-related osteonecrosis of the jaw in patients with cancer. In: Post TW, ed. UpToDate. Waltham, MA: UpToDate; 2020. https://www.uptodate.com/contents/medication-related-osteonecrosis-of-the-jaw-in-patients-with-cancer?search=mronj&source=search_result&selectedTitle=1~74&usage_type=default&display_rank=1. Accessed July 15, 2020.

45. Palaska PK, Cartsos V, Zavras AI. Bisphosphonates and time to osteonecrosis development. *Oncologist.* 2009; 14:1154–1166.

46. Khan AA, Morrison A, Hanley DA, et al. Diagnosis and management of osteonecrosis of the jaw: a systematic review and international consensus. J Bone Miner Res. 2015;30:3–23.

47. Arce K. Osteoradionecrosis. In: *Current Therapy in Oral and Maxillofacial Surgery.* Philadelphia, PA: Elsevier/Saunders; 2012:473–482.

48. Galloway T, Amdur RJ. Management of late complications of head and neck cancer and its treatment. In: Post TW, ed. UpToDate. Waltham, MA: UpToDate; 2020. https://www.uptodate.com/contents/management-of-late-complications-of-head-and-neck-cancer-and-its-treatment?search=osteoradionecrosis%20of%20jaws&source=search_result&selectedTitle=1~65&usage_type=default&display_rank=1. Accessed July 15, 2020.

49. Neville BW, Damm DD, Allen CM, Chi AC. Physical and chemical injuries. In: Neville BW, Damm DD, Allen CM, Chi AC, eds. *Oral and Maxillofacial Pathology.* 4th ed. St. Louis, MO: Elsevier; 2016:259–302.

50. Ruggiero SL, Dodson TB, Fantasia J, et al. American Association of Oral and Maxillofacial Surgeons position paper on medication-related osteonecrosis of the jaw—2014 update. *J Oral Maxillofac Surg.* 2014;72:1938–1956.

51. Allen MR, Ruggiero SL. A review of pharmaceutical agents and oral bone health: how osteonecrosis of the jaw has affected the field. *Int J Oral Maxillofac Implants.* 2014;29:e45–e57.

52. Thorn JJ, Hansen HS, Specht L, Bastholt L. Osteoradionecrosis of the jaws: clinical characteristics and relation to the field of irradiation. *J Oral Maxillofac Surg.* 2000;58:1088–1093.

53. Fedele S, Porter SR, D'Aiuto F, et al. Nonexposed variant of bisphosphonate-associated osteonecrosis of the jaw: a case series. *Am J Med.* 2010;123:1060–1064.

54. Pitak-Arnnop P, Sader R, Dhanuthai K, et al. Management of osteoradionecrosis of the jaws: an analysis of evidence. *Eur J Surg Oncol.* 2008;34:1123–1134.

55. Delanian S, Chatel C, Porcher R, Depondt J, Lefaix J-L. Complete restoration of refractory mandibular osteoradionecrosis by prolonged treatment with a pentoxifylline-tocopherol-clodronate combination (PENTOCLO): a phase II trial. *Int J Radiat Oncol.* 2011;80:832–839.

56. Kwon Y-D, Kim D-Y. Role of teriparatide in medication-related osteonecrosis of the jaws (MRONJ). *Dent J.* 2016;4:41.

57. Lo Russo L, Lo Muzio L, Buccelli C, Di Lorenzo P. Bisphosphonate-related osteonecrosis of the jaws: legal liability from the perspective of the prescribing physician. *J Bone Miner Metab.* 2013;31:601–603.

58. Lo Russo L, Ciavarella D, Buccelli C, et al. Legal liability in bisphosphonate-related osteonecrosis of the jaw. *Br Dent J.* 2014;217:273–278.

59. Wang TJC. Fundamentals of patient management. In: Chao KSC, Perez CA, Wang TJC, eds. *Radiation Oncology: Managment Decisions.* 4th ed. Philadelphia, PA: Lippincott Williams & Wilkins; 2019:1–14.

60. Prabhu AV, Quang TS, Funahashi R, et al. A national WestlawNext Database analysis of malpractice litigation in radiation oncology. *Fed Pract.* 2018;35:S44–S52.

61. *Ann Streimer v Ronald Biondo, DDS and William Grace, MD,* 2008, 21 Misc 3d 1124(A), 52164(U) (NY Slip Op 2008).

62. Jury awards plaintiff $8 million in Fosamax lawsuit. Litigation Blog. LexisNexis Legal Newsroom. https://www.lexisnexis.com/legalnewsroom/litigation/b/litigation-blog/posts/jury-awards-plaintiff-8-million-in-fosamax-lawsuit. Accessed July 29, 2020.

63. $8M Fosamax verdict remitted by MDL judge to $1.5M or new damages trial. Litigation Blog. LexisNexis Legal Newsroom. https://www.lexisnexis.com/legalnewsroom/litigation/b/litigation-blog/posts/8m-fosamax-verdict-remitted-by-mdl-judge-to-1-5m-or-new-damages-trial. Accessed July 29, 2020.

64. Jury awards plaintiff $10.4 million for injuries, punitive damages linked to Novartis' Zometa. Litigation Blog. LexisNexis Legal Newsroom. https://www.lexisnexis.com/legalnewsroom/litigation/b/litigation-blog/posts/jury-awards-plaintiff-10-4-million-for-injuries-punitive-damages-linked-to-novartis-zometa. Accessed July 29, 2020.

65. Merck to settle suits alleging jaw damage from osteoporosis drug. Litigation Blog. LexisNexis Legal Newsroom. https://www.lexisnexis.com/legalnewsroom/litigation/b/litigation-blog/posts/merck-to-settle-suits-alleging-jaw-damage-from-osteoporosis-drug. Accessed July 29, 2020.

66. National Institute of Dental and Craniofacial Research, National Institutes of Health, US Department of Health and Human Services. *Dental Provider's Oncology Pocket Guide.* 2009. https://www.nidcr.nih.gov/sites/default/files/2017-09/oncology-guide-dental-provider_0.pdf. Accessed July 29, 2020.

67. National Institute of Dental and Craniofacial Research, National Institutes of Health, US Department of Health and Human Services. *Oncology Pocket Guide to Oral Health.* 2009. https://www.nidcr.nih.gov/sites/default/files/2020-06/oncology-guide-oral-health.pdf. Accessed July 29, 2020.

CHAPTER 16

Integrative Oncology

Markus Ploesser, MD, LLM

INTRODUCTION

In discussing the legal issues pertaining to integrative and alternative healing methods in oncology, with a focus on the liability concerns of medical practitioners in this field, there are a number of matters to consider. First, the nature of alternative therapies used in oncologic treatment must be considered, with particular reference to the reasons for which cancer patients choose them and how they are used and whether these therapies are combined with conventional cancer treatments or used on their own. These alternative treatments must also be investigated; there are specific claimed benefits for each treatment, and these have been medically proven to a greater or lesser degree. In particular, it is necessary to distinguish alternative treatments from experimental treatments and to discuss the legislation pertaining to the provision of these on the market, as well as the potential medical liability of treating physicians. The reasons motivating cancer patients to choose to be treated with these alternative treatments will also be discussed, including discussion of whether treating oncologists oversee the administration of these treatments or whether patients choose to undergo alternative treatment without the endorsement of their treating physician. In addition to these issues, there are also concerns pertaining to consent that must be considered. These matters are complicated and interlinked, and ultimately, the primary aim of oncologists is to treat their patients to the best of their ability and comply with the law. Thus, this chapter seeks to clarify the aforementioned issues.

ONCOLOGY TREATMENT AND ALTERNATIVE THERAPIES

The use of complementary and alternative medicine (CAM) has become increasingly popular among patients diagnosed with cancer over the course of the past two decades.[1]

Although these therapies can be effective, they often have a number of toxic side effects that are unpleasant for patients, especially when they are already dealing with a serious and life-threatening illness.[1] Patients may use CAM therapies to cope with the toxic effects of conventional treatments such as radiation or chemotherapy.[2]

Furthermore, in comparison to the perceived toxicity of conventional medicine, CAMs are often perceived by many cancer patients to be natural and thus more beneficial. However, proof of the benefits of these treatments is lacking.[3]

There are wide variety of CAMs, and the term is used primarily to refer to substances and treatments that are considered to be "outside of the American medical mainstream" and that oncologists do not generally recommend.[4] It is necessary to distinguish between alternative and complementary treatments or medicines; alternative treatments are ones that are used in place of conventional medicine, whereas complementary treatments are used in addition to conventional medicine.[4] Research has found that as cancer patients find themselves being forced to deal with the long-term effects of the disease and the toxicity of conventional treatments, they become more likely to use CAMs.[4] There are a large number of CAMs available for patients to choose from, from nutritional supplements to mind-body approaches to the total overhaul of conventional treatment by clinics such as the Burzynski Clinic. Of note, the Burzynski Clinic has been subject to a huge amount of controversy and litigation and has been both reviled and lauded by cancer patients in equal measure.[5] Even the most seemingly innocuous CAMs have side effects. Some of these are discussed in the following sections.

NUTRITIONAL THERAPIES

Nutritional supplements, such as vitamins C and E and selenium, might seem harmless; however, they have the potential to adversely interact with radiation therapy and chemotherapy. Thus, they can damage the efficacy of the treatment a cancer patient is receiving.[4] Another alternative treatment that is used is insulin potentiation therapy; this treatment involves the injection of insulin together with a reduced dose of conventional chemotherapy medication.[6] There is proof that the use of insulin potentiation therapy can cause temporary reduction of the size of tumors in some patients; however, there is absolutely no evidence that its use can improve survival for cancer patients.[7]

Another example of a nutritional CAM is the restrictive Kousmine diet, which emphasizes a natural vegetarian diet and the use of vitamin supplements.[8] Although eating a clean and vegetarian diet may certainly have some minor health benefits in general, absolutely no evidence exists that this diet is in any way an effective treatment for cancer.[8] Another treatment that has appealed to patients is the use of mistletoe, which was posited as an actual cure for cancer by the spiritualist Rudolf Steiner. Moreover, Steiner maintained that its harvesting was necessary at the time of the most advantageous planetary alignment in order to improve its efficacy. The American Cancer Society[9] has explicitly stated that "available evidence from well-designed clinical trials does not support claims that mistletoe can improve length or quality of life."

In addition to the provision of false hope to patients, many of the treatments that are marketed to patients have absolutely no beneficial effect at all.

MIND-BODY HEALING APPROACHES

Mind-body healing approaches are also extremely popular; although support groups and mental and spiritual guidance certainly have the potential to help struggling patients, they also may offer false hope to patients, as well as potentially negatively impact on the relationship between a patient and a physician. This is common in cases where the influence of the alternative practitioner is excessively strong.[4] This is also the situation with regard to special cancer clinics such as the Burzynski Clinic.[4]

CASE LAW # 1

The Burzynski Clinic has been the subject of extensive controversy. Founded in 1976 in Texas, it is most well known for its provision of "antineoplaston therapy." This therapy involves the use of mixtures and peptide derivatives that the practitioner Burzynski used in his alleged treatment for cancer.[10] As will be discussed, Burzynski and his treatments have been the subject of government-directed lawsuits on numerous grounds, including the costs that cancer patients participating in his trials are expected to bear, problems with the ways in which these trials are performed, and the sale of treatments at the clinic that have not been subject to the approval of the state board. Lawyer Richard Jaffe has acted extensively in the defense of Burzynski and chronicled this defense in his 2008 book on Burzynski's work and legal battles, *Galileo's Lawyer*.[11] In 1997, Jaffe testified to the US Congress in their investigation of abuses of authority by the US Food and Drug Administration (FDA) that although the drug used by Burzynski was never approved by the FDA for interstate marketing, "there has never been an allegation, concern or a whisper that his treatment is harmful or toxic, unlike many conventional drugs."[10] It is notable, however, that in 2015, Jaffe withdrew from acting as Burzynski's defense lawyer in his hearing with the Texas State Office of Administrative Hearings, as he was himself pursuing an action against Burzynski in the bankruptcy court.[11]

Burzynski began providing his treatment in 1984, and he has attracted both condemnation and praise. Specifically, the offering of his antineoplaston therapy as an experimental treatment has resulted in him being the subject of a huge amount of controversy in the media. Moreover, he has been accused of "unethical conduct," as well as of being a "merchant of false hope."[5] Furthermore, the scientific papers he has published on the treatment he has developed have been the subject of academic controversy, and the scientific validity of the trials he has conducted and their published results have been disputed.[12] The case of Burzynski is extremely complicated and illustrates the complexity of the US laws on the provision of CAMs in cancer treatment and the liability that medical practitioners outside of the conventional medical system may leave themselves open to. It should be noted that the antineoplaston therapy offered by Burzynski from 1984 was never approved for general use either in the state of Texas or federally by the FDA.[13] In fact, the compounds Burzynski used were never licensed as drugs, despite the fact that Burzynski administered them in return for payment at his clinic. In 2011, the Burzynski Clinic attracted further controversy as it began to market the provision of "personalised gene-targeted cancer therapy."[13] The key problem with this, however, is that Burzynski's treatment bears almost no similarity to targeted therapy, which is the primary treatment used in cancer therapy.[14]

The case of Burzynski and his clinic has been extensively documented, and it is necessary to outline the main issues that can provide instruction for medical practitioners seeking to avoid liability in relation to integrative or healing methods in their own practices. First, the clinical trials conducted by Burzynski were a major problem and attracted the attention of the authorities. The FDA Regulations Relating to Good Clinical Practice and Clinical Trials detail the FDA regulations that govern the protection of participating human subjects and the way in which such trials should be conducted.[15] However, the trials conducted by Burzynski have been criticized; the National Cancer Institute (NCI)[16] has noted that "no phase III randomized, controlled trials of antineoplastics as a treatment for cancer have been conducted. Publications have taken the form of case reports, phase I clinical trials, toxicity studies, and phase II clinical trials." In addition, the NCI notes that these studies "often report remissions" and that "other investigators have not been successful in duplicating these results."[16]

As a result of numerous other anomalies pertaining to the clinical trials conducted by Burzynski, in 2013, the FDA began a series of investigations into the trials, which were paused, and the FDA identified a number of issues with the institutional review board established by Burzynski, as well as issues pertaining to both the conduct of the Burzynski Clinic as well as the role of Burzynski himself as the principal investigator of the trials.[17]

In addition to the problems pertaining to the clinical trials conducted by Burzynski, there are serious problems with the efficacy of the antineoplaston therapy that he has developed and pioneered. The professional medical community is of the opinion that there is simply "not enough reliable evidence to use it as a cancer treatment."[18] Randomized controlled trials conducted on antineoplaston therapy have found that it is not a useful cancer treatment.[18] The problem is that there are a number of former patients of Burzynski who have been adamant regarding the benefits of his treatment and have testified on his behalf before the US Congress. In particular, one patient, David Smith, was adamant that the treatment provided by Burzynski was responsible for improving his cancer to the extent that his symptoms began to improve to the point that he was able to discontinue his narcotic pain medication.[10] The former patient recounted to the Congress subcommittee his despair on discovering that the FDA had denied the right to Burzynski to continue the provision of his treatment.[10] This conflict between the FDA and Burzynski impinged upon the right of this patient to choose his own therapy on the grounds of informed consent, which will be discussed later. As David Smith noted to the US Congress, "there is something very wrong when I cannot choose my own medical treatment; when I am forced to accept the dictates of the FDA and have no legal rights to pursue an experimental therapy with informed consent."[10] This separate issue is certainly problematic; however, it might be questioned as to how far the consent of such a patient is truly "informed" when the information on which he is basing his decision is alleged to be so flawed. Furthermore, the government, through the medium of the FDA, has a duty to protect citizens from sham and potentially detrimental treatment.

This is certainly an unfortunate situation for patients such as David Smith, who have been convinced of the benefits they were receiving from the antineoplaston treatment. However, it is notable that since 1993, the American Cancer Society[19] has been adamant that there a complete lack of evidence that antineoplaston therapy has any beneficial effect; in addition, it recommends that this therapy should not be purchased because there may actually be detrimental health effects. In addition to the ethical concerns regarding the conduct of the clinical trials and their accuracy, another concern to be considered is the cost of the treatment at the Burzynski Clinic, which desperate patients were forced to bear. The American Cancer Society noted that treatment at the Burzynski Clinic could cost between $7000 and $9500 per month. Moreover, given the alternative and unproven nature of the therapy, which is quite firmly outside of conventional medicine, health insurance companies are unwilling to cover the costs.[18] The huge cost of the treatment and the refusal of medical insurance companies to cover the treatment meant that patients were often forced to resort to crowdfunding to raise money for the alternative cancer treatment.[20]

The case of Burzynski brings up a number of important legal issues. The first is that the use of antineoplaston therapy by Burzynski, the marketing of this treatment, and its administration were deemed to be illegal by both the FDA and the Texas attorney general.[21] In fact, the FDA kept a close eye on the work of Burzynski and his clinic for a number of years. Furthermore, over the years, he was fined and his activities were curbed, but the FDA found it very difficult to shut him down completely. In 2013, the FDA contacted Burzynski regarding the objectionable conditions that had been observed regarding the clinical investigations of antineoplaston medications. The FDA was explicit in its criticisms of Burzynski, stating that his failure to conduct his research in accordance with the "protocol requirements jeopardizes subject safety and welfare and raises concern about the validity and integrity of the data collected at [his] site."[22] The 2013 warning letter to Burzynski from the FDA details his breaches of medical ethics and regulations, which had been repeated over the years and indeed would continue to be repeated until the Texas Medical Board finally recommended that his license to practice medicine be revoked. Although Burzynski was ultimately permitted to keep his license, he was severely fined and sanctioned for over 130 violations of medical law.[23]

The 2013 FDA warning letter detailed a number of breaches by Burzynski, including his failure to ensure that the clinical studies were conducted in accordance with the investigational plans. In addition, he failed to protect the rights, safety, and welfare of the human subjects in the trials and failed to obtain their informed consent, specifically because the documents he used did not contain all the necessary elements for informed consent to be possible, nor did they contain a statement concerning billing and research subjects were handed billing agreements only after the provision of their consent. The FDA detailed the specific legislation pertaining to these breaches, under the Code of Federal Regulations. However, despite the fact that the FDA detailed the continuous breaches made by Burzynski of a number of federal laws over many years, it failed to properly close his business and stop him from selling false treatments and providing patients with false hope. As Gorski[24] wrote, authorities such as the FDA are "supposed to protect the public from practitioners like Burzynski, but all too often they fail at their charges, in this case spectacularly." In fact, when examining the breaches committed by Burzynski over the years, along with the numerous actions taken by the authorities against him, including a 20-day trial on fraud in 1994[25] and a complaint against him by the Texas State Board of Medical Examiners in 2012 for his alleged failure to meet medical standards, it is quite incredible that it took so long for the FDA to properly reprimand him, and he has still been permitted to keep his medical license.

Furthermore, not all of Burzynski's former patients are convinced by his work. In 2012, he was sued by an elderly cancer patient on the grounds that he had "swindled" his patients out of hundreds of thousands of dollars by "using false and misleading tactics."[26] Burzynski also hired a representative for his clinic who intimidated and threatened bloggers in the United Kingdom who questioned the treatments offered by his clinic, stating that the intention was to halt the "dissemination of false and inaccurate information concerning Dr. Burzynski and the Clinic."[27] The threatening behavior of Burzynski's representatives toward his critics reflects extremely badly on him and his work, as all medical treatment should be open to questioning. It is certainly an unethical way for a doctor to behave, and it is not behavior that should be emulated. In his extensive study of Burzynski and his work, Smith[5] asked whether the doctor is a "charlatan or a major innovator, a common swindler or a courageous pioneer." Whatever the truth may be, the Burzynski case provides numerous lessons for medical practitioners as to how they may avoid medical liability, simply by ensuring that they do not commit the same infractions as Burzynski. Furthermore, there is evidence that Burzynski did not start out with the intention of defrauding vulnerable cancer patients of their money and providing them with false hope. Rather, it is clear that he was genuinely convinced of the potential for antineoplastons to cure cancer and that, once he found himself ostracized by the conventional medical community and subjected to "a campaign of damaging innuendo," he found himself with no other option than to "aggressively" pursue terminally ill cancer patients for treatment.[5] Burzynski then found himself subjected to battles with the FDA and insurance companies, which refused to cover the costs of his patients due to the unrecognized status of his treatments.[5] However, it should be noted that the courts were generally favorable to Burzynski in these battles, and it is posited that this is primarily because they recognized the right of patients to choose their own treatment.

Interestingly, Smith[5] has adopted a highly sympathetic approach to Burzynski, asserting that the "dominant position enjoyed by biomedicine over health care delivery" is ultimately dependent upon the ability of the medical profession to "exercise strict and hierarchically structured control over professional activities pertaining to research, the deployment of new drugs or other treatment modalities, relations with the state, and relations with the pharmaceutical industry." This approach paints Burzynski as a victim of conventional medicine because he challenged their authority. However, it may be argued that such an approach harms patients. Legislation pertaining to the actions of medical professionals exists for the protection of patients. Thus, it may be argued that the actions of Burzynski were not those of a renegade acting in the best interests of cancer patients, but those of a doctor who willfully ignored the regulations that had been put in place to protect patients. Burzynski was acutely aware of the FDA requirements and the Code of Federal Regulations; however, he was sufficiently arrogant so as to imagine that these rules did not apply to him.

The key issues with regard to liability, therefore, concern the failure of Burzynski to comply with federal regulations and the basic principles of medical ethics, particularly with regard to the vital importance of the protection of patients, as stated in the Nuremberg Code, which established that, for research to be ethical, the welfare and rights of the human subjects must be the priority.[28] The crimes documented at Nuremberg and other horrors that were committed in the Second World War gave rise to the Declaration of Helsinki,[29] which states: "It is the duty of physicians who are involved in medical research to protect the life, health, dignity, integrity, right to self-determination, privacy, and confidentiality of personal information of research subjects. The responsibility for the protection of research subjects must . . . never rest with the research subjects, even though they have given consent."

The numerous charges that were brought against Burzynski highlight the fact that he breached this most basic principle of medical ethics numerous times in his eagerness to prove the veracity of his treatments. The main charges that have been brought against Burzynski concern his failure to act in accordance with the regulations on medical trials, his failure to meet the necessary standard of care, his negligence, his failure to conduct proper due diligence, breaches of professional conduct (e.g., with the bloggers), and his insistence on prescribing medications that had not been approved by the FDA. The main lessons here for practitioners of both conventional medicine and CAMs are that to avoid liability for such breaches, they must act at all times in accordance with the basic rules of medical ethics and the legislation. They are advised to conduct clinical trials in accordance with the regulations, document all results and data accurately, and place the needs of the test subjects first. The issue with regard to the requirement to raise money is unfortunately a necessary factor in light of the limitations of insurance provision for health care treatment. However, the argument that Burzynski was taking money in return for the provision of false hope is valid. Furthermore, his behavior toward the bloggers who challenged him is reprehensible; the silencing of critics by medical professionals is unacceptable. FDA pursued Burzynski for years, and yet his medical license remains intact. However, full compliance with legislation and regulations is necessary; even though the difficulty with which the FDA pursued Burzynski highlights the inefficacy of the legislation, it exists in order to protect citizens and therefore must be fully complied with.

THE ISSUE OF CONSUMER PROTECTION

The issue of consumer protection conflicts with the right to have a freedom of choice in alternative oncologic treatment. The laws imposed by the FDA and the Federal Food, Drug, and Cosmetic Act (FDCA) mean that, prior to their approval for sale to the market, medications must meet efficacy and safety standards.[30] Furthermore, these laws are vital in ensuring that medications are effective and safe, whereas the laws that regulate the marketing of these same products are crucial in order to prevent crimes such as false advertising and mail fraud.[30] One of the reasons for the existence of the California Health and Safety Code, for example, is to place restrictions on physicians providing unconventional treatments for cancer.

CASE LAW # 2

In the case of *The People v Privitera* (1976), in which Privitera had been discovered marketing Laetrile as a treatment for cancer, it was alleged that the right to take laetrile is a right of privacy.[31] However, as noted earlier, laws exist for the purpose of the protection of the wider population, and the court held that the federal statutory law is necessary even in breaching privacy as it bears a "reasonable relationship to the achievement of the legitimate state interest in the health and safety of its citizens."[31] Ultimately, the legal standard of care for medical liability and a finding of malpractice require that the provision of treatment falls below that provided by physicians that meets the "knowledge, skill and care ordinarily possessed and employed by members of the profession in good standing" in the circumstance concerned.[32]

For a medical professional to fall below this standard, the circumstances must be dire; indeed, there is evidence that only a very small percentage of patients are compensated for medical malpractice.[33]

The use of CAMs by patients as well as the increasing administration of unconventional treatment by both medical physicians and practitioners of alternative medicine have the potential to cause serious problems for cancer patients. It is possible that the use of CAMs may disrupt their treatment and potential recovery, providing patients with false hope and violating medical ethics and the federal and state laws of the United States. In an ideal scenario, the lines of communication between patient and medical practitioner would be open and honest; however, research has revealed that this is not always the case.[1] This situation is detrimental for cancer patients, who, research has revealed, often have good reasons for their attraction to the use of CAM.[1] However, an integrative approach to treatment will always be in the best interests of patients, so that they can realize the beneficial effects of both CAMs and conventional medicine.[1] When a conventional medical practitioner is aware of the patient's interest in CAM, the practitioner can either encourage the appropriate use of the treatment or discourage it when the effects have been proven to be negative.[34]

There are reasons why cancer patients do not disclose their use of CAMs to their conventional physicians; one such reason is simply the fact that they were not asked or the topic was not brought up by the treating physician.[35] Indeed, there is evidence to suggest that as many as 60% of cancer patients fail to disclose their use of CAMs to their primary care providers.[36] This may partly be due to the failure to educate patients on the requirement to share such relevant information with their treating physicians. In fact, it has been posited that many patients may not realize that their use of CAMs has any medical relevance.[4] Indeed, many patients may consider some CAMs to merely consist of the adoption of a certain diet or a type of lifestyle and that their choice in these matters does not require medical approval.[4] However, in light of the popularity of the use of CAMs among cancer patients, it might be suggested that the failure of any member of a health care team to bring this issue up is a failure of care. There is also evidence that patients often fear the disapproval of their physicians and thus feel they need to keep their use of CAMs secret.[37] Furthermore, the use of CAMs can cause a patient to become ineligible for clinical trials.[36] Medical investigators are particularly concerned about the undisclosed use of CAMs by patients undergoing clinical trials; many patients consciously choose not to disclose this information because they are aware that the use of CAMs would render them ineligible for such trials. Indeed, one survey found that 63% of patients on a clinical trial failed to disclose their use of CAMs,[38] despite the fact that the undisclosed use of such CAMs would inevitably skew the results of such clinical trials.

Another problem is that conventional medicine and CAM continue to be regarded as two different fields. The use of integrative medicine in conventional medical settings remains a rarity; as a result, many oncologists and nursing specialists lack expertise in CAMs and thus avoid discussing them with patients.[39] A key point must be made on this issue in terms of potential liability for health professionals; while the failure to ask a patient whether they are using CAMs would be highly unlikely to meet the criteria required for negligence, in light of the popularity of their use, it should be noted that it would certainly be an oversight on the part of treating physicians. CAMs are biologic products or involve their use; as such, it is crucial that physicians are aware of their use.[1] Therefore, doctors and nurses should ensure that they check whether their patients use CAMs or are undergoing such treatment and should also educate themselves on the products and treatments available. As such, they would then have the ability to educate their patients on their use and interactions with conventional treatments and even, where appropriate, suggest the CAMs that could be most useful for their patients.

CLINICAL VIGNETTE # 1

Dr. Smith is a naturopathic doctor who runs a small clinic in downtown Seattle. She routinely sees patients who have "lost all hope" because of metastatic cancer. In her clinic, she offers elderflower and alkaline baking soda tinctures to patients to make them feel better. In fact, testimonies from many patients on Yelp showed that they have been very satisfied with Dr. Smith's compassionate approach. When approached by a medical oncologist claiming that Dr. Smith is selling snake oil to patients, Dr. Smith fires back saying that, "If my tinctures are making patients feel better near the end of their lives, I do not see why that is a problem. Yes, I do sell them for $500 a vial, but given how much chemotherapy costs, this is just a drop in the bucket."

Because a tincture is defined by the *Cambridge English Dictionary*[40] as "a *medicine* that consists of a *mixture* of *alcohol* and a *small amount* of a *drug*," can Dr. Smith's tinctures be classed as CAM, and if so, is she operating within the law and complying with medical ethics and legislation or merely profiting from her patients' mental and medical conditions?

Herbs and other botanicals are considered to be dietary supplements under the US Dietary Supplement Health and Education Act of 1994 (DSHEA). These may be extracts or concentrates, and their manufacture in any form, for instance, as liquids and tablets, is regulated under DSHEA.[41,42] Any manufacturer, including small businesses, must comply with the FDA's Good Manufacturing Practices, and labeling and advertising are also regulated by the FDA and the Federal Trade Commission (FTC). However, manufacturers of dietary supplements do not have to register their products.[42] The treatment offered by Dr. Smith is classed as a CAM used in the treatment of cancer patients. Although the description of the treatment suggests that patients are provided with apparently natural ingredients, there appears to be no evidence of their efficacy. There is little information as to how they are prepared and on their purity, although this is not required legally.

A scientific study of tinctures states that they "consist of water, from 25% to 90% alcohol and from about 2% to about 20% dissolved plant components"[43] but that there is very wide variation in the proportions, which are dependent on the species of plant, the initial reagents, and the formula employed. The plant-based tinctures can vary considerably in terms of shelf life, potency, and efficacy, even if made using a standard formula, and sediment may appear immediately or months after manufacture.[43,44] Therefore it is difficult to distinguish a good batch from a poorer one. The herbal quality is related to the intrinsic vitality or energy according to herbalists, but Chenery[43] suggests it may be related to the concentration of active substances in the batch concerned. However, there is inexact knowledge about the relationship between dosage and tincture concentration and the clinical difference this implies, and too high of a plant weight–to–liquid volume ratio may cause tinctures to be toxic.[44] Therefore, specific weight-to-volume ratios for tincture manufacture cannot be recommended, but the assumption is that appropriate standards and specifications, including use of high-quality initial reagents, will be employed by professionals.[44] Because Dr. Smith does not make any claims about the tincture other than it is designed to make the patient "feel better," the potential variation in the dosage of the plant and its efficacy do not appear to be relevant to this case. However, the use of the word *patient* rather than *client* infers that diagnosis and treatment are taking place, which is contrary to FDA rules on the permitted activities of herbal practitioners.[41,42]

Manufacturers of dietary supplements are compelled by law to monitor for adverse effects and to report them, whereas consumers and health care professionals may voluntarily report adverse effects.[41] There is no evidence that Dr. Smith has monitored for adverse effects. In fact, some consumers have expressed their satisfaction, but this feedback is limited to a single social media site, so no firm conclusions can be drawn about the effectiveness or harmful effects of the tincture. Although an oncologist accuses Dr. Smith of selling snake oil, he has not gathered any facts to prove that she is providing any potentially harmful substance to clients.

In the United States, medical practice is regulated at the state level, and generally, only qualified doctors can prescribe, treat, and cure disease. In alignment with FDA[41] rules, the American Herbalists Guild (AHG)[42] warns that anyone providing herbs to clients must avoid using language that infers that they are acting in a medical context, such as providing diagnosis, treatment, or cures, because the implication is that the herbal remedy is an approved drug. This would violate FDA and FTC regulations that are formulated to protect consumers from unfair, deceptive, or fraudulent practices by suppliers.[45] The FDA[41] also recommends that individuals should consult a qualified medical professional before taking dietary supplements; it advises that taking dietary supplements may interfere with medical treatment and that some supplement ingredients, including plant components, may be contaminated. Therefore, the AHG recommends that all herbal practitioners should use an informed consent and disclosure form with those they are supporting.[42]

As a qualified medical practitioner, Dr. Smith appears to be working within the law because there is no evidence she is claiming to treat or cure any client. However, she refers to her clients as patients twice, and the vignette does not provide any details regarding whether she recommends clients seek independent medical advice before taking the CAM. If the informed consent procedure is not being employed, and there is no evidence that it is, Dr. Smith could be subject to legal action if a client reports that they have not been advised to speak to their physician about possibly taking her tincture and/or it is toxic. In any case, Dr. Smith is acting outside the ethical code of the AHG, which recommends the use of an informed consent and disclosure form. Therefore, legal action is possible on two grounds: for allegedly providing diagnosis and treatment and for possible lack of informed consent and disclosure regarding the potential effects of taking the tincture. Either would need a complaint to be lodged with the FDA or FTC. The AHG might also take action against Dr. Smith based on lack of compliance with its ethical code.

However, Dr. Smith could also be reprimanded or temporarily suspended for her lack of compliance with the Code of Medical Ethics. Sections 3 to 7 of the Code of Medical Ethics of the American Medical Association[46] specify that physicians should practice scientifically based healing and expose colleagues who do not, without hesitation; ensure that the profession is not brought into disrepute by illegal or unethical conduct of other physicians demonstrating moral deficiencies or professional incompetence; be able to freely choose whom they serve; not provide services that could cause deterioration of medical care; limit their professional income to medical services actually rendered and ensure their fee is appropriate for services rendered and the patient's financial situation; and dispense or supply remedies in the best interest of the patient. In relation to these guidelines, the oncologist could report Dr. Smith for violation of these principles as is his duty under the ethics of his profession. First, he might formally claim that her practices are not scientifically proven, but this would probably not be a very strong case unless he were able to prove that the tincture was toxic and/or would negatively interfere with her medical treatment for cancer. These aspects of practice would be classed as professional incompetence. Second, Dr. Smith's remark, "Yes, I do sell them for $500 a vial, but given how much chemotherapy costs, this is just a drop in the bucket," is contrary to professional ethics, regarding both professional income and charging a fee that is appropriate to the services provided. The apparent lack of ethical procedure with both the use of the word *patient* in Dr. Smith's herbal practitioner context and her service, which could be considered to cause deterioration to the individual's medical condition, are additional grounds for action by the American Medical Association.

This clinical vignette demonstrates that qualified physicians practicing in a CAM context have responsibilities to their clients to conform with FDA and FTC legislation regarding the solutions they offer to clients suffering from cancer. Despite being medical professionals in the traditional sense, they must still follow the recommendations made earlier, particularly regarding referring clients for prior consultation with their physicians and providing informed consent and disclosure regarding the herbal dietary supplement. They must also shape their language to the herbal practitioner role, so that any accusation of physician-patient relationship is avoided. Qualified physicians operating in the CAM context must also be constantly aware of the professional ethics that are required of them as qualified medical practitioners; noncompliance with medical practitioner ethics is also subject to legal action, and in this case, contravening the ethics of the AHG may also result in negative consequences.

CONCLUSION

There is good reason for physicians to be concerned about the negative impact the use of CAMs may have on cancer patients; for example, some treatments have been proven to have toxic effects on the liver and kidneys.[47] This is not to say, however, that all CAMs are fraudulent or ineffective; this is certainly not the case. In fact, there is mounting evidence that the use of certain CAMs can be highly beneficial for cancer patients.

KEY POINTS:

- To avoid medial liability, doctors must always first consider the requirements and dignity of their patients, as required by the Declaration of Helsinki.
- Physicians must also ensure full compliance with medical legislation, especially with regard to the provision of treatments and their marketing.
- Finally, physicians must make a point of asking patients about their use of CAMs and encourage them to be open about their use of such alternative medicine. As discussed, the heavy use of such complementary treatment, if only for several weeks, can have extremely negative results in terms of drug interactions and can potentially derail conventional treatment.
- In order for integrative treatment to be possible, patients must be encouraged to be as open with their doctors as possible, so that they can be fully apprised of the risks and the most appropriate course of action.

References:

1. Buckner C, Lafrenie R, Dénommée B, Caswell J, Want D. Complementary and alternative medicine use in patients before and after a cancer diagnosis. *Curr Oncol.* 2018;25(4):e275–e281.
2. Zaid H, Silbermann M, Amash A, Gincel D, Abdel-Sattar E, Sarikahya, N. Medicinal plants and natural active compounds for cancer chemoprevention/chemotherapy. *Evid Based Complement Alternat Med.* 2017;2017:7952417.

3. Fouladbakhsh J, Stommel M. Gender, symptom experience, and use of complementary and alternative medicine practices among cancer survivors in the U.S. cancer population. *Oncol Nurs Forum*. 2010;37:E7–E15.

4. Kronenberg F, Mindes J, Jacobson J. The future of complementary and alternative medicine for cancer. *Cancer Invest*. 2005;23:420–426.

5. Smith M. The Burzynski controversy in the United States and in Canada: a comparative case study in the sociology of alternative medicine. *Can J Sociol*. 1992;17(2):133–160.

6. Insulin potentiation therapy. Cam-Cancer. https://cam-cancer.org/en/insulin-potentiation-therapy. August 16, 2021.

7. Wider B. What cancer care providers need to know about CAM: the CAM-Cancer project. *Focus Altern Complement Ther*. 2023;18(2):95–100.

8. Abgrall J. *Healing or Stealing? Medical Charlatans in the New Age*. New York, NY: Algora Publishing; 2000.

9. More information on complementary and alternative medicine. 2013. American Cancer Society. https://www.cancer.org/treatment/treatments-and-side-effects/complementary-and-alternative-medicine/more-cam-info.html. Accessed May 24, 2020.

10. US Congress. *Adequacy of Access to Investigative Drugs for Seriously Ill Patients: Hearing Before the Subcommittee on Oversight and Investigations of the Committee on Commerce, House of Representatives, One Hundred Fifth Congress Volume 4*. Washington, DC: Government Printing Office; 1997.

11. Jaffe R. *Galileo's Lawyer: Courtroom Battles in Alternative Health, Complementary Medicine and Experimental Treatments*. Nashville, TN: Thumbs Up Press; 2008.

12. Vickers A. Alternative cancer cures: "unproven" or "disproven"? *CA Cancer J Clin*. 2004;54(2):110–118.

13. Tweddle S, James N. Lessons from antineoplaston. *Lancet*. 1997;349:1481.

14. Gorski D. Dr. Stanislaw Burzynski's "personalized gene-targeted cancer therapy": can he do what he claims for cancer? https://sciencebasedmedicine.org/stanislaw-burzynskis-personalized-gene-targeted-cancer-therapy/. Accessed May 24, 2020.

15. The FDA regulations relating to good clinical practice and clinical trials. US Food and Drug Administration. https://www.fda.gov/science-research/clinical-trials-and-human-subject-protection/regulations-good-clinical-practice-and-clinical-trials. Accessed May 24, 2020.

16. Antineoplastons (PDQ®)–Health Professional Version. National Cancer Institute. Updated August 15, 2019. https://www.cancer.gov/about-cancer/treatment/cam/hp/antineoplastons-pdq#section/all. Accessed May 24, 2020.

17. Szabo L. Doctor accused of selling false hope to families. May 15, 2015. https://eu.usatoday.com/story/news/nation/2013/11/15/stanislaw-burzynski-cancer-controversy/2994561/. Accessed May 24, 2020.

18. Antineoplaston therapy. Cancer Research UK. https://www.cancerresearchuk.org/about-cancer/cancer-in-general/treatment/complementary-alternative-therapies/individual-therapies/antineoplaston-therapy. Accessed May 24, 2020.

19. Antineoplaston therapy. American Cancer Society. 2008. http://www.cancer.org/Treatment/TreatmentsandSideEffects/ComplementaryandAlternativeMedicine/PharmacologicalandBiologicalTreatment/antineoplaston-therapy. Accessed May 24, 2020.

20. Newman M. Is cancer fundraising fuelling quackery? *BMJ*. 2018;362:k3829.

21. *Texas State Board of Medical Examiners v Stanislaw R. Burzynski, MD, PhD*, Appeal from 353rd District Court of Travis County. Justia Law. February 7, 1996. https://law.justia.com/cases/texas/third-court-of-appeals/1996/847.html. Accessed May 12, 2021.

22. Warning letter. US Food and Drug Administration. December 18, 2013. http://www.circare.org/info/bri/burzynski-ci-fdawl_20131203.pdf. Accessed May 24, 2020.

23. Malislow C. Unorthodox doc Stanislaw Burzynski faces $360,000 fine and probation. February 17, 2017. https://www.houstonpress.com/news/unorthodox-doc-stanislaw-burzynski-faces-360-000-fine-and-probation-9206755. Accessed May 24, 2020.

24. Gorski D. Stanislaw Burzynski: four decades of an unproven cancer cure. March 2014. https://skepticalinquirer.org/2014/03/stanislaw-burzynski-four-decades-of-an-unproven-cancer-cure/. Accessed May 24, 2020.

25. Maxwell L, Mayo T. Health care law. *SMU Law Rev.* 1997;50(2):1291–1292.
26. Langford C. Cancer patient says doc used her as ATM. January 19, 2012. https://www.courthousenews.com/cancer-patient-says-doc-used-her-as-atm/. Accessed May 4, 2020.
27. McCartney M. Texan clinic threatens UK bloggers with legal action over criticisms of its treatments. *BMJ.* 2011;343:d7865.
28. Gallin J, Ognibene F. *Principles and Practice of Clinical Research.* Philadelphia, PA: Elsevier; 2011.
29. WMA Declaration of Helsinki: Ethical Principles for Medical Research Involving Human Subjects. World Medical Association. October 2013. https://www.wma.net/policies-post/wma-declaration-of-helsinki-ethical-principles-for-medical-research-involving-human-subjects/. Accessed May 12, 2021.
30. Unconventional cancer treatments: a summary. Chapter 10: laws and regulations affecting unconventional cancer treatments. US Congress. September 1990. https://ota.fas.org/reports/9044.pdf. Accessed May 12, 2021.
31. *People v Privitera.* Justia Law. https://law.justia.com/cases/california/supreme-court/3d/23/697.html. Accessed May 12, 2021.
32. Prosser W, Keeton W, Dobbs D, Keeton R, Owens D. *Prosser and Keaton on the Law of Torts.* 5th ed. Eagan, MN: West Publishing Company; 1984.
33. Sage W, Kersh R. *Medical Malpractice and the U.S. Health Care System.* Cambridge, United Kingdom: Cambridge University Press; 2006.
34. Lopez G, McQuade J, Cohen L, et al. Integrative oncology physician consultations at a comprehensive cancer center: analysis of demographic clinical and patient reported outcomes. *J Cancer.* 2017;8:395–402.
35. Ezeome E, Anarado A. Use of complementary and alternative medicine by cancer patients at the University of Nigeria Teaching Hospital, Enugu, Nigeria. *BMC Complement Altern Med.* 2007;7:28.
36. Lazar J, O'Connor B. Talking with patients about their use of alternative therapies. *Prim Care.* 1997;24:699–714.
37. Quandt S, Chen H, Grzywacz J, Bell R, Lang W, Arcury T. Use of complementary and alternative medicine by persons with arthritis: results of the national health interview survey. *Arthritis Rheum.* 2005;53:748–755.
38. Culy C, Spencer C. Amifostine: an update on its clinical status as a cytoprotectant in patients with cancer receiving chemotherapy or radiotherapy and its potential therapeutic application in myelodysplastic syndrome. *Drugs.* 2001;61:641–684.
39. Astin J. Why patients use alternative medicine: results of a national study. *JAMA.* 1998;279:1548–1553.
40. Tincture. *Cambridge English Dictionary.* https://dictionary.cambridge.org/dictionary/english/tincture. Accessed May 11, 2021.
41. FDA 101: dietary supplements. US Food and Drug Administration. https://www.fda.gov/consumers/consumer-updates/fda-101-dietary-supplements. Accessed May 11, 2021.
42. Legal and regulatory FAQs. American Herbalists Guild. 2021. https://www.americanherbalistsguild.com/legal-and-regulatory-faqs. Accessed May 11, 2021.
43. Chenery P. *Plants, Colloids and Tinctures: Nature's Pharmaceutics.* 2nd ed. Rutland, United Kingdom: Herbal Research Notes; 2009.
44. Romm A, Hardy M, Mills S. *Botanical Medicine for Women's Health.* London, United Kingdom: Churchill Livingstone; 2010.
45. What we do. Federal Trade Commission. https://www.ftc.gov/about-ftc/what-we-do. Accessed May 11, 2021.
46. Riddick F. The Code of Medical Ethics of the American Medical Association. *Ochsner J.* 2003;5(2):6–10.
47. Pinn G. Adverse effects associated with herbal medicine. *Aust Fam Physician.* 2001;30(11):1070–1075.

PART III

Cogent Issues in Oncology

CHAPTER 17

Pain Management and Opioids

Danial Laird, MD, JD, Lauren Price, and Sarah Fagan, MPH, MA

INTRODUCTION

Oncologists and other physicians frequently and appropriately use opioid analgesics to manage cancer pain. Recently, however, in the context of a national opioid epidemic, the use of opioids has become increasingly controversial, and clinicians must consider a number of important legal issues when prescribing opioid pain medication to patients with cancer pain.

Prescribing opioids to cancer patients can create civil liability issues related to overdose, addiction, suicide, inadequate analgesia, and adverse unintended consequences of avoiding opioids in favor of other types of medication. Alleged inappropriate prescribing by physicians can lead to action against a prescriber's license by state boards of medicine, nursing, or pharmacy. Clinicians can face criminal charges from state governments and can face legal action by the Department of Justice (DOJ) or the Drug Enforcement Administration (DEA) for alleged inappropriate opioid prescribing. Some brief clinical vignettes will help the reader appreciate the various legal issues associated with prescribing opioids.

KEY LIABILITY ISSUES WHEN PRESCRIBING OPIOID ANALGESICS

Civil liability for opioid prescribing

Opioids have long been recognized as a safe and reliable way to treat cancer pain, are easily titrated to the appropriate analgesic effect, and can be administered by multiple routes.[1] Nonetheless, more than half of cancer patients experience pain while undergoing treatment, with 39.3% of patients still experiencing pain after curative therapy.[2] Among those treated for their pain, approximately one-third of patients report untreated or undertreated pain related to their cancer.[2] Cancer patients may experience somatic, visceral, and neuropathic pain, as well as various pain syndromes.[3] Opioids have long been appropriately used by clinicians in the management of cancer pain.

Chronic cancer pain has been defined by the International Association for the Study of Pain (IASP) as including "pain caused by the primary cancer itself or metastases (chronic cancer pain) or its treatment (chronic post-cancer treatment pain)."[4] While some authors have attempted to make a physiologic distinction between cancer pain and noncancer pain, the distinction has not been recognized by many medical authorities, including the US Food and Drug Administration (FDA), since the physiologic mechanisms for both types of pain are similar.[5,6]

From the standpoint of civil liability with regard to prescribing of opioids, clinicians may have liability risk for purportedly overprescribing opioids, thereby putting patients at risk for addiction and fatal overdose. Less commonly, physicians may encounter legal risk at the other extreme, by allegedly failing to treat cancer pain appropriately. In the current medical and political environment where the utility of opioids is being widely questioned vis-à-vis the current opioid crisis, the perceived liability for purportedly overprescribing is likely the most significant concern.

For the purposes of professional negligence, the physician is held to the standard as to what a reasonably prudent clinician would have done in the same or similar circumstances. Physicians prescribing opioids for cancer-related pain may have more protection against liability than those prescribing opioids for chronic nonmalignant pain.

Although opioid prescribing in the United States reached record levels in the 1990s and increased through approximately 2010, opioid prescribing has subsequently steadily decreased over the past ten years in response to efforts by the Centers for Disease Control and Prevention (CDC) and other federal and state interventions.[7] At the same time, the number of people dying of opioid overdose in the United States has continued to increase, particularly during the coronavirus disease 2019 (COVID-19) pandemic.[8,9] Over the past several years, most opioid deaths have been due to illegal opioids, including illicit fentanyl and heroin.[10] Nonetheless, the narrative that physicians generally overprescribe opioids is still widely publicized by the media.

Perceived overprescribing

The overprescribing of opioids has been associated with addiction, unintended overdose, and suicide.[11] Physicians may encounter professional liability for any of these issues, although the incidence may be less than that commonly perceived by clinicians. Most current opioid-related deaths involve nonprescribed opioids, including stolen or diverted prescription medications, illicit fentanyl, illicit fentanyl analogues, and heroin.

Addiction to opioids

The American Society of Addiction Medicine (ASAM) defines addiction as a "treatable, chronic medical disease involving complex interactions among brain circuits, genetics, the environment, and an individual's life experiences."[12] The ASAM definition of addiction further specifies that "people with addiction use substances or engage in behaviors that become compulsive and often continue despite harmful consequences."[12] Addiction, therefore, likely involves a genetic predisposition combined with certain environmental factors and life experiences that may predispose a patient to addiction.

Addiction to opioids usually involves physical dependence combined with use that is compulsive and continues even in the face of harmful consequences. A cancer patient who has a genetic and environmental basis to develop addiction may begin compulsive, harmful use of opioids without substandard care on the part of the oncologist or other clinician. However, oncologists and other providers who prescribe opioids must be constantly vigilant for the signs and symptoms of opioid addiction and appropriately treat addiction if it develops.

As discussed later, there are numerous tools available to clinicians that can help to identify addiction when prescribing opioids. Referral to addiction medicine specialists should be made as indicated.

Lawsuits that allege that a physician caused a patient to become "hooked" or addicted to pain medication do occur,[13] but the frequency is probably less than is commonly perceived. An examination of autopsy toxicology results, prescription database entries, and clinical data reveals that patients who develop opioid addiction often have preexisting addictive behaviors that started prior to the time that the opioids were prescribed.[14] Toxicology results often reveal the presence of nonprescribed opioids, illicit opioids, polypharmacy, and diverted opioids.[15] These findings accentuate the need to screen patients for substance use disorder early in the physician-patient relationship.

For patients with cancer pain, there is often no practical alternative to opioids for pain, even in those with risk factors for addiction and in patients with a known history of addiction. In these situations, it is important for the clinician to document that the addiction history was known, that the potential risks and benefits were discussed with the patient, that informed consent was obtained, and that the decision to prescribe was made in collaboration with the patient.

Unintended overdose and suicide

Despite aggressive interventions on the part of federal and state authorities, opioid overdoses in the United States continue to trend upward. Most recently, a larger proportion of these deaths have been due to illicit fentanyl, illicit fentanyl analogues, and heroin. The situation in which a patient with a legally prescribed opioid overdoses on his or her own prescribed medication may be less common. In a recent study, state-level drug policy interventions were shown to be associated with fewer opioid prescriptions, but these interventions may have the unintended consequence of motivating patients with opioid use disorder to access illicit opioids, potentially leading to a higher rate of opioid overdose deaths.[16]

Nonetheless, clinicians who prescribe opioids may be involved in litigation wherein a patient is injured or dies due to respiratory depression from opioids or from an interaction between opioids and other medications. For several decades, physicians have been aware of the synergistic interaction of opioids and benzodiazepines that can cause respiratory depression. However, in 2016, the FDA mandated a black box warning on both opioids and benzodiazepines, and thus, the interaction has become more widely known and the incidence of prescribing opioids and benzodiazepines concurrently has decreased.[17] Nonetheless, civil suits for wrongful death against a physician may result from the failure to recognize the interaction between opioids and other medications.

Patients with cancer may develop depression, anxiety, and other psychiatric comorbidities. Therefore, it is important for clinicians to be aware that opioids might be a logical choice for patients contemplating suicide. Fortunately, most oncologists are proficient at diagnosing and treating depression and other psychiatric illnesses. Nonetheless, clinicians should be aware that opioids can be used as a means of suicide and take appropriate steps to screen for depression and suicidal ideation. Occasionally, patients with cancer and other serious illnesses may complete suicide even after having been appropriately screened for psychiatric comorbidities and even when opioids were prescribed pursuant to the standard of care.

Liability for inadequate analgesia

In the 1990s, several health care organizations, including The Joint Commission, placed an emphasis on the importance of pain management. In recent years, this has subsided with the belief that overemphasis on pain relief may have been a driving factor behind opioid overprescribing in the 1990s and early 2000s. With a new lack of emphasis on pain management, reports are now appearing in the medical literature of patients being unable to access adequate pain management.[18] For example, a recently published study indicated that up to one-half of primary care patients taking opioids for chronic pain had difficulty accessing a primary care provider.[19] There are multiple media and other anecdotal reports of patients with postsurgical pain, trauma-related pain, cancer pain, and sickle cell disease pain who were not able to obtain adequate pain medication.

Legal causes of action for inadequate pain relief may become more common as physicians fear legal and disciplinary action for overprescribing opioids. There were some well-publicized lawsuits in the 1990s for inadequate analgesia. At least two such cases involved cancer patients.[20]

CASE LAW # 1

The case of *Estate of Henry James v Hillhaven Corporation*[21] reportedly involved an elderly nursing home patient who died of metastatic prostate cancer. A nurse employee of the nursing home allegedly failed to administer opioid pain medications because she was afraid the patient would become addicted. A jury found in favor of the estate and James family on the basis that failure to provide opioid analgesics for metastatic prostate cancer was a breach in the standard of care.

CASE LAW # 2

In *Bergman v Wing Chin, MD and Eden Medical Center* (No. H205732-1 [Cal App Dept Super Ct 1999]), a patient died of what was believed to be lung cancer. The medical records reportedly recorded the patient's pain as being either seven or ten on a ten-point scale while at the nursing home. The patient was later transferred to hospice case where he died. The family filed suit against the nursing home for elder abuse, and a jury returned a verdict in which it found that the failure to appropriately treat the patient's pain was grossly negligent or reckless. The nursing home settled the case; however, a jury verdict found against the physician and in favor of the estate of the deceased patient.[22]

As shown from Case Law Nos. 1 and 2, liability for inadequate analgesia may involve allegations of professional negligence or, in some cases, allegations of gross negligence or even recklessness. It is important for clinicians to remember that it may be considered below the standard of care to refuse to prescribe opioids to cancer patients if a reasonably prudent provider in the same or similar circumstances would have used opioids to relieve pain. While there are often numerous alternatives to treat pain, in cases of severe intractable pain such as that associated with metastatic cancer, the standard of care may require opioids to be prescribed.

Unintended consequences of avoiding opioids

An emerging area of liability for clinicians treating pain is that of unanticipated and unintended consequences of avoiding opioids in clinical practice. In general, physicians are taught to use opioid analgesics as a last resort, only after other nonopioid medications have failed. This approach is widely followed by clinicians due to the complications of opioid therapy, including the most feared complications, respiratory depression and death. However, as noted earlier, in certain cases of severe pain, the standard of care may require the use of opioid analgesics when other modalities prove ineffective or are not available.

Some recent legal cases have involved situations in which clinicians made a good faith effort to avoid opioids but failed to recognize the consequences of overuse of nonopioid therapy. Nonsteroidal anti-inflammatory drugs (NSAIDs) are appropriately commonly used as a first-line treatment against various types of pain in an effort to avoid or reduce reliance on opioid analgesics. Unless there are contraindications, NSAIDs can sometimes provide adequate relief for certain types of pain, including cancer pain.

As most physicians are aware, NSAIDs carry an FDA-mandated Black Box Warning in the dosage and administration prescribing instructions. For example, the FDA-mandated black box warning on ketorolac tromethamine (Toradol) injection carries black box warnings regarding gastrointestinal bleeding and perforation, myocardial infarction, bleeding, and other complications. Additionally, the black box warning advises against the concomitant use of two or more NSAIDs. Many NSAIDs require the clinician to reduce the dose in patients who are elderly or have decreased renal function.

In recent years, there have been professional negligence lawsuits related to the overuse or inappropriate use of NSAIDs in patients with preexisting medical conditions that were contraindications to the use of NSAIDs. Examples include wrongful death due to fatal gastrointestinal bleed allegedly due to concomitant NSAID use and multiorgan failure allegedly due in part to NSAID overuse.[23] Although NSAIDs do have an opioid-sparing effect, the potential benefits of NSAIDs must be weighed against the potential risks, as is the case with opioids.

State and federal action against physicians

Civil litigation related to prescribing opioids usually involves allegations of medical malpractice by a patient or family against a clinician. Far more serious but less common are allegations of inappropriate opioid prescribing that lead to disciplinary actions taken by state boards of medicine, criminal charges, or actions taken by the federal DEA.

In the current environment where opioid prescribing is strongly discouraged, every clinician who prescribes opioids should have a contingency plan in effect in the event that his or her opioid-prescribing practices are called into question. In a civil matter, such as a medical malpractice case, the physician's professional liability insurance carrier will usually hire a civil defense law firm to defend the case. A physician who is served with a medical malpractice lawsuit should immediately contact his professional liability insurance carrier to obtain a medical malpractice defense attorney.

On the other hand, if the physician's opioid-prescribing practices are being called into question by a governmental entity such as a state board of medicine or a division of state government such as a district attorney's office, professional liability insurance policies may not provide coverage to defend these types of legal matters. The same is true for legal actions involving the federal government, including the DEA. In the event a physician is notified of an investigation by a state board of medicine related to prescribing opioids, he or she should contact a civil attorney with significant experience defending physicians in matters before state boards of medicine. Generally, a physician should not surrender his medical license except on the advice of legal counsel.

In a circumstance where a physician is charged with criminal conduct related to the prescribing of opioids, he or she should immediately contact a criminal defense attorney with significant experience defending health care providers in such matters. It is almost never in the best interest of a physician to surrender his DEA license or medical license on the spot except on the advice of legal counsel.

Legal risk mitigation strategies when prescribing opioids

There are a number of widely used interventions clinicians can incorporate into their practices to minimize the risk of adverse patient outcomes from opioid prescribing and hopefully decrease the likelihood of legal action against the prescriber on the part of governmental authorities. Such steps include following clinical practice guidelines, obtaining informed consent, monitoring state prescription database programs, using patient contracts for opioids, ordering urine drug testing, providing naloxone to patients as an opioid antidote, referring patients to pain management, and screening patients on an ongoing basis for mental illness, substance use disorders, diversion, and medication interactions.

Clinical practice guidelines, legislation, and regulation

Many organizations, including both public and private entities, have issued clinical practice guidelines, recommendations, and parameters that are arguably applicable to prescribing opioids for cancer pain. The World Health Organization (WHO) has issued "Guidelines for the Pharmacological and Radiotherapeutic Management of Cancer Pain in Adults and Adolescents."[24] In 2016, the CDC issued its "Guideline for Prescribing Opioids for Chronic Pain—United States."[25] These guidelines were intended for use by primary care providers, yet they have been widely applied to specialist practice. Additionally, the National Cancer Institute and the Oncology Nursing Society have published documents addressing the issue of cancer pain management. The American Society of Clinical Oncology (ASCO) has published guidelines on palliative care and also on chronic pain among adult survivors of cancer. A number of other organizations have also published position statements and clinical guidelines on the management of cancer pain. Reading and following various clinical guidelines may help clinicians understand and follow the standard of care, but it is important to appreciate that given the number of clinical guidelines by various organizations, there are sometimes discrepancies between various recommendations, and comprehending all of the recommendations can be an arduous task. Care for each patient must be individualized, and prescribing opioids or other analgesics in a manner that is not consistent with various recommendations or clinical guidelines may be appropriate given the unique needs of the cancer patient.

In response to the opioid crisis, several state legislatures have enacted statutes or administrative code that governs the prescribing of opioids to patients in various states. Additionally, some state boards of health, nursing, and medicine have enacted regulations that govern the prescribing of opioids by providers. In most instances, the standard of care requires that clinicians know and understand the local, state, and federal regulations that apply to prescribing opioids. Clinicians who do not comply with such regulations may be subject to disciplinary action by governmental authorities.

Informed consent

Opioid therapy in the cancer patient is associated with known complications that are similar to those when prescribing opioids in other clinical settings. Tolerance, dependence, addiction, oversedation, medication interactions, and overdose, intentional or unintentional, are known risks of opioid therapy. Many authorities recommend that clinicians who prescribe opioids initially discuss the various risks and potential benefits of opioid therapy with the patient and have the patient sign a written informed consent form.[26] Several professional organizations offer exemplars of such forms.

Consultation with pain management specialists

Cancer patients may occasionally require high-dose opioid therapy, and most oncologists are familiar with and skilled in prescribing opioids for cancer pain. In some circumstances, however, consultation with a pain management specialist or another oncologist may be beneficial in ensuring that opioid therapy at the prescribed doses is appropriate. Interventional pain management specialists may also be able to recommend blocks or other procedures that could reduce the need for opioid therapy and, in some circumstances, reduce the risk of adverse events.

Prescription drug monitoring programs

Nearly all states in the United States now participate and share data in prescription drug monitoring programs (PDMPs). Such databases typically list a patient's prescribed controlled substances by date, including opioids, the prescriber, the date filled, the dispensing pharmacy, and the quantity of medication filled. Various states, including Florida and Nevada, require that clinicians prescribing opioids consult the database on a regular basis. Consulting a PDMP database can tell an opioid-prescribing clinician whether the patient is receiving prescribed opioids from other providers, whether the patient is using multiple pharmacies, whether the patient is receiving early refills, and other information that could indicate issues with patient misuse of opioids. Physicians are cautioned that PDMP databases are sometimes reliant on retail pharmacy–entered data, and clerical errors in such databases are not rare. Additionally, clinicians must use caution in the way they use and store PDMP data because federal and state privacy laws may be implicated. For legal purposes, primary source verification of opioid prescriptions, such as pharmacy and medical records, is considered a more reliable source of admissible evidence.

The use of opioid contracts

For several years, some authorities have recommended "opioid contracts" or other written agreements between clinicians prescribing opioids and the patient. Some state laws and regulations mandate the use of such agreements. These agreements usually specify conditions of opioid prescribing, such as the condition that the patient receive all opioids from a single medical practice or that early refills are not permitted, or they may specify the conditions under which lost or stolen medication will be replaced. Some patients object to such contracts as being unilateral or contracts of adhesion. There are limited data demonstrating the effectiveness of patient agreements and contracts.

Intermittent urine drug screening

Many physicians who prescribe long-term opioid therapy for chronic pain use intermittent urine drug screening as a means of detecting either use of nonprescribed controlled substances or diversion of prescribed substances. The extent to which oncologists use urine drug testing and the extent to which this benefits cancer patients prescribed opioids are largely unknown.

Offering opioid tapers where appropriate

Due to the risks associated with opioid prescribing, a general principle of opioid therapy for both malignant and nonmalignant pain is that the lowest effective dose should always be prescribed. In cancer patients with advancing disease, it is often necessary to continually increase the opioid dose due to both the development of opioid tolerance and the progression of disease. However, some cancer patients with chronic pain resulting from cancer or its treatment may be on long-term opioid therapy for a period of months or even years. In those patients, intermittent trials of tapering the medication may help ensure that the patient is using the lowest effective dose of opioid medication. For example, a patient receiving a pain tablet four times per day as needed might be dispensed 120 tablets per month. With the patient's consent and cooperation, decreasing the number of tablets dispensed by 5% to 10% may assist the patient and prescriber in determining whether it would be possible to dispense fewer tablets per month on an ongoing basis. Involuntary opioid tapers, undertaken without the consent and cooperation of the patient, are rarely if ever justified and raise ethical issues.[27]

Prescribing and dispensing naloxone

Prescribing and dispensing naloxone as an antidote to opioid overdose has been credited with saving lives due to respiratory depression from opioid overdose. For patients receiving opioid therapy, it may be useful to document in the medical record that a naloxone prescription was offered and that it was either prescribed or declined by the patient.

Minimizing risks of polypharmacy

Opioid death statistics indicate that, in many cases, opioid overdose deaths involve polypharmacy or the concomitant prescribing of several drugs with sedative-hypnotic properties. As discussed earlier, opioids can interact with benzodiazepines, resulting in a synergistic effect of respiratory depression. Additionally, other noncontrolled substances, such as antiseizure medications and centrally acting muscle relaxants, can also have sedating properties that may increase the risk of oversedation from polypharmacy. Where possible, it is important for clinicians to minimize the concomitant prescribing of multiple sedating medications.

Screening for opioid use disorder

A clinician prescribing opioids should complete a substance use history including eliciting any history of alcoholism, smoking, recreational drug use, illicit drug use, and prescription drug use. One commonly used screening device for detecting aberrant behavior with regard to opioids is the Opioid Risk Tool questionnaire.[28] This questionnaire has been used by clinicians prescribing opioids for both cancer and benign painful conditions. Recognizing risk factors for opioid misuse early in the therapeutic relationship can often help avert adverse outcomes.

Screening for mental health disorders

Most oncologists are likely very familiar with the diagnosis and treatment of psychiatric comorbidities in cancer patients, and screening for such disorders is often already part of the initial oncology workup. In patients who are prescribed opioids, recognizing depression and suicidal ideation is particularly important. At times, it may be necessary for the clinician to prescribe smaller quantities of opioids on a more frequent basis if there is concern about self-harm. For example, in a patient with severe pain and possible suicidal ideation, prescribing a two-week supply of opioid pain medication, rather than a full month of medication, may be an effective risk mitigation strategy.

CLINICAL VIGNETTE # 1

Patient A is a 47-year-old woman who underwent platinum-based chemotherapy and a double mastectomy nine years previously for breast cancer. She has struggled for several years with severe chemotherapy-induced peripheral neuropathy (CIPN). The patient believes her pain is effectively treated using physical therapy combined with duloxetine, pregabalin, and 10-mg hydrocodone tablets dosed orally, three times daily, on an as-needed basis. She wishes to establish care with a physician for long-term pain management of her CIPN.

When planning long-term opioid therapy for cancer-related pain, a clinician should screen for both mental health disorders as well as substance use disorders. Prudent steps should be taken to minimize the risk of adverse events from prescription opioids, and the opioid dosage should usually not be escalated over time.

Patient A is initially seen in clinic after completing a medical history questionnaire and authorization for release of medical records. Previous medical records are obtained, which confirm the history of breast cancer and treatment of the cancer with platinum-based chemotherapeutic agents.

The diagnosis of CIPN is confirmed. At her first visit, the patient reviews and signs an informed consent for long-term opioid therapy and a pain contract after the potential risks and benefits of long-term opioid therapy are discussed. The patient is screened for depression using the Beck Depression Inventory. Her risk of opioid misuse is assessed using the Opioid Risk Tool, and she is determined to be at low risk for opioid misuse.

Following her initial intake, patient A is seen monthly and prescribed duloxetine 60 mg/d orally, pregabalin 50 mg three times per day orally, and hydrocodone/acetaminophen 10/325 mg three times per day orally as needed. She undergoes urine drug testing at her initial visit and then intermittently every few months. The patient's PDMP report is run intermittently, and there is no evidence of opioid diversion or misuse. The patient's opioid dose does not escalate over time, and her medication, combined with intermittent physical therapy, provides increased function and quality of life. Her CIPN is successfully treated for several years using this approach. There are no legal issues of concern.

CLINICAL VIGNETTE # 2

Patient B is a 58-year-old man who was diagnosed with stage II colon cancer two years ago. After his initial surgical resection, he was prescribed 10-mg oxycodone tablets 6 times per day on an as-needed basis. Because of ongoing abdominal pain, his medical oncologist continued to write prescriptions for opioids for the following 20 months. As the patient developed tolerance to opioids, he requested higher doses of oxycodone as well as more tablets per month. At his most recent oncology office visit, the oncologist prescribed oxycodone 15 mg six times per day as needed and wrote a prescription for 180 tablets to be dispensed each month. Although not disclosed to the oncologist, over the previous six months, the patient had also been seeing his primary care physician for severe anxiety related to his cancer diagnosis and the loss of his job. The primary care physician has been treating the patient's anxiety with lorazepam, 2-mg tablets orally three times per day as needed, and writing for 90 tablets to be dispensed as a month's supply. Neither the oncologist nor the primary care physician realizes that an opioid and benzodiazepine have been prescribed concurrently. Two days after filling the prescription for the 15-mg oxycodone tablets, patient B is found unconscious and unresponsive in his bed. Paramedics are unable to resuscitate patient B, and he is declared dead. An autopsy with toxicology establishes the cause of death as respiratory depression secondary to coadministration of opioids and benzodiazepines. Patient B's family files a lawsuit for wrongful death against the medical oncologist and primary care physician.

When prescribing opioids or benzodiazepines, clinicians are required to undertake risk mitigation strategies that a reasonably prudent clinician would take in the same or similar circumstances. Here, neither the oncologist nor the primary care physician was aware of the fact that another physician was prescribing a medication that could potentially interact with the medication the other was prescribing. There are several ways in which this outcome could arguably have been prevented. A pain management agreement with the oncologist might have made it clear that all controlled substances were to be prescribed by a single medical practice. Routine intermittent urine drug screening by either office might have detected the presence of both opioids and benzodiazepines, alerting the clinicians to make inquiries regarding the source of the other medication. Finally, inquiry of the PDMP would likely have revealed that the patient was receiving controlled substances from more than one provider, and either provider could have taken corrective action.

CLINICAL VIGNETTE # 3

Patient C is a 26-year-old man with osteosarcoma of the femur who is admitted to an acute care hospital in order to receive intravenous antibiotics for a soft tissue and bone infection. The infected limb is quite painful, and in order to minimize the use of opioids, intravenous ketorolac tromethamine is ordered, 30 mg intravenously as needed every six hours for up to five days. The nursing staff is instructed to use NSAIDs prior to using opioids for pain management. The hospital's medication administration policy allows medications to be administered up to one-half hour early, and several of the doses are administered by the nursing staff early because of the patient's severe pain. On his third day of admission, patient C develops acute renal failure due to NSAID toxicity. His serum potassium level climbs dangerously high to 7.9 mEq/dL, and before hemodialysis can be arranged, he suffers cardiac arrest due to hyperkalemia. The code blue team is unable to resuscitate the patient. The cause of death is hyperkalemic cardiac arrest secondary to acute renal failure. His family files a wrongful death lawsuit against the hospital and prescribing physicians.

Because of the risks of respiratory depression and the potential for misuse, nonopioid medications should be used as first-line treatment for most types of pain when possible. However, when nonopioids, especially NSAIDs, are used in lieu of opioids, a prudent clinician must consider the potential adverse effects of the alternatives. Here, an NSAID (ketorolac tromethamine) was an acceptable alternative to opioids alone to treat pain associated with osteosarcoma. However, pursuant to the manufacturer's FDA-approved dosage and administration instructions, repeat doses of ketorolac should not be administered more often than every six hours. Additionally, when NSAIDs are used as the primary analgesic in ill patients, the patient's renal function must be monitored and abnormalities treated in a timely fashion.

CONCLUSION

Opiates in one form or another have been used to relieve human suffering for thousands of years. On one hand, clinicians prescribing opioids may face medicolegal risk from purportedly overprescribing opioids, leading to addiction, overdose, or death. On the other hand, in an age of antiopioid sentiment due to an ongoing opioid epidemic, physicians may face liability for failing to provide adequate analgesia or for unintended consequences associated with avoiding opioids. Clinicians have numerous tools available to mitigate the risk of adverse events associated with prescribing opioids.

KEY POINTS:

- It is important to document medical necessity when prescribing opioids.
- It is important to document a discussion of the alternatives, risks, and potential benefits of opioid therapy.
- It is important to obtain and document patient informed consent when prescribing opioids.
- When a physician or other provider is accused of inappropriate opioid prescribing, the provider should not surrender his or her medical or DEA license on the spot without first consulting qualified legal counsel.
- It is often a good idea to consult the state's PDMP when prescribing opioids so problems can be detected early.
- Screening patients for substance use disorder and psychiatric comorbidities is often recommended when prescribing opioids.
- Intermittent urine drug screening may be useful when prescribing opioids.
- It is important to remember that failure to provide adequate analgesia can also be a source of clinician liability.
- When avoiding opioids, it is important to consider the unintended consequences of nonopioid pain medication alternatives such as NSAIDs.

References:

1. Portenoy RK, Mehta Z, Ebtesam A. Cancer pain management with opioids: optimizing analgesia. In: UpToDate. 2021. https://www.uptodate.com/contents/cancer-pain-management-with-opioids-optimizing-analgesia?search= how%20do%20i%20use%20opioids%20for%20cancer%20pain%3F&source=search_result&selectedTitle=1~150& usage_type=default&display_rank=1. Accessed March 2, 2021.
2. van den Beuken-van Everdingen MHJ, Hochstenbach LMJ, Joosten EAJ, Tjan-Heijnen VCG, Janssen DJA. Update on prevalence of pain in patients with cancer: systematic review and meta-analysis. *J Pain Symptom Manageme*. 2016;51(6):1070–1090.e9.
3. Caraceni A, Shkodra M. Cancer pain assessment and classification. *Cancers*. 2019;11(4):510.
4. Bennett MI, Kaasa S, Barke A, et al. The IASP classification of chronic pain for ICD-11: chronic cancer-related pain. *Pain*. 2019;160(1):38–44.
5. Kolodny A. FDA/CDER response to physicians for responsible opioid prescribing: partial petition approval and denial. Regulations.gov. September 2013. https://beta.regulations.gov/document/FDA-2012-P-0818-0793. Accessed April 2, 2020.
6. Peppin JF, Schatman ME. Terminology of chronic pain: the need to "level the playing field." *J Pain Res*. 2016;9:23–24.
7. Prescribing practices. Centers for Disease Control and Prevention. Published August 20, 2019. https://www.cdc .gov/drugoverdose/data/prescribing/prescribing-practices.html. Accessed March 2, 2021.
8. Holland KM, Jones C, Vivolo-Kantor AM, et al. Trends in US emergency department visits for mental health, overdose, and violence outcomes before and during the COVID-19 pandemic. *JAMA Psychiatry*. 2021;78(4):372–379.

9. Rodda LN, West KL, LeSaint KT. Opioid overdose–related emergency department visits and accidental deaths during the COVID-19 pandemic. *J Urban Health*. 2020;97(6):808–813.

10. Fentanyl. Opioid overdose. Centers for Disease Control and Prevention. Published February 16, 2021. https://www.cdc.gov/drugoverdose/opioids/fentanyl.html. Accessed March 2, 2021.

11. Guy GP Jr, Zhang K, Bohm MK, et al. Vital signs: changes in opioid prescribing in the United States, 2006-2015. *MMWR Morb Mortal Wkly Rep*. 2017;66(26):697–704.

12. ASAM definition of addiction. American Society of Addiction Medicine. Published September 15, 2019. https://www.asam.org/Quality-Science/definition-of-addiction. Accessed March 2, 2021.

13. Barnes M, Sklaver S. Active verification and vigilance: a method to avoid civil and criminal liability when prescribing controlled substances. *DePaul J Health Care Law*. 2013;15(2):93.

14. Singer JA, Sullum JZ, Schatman ME. Today's nonmedical opioid users are not yesterday's patients; implications of data indicating stable rates of nonmedical use and pain reliever use disorder. *J Pain Res*. 2019;12:617–620.

15. Persico AL, Wegrzyn EL, Fudin J, Schatman ME. Fentalogues. *J Pain Res*. 2020;13:2131–2133.

16. Lee B, Zhao W, Yang K-C, Ahn Y-Y, Perry BL. Systematic evaluation of state policy interventions targeting the US opioid epidemic, 2007-2018. *JAMA Network Open*. 2021;4(2):e2036687.

17. Zhang V, Olfson M, King M. Opioid and benzodiazepine coprescribing in the United States before and after US Food and Drug Administration boxed warning. *JAMA Psychiatry*. 2019;76(11):1208–1210.

18. Inserro A. Oncologists, hematologists welcome CDC clarification on opioid therapy for chronic pain. AJMC. April 2019. https://www.ajmc.com/view/oncologists-hematologists-welcome-cdc-clarification-on-opioid-therapy-for-chronic-pain. Accessed August 13, 2020.

19. Lagisetty P, Macleod C, Thomas J, et al. Assessing reasons for decreased primary care access for individuals on prescribed opioids: an audit study. *Pain*. 2021;162(5):1379–1386.

20. Rich BA. Physicians' legal duty to relieve suffering. *West J Med*. 2001;175(3):151–152.

21. *Estate of Henry James v Hillhaven Corporation*, 89 CVS 64 (NC Super Ct 1991).

22. Ling W. Prescription opioid addiction and chronic pain: more than a feeling. *Drug Alcohol Depend*. 2017;173(suppl 1):S73–S74.

23. Bekker J. Man awarded $43M for wife's death in Las Vegas hospital hopes for change. *Las Vegas Review Journal*. Published January 29, 2019. https://www.reviewjournal.com/local/local-las-vegas/man-awarded-43m-for-wifes-death-in-las-vegas-hospital-hopes-for-change-video-1585075/. Accessed March 2, 2021.

24. WHO guidelines for the pharmacological and radiotherapeutic management of cancer pain in adults and adolescents. World Health Organization. 2019. https://www.who.int/publications/i/item/who-guidelines-for-the-pharmacological-and-radiotherapeutic-management-of-cancer-pain-in-adults-and-adolescents. Accessed March 2, 2021.

25. Dowell D, Haegerich TM, Chou R. CDC guideline for prescribing opioids for chronic pain—United States, 2016. *JAMA*. 2016;315(15):1624–1645.

26. Sandbrink F, Oliva EM, McMullen TL, et al. Opioid prescribing and opioid risk mitigation strategies in the Veterans Health Administration. *J Gen Intern Med*. 2020;35(3):927–934.

27. Darnall BD, Juurlink D, Kerns RD, et al. International stakeholder community of pain experts and leaders call for an urgent action on forced opioid tapering. *Pain Med*. 2019;20(3):429–433.

28. Webster LR, Webster RM. Predicting aberrant behaviors in opioid-treated patients: preliminary validation of the Opioid Risk Tool. *Pain Med*. 2005;6(6):432–442.

CHAPTER 18

Cannabinoids, Oncology, and the Law

Christopher Anderson, MA, JD

INTRODUCTION

This chapter may be unlike the other chapters in this book because of the distinctive uncertainties prevailing at the intersection of medicine and the law surrounding cannabis in the United States. Other chapters in this book discuss issues concerning oncology and law with the benefit of an extensive historical system of laws, regulations, and precedential case law. The legal issues involving medical malpractice standards or insurance controversies may vary from state to state, but in most such states, there is a significant practical history and body of law from which to distill reliable guidance and recommendations. However, the pertinent history of cannabis law and cannabis's application in oncology are developing at an almost daily pace and within a complicated context, which the Massachusetts Supreme Court recently pithily characterized as "a hazy thicket":

> [T]he current legal landscape of medical marijuana law may, at best, be described as a hazy thicket. Marijuana is illegal at the Federal level and has been deemed under Federal law to have no medicinal purposes, but Massachusetts, as well as the majority of States, have legalized medical marijuana and created regulatory schemes for its administration and usage. Complicating and confusing matters further, Congress has placed budgetary restrictions on the ability of the United States Department of Justice to prosecute individuals for marijuana usage in compliance with a State medical marijuana scheme, and the Department of Justice has issued, revised, and revoked memoranda explaining its marijuana enforcement practices and priorities, leaving in place no clear guidance.[1]

This haze is thickened by the fact that the majority of all medicinal cannabis programs in the United States have come into existence in the last eight years—a very short period of time for controversies to have arisen and been resolved into legal precedent. From the perspective of an individual practitioner considering medicinal cannabis's application to oncology, the ongoing reform of cannabis law and the remarkable expansion of regulated medicinal cannabis programs simply have not yet generated much case law from which practitioner-focused counsel can be derived.

As of this writing, cannabis (or, in the official language of US federal law, "marihuana" and "tetrahydrocannabinols, except for tetrahydrocannabinols in hemp") remains listed on Schedule I of the Controlled Substances Act (CSA), such that cannabis remains federally illegal in all instances.[2] By an unusual sort of reverse definition, because of its Schedule I status, cannabis is functionally deemed by the federal government to "have no currently accepted medical use in the United States, a lack of accepted safety for use under medical supervision, and a high potential for abuse."[3] But this assertion is directly contravened both by the laws of at least 34 states and by the existence (since 1976) of the federal Compassionate Investigational New Drug program, through which a small number of qualified patients have obtained medical cannabis directly from the US government.

CASE LAW # 1

In *Gonzales v Raich*, the US Supreme Court affirmed the constitutionality of the CSA's criminalization of cannabis.[4] The *Raich* decision found that home growing of medicinal cannabis might affect interstate commerce and that the federal government therefore had the constitutional authority to criminalize cannabis production even where the cannabis at issue was, ostensibly, part of a regulated and entirely intrastate program. The *Raich* majority reviewed the long history of cannabis regulation and the status of cannabis as a Schedule I controlled substance and noted that that the evidence offered in support of medical efficacy of cannabis might "cast serious doubt on the accuracy of the findings that require marijuana to be listed in Schedule I."[4]

Since the *Raich* decision in 2005, a supermajority of all the United States and its territories have determined that, at least within their borders, cannabis does have currently accepted medical uses and should be legal for some purposes. As of 2021, cannabis is still a Schedule I controlled substance, but the mounting scientific evidence and political support for cannabis legalization seem likely to result in some kind of change to that Schedule I status.

Because the possibility of a federally approved standardized model is foreclosed by cannabis's Schedule I status and federal illegality, each state that has legalized medicinal cannabis has implemented its own distinctive regulatory program. These programs evolve from one to the next, building on the successes and frameworks of previous programs, but they still have material idiosyncrasies from state to state. Consequently, any discussion of the utility of cannabis in the oncology domain involves too many variables for definitive answers to the question of what the law is regarding cannabis and oncology.

All of this leads to the "cannabis caveat," which should always be kept in mind when considering issues involving cannabis and oncology (or any practice area). Cannabis remains an "illegal" Schedule I controlled substance; every cannabis-legal state has its own regulatory approach, which is, by current definition, essentially at odds with federal law. The cannabis caveat, then, is a reminder that careful attention must be paid to the specific context and circumstances involved. Even a detailed 50-state survey of the laws, case law, and practical implications could not provide a concrete answer because (1) these state-by-state regulatory regimes are practically evolving all the time[5] and (2) the circumstances of the individual patient and potential application are critically important to understand.

CANNABIS AND CANCER TREATMENT

Cannabis and oncology

Cannabis's pain-relieving, antinausea, and appetite-inducing characteristics contributed to its early medicinal popularity in the oncology domain. Some researchers have proposed that a connection between cannabis and cancer management dates back to the earliest stages of modern humanity. Magnetic resonance imaging of the Siberian Ice Maiden, a 2500-year-old individual discovered in 1993 in possession of a stash of cannabis, "revealed she had a primary tumor in her right breast along with metastatic disease. It was speculated that she could have used cannabis to manage her pain or treat her malignant disease."[6] The application of cannabis to oncology issues has been widely understood for some time: a 1991 Harvard Medical School study indicated that nearly half (44%) of US oncologists were already recommending cannabis use as a palliative or mitigating therapeutic to combat the side effects of cancer treatments. This was five years before California became the first state (in 1996) to authorize the medical use of cannabis.[7] The Americans for Safe Access Foundation noted that:

> In 2001, a review of clinical studies conducted in several states during the past few decades revealed that, in nearly 2,000 individuals with cancer, inhaled cannabis and oral cannabinoids were effective anti-emetics. Other studies have concluded that the active components in cannabis produce palliative effects in cancer patients by preventing nausea, vomiting, and pain and by stimulating appetite.[8]

That report and other surveys of contemporary research also note the potential that cannabis may not only ameliorate side effects but also battle tumors:

> The tumor-fighting properties of cannabinoids have also been demonstrated in numerous laboratory studies and investigated in a successful Phase I clinical study looking at the safety of THC (tetrahydrocannabinol) in patients with recurrent brain cancer. Researchers have observed that "these compounds have been shown to inhibit the growth of tumor cells in culture and animal models by modulating key cell-signaling pathways. Cannabinoids are usually well tolerated, and do not produce the generalized toxic effects of conventional chemotherapies."[9]

Other researchers have concluded that cannabinoids "have a direct effect on cancer and the side effects of chemotherapy. They have been shown to inhibit tumor growth in multiple cell lines. Animals treated with cannabinoids had a slower tumor growth than control animals, and cannabinoids do not harm healthy cells at the same dose that is needed to kill cancer cells."[10]

This chapter is not intended to endorse or advance scientific conclusions regarding the oncologic applications of cannabis. Rather, it is an operating assumption of this chapter that there are already widely recognized medicinal applications for cannabis (in oncology specifically) and that readers are health care professionals who are interested in understanding the legal issues involved in applying medicinal cannabis to their practice domain.

Can health care professionals legally apply cannabis in their patient-care regimens?

The starting point for any health care professional (HCP) considering cannabis applications in the oncology domain might be the simple question, "Is cannabis legal in [insert state of practice]?" But the CSA Schedule I status of cannabis and the "hazy thicket" that the Massachusetts Supreme Judicial Court noted in late 2020 are stark reminders that:

> [A]n individual who "aids, abets, counsels, commands, induces or procures" the commission of a Federal offense, including a violation of the CSA, may be subject to the same penalties as the principal . . . Accordingly, regardless of the legal status of marijuana at the State level, marijuana users, and those who aid or abet the distribution or possession of marijuana, "remain potentially subject to Federal criminal prosecution."[11]

So, even if cannabis is legal within an HCP's state, cannabis use or possession is prohibited by federal law, and the penalties for violation can be severe. However, the actual in-fact enforcement of those federal laws is—at best—remarkably *de minimis*.

The Massachusetts Supreme Judicial Court had noted that congressional actions have "placed budgetary restrictions" on the federal government's ability to interfere with state-managed medicinal cannabis programs, and the Department of Justice (DOJ) has "issued, revised, and revoked memoranda explaining its marijuana enforcement practices and priorities."[11] These funding and priority-based controls were attempts to provide states with some reliable confidence that the federal government would not intervene to disrupt state-based cannabis regulatory programs. The Rohrabacher-Farr Amendment (also known as the Rohrabacher-Blumenauer Amendment) prohibits the DOJ (the parent agency to the Drug Enforcement Administration [DEA]) from using federal funds to interfere with the implementation of state medical cannabis laws.[12] This budgetary rider was passed in 2014 and has been routinely renewed. The DOJ has issued various guidance memoranda, most notably the Ogden (2009) and Cole (2013) Memoranda, the latter of which outlined the DOJ's eight principal enforcement priorities that shaped the federal government's scrutiny of state-based cannabis activity. In 2018, these memos were formally rescinded by Attorney General Jeff Sessions. Despite that formal rescission, there has been no appreciable change in the enforcement efforts of the DOJ; the current administration has indicated no intention to crack down on state-based cannabis legalization.

In addition to the encouraging facts of congressional budgetary restrictions and tolerant enforcement priorities of the DOJ, there are simple facts regarding federal criminal charges being leveled against HCPs who operate in compliance with a state-regulated medicinal cannabis program. A reporting table maintained by the DEA, "Cases Against Doctors," indicates only 22 criminal cases brought against doctors since 2012, with circumstances generally involving opiates.[13] The DEA reporting reflects two cases involving cannabis as the pertinent controlled substance. Similarly, the Americans for Safe Access Foundation "2020 State of the States Report" notes that between 2014 and 2020, there were only two federal raids relating to medicinal cannabis programs.[14]

The state law enforcement actions against HCPs operating in the medicinal cannabis domain generally involve situations where the HCPs use a state's regulatory system as a façade to enable "obvious" criminal activity such as fraudulent authorizations or knowing participation in schemes by which "patients" obtain medicinal cannabis in order to divert into the illicit market-place. For example, in Michigan in 2011, prosecutors brought criminal charges against a Detroit doctor who was allegedly participating in a for-profit medical marijuana operation involving the sale of falsified medical marijuana physician certifications.[15] In Colorado in 2014, a doctor faced felony charges after admitting to writing more than 7000 medical marijuana recommendations without actually seeing many of those patients in any actual capacity.[16]

In addition, because the HCP is merely permissively recommending, not prescribing, canna-bis, that risk is insulated by the principles of the doctor-patient privilege and the First Amend-ment to the US Constitution. If an HCP is practicing in a state where cannabis is legal, it is difficult to envision practical circumstances in which that HCP's counseling about cannabis, including a recommendation for use in compliance with state law, would result in federal author-ities seeking criminal charges against the HCP. Addressing patients' inquiries about cannabis is constitutionally protected speech that should not be chilled by federal authorities.

CASE LAW # 2

In *Conant v Walters*, the Ninth Circuit Court of Appeals invoked First Amendment freedom of speech principles to determine that a physician was protected from federal government actions related to the physician's recommendation of cannabis as a medicinal option.[17] The *Conant* case resulted in an injunction against the federal government, prohibiting it from both (a) revoking an HCP's license to prescribe controlled substances and (b) even conducting an investigation of the HCP that might result in such a revocation. The *Conant* court noted that open and confident com-munication between patients and their doctors was an integral component of medical practice and a necessity that gave rise to the doctor-patient privilege:

> The doctor-patient privilege reflects "the imperative need for confidence and trust" inherent in the doctor-patient relationship and recognizes that "a physician must know all that a patient can articulate in order to identify and to treat disease; barriers to full disclosure would impair diag-nosis and treatment." . . . The Supreme Court has recognized that physician speech is entitled to First Amendment protection because of the significance of the doctor-patient relationship.[17]

An HCP's discussion of cannabis issues, including a recommendation to their patient of cannabis use, was deemed to be a provision of useful information and quite different from the actual dispens-ing of a controlled substance. The risk of even an investigation by federal authorities would, accord-ing to the *Conant* court, have an unconstitutional chilling effect on the physician's right to speak about matters of tremendous professional importance.[17]

This case is widely understood as sufficient protection to cover HCPs across the country with respect to their discussions or recommendations regarding the medicinal value of cannabis. Maryland's Medical Cannabis Commission cites *Conant* within its frequently asked questions addressing the issues of whether providers have a constitutional defense against "interference from federal authorities for advising patients about medical marijuana."[18]

Similarly, in 2011, a Colorado court found a state constitutional protection that resulted in a physician who had been accused of writing fraudulent medical marijuana recommendations having all criminal charges against him dismissed. The doctor had been chosen completely at random; there were no medical cannabis–related complaints lodged against the doctor. The judge ruled that the doctor's recommendation of medical cannabis to an undercover police officer complaining of severe pain was protected by Colorado's constitutional amendment that guaranteed physicians an exception from the state's criminal laws when making medical marijuana recommendations to qualified patients.[19]

For an HCP who is discussing or even recommending the application of cannabis for bona fide oncology issues, there is an almost infinitesimal likelihood of state or federal criminal consequence.

Jurisdiction matters

As of Spring 2021, only two states, Idaho and Nebraska, maintain a strict prohibition against any form of cannabis use or possession. Twelve other states (Alabama, Georgia, Indiana, Iowa, Kansas, Kentucky, North Carolina, South Carolina, Tennessee, Texas, Wisconsin, Wyoming) permit *some* medicinal use of *some* mode of cannabis product while still prohibiting products that contain more than a negligible amount of THC. However, prohibitionist states are a distinctive (and shrinking) minority.

A total of 36 states and five US jurisdictions have legalized (and generated regulatory programs for) the medicinal use of cannabis: Alaska, Arizona, Arkansas, California, Colorado, Connecticut, Delaware, Florida, Hawaii, Illinois, Louisiana, Maine, Maryland, Massachusetts, Michigan, Minnesota, Mississippi, Missouri, Montana, Nevada, New Hampshire, New Jersey, New Mexico, New York, North Dakota, Ohio, Oklahoma, Oregon, Pennsylvania, Rhode Island, South Dakota, Utah, Vermont, Virginia, Washington, and West Virginia, plus the District of Columbia, Guam, the Northern Mariana Islands, Puerto Rico, and the US Virgin Islands.[20]

The Americans for Safe Access Foundation State of the States Report is an immensely valuable tool for any HCP seeking to understand the specific context and practicalities of medicinal cannabis applications in their practice. This report not only provides a scorecard for each state—calculated based on more than 50 dimensions of utility, patient safety, supply-chain issues, and patient rights—but also delivers longitudinal analyses of a given state's evolution on medicinal cannabis issues. This report is an intensely researched and carefully presented resource and can be relied on to supplement the official agency-managed materials that every state authority publishes to educate the public, patients, caregivers, and the medical professional community regarding the state-managed program.

From a statistical standpoint, it is more likely than not that an HCP reading this book is practicing medicine in a state in which adult or patient use has been deemed legal by the state authorities. In November 2020, voters in four states voted to legalize recreational (or adult-use) cannabis, and the state of Virginia will implement adult-use legalization by 2024. As a result, 16 states and three US jurisdictions will permit adults to use cannabis without *any* required medical authorization: Alaska, Arizona, California, Colorado, Illinois, Maine, Massachusetts, Michigan, Montana, Nevada, New Jersey, Oregon, South Dakota, Vermont, Virginia, and Washington, as well as the District of Columbia, the Northern Mariana Islands, and Guam. The growing list of adult-use states and territories is such that the "average" HCP reading this chapter is likely to be practicing in a location where cannabis is not only a potential medicine but perhaps also an ordinary part of the patient's lifestyle.

The net-net conclusion amounts to this: there is an extremely attenuated risk quotient surrounding good faith recommendations of cannabis offered to legitimately needy patients by professionally informed HCPs. But even so, and with the cannabis caveat firmly in mind, HCPs considering the application of cannabis in patient care must thoroughly understand the regulatory mechanisms that compose their state's cannabis regime.

HIGHEST COMMON DENOMINATORS ACROSS MEDICINAL CANNABIS PROGRAMS

Medicinal cannabis programs have evolved significantly from the initial gauzy permissiveness of California's Compassionate Use Act of 1996. The programs operating across 41 US jurisdictions share similar structural frameworks and critical components that can be abstracted to reveal "highest common denominator" patterns. A given medicinal cannabis program is almost certain to include the following: (1) a set of **qualifying conditions** deemed by the state authorities to potentially benefit from the application of cannabis and (2) a requirement that there be a (a) **bona fide patient-doctor relationship**, within which there is (b) **an assessment of the patient** by a medical professional, leading to (3) that assessing medical professional providing a **formal "recommendation" or "authorization"** for the patient's use of cannabis to treat the qualifying condition.

How these three programmatic elements [(3) an HCP recommendation to (2) a bona fide patient that the patient use medicinal cannabis to treat their (1) qualifying condition] are presented, defined, and operationalized in a medicinal cannabis program will vary from state to state. For instance, Michigan defines what is required for a medical professional to secure "safe harbor" protection from state penalties when authorizing medicinal cannabis applications (bracketed numbers have been inserted to correlate to the common denominators identified above):

> (g) A physician shall not be subject to [regulatory or licensure penalties], solely for providing [3] written certifications, in the course of a [2] bona fide physician-patient relationship and after the physician has completed a full assessment of the qualifying patient's medical history, or for otherwise stating that, in the physician's professional opinion, a patient is likely to [1] receive therapeutic or palliative benefit from the medical use of marihuana to treat or alleviate the patient's serious or debilitating medical condition or symptoms associated with the serious or debilitating medical condition.[21]

In addition to those three broad common denominators, state programs generally impose additional oversight controls designed to prevent diversion (i.e., leakage from the legal system into the illicit markets). These regulatory rigors include (4) strict supply-chain and tracking obligations on the manufacturers and distributors of cannabis products and (5) a limit on the amount of cannabis that a qualified patient can procure in a given period of time.

Because HCPs do not actually produce, possess, or distribute cannabis to their patients themselves, this chapter does not address these two components of states' cannabis regulatory programs in depth. However, the section "Landscape of Medicinal Cannabis Marketplace Actors" outlines the general actors involved in a state-regulated supply chain and the section "Restrictions on Form and Amount" discusses the purchase or possession limits that regulate how much cannabis a patient may procure.

Qualifying or debilitating conditions

The central gate-keeping element of any medicinal cannabis program is the state-generated list of qualifying or debilitating conditions for which cannabis can be authorized. Generally, such conditions are explicitly enumerated and defined within the state's medicinal cannabis statutes or rules. Consistent with the "it depends" theme of this chapter, the legalistic definitions of "qualifying" or "debilitating" conditions and the enumerated list of conditions will vary from state to state. However, for the purposes of this chapter, it is almost certainly the case that if medicinal cannabis is legal, then the state regulations establishing such legality will either (1) explicitly include cancer or (2) recognize some cancer-related circumstance as a qualifying condition.

For instance, Maryland regulations eschew enumerated qualifying conditions in favor of permitting cannabis use to remedy symptoms such as cachexia, anorexia, wasting syndrome, severe or chronic pain, severe nausea, seizures, severe or persistent muscle spasms, glaucoma, posttraumatic stress disorder, or another chronic medical condition that is severe and for which other treatments have been ineffective.[14,18] Similarly, in Michigan, medicinal cannabis applications are approved not only for certain debilitating medical conditions but also to ameliorate symptoms resulting from pathologies, including symptoms resulting from treatment:

> (b) "Debilitating medical condition" means one or more of the following: (1) Cancer, glaucoma, positive status for human immunodeficiency virus, acquired immune deficiency syndrome, hepatitis C, amyotrophic lateral sclerosis, Crohn's disease, agitation of Alzheimer's disease, nail patella, or the treatment of these conditions. (2) A chronic or debilitating disease or medical condition or its treatment that produces one or more of the following: cachexia or wasting syndrome; severe and chronic pain; severe nausea; seizures, including but not limited to those characteristic of epilepsy; or severe and persistent muscle spasms, including but not limited to those characteristic of multiple sclerosis.[22]

The bona fide doctor-patient relationship

Doctor and patient

Doctor

The central actor in the medicinal application of cannabis is, of course, the doctor who is (1) in good standing with the state's medical board and (2) has no restrictions on their ability to prescribe. The scope of "doctor" will, like so much else, vary from state to state. Missouri only allows MDs or osteopaths to certify patients as have qualifying medical conditions. However, many states have expanded the scope to include other HCPs. In Illinois, for instance, nurse practitioners and physician assistants are now permitted to certify patient-applicants for medicinal cannabis. In Massachusetts, both physicians and certified nurse practitioners (CNPs) are eligible to participate in the state's medicinal cannabis program if they (1) hold an active full license with no prescribing restrictions, (2) hold a Massachusetts Controlled Substances Registration (MCSR), and (3) have at least one established place of practice in Massachusetts. CNPs must also (4) hold a board authorization by the Massachusetts Board of Registration in Nursing to practice as a CNP in Massachusetts. In Maryland's medical cannabis program, physicians, nurse practitioners, dentists, podiatrists, and nurse-midwives may potentially certify patients as eligible for medicinal cannabis.[23]

Registered provider

HCPs must also register themselves with the state regulator in order to participate in their state's medicinal cannabis program. The mechanics of such registration and ongoing maintenance will vary from state to state. In Maryland, for instance, providers must register themselves on the state program's website and renew such registration every two years in order to provide patient certifications. That registration involves providing their Maryland board license number, their Controlled Dangerous Substances number, and a succinct specification of (1) the conditions or diseases the HCP intends to treat with cannabis and (2) any criteria for including or excluding patients from cannabis authorizations. In Massachusetts, health care providers must register only once with the state regulator and will retain the ability to certify a patient indefinitely, unless:

- They surrender their registration.
- Their license or board authorization to practice medicine or nursing in Massachusetts is suspended, revoked, or restricted with regard to prescribing, or their MCSR is revoked or suspended.
- They voluntarily agree not to practice medicine or nursing in Massachusetts.
- They are determined to have fraudulently issued a written certification or to have certified a qualifying patient without completing the required professional development credits, as described in the regulations.

Every state regulator has the power to suspend revoke, or restrict an HCP's ability to issue medicinal authorizations, and while the act of authorizing cannabis is not a "prescription," it would behoove an HCP to consider cannabis authorization as quite similar to prescribing rights in terms of stringent attention toward regulatory compliance.

The requirement that HCPs obtain or maintain some degree of professional development credits relating to medicinal cannabis is not uncommon. In Florida, for instance, a two-hour course and examination are required in order for an HCP to gain access to the state's Medical Marijuana Use Registry. The Florida Medical Association and the Florida Osteopathic Medical Association administer the course and exam, and successful completion is required each time a physician renews their medical license.

Registered qualifying patient or caregiver

The "patient" side of the doctor-patient relationship is fairly straightforward: this is the individual suffering from the qualifying or debilitating medical condition that may be eased through the use of medicinal cannabis. A patient will present themselves to be assessed and will receive some formal authorization to procure (and possess) medicinal cannabis. The abstracted rule of thumb is that patients who are over 18 and capable of procuring their own medicine will do so; for qualified patients who are either under 18 or incapable of procuring their medicinal cannabis themselves, the role of caregiver comes into play.

Caregivers are authorized to procure (and possess for the purposes of transporting or administering) medicinal cannabis on behalf of a qualifying authorized patient. For instance, in general, the term *primary caregiver* or *caregiver* means a person who is at least 21 years old and who has agreed to assist with a patient's medical use of cannabis. States typically impose restrictions on who can act as a caregiver (e.g., only those who have not been convicted of any felony within the past ten years and have never been convicted of a felony involving illegal drugs or a felony that is an assaultive crime).[24] States also often impose restrictions on the number of qualifying patients that a single caregiver may represent in order to avoid giving one individual a lawful right to possess very large quantities of cannabis.

Both patients and their designated caregivers must be registered with the state regulator before being permitted to procure medicinal cannabis. The patient's application to and registration with the state regulator may be required before the patient can properly consult with an HCP to obtain an authorization. For instance, in Maryland, a patient must complete and submit an online application, during which they provide: (1) a valid e-mail account; (2) the last four digits of their Social Security number; (3) an electronic copy of a specific form of government-issued photo ID; and (4) proof that the applicant lives in Maryland. After receiving approval from the state regulator, a Maryland patient can then visit a registered HCP to obtain a valid certification. After being both (1) fully registered and (2) in possession of a valid certification, the patient is able to print their patient ID card and then use that card to purchase medicinal cannabis from a licensed dispensary.

In Florida, a would-be patient must first seek treatment from a qualified physician or osteopath registered in the state program. That registered physician must enter the patient's information into the state's Medical Marijuana Use Registry, which would then permit the patient to apply for and be approved to receive a Medical Marijuana Use Registry identification card. After being approved by the regulator, the patient may procure medicinal cannabis only at an approved medical marijuana treatment center or via delivery.

Patient assessment

The other requirement in any medicinal cannabis authorization is that there be an actual assessment of the patient, which generally involves: (1) that there be a bona fide doctor-patient relationship, (2) within which the HCP performs an in-fact assessment of the patient and (3) determines that the patient has a qualifying condition that might benefit from medicinal cannabis application.

An exemplary statutory definition can be found at Michigan Compiled Laws (§ 333.26423), which includes requirements for a "relevant, in-person, medical evaluation of the patient" and the capacity for the physician to "monitor the efficacy of the use" of the recommended cannabis application. The Michigan Supreme Court was obliged to interpret the statutory language (which it is worth noting was impractically presented as a single sentence) regarding the "bona fide physician-patient relationship." In its decision, that court "reduced" the legalese of the statutory provision to "three elements" that were necessary to establish the "Imprimatur of the Physician-Patient Relationship"[25]:

1. The existence of a bona fide physician-patient relationship,
2. in which the physician completes a full assessment of the patient's medical history and current medical condition, and
3. from which results the physician's professional opinion that the patient has a debilitating medical condition and will likely benefit from the medical use of marijuana to treat the debilitating medical condition.[25]

The Michigan Supreme Court's three elements are a useful guide for understanding the prerequisites of a patient assessment leading to the certification that the patient might benefit from medicinal cannabis. However, any HCP considering medicinal cannabis authorization must review the specific statutory language governing their state. For instance, in Maryland, it may be necessary for other treatments to have first proven ineffective before medicinal cannabis can be authorized.

It is important to point out that there is no provision in any state law that obligates an HCP to authorize or qualify a patient for medicinal cannabis. HCPs are expected to assess the patient's medical history, medical condition, and general circumstances and to recommend the treatment options that they think are appropriate to that patient. A patient is not entitled to a medicinal cannabis authorization; there may be significant reasons why even patients suffering from qualifying conditions might be found to be inappropriate candidates for medicinal cannabis application.

Telemedicine

In Missouri, their recently implemented medicinal cannabis program does permit for authorizations via telemedicine if the "standard of care does not require an in-person encounter, and if the physician can conduct an exam via telemedicine in a manner that allows that physician to truthfully answer all attestations on the physician certification form in the affirmative." By contrast, Florida law requires that the HCP conduct a physical examination while physically present in the same room as the patient and after a full assessment of the patient's medical history. Consequently, in Florida, there is no possible certification through telemedicine.

CLINICAL VIGNETTE # 1

Tim Jones is a 70-year-old man who was recently diagnosed with local non–small-cell lung cancer. He is currently on week four of his chemoradiation therapy. He has confluent mucositis, and the opioid pain regimen does not appear to give him any relief. He is anxious, stressed out, and in moderate pain. He lives in Alabama, and the closest medical center is two hours away. He schedules a telemedicine consult with his oncologist, Dr. Joseph Scrippaway, and wants to know if the doctor can call in some marijuana for him that he can pick up at a local dispensary to calm his nerves. Should Dr. Scrippaway just call in a script to the dispensary?

The patient, Mr. Jones, lives in Alabama, which has some of the strictest cannabis-related laws in the United States. While Alabama does permit some use of medicinal cannabis, that permission is limited to cannabidiol (CBD) applications for epileptic seizures (and Alabama's medicinal cannabis law merely provides an affirmative defense to the individual against possession charges; there is no regulated mechanism under which Dr. Scrippaway could affirmatively authorize cannabis, even for a seizure patient).[26,27] As of this writing, Alabama is considering broadening its medical cannabis program to include products containing THC, but this is still before the legislature and has not been signed into law, much less rolled out as a formal regulatory program.

Based on the facts presented in this vignette, there is likely no legitimate opportunity for the Alabama physician, Dr. Scrippaway, to authorize cannabis for use by Mr. Jones. Alabama does not currently permit medicinal cannabis applications in oncology situations.

If we shifted the location of the proposed vignette from Alabama to, say, Louisiana, then the analysis changes, because Louisiana does have a regulated medical cannabis program that includes cancer among the qualifying conditions.[28] Louisiana's program is still in its early stages, and the bureaucratic processes must be carefully and diligently followed. An HCP interested in securing a Therapeutic Marijuana Registration (TMR) permit would start their qualification process with the Louisiana State Board of Medical Examiners.[29] The board determines the qualifications for HCPs and notes that a recommending physician must:

- Hold a current, unrestricted license to practice medicine issued by the board
- Obtain a Schedule I authority or such other authority as may be designated for therapeutic marijuana by the Louisiana Board of Pharmacy (recommending therapeutic marijuana without obtaining this will put the licensee at risk for disciplinary action)
- Practice at a physical practice location in Louisiana
- Have completed the Therapeutic Marijuana Rules Review Course

If Dr. Scrippaway is qualified to participate in Louisiana's program, then he could recommend cannabis for Mr. Jones without Mr. Jones even registering himself with the state regulator: Louisiana does not require that qualifying patients join a state registry or get a medical marijuana card at any point.

However, significant hurdles still remain in the scenario. First, Louisiana does not permit medicinal cannabis recommendations via telemedicine consultations. Second, Louisiana only has ten medicinal cannabis dispensaries throughout the state that are dispensing cannabis grown by only two authorized cultivators. Finally, in Louisiana's program, only certain forms of medical cannabis are permitted: oils, pills, liquids, topical applications, and inhaled via a device similar to an inhaler (but not one that combusts raw cannabis flower; cannabis flower is not available in Louisiana). As a result, it may be quite difficult, though not impossible, for Mr. Jones to procure cannabis in Louisiana.

Monitoring of patient condition or renewal of authorization

In most states, a patient's authorization for medicinal cannabis must be renewed annually; the patient's program ID card will expire without (1) a renewed assessment and (2) affirmative action to secure reauthorization. However, some states impose an affirmative obligation not only on patients to periodically renew their authorization but also on the authorizing HCP to monitor the patient's application of medicinal cannabis. In Illinois, for instance, an authorizing HCP must "have responsibility for the ongoing care and treatment of the qualifying patient's debilitating condition, provided that the ongoing treatment and care shall not be limited to or for the primary purpose of certifying a debilitating medical condition or providing a consultation solely for that purpose." That is to say, the bona fide relationship must be more expansive and sustained than merely the acquisition and renewal of the medicinal cannabis authorization. In Maryland, the bona fide relationship is statutorily defined as one in which the HCP (1) will create and maintain medically standardized records and (2) expects to monitor the patient's cannabis application program and take any medically indicated actions.

The authorization

Authorization on file with the state

The HCP's determination that medical cannabis could be therapeutic or palliative for a patient with a qualifying condition is then documented as an "authorization," "recommendation," or "certification" (each state will have its own nomenclature for the authorizing document), and this fact is relayed to the state regulatory agency in order to enable the patient to procure such medicinal products. It is vitally important to note that this is not a prescription to the patient; because cannabis remains on Schedule I of the CSA, there is at present no situation where cannabis is prescribed to a patient. Rather, a qualified HCP can offer a recommendation to a qualifying patient and that patient can use the recommendation to procure medicinal cannabis from a qualified dispensary (which is not a pharmacy and will generally deal exclusively in cannabis products).

The final form certification (or authorization or recommendation), which will be on file with the state program, will generally include information such as the following:

- Patient's name, address, and date of birth
- Patient's medical condition(s)
- HCP's name
- Date of patient qualification
- HCP's signature or attestation

The registries for states' medicinal cannabis programs are near universally maintained in dedicated digital traceability systems that enable the states to track cannabis patients and producers, monitor in near real time the cannabis marketplace, and generally ensure against oversupply or diversion.

After the state regulator has received the HCP's authorization and after patients have properly enrolled themselves in the state program, then patients will generally be able to secure some type of registration card or program ID.

CLINICAL VIGNETTE # 2

Jane Potter is a 55-year-old woman who was recently diagnosed with metastatic ovarian cancer. She lives in San Mateo, California. She is recently divorced and lives by herself. Her oncologist, Dr. Edith Edible, recently prescribed her oxycodone five mg as needed and morphine 30 mg orally every 12 hours. Her pelvic pain level goes from ten to about a seven. She can barely perform the activities of daily living. She purchased some edibles at a cannabis retail store down the street, and after taking a few bites, her pain level went down to three. Because she wants to visit her sister in New Orleans, Louisiana, she wants to buy five boxes of the edibles but fears that she may get in trouble bringing them on the flight. She calls her Dr. Edible for advice. What should Dr. Edible tell her?

Dr. Edible is free, under the precedent established by the *Conant* case, to discuss medicinal cannabis applications with Ms. Potter. Because California has legalized adult-use cannabis, Ms. Potter does not need to obtain a medical authorization from Dr. Edible, but she may wish to participate in the state's medical program in order to lawfully avoid the sales and use tax applied to commercial cannabis sales.

While a California-based medical authorization might also be useful for Ms. Potter if she elects to transport her medicinal cannabis products with her to Louisiana, that authorization is not a definitive protection for her against actions by the Transportation Security Administration or law enforcement officials in Louisiana. And in this regard, it would likely be unwise for Dr. Edible to offer any more information than the reminder that cannabis remains federally illegal and that cannabis lawfully purchased in one state *cannot* be lawfully transported to another state, under any circumstances (at present).[30]

While the likelihood of intrusion by either the Transportation Security Administration or Louisiana law enforcement might be quite low (particularly with edibles, which might be difficult to identify as cannabis products), Dr. Edible should not counsel her patient about her legal rights or the legality of her planned conduct.

Patient ID card

The patient's authorization is then presented by the patient (or caregiver) to gain access to and procure medicinal cannabis from authorized dispensaries. The authorization card can also be used to justify the patient's (or caregiver's) possession or use of medicinal cannabis if queried by law enforcement authorities or other parties (such as an employer).

Some states offer reciprocal recognition of a patient's medicinal cannabis authorization card from another state, including Alaska, Arizona, Arkansas, California, Colorado, Maine, Massachusetts, Michigan, New Hampshire, Nevada, Oklahoman, Oregon, Pennsylvania, Rhode Island, Washington, and Washington, DC. Reciprocity is not assured, however, and as with everything in this area, it should be investigated and determined in the specific circumstances.

Landscape of medicinal cannabis marketplace actors

The statutes that generate medicinal cannabis regulations generally define the actors who operate in that marketplace, and although the specific terms may vary from state to state, the categorical types are broadly similar. The roles of HCPs, patients, and caregivers have been discussed previously. Other critical operators that compose the medicinal cannabis industry are discussed in the following sections.

Producers, cultivators, or growers

The starting point of any cannabis market supply chain are state-licensed farms that grow and harvest cannabis plants. Cannabis crops can be grown fully outdoor, entirely indoor, or in a hybrid situation such as a greenhouse.

Processors or manufacturers

These are the state-licensed operators that receive harvested cannabis from the grower and process that raw biomass into other formats for end-user consumption, such as edibles, tinctures, capsules, or concentrates.

Dispensaries, retail stores, or delivery providers

These are the state-licensed businesses that sell cannabis (and sometimes ancillary paraphernalia) to authorized patients or their caregivers. The specific nomenclature for such entities varies across state programs, although the default colloquial term applicable in medicinal contexts remains *dispensary*. In Florida, they are called *medical marijuana treatment centers*, and in New Jersey, they are called *alternative treatment centers*. In Massachusetts, they were initially known as *registered marijuana dispensaries* but became *medical marijuana treatment centers* in 2019. In Missouri, they are simply known as *dispensaries*, which is one category of licensed medical marijuana facility. In some states where cannabis has been legalized for adult use, the point-of-sale facility will simply be a licensed cannabis retail store, and such retailers may sell both medicinal and adult-use cannabis.

Because the dispensary is the business from which patients will secure their authorized medicinal cannabis, it may behoove HCPs to cultivate some familiarity with the various stores in their area since the patient will be relying on such stores to fulfill the recommendation.

In some states, delivery services may enable qualifying patients to receive their authorized medicinal cannabis without necessarily visiting a dispensary in person each time.

Transportation licensees

These state licensees are granted permission to possess and transport volumes of cannabis between other licensees. They are generally not licensed to deliver directly to the consumer (although some states do have delivery services, but those services are more akin to the retail or dispensary licensees from a regulatory perspective), but rather focus on transporting cannabis products to testing or research facilities and delivering product between the supply-chain operators.

Testing labs

Every state imposes significant health, safety, and product quality assurance requirements for legalized cannabis products. To provide this quality control, states will issue specialized licenses to independent testing laboratories that are thereby authorized to possess and test cannabis samples to ensure the products conform to the program's safety, potency, and general quality requirements.

Research institutions
Some states (e.g., Pennsylvania) have licensed specific research institutions to perform targeted scientific research on cannabis.

State regulatory agencies
The agencies charged with administering the state's medicinal cannabis program are often a division of the state health regulator. The Florida Department of Health has an Office of Medical Marijuana Use (OMMU), which: writes and implements medical cannabis rules; oversees the Medical Marijuana Use Registry; licenses Florida businesses to cultivate, process, and dispense medical cannabis to qualified patients; and certifies cannabis testing laboratories. In Missouri, the Section for Medical Marijuana Regulation (SMMR) was created within the Missouri Department of Health and Senior Services to oversee the Medical Marijuana Regulatory Program (MMRP).

In states where cannabis is legal for adult use, cannabis regulators may be aligned with the state's alcohol regulator or may be responsible for overseeing both the adult-use market and medicinal programs. In Washington State, the Liquor and Cannabis Board (LCB) regulates all cannabis products, with special "endorsements" available to enable patients to procure medicine without the same excise tax imposed on adult-use cannabis. In Oregon, the Oregon Liquor Control Commission (OLCC) handles all cannabis regulation, but the Oregon Medical Marijuana Program (OMMP) is administered by the Oregon Health Authority, which is advised by the Oregon Cannabis Commission (OCC). In Massachusetts, the Cannabis Control Commission (CCC) governs both the commonwealth's medicinal cannabis program and the adult-use marketplace. The Michigan Medical Marijuana Program (MMMP) is a state registry operating under the authority of Michigan's Marijuana Regulatory Agency.

In California, the longtime medicinal cannabis industry was brought into coordination with the adult-use marketplace through the Medicinal and Adult-Use Cannabis Regulation and Safety Act (MAUCRSA). Under MAUCRSA, a single regulatory system now governs both the medical and adult-use cannabis industry in California; the Office of Administrative Law manages the cannabis regulations enforced by the (1) Bureau of Cannabis Control, (2) California Department of Food and Agriculture, and (3) California Department of Health.

Restrictions on form and amount

Product purchase or possession limits
Every state imposes a limitation on the amount of cannabis that a person, whether a patient or an ordinary adult, can lawfully possess at a given time. In addition, patients are generally only permitted to purchase limited amounts over a given period. For instance, in Illinois, a registered qualifying patient may purchase up to 2.5 oz of medicinal cannabis during a 14-day period. This "adequate supply" is defined by Illinois statute and can only be procured from licensed medical

cannabis dispensaries. In Missouri, a registered HCP may certify the patient to procure up to four oz of dried cannabis (or its equivalent) over a 30-day period. Amounts in excess of four oz can be justified by attestation of two independent physicians certifying to the department a compelling reason that specifies what other amount the qualifying patient needs. In Maryland, the certification issued by the HCP to the patient will identify the amount of dried flower and THC that the patient may purchase over a rolling 30-day period.

In states where adult-use cannabis is legal, a possession limit of one oz (when "out in public") is something of a default standard, although some states permit increased quantities held at home (e.g., Massachusetts permits adults to possess up to ten oz at home). It is perhaps worth pointing out that different cannabis formats will implicate different weights; states have addressed this through category-specific permissions. For instance, in Washington State, adults may possess one oz of usable marijuana, 16 oz of marijuana-infused product in solid form, 72 oz of marijuana-infused product in liquid form, or seven g of marijuana concentrate.

Product format restrictions

Cannabis begins as raw flower, but various extraction and reformulation processes allow for a wide range of end-product formats, including food-based edibles, lozenges (generally also considered an edible), tinctures, topical salves, and concentrates (including a wide range of oils and crystalline "dabs"). Table 18-1 provides a basic primer on the potentially available categories of cannabis products.

Table 18-1. Basic Primer on Available Categories of Cannabis Products

Format and Administration Route	Advantages	Disadvantages
Smoked cannabis	Fast acting; strong effects may be achieved immediately	Combustion of plant material creates carcinogenic chemicals; smoking is considered an antisocial act; accurate dosing can be problematic; short-term effect duration; many potentially therapeutic substances are destroyed in the combustion process
Vaporized cannabis	Fast acting; clean of carcinogens; no combustion of plant material and therefore preservation of many potentially therapeutic substances	Short-term effect duration, and redosing may be required frequently
Topical preparations	Beneficial mostly for specific skin-related indications; easy and local administration method	Low level of bioavailability; may be inadequate for most indications in which systemic cannabinoid exposure is sought
Edible products	Easy oral administration; full preservation of beneficial active ingredients; longer effect relative to smoking and vaporizing	Relatively long time before initiation of therapeutic effects; variable bioavailability levels and therefore difficult to dose properly
Sublingual administration	Easy administration with no toxic carcinogens	Short-term effect; redosing may be required frequently

States often impose "format" restrictions that prohibit certain forms of cannabis consumption. Generally, this involves a prohibition against raw cannabis such that patients cannot ingest cannabinoids through smoking flower. However, programs that prohibit raw flower usually permit the consumption of cannabis concentrate (e.g., oil) through vaporization.

SUMMARY OF CANNABIS SCIENCE

Even with the presumption of an active awareness of medicinal cannabis, an HCP may find the following succinct and of-the-moment primer on the "state of the science" of medicinal cannabis to be useful. HCPs are as instrumental as research scientists, legislators, and administrators in the evolution of societal attitudes about cannabis. Attention to the dangers associated with cannabis as a drug should be paralleled by practitioner awareness of the scientific discoveries about the potential medicinal values and applications that *Cannabis*, its constituent compounds (particularly cannabinoids and terpenoids), and its various forms and modalities may have. The pace of the developments, in terms of understanding the compounds as "medicine" and the plant breeding and genotype manipulations that enable targeted production of specific compounds, requires that everyone, particularly science-minded HCPs, begin to reassess the domain. It is not just cannabis that has utility in oncology applications but potentially a whole host of distinctive *cannabinoids*.

The plant

As an annual herbaceous plant in the Cannabaceae family, *Cannabis* is one of 11 genera in a family that includes hops (*Humulus*) and hackberries (*Celtis*). As the plant was carried alongside human expansion into a diverse range of climates, its growth patterns, chemical expressions, and human uses have changed dramatically, resulting in an increasing diversity of genetic expressions. Horticulture techniques, both modern and ancient, have enabled the many different subspecies to be bred back together to create entirely new possibilities for the plant: it has utility as a fiber, as a nutritional resource, and in religious and pharmacologic applications. With respect to the pharmacologic applications, the most remarkable and critical components of the plant are the chemical compounds that it produces, broadly classified as cannabinoids and terpenoids.

Cannabinoids

Cannabinoids can be divided into three categories: phytocannabinoids, endocannabinoids, and synthetic cannabinoids. Phytocannabinoids refer to the chemical compounds produced by and in the plant; endocannabinoids are compounds produced endogenously by the human body, in the human body[31]; and synthetic cannabinoids are produced by human processes to circumvent the CSA's legal prohibitions against cannabis while also mimicking the structure and effects of phyto- and endocannabinoids.[32]

Phytocannabinoids

Research continues to reveal important properties regarding phytocannabinoids: the current state of the science believes that at least 100 phytocannabinoids exist in the cannabis plant, including practically impactful chemical differentiations such as acids and varins. These are generally grouped into certain structural categories, the central ones being THC, CBD, cannabigerol (CBG), and cannabichromene (CBC). Cannabinol (CBN) is not produced by the plant itself, but rather is formed as THC breaks down through oxidation.[33] The "major cannabinoids"—THC and CBD—are called such because they (or, more accurately, their precursor acid forms) appear in relatively high concentrations in cannabis and are most closely associated with the effects of cannabis and its medicinal applications. The "minor cannabinoids" are those that are produced by, or can be extracted from, the plant in lesser concentration: CBN, CBG, CBC, and cannabicyclol (CBL). In addition, there are precursor acid forms, such as cannabigerolic acid (CBGA) and tetrahydrocannabinolic acid (THC-A), and varins, such as cannabidivarin (CBDV) and tetrahydrocannabivarin (THCV).

The phytocannabinoids are generally found in their highest concentrations in the cannabis plant's trichomes, which are resinous glands that form most densely on the inflorescence (flower) of the female cannabis plant. Trichomes are formed on other parts of the plant as well, in lesser density, most notably the "sugar leaves" that frame the flowering parts of the plant. The lower fan leaves carry far fewer trichomes, and in the earlier stages of "commercial" cannabis production, they were often discarded altogether. However, in the modern cannabis industry, nearly every part of the plant can be processed using solvents and machinery to extract the critical compounds from the mere plant matter.

Synthetic cannabinoids

Synthetic cannabinoids include Marinol/Dronabinol, Sativex (which is characterized by a THC-to-CBD ratio of 1:1), and Epidiolex (which is characterized as a high-CBD product). Because these can be prescribed and are regulated by US Food and Drug Administration (FDA) guidelines, this chapter does not address their application in oncology.

Terpenoids

Widely known as "essential oils," terpenoids (also called "terpenes") appear throughout the plant world, delivering color, smell, and flavor. Over 30,000 terpenoids have been identified in plants; *Cannabis* produces more than 200.[34] Some of the most prominent terpenes and their appreciable effects are as follows:

1. Limonene: This is the prototypical "citrus" chemical. Limonene results in fast-acting stimulation and mood elevation and consequently may be an effective antidepressant.
2. β-Caryophyllene: This chemical, also found in black pepper, has anti-inflammatory properties.
3. Linalool: This is the chemical that gives lavender its lavender smell. It is believed to be mildly psychoactive and is associated with analgesic, anesthetic, and sedative effects.
4. Myrcene: This is also found in hops and is the most concentrated terpene generally found in cannabis. Myrcene is associated with relaxation and sedation.
5. Humulene: This is also found in hops, although it is more subtle (and in lesser concentrations) than myrcene.
6. Pinene (α and β): As the name reflects, this is the chemical that makes something smell like a pine tree. Pinene impacts enzymes that inhibit short-term memory; high-pinene cultivars have been reported to avoid the short-term memory issues caused by high-THC cultivars.[35]

Cannabis strains: indica, sativa, and hybrid

Cannabis sativa is generally divided into three distinct subspecies: *C sativa* ssp *ruderalis*, *C sativa* ssp *sativa*, and *C sativa* ssp *indica*. Ruderalis, now commonly called hemp, was cultivated primarily for its tall, fibrous stalks and contains little to no amounts of THC and slightly higher levels of CBD. Landrace (i.e., semi-natural cultivars that have persisted as distinctive strains with minimal human manipulation) sativa grows very tall and lanky, with long internodal length covered with wispy flowers (generally) high in THC and low in CBD. Indica landraces are characterized by short structure and growth cycle and dense flower clusters covered in resinous trichomes that contain high concentrations of cannabinoids, including greater amounts (relative to sativa) of CBD. Because each cannabis cultivar has distinctive chemical composition and crop characteristics, cannabis breeders were able to selectively optimize sought-after characteristics through structured breeding programs. However, the traits often ascribed to the subspecies, likely a result of the general chemical compositional differences (e.g., *C sativa* ssp *indica* contains higher concentrations of CBD), persisted even as interbreeding blurred the lines of the subspecies.

Over the years, and particularly once cannabis became a global cash crop, *Cannabis* breeders have created thousands of "strains," and colloquial taxonomies generally refer to such cultivars as (1) a sativa, (2) an indica, or (3) a hybrid composed of cross-bred subspecies. Generally, this is not a definitive assertion of scientific nature and type, but an approximation of the genetic provenance and a shorthand implication as to subjective experience. For example, the experiential effect of "sativas" is often characterized as high energy, whereas "indicas" are sedative and relieve pain. In plain truth, from a scientific taxonomy perspective, there are very few "pure" sativas or pure indicas; the nomenclature is relied on for subjective characterization, but that reliance (particularly in a medicinal context) perpetuates confusion and misunderstanding. While the "indica" versus "sativa" nomenclature and colloquial presumptions may be useful to some patients and the genealogic history of cannabis cultivation and breeding is fascinating to investigate, the best way to assess the effect and utility of cannabis as a medicinal product is to understand the specific chemical composition of the material that is being ingested—specifically, a cultivar's (i.e., strain's) unique cannabinoid and terpenoid combination or a manufactured product's specific cannabinoid profile. These are components that will interact with the "lock-and-key mechanisms" of the human body's endocannabinoid system and therefore create a measurable effect in the patient.

The endocannabinoid system

Within humans and other animals, there exist natural internal (endogenous) systems that appear to be designed to receive and/or process specific chemicals.[36] As Betty Wedman St. Louis explains, "the endocannabinoids system (ECS) is a natively produced biological system for regulating cell function through paracrine (cell-to-cell) and autocrine (within a cell) activity."[37] The ECS is "a group of ligands (including anandamide), their receptors, and signaling pathways involved in regulating a variety of physiological processes including movement, mood, memory, appetite, and pain."[38] The discovery and investigation of the ECS grew out from Dr. Raphael Mechoulam's isolation of THC, the main psychoactive compound in cannabis, in 1964. In 1973, scientists discovered the brain receptors that interacted with opiates such as opium, heroin, and morphine. By 1988, Dr. Allyn Howlett had discovered the receptor with which THC interacted.[39] In 1992, a specific endocannabinoid—a compound produced within the human body—was discovered: anandamide. By 1995, a second such endocannabinoid, 2-arachidonlygylycerol (2-AG), was discovered.[40] Subsequent research has revealed five endogenous cannabinoids.[40]

Dr. Ethan Russo offers an extensive description of the ECS and its importance in a variety of physiologic functions:

> THC and other cannabinoids exert many actions through cannabinoid receptors, G-protein-coupled membrane receptors that are extremely densely represented in central, spinal, and peripheral nociceptive pathways. Endogenous cannabinoids (endocannabinoids) even regulate integrative pain structures such as the periaqueductal gray matter. The endocannabinoid system also interacts in numerous ways with the endogenous opioid and vanilloid systems that that can modulate analgesia and with a myriad of other neurotransmitter systems such as the serotonergic, dopaminergic, glutamatergic, etc., pertinent to pain. Research has shown that the addition of cannabinoid agonists to opiates enhances analgesic efficacy markedly in experimental animals, helps diminish the likelihood of the development of opiate tolerance, and prevents opiate withdrawal.[41]

The operation of the ECS and cannabinoids is often analogized as a "lock-and-key mechanism": the endogenous system is the lock, and the chemical compounds (whether endogenous or exogenous) are the keys. At present, there are five identified endocannabinoids and two confirmed receptors, with a third suspected.[42] Research suggests that the ECS is "switched on" when the body needs "protection" in response to pathology, a list of which potentially includes "cancer, neuropathic and inflammatory pain, multiple sclerosis, post-traumatic stress disorder, traumatic brain injury, hemorrhagic, septic, and cardiogenic shock, hypertension, atherosclerosis, and Parkinson's disease."[43] Current research indicates that, more broadly, the ECS plays an important role in homoeostasis, or maintaining internal balance within important physiologic systems, including:

- Gastrointestinal activity
- Cardiovascular activity
- Perception of pain
- Bone mass
- Metabolism
- Inflammation
- Hormone regulation
- Immune system function
- Inhibition of tumor cell growth

Research and anecdotal reportage regarding cannabis use indicate that the ECS and the individual's experience with cannabis compounds are highly idiosyncratic. The intricate relationships among the ECS, the body's biochemistry, and external cannabinoids/terpenoids are not readily susceptible to reliable prediction, from person to person. This is another variation of the cannabis caveat: the context, including even the specific biochemistry of a patient, is a critical element in the overall efficacy of medicinal cannabis applications.

Two cannabinoid receptors have been positively identified in the human body—CB1 and CB2—and research suggests the existence of a third receptor.[42] CB1 receptors are found in the brain, lungs, vascular system, muscles, gastrointestinal tract, and reproductive organs. Particular areas of brain function that are affected by CB1 receptors include:

- Pain
- Cognition: memory, learning, decision making
- Emotion: anxiety, depression, fear
- Motor skills
- Appetite
- Nausea

Early investigations of CB2 receptors identified them in the peripheral tissue of the immune system and in the spleen, tonsils, thymus gland, bones, and skin. CB2 receptors affect the release of cytokines relating to inflammation and general immune function.

CB1 and CB2 receptors are co-located in the immune system, liver, bone marrow, pancreas, and heart.

With respect to the ECS and specific oncology issues, Wedman notes that "many cancer patients have increased amounts of CB1 and/or CB2, which researchers believe is the body's effort to combat the disease . . . The phytocannabinoid CBD has been reported to reverse or prevent many of the cancer cell growths in experiments. In addition to cell growth management, cannabinoid treatment may have additional benefits in pain, nausea, sleep, depression, and anxiety associated with cancer."[44]

Notably, there are no cannabinoid receptors in the respiratory control areas of the brain or brainstem. This is in stark contrast to the abundance of opioid receptors in the brain's respiratory control areas. An overdose of opioids can lead to respiratory suppression and arrest; there is no evidence of any fatal overdose from phytocannabinoids, which do not interact with the brain's respiratory control area. The Centers for Disease Control and Prevention, which compiles annual mortality data regarding alcohol, tobacco, and other substances, no longer has a category for cannabis-related fatalities because there are none reported.

CONCLUSION

HCPs are pivotal "influencers" in the implementation, efficacy, and continuous improvement of the scientific and societal awareness of the utility of cannabis (and more accurately, cannabinoids). HCPs deserve concrete, reliable, actionable guidance so that they can perform their vital clinical work efficiently and confidently. This chapter aims to provide oncology practitioners with information, awareness, and resources that will enable them to understand the common denominator issues arising in this domain. Such information should enable them to responsibly and confidently interact with patients for whom cannabis is potentially relevant and give them some sense of the issues that will require additional research to resolve the more contingent circumstances. This chapter focused primarily on the applications and regulatory regimes for medicinal cannabis, which are the topics most likely to arise at the intersection of oncology and legalized cannabis. However, given the rapidly changing social mores and laws regarding adult-use cannabis and because of the normalization halo that accompanies legalization and decreased stigma, HCPs may see an increase in patients acknowledging recreational use and seeking guidance about impacts or interactions with prescription medicines, treatment regimens, or general health issues. It is advisable that an HCP be familiar with cannabis, not merely as a medicinal option, but as a substance that more and more patients may acknowledge using for nonmedicinal (i.e., recreational) purposes. Overall, cannabis is a low-risk product, but patient information withheld is patient risk compounded.

KEY POINTS:

- As pivotal "influencers," HCPs should educate themselves on the medicinal applications of cannabis in their field.
- HCPs should learn their state's regulatory regime.
- HCPs who want to participate in authorizing cannabis use should register with their state's regulatory agency.
- HCPs should adhere to and comply with their state's regulatory regime, including regular renewal of authorizing privileges.
- HCPs should stay abreast of developments at the federal level: FDA, DEA (and DOJ more broadly), and Congress.
- HCPs who counsel patients on cannabis would benefit from familiarity with the marketplace for medicinal cannabis in their state.
- HCPs should be familiar with and understand the range of cannabis products and their various advantages and disadvantages.
- HCPs should educate themselves on the risks of cannabis substance abuse or potential for diversion by their patients.

References:

1. *In re Wright*, SJC-12873, at *2-3 (Mass 2020).
2. Specifically, "any material, compound, mixture, or preparation, which contains any quantity of [marihuana or tetrahydrocannabinols not from hemp], or which contains any of their salts, isomers, and salts of isomers whenever the existence of such salts, isomers, and salts of isomers is possible within the specific chemical designation" (Controlled Substances Act, 21 USC § 812).
3. Controlled substance schedules: marijuana. Drug Enforcement Administration. https://www.deadiversion.usdoj.gov/schedules/. Accessed August 18, 2021.
4. *Gonzalez v Raich,* 125 SCt 2195, 2205, 2211 n 37 (2005).
5. On November 3, 2020, 4 states voted to legalize cannabis for adult use. Mississippi and South Dakota each voted to legalize cannabis for medicinal uses (and, unusually, South Dakota simultaneously legalized cannabis for adult use). In February 2021, Virginia passed legislation legalizing adult-use cannabis, but this legalization will not occur until 2024.
6. Wedman-St. Louis B. *Cannabis: A Clinician's Guide*. Boca Raton, FL: CRC Press; 2018:8; citing Mosbergern D. Now we know what killed the ancient 'ice princess' and why she had that marijuana. The Huffington Post. 2014. www.huffingtonpost.com/2014/10/16/siberian-ice-princess-cancer-cannabis. Accessed August 18, 2021.

7. Machado Rocha FC, Stefano SC, De Cassia Haike R, Rosa Oliveiria LMQ, Da Silveira DX. Therapeutic use of *Cannabis sativa* on chemotherapy-induced nausea and vomiting among cancer patients: systematic review and meta-analysis. *Eur J Cancer Care (Engl)*. 2008;17:431–443; cited in Americans for Safe Access Foundation. *A Patient's Guide to Medical Cannabis*. Washington, DC: Americans for Safe Access Foundation; 2016:9.

8. Americans for Safe Access Foundation. *A Patient's Guide to Medical Cannabis*. Washington, DC: Americans for Safe Access Foundation; 2016:9.

9. Americans for Safe Access Foundation. *A Patient's Guide to Medical Cannabis*. Washington, DC: Americans for Safe Access Foundation; 2016:9, citing Guzmán M. Cannabinoids: potential anticancer agents. *Nat Rev Cancer*. 2003;3:745–755.

10. Wedman-St. Louis B. *Cannabis: A Clinician's Guide*. Boca Raton, FL: CRC Press; 2018:35, citing Chakravarti B, Ravi J, Ganju RK. Cannabinoids as therapeutic agents in cancer: current status and future implications. *Oncotarget*. 2014; 5(15):5852–5872.

11. *In re Wright*, SJC-12873, at *6-7 (Mass 2020).

12. Pub L No. 113-235, § 538, 128 Stat 2130, 2217 (2014).

13. Cases against doctors. Drug Enforcement Administration. https://apps2.deadiversion.usdoj.gov/CasesAgainst Doctors/spring/main?execution=e1s1. Accessed August 18, 2021.

14. 2020 State of the States Report. Americans for Safe Access Foundation. https://www.safeaccessnow.org/sos. Accessed August 18, 2021.

15. Schuette, Smith announce criminal charges against doctor, appliance store owner for sale of falsified medical marijuana physician certificates. Michigan Department of Attorney General. https://www.michigan.gov/ag/0,4534, 7-359-92297_47203-258589--,00.html. Accessed August 18, 2021.

16. Ingold J. Colorado medical-marijuana doctor facing felony charges. *The Denver Post*. December 1, 2014. https:// www.denverpost.com/2014/12/01/colorado-medical-marijuana-doctor-facing-felony-charges/. Accessed August 18, 2021.

17. *Conant v Walters*, 309 F3d 629, 638-639 (9th Cir 2002) (internal citations omitted).

18. Provider FAQ. Maryland Medical Cannabis Commission. https://mmcc.maryland.gov/Pages/physicians_faq.aspx. Accessed August 18, 2021. ("Do providers have a state and federal constitutional defense to any interference from federal authorities for advising patients about medical marijuana?")

19. Colorado court dismisses charges against medical marijuana doctor. Salem-News.com. http://www.salem-news .com/articles/may132011/marijuana-doctor.php. Accessed August 18, 2021.

20. State medical marijuana laws. National Conference of State Legislatures. July 14, 2021. https://www.ncsl.org/ research/health/state-medical-marijuana-laws.aspx. Accessed August 18, 2021.

21. Mich Comp Laws § 333.26424.

22. Mich Comp Laws § 333.26423.

23. Witte B. Maryland, after delays, begins the sale of medical marijuana. Associated Press. December 2, 2017. https:// apnews.com/article/fda24f32af7d430c8f6a10ce2cd064f2. Accessed August 18, 2021.

24. In Pennsylvania, as defined in section 9a of chapter X of the code of criminal procedure, 1927 PA 175, MCL 770.9a.

25. *People v Hartwick*, 870 NW2d 37, 56-57 (Mich 2015).

26. Alabama marijuana laws. FindLaw. https://statelaws.findlaw.com/alabama-law/alabama-marijuana-laws.html. Accessed August 18, 2021.

27. Cannabis in Alabama. Wikipedia. https://en.wikipedia.org/wiki/Cannabis_in_Alabama. Accessed August 18, 2021.

28. Medical marijuana. Louisiana Department of Agriculture and Forestry. https://www.ldaf.state.la.us/medical-marijuana/. Accessed August 18, 2021.

29. Application instructions for initial licensure therapeutic marijuana registration permit. Louisiana State Board of Medical Examiners. https://www.lsbme.la.gov/content/application-instructions-initial-licensure-therapeutic-marijuana-registration-permit. Accessed August 18, 2021.

30. The Transportation Security Administration (TSA) continues to list medicinal cannabis as a prohibited material, although it notes: "Accordingly, TSA security officers do not search for marijuana or other illegal drugs, but if any illegal substance is discovered during security screening, TSA will refer the matter to a law enforcement officer." See Medical marijuana. TSA. https://www.tsa.gov/travel/security-screening/whatcanibring/items/medical-marijuana. Accessed August 18, 2021.

31. Endocannabinoids are compounds produced endogenously by the human body, in the human body. See Wedman-St. Louis B. *Cannabis: A Clinician's Guide*. Boca Raton, FL: CRC Press; 2018:16; Goldstein B. *Cannabis Revealed*. Self-published; 2016:13.

32. Wedman-St. Louis B. *Cannabis: A Clinician's Guide*. Boca Raton, FL: CRC Press; 2018:23, 109.

33. Backes M. *Cannabis Pharmacy: The Practical Guide to Medical Marijuana*. New York, NY: Black Dog & Leventhal; 2014:42–43.

34. Wedman-St. Louis B. *Cannabis: A Clinician's Guide*. Boca Raton, FL: CRC Press; 2018:20; Goldstein B. *Cannabis Revealed*. Self-published; 2016:14.

35. Backes M. *Cannabis Pharmacy: The Practical Guide to Medical Marijuana*. New York, NY: Black Dog & Leventhal; 2014:47, citing Miyazawa M, Yamafuji C. Inhibition of acetylcholinesterase activity by bicyclic monoterpenoids. *J Agric Food Chem*. 2005;53(5):1765–1768.

36. Wedman-St. Louis B. *Cannabis: A Clinician's Guide*. Boca Raton, FL: CRC Press; 2018:16; Goldstein B. *Cannabis Revealed*. Self-published; 2016:25.

37. Wedman-St. Louis B. *Cannabis: A Clinician's Guide*. Boca Raton, FL: CRC Press; 2018:30.

38. Americans for Safe Access Foundation. *A Patient's Guide to Medical Cannabis*. Washington, DC: Americans for Safe Access Foundation; 2016:5, citing Hanuš LO. Pharmacological and therapeutic secrets of plant and brain (endo) cannabinoids. *Med Res Rev*. 2009;29:213–271.

39. Goldstein B. *Cannabis Revealed*. Self-published; 2016:25.

40. Goldstein B. *Cannabis Revealed*. Self-published; 2016:26.

41. Americans for Safe Access Foundation. *A Patient's Guide to Medical Cannabis*. Washington, DC: Americans for Safe Access Foundation; 2016:5, citing Russo EB. Clinical endocannabinoid deficiency (CECD): can this concept explain therapeutic benefits of cannabis in migraine, fibromyalgia, irritable bowel syndrome and other treatment-resistant conditions? *Neuro Endocrinol Lett*. 2008;29:192–200.

42. Goldstein B. *Cannabis Revealed*. Self-published; 2016:26–27.

43. Goldstein B. *Cannabis Revealed*. Self-published; 2016:30.

44. Wedman-St. Louis B. *Cannabis: A Clinician's Guide*. Boca Raton, FL: CRC Press; 2018:31.

ADDITIONAL RESOURCES

Additional resources that provide up-to-the-moment information on state regulatory programs include the following:

- Wikipedia: https://en.wikipedia.org/wiki/Legality_of_cannabis_by_U.S._jurisdiction. *Wikipedia is a fine site for initial research and slightly deeper dives into state-specific issues.*
- NORML: https://norml.org/; and its state chapter sites: https://norml.org/find-a-chapter/
- Americans for Safe Access: https://www.safeaccessnow.org/
- Marijuana Policy Project: https://www.mpp.org/
- FAQ weblink: https://health.mo.gov/safety/medical-marijuana/faqs-patient.php
- State-specific medicinal cannabis program websites, such as:
  - Alaska: http://dhss.alaska.gov/dph/VitalStats/Pages/marijuana.aspx
  - Arkansas: https://www.healthy.arkansas.gov/programs-services/topics/medical-marijuana

- California: https://cannabis.ca.gov/
- Florida: https://knowthefactsmmj.com/registry/#instructional-guides
- Illinois: http://dph.illinois.gov/topics-services/prevention-wellness/medical-cannabis
- Illinois regulations § 946.300: http://www.idph.state.il.us/rulesregs/2014_Rules/Adopted/77_IAC_946_7-29.pdf
- Louisiana: https://www.ldaf.state.la.us/medical-marijuana/
- Maryland: https://mmcc.maryland.gov/Pages/home.aspx
- Missouri: https://health.mo.gov/safety/medical-marijuana/index.php
- New Mexico: https://www.nmhealth.org/about/mcp/svcs/
- Oregon: https://www.oregon.gov/oha/ph/diseasesconditions/chronicdisease/medicalmarijuanaprogram/Pages/physicians.aspx
- Washington: https://www.doh.wa.gov/YouandYourFamily/Marijuana/MedicalMarijuana

CHAPTER 19

The US Food and Drug Administration

Amirala S. Pasha, DO, JD

INTRODUCTION

The US Food and Drug Administration (FDA), an agency within the US Department of Health and Human Services (HHS), traces its roots to the 1906 Pure Food and Drug Act. The FDA is responsible for protecting the public health by assuring food (except for meat from livestock, poultry, and some egg products, which are regulated by the US Department of Agriculture) safety and proper labeling; ensuring safety and effectiveness of human and veterinary drugs, vaccines, other biological products, and medical devices; protecting the public from electronic product radiation; ensuring safety and proper labeling of cosmetics and dietary supplements; regulating tobacco products; and finally helping to speed product innovations.[1]

The federal law establishing the legal framework within which the FDA operates, the Federal Food, Drug, and Cosmetic Act (FDCA), can be found in the US Code (USC) beginning at 21 USC 301. The FDA, similar to other federal agencies, develops regulations based on various laws under which it operates. This process follows the typical procedures required by the Administrative Procedure Act, including "notice and comment rulemaking" allowing public input on the proposed regulation before it is finalized. FDA regulations are also considered federal laws and can be found in Title 21 of the Code of Federal Regulations (CFR). The FDA also issues guidance that is not legally binding on the public or the FDA but describes the agency's current thinking on regulatory issues.[2,3]

As evident from the previous description, the FDA is involved in a large portion of the economy. Based on 2019 figures, the FDA is responsible for the oversight of more than $2.6 trillion in consumption, which accounts for about 20 cents of every dollar spent by US consumers.[4] Multiple volumes of books have been written on FDA law analyzing every aspect of its function in detail. However, in this chapter, in keeping with this book's overall theme, the discussion will be limited to the cross section of FDA law that directly affects clinicians. In particular, off-label use, off-label promotion, and preapproval access will be explored in detail. One recurring concept within the scope of this discussion will be that the FDA is not involved in regulating the practice of medicine.

Of note, although within the legal framework of the FDA, *drugs* and *biologics* are defined and treated somewhat differently, for the purposes of this chapter, they are used interchangeably. Furthermore, the term *medical product* will be used in this chapter to describe collectively one or more drug, biologic product, and/or medical device.

OFF-LABEL USE

Once a drug or device is approved (or cleared) for any specific use, it can be prescribed for any patient and any use as deemed appropriate by the prescriber. Such approach can be used to conduct additional research on that drug or device. It is also commonly done in the regular course of practicing medicine—a practice commonly known as off-label use. The former falls under the jurisdiction of the FDA, whereas the latter is outside of the scope of the FDCA and the FDA's purview.[5] The FDA defines off-label use as "use for indication, dosage form, dose regimen, population or other use parameter not mentioned in the approved labeling."[6] Combination chemotherapy that includes a combination of drugs that have not been approved to treat the type of cancer for which it is being used (e.g., folinic acid [leucovorin], fluorouracil, and oxaliplatin [FOLFOX] to treat colon cancer) also fall under this definition of off-label use as the FDA generally only approves individual drugs that form the combination chemotherapy. Often, the lines can be blurred between research and clinical care, especially in the setting of more novel therapeutics. The most basic test suggested to differentiate between the two uses has been to focus on the prescriber's motivations and goals in prescribing the medication. If the medical product is being prescribed to prevent, diagnose, or treat a disease or condition in a particular patient, then it is more likely to be classified as an off-label use. However, if the aim is to gather more data for assessment of effectiveness and safety, then it is more likely to be classified as an experimental or research use. If such use falls under experimental research, then the necessary safeguards and oversights of a formal study must be in place to avoid legal liability (see Chapter 20 on clinical trials). Alternatively, if the use is limited to off-label use as part of the practice of medicine, then the clinicians must take due care to avoid malpractice liability associated with off-label use, typically brought under a negligence (including informed consent) cause of action.[6,7] The specific legal elements to succeed in such cases and available defenses are discussed elsewhere in this book.

Despite what has been advocated in academia and by some commentators,[5,8] many courts have held that there is no duty on behalf of the clinician to disclose that the proposed use of the medical product is considered off-label. For instance, two separate appellate cases involving the off-label use of medical devices in spinal surgeries in Minnesota and Ohio found that off-label use on its own is not a materially inherent risk that requires disclosure.[7,9,10] Rather, in malpractice claims involving informed consent as the cause of action, the focus of analysis is typically on the adequacy of disclosure of material risks associated with a treatment's use. The adequacy of disclosure is determined based on applicable state laws and precedent; typically, courts use one of the following standards to assess the adequacy of the informed consent: (1) what another reasonable physician would have disclosed; (2) what information a reasonable patient would have regarded as important; or less frequently, (3) what the actual patient would have wanted to know.[11] The FDA-approved labeling, any applicable warnings (e.g., black box warning), and prescribing guidelines in the *Physician's Desk Reference* are examples of legitimate sources of such information.[11,12]

Although courts have widely held that, generally, off-label use alone is not sufficient to establish presumption of breach of duty, the off-label nature of the use can be introduced as evidence in support of such claims. Typically, the more information the clinician discloses to the patient as part of obtaining informed consent, the less likely such claims would succeed.[6] Consequently, when possible, disclosure of off-label nature of use, especially with high-risk treatments or procedures, provides an additional layer of protection against malpractice liability. Accordingly, proper documentation of all discussions regarding risks and benefits is of vital importance for raising any potential defenses in a malpractice case.

OFF-LABEL PROMOTION

Similar to off-label use, off-label promotion involves promotion of an approved (or cleared) medical product for a use other than those approved by the FDA. This also applies to combination chemotherapy, discussed earlier. Unlike off-label use, off-label promotion may lead to legal liability, including penalties under state consumer protection acts; state product liability; liability under the False Claims Act, which is usually brought against a manufacturer and is outside of the FDA's jurisdiction; and misbranding actions, including criminal prosecution under the FDCA.[13] The focus will remain on the FDA's role and the FDCA in this chapter. The FDCA prohibits the "introduction or delivery for introduction into interstate commerce any . . . drug [or] device . . . that is adulterated or misbranded."[14] If a drug or device has inadequate direction to allow a layperson to use the drug safely and for the purposes for which it is intended, then it is considered to be misbranded. The FDA considers off-label promotion, which by definition involves promotion of an unapproved use, to be potentially a violation of misbranding regulations because the label lacks instructions on how to safely use the drug or device for such unapproved use.[14] The discussion in this section focuses on off-label promotion of an approved medical product and does not apply to promotion of an unapproved medical product.

Traditionally, the FDA has been mainly concerned with regulating off-label promotion by manufacturers. Typically, the concern for off-label promotion is raised for clinicians in the setting of professional presentations such as speaking at continuing medical education (CME) programs.[15] Activities (programs and materials) that are not supported by the industry are exempt from FDA regulations. For activities that are in some way supported by the industry, the FDA differentiates between (1) activities performed by, or on behalf of, the companies that market the products and (2) activities, supported by companies, that are otherwise independent from the promotional influence of the supporting company. The former is subject to FDA regulations, whereas the latter is exempt. To determine whether an activity is truly independent and thereby exempt from FDA regulations, the agency considers multiple factors, including (1) who is in control of the content as well as selection of presenters and moderators, (2) presence of meaningful disclosures, (3) focus of the program, (4) relationship between provider and supporting company, (5) provider's involvement in sales or marketing, (6) provider's demonstrated failure to meet standards, (7) multiple presentations of the same program, (8) audience selection methods, (9) opportunities for discussion, (10) dissemination, (11) ancillary promotional activities, and (12) complaints.[16]

For activities deemed to fall under the FDA's jurisdiction, the rules and regulations surrounding off-label promotion have been in flux for many years. Prohibitions on off-label promotion involve restricting commercial speech, which is afforded qualified protection under the First Amendment of the US Constitution. When evaluating constitutional limitations on restricting commercial speech, the court must first determine whether the restrictions involve otherwise unlawful activity or the speech is false or misleading. If so, it can be prohibited. If not, then the court must evaluate the prohibition under a complex three-prong test to determine whether the prohibition involves a substantial government interest, the prohibition advances such interest, and the prohibition is not more extensive than necessary.[14,17] Over the years, the courts have found that off-label promotion involves promoting a legal activity (i.e., off-label use), and as long as the promotion is truthful and not misleading, it cannot be prohibited (the full legal analysis is detailed later in the Case Law examples that follow). In part, as a consequence of this evolving precedent on First Amendment commercial speech doctrine, it appears that now the FDA's stance on this issue has shifted to generally refrain from bringing misbranding actions against truthful, non-misleading off-label promotion.[13] It must be noted that since courts have not clarified the threshold for determining what is considered truthful and non-misleading, clinicians should take extra care to ensure that their promotion meets such standard even under extra scrutiny.

CASE LAW # 1

In the case of *Klein v Biscup,* Ms. Klein underwent spinal fusion performed by Dr. Biscup using bone plates and screws that were approved by the FDA for long and flat bones but not for spinal surgeries (i.e., off-label use). Although an informed consent with its typical features was obtained from Ms. Klein, she was never informed regarding the off-label nature of the bone plates and screws used in her surgery. After the surgery, Ms. Klein continued to suffer from pain and underwent an additional surgery by Dr. Biscup, where the original device was removed and a new device was implanted. Ms. Klein brought a malpractice suit in Ohio against Dr. Biscup for failure to obtain informed consent in relation to nondisclosure of the off-label use and alleging negligence for deviation from the standard of care. Ms. Klein also brought suit against the manufacturer; however, that element is beyond the scope of this chapter. The trial court granted partial summary judgment in favor of Dr. Biscup on the claim related to the informed consent and off-label use. The negligence claim was tried by a jury, which returned a verdict in favor of Dr. Biscup.[10]

On appellate review of the partial summary judgment regarding the informed consent element, the court noted that an informed consent requires disclosure of material risks. The central question was whether off-label use alone constituted such material risk. On review of the legislative history of the FDCA, the court observed that congress recognized that the act is "not intended as a medical practices act and [would] not interfere with the practice of the healing art." Additionally, the FDA had previously acknowledged in a bulletin that the FDCA does not limit the manner in which a physician may use an approved medical product. Therefore, the court concluded that off-label use of a medical device is a matter of medical judgment and "off-label use of a medical device is not a material risk inherently involved in a proposed therapy which a physician should disclose to a patient prior to the therapy."[10] The summary judgment was affirmed.[10]

CASE LAW # 2

In *United States v Caronia*, Alfred Caronia, a pharmaceutical sales consultant, was criminally charged and convicted under the FDCA for conspiracy to introduce a misbranded drug into interstate commerce for his off-label promotion of Xyrem. The Second Circuit vacated his conviction and remanded the case. Central to the appeals court's decision was whether criminal prohibition of off-label promotion violated Caronia's right to free speech under the First Amendment. The court noted that off-label promotion in its essence is a form of commercial speech and, under the *Central Hudson* test, such speech is protected by the First Amendment if it involves a lawful activity and is truthful and not misleading. However, the government can restrict such speech if (1) the government has asserted a substantial interest, (2) the restrictions directly and materially advance the government's substantial interest, and (3) the restrictions are narrowly tailored.[18,19]

In this case, it was held that off-label promotion does involve promotion of a legal activity (i.e., off-label use) and Caronia's statements were not false or misleading; therefore, he was afforded qualified protection under the First Amendment. Conversely, the government's interest in preventing unsafe prescribing and usage of drugs was found to be a substantial interest. However, prohibition on off-label promotion was not found to be advancing the government's substantial interest since the outcome that this prohibition was aimed to prevent (i.e., off-label use) remained legal. Finally, it was found that a complete and criminal ban on off-label promotion was not narrowly tailored. Therefore, the government's construction of the misbranding provision of the FDCA by complete and criminal ban of off-label promotion was held to be unconstitutional. Furthermore, the court held that the "the government cannot prosecute pharmaceutical manufacturers and their representatives under the FDCA for speech promoting the lawful, off-label use of an FDA-approved drug." The FDA opted not to appeal this decision.[18]

CASE LAW # 3

The case of *Amarin v FDA* involved the drug Vascepa, a cholesterol-lowering drug, which was already approved for severe hypertriglyceridemia but was denied approval for its broader indication of hypertriglyceridemia (as opposed to severe form of the condition) in patients already on statin therapy despite favorable clinical trials. In its denial, the FDA warned the manufacturer that it would consider Vascepa misbranded if the drug was marketed for its second (unapproved) broader indication by disseminating peer-reviewed publications and other associated material. The manufacturer, Amarin Pharmaceuticals, Inc., brought a civil suit against the FDA in federal district court arguing that threat of criminal action for its truthful and non-misleading off-label promotion violated its commercial speech rights.[20,21]

The district court, after reaffirming the analysis in *United States v Caronia* regarding off-label promotion and commercial speech (see Case Law # 2), held that the FDA is prohibited from bringing misbranding action "based on truthful promotional speech alone" and provided the manufacturer with preliminary relief. Subsequently, the case was settled between the parties, and the FDA did not seek appellate review of the preliminary relief. The parties agreed in part that the manufacturer may engage in truthful and non-misleading off-label promotion of Vascepa and that such speech will not serve as the basis for any criminal prosecution for misbranding. Technically, the settlement only applies to this case, but the preliminary injunction remained intact, and although not binding on any other court, it will likely have persuasive value. Furthermore, being that this is the first case where the FDA has voluntarily agreed to allow a company to engage in truthful and non-misleading off-label promotion outside of a previously allowed narrow scope, it is likely that it will serve as a blueprint on FDA's regulation of off-label promotion of previously approved (or cleared) medical products.[20,21]

CLINICAL VIGNETTE # 1

Medication X is a chemotherapy drug previously approved by the FDA for the treatment of non–small-cell lung cancers (NSCLCs) with a certain mutation. In a multicenter clinical trial conducted by the manufacturer of medication X, it was found that medication X is also effective in treatment of NSCLC with a different mutation than previously approved by the FDA. The clinical trial has ended, and the favorable results have been published in peer-reviewed medical journals. The manufacturer is in the process of submitting required application to obtain FDA approval for the new indication (i.e., NSCLC with a different mutation). In the interim, the manufacturer has invited Dr. Jones, a well-regarded clinician and researcher in the field of NSCLC, who was one of the site leads in the recently concluded clinical trial, to speak to other oncologists on behalf of the company at various events sponsored by the manufacturer to discuss the findings of the trial. She will be compensated by the manufacturer for her participation in these events. Dr. Jones has also been invited by her state's medical society to discuss the findings of the clinical trial at their annual meeting as part of the society's CME offerings. The medical society prides itself on conducting its meetings free from the influence of commercial interest and follows applicable rules to award CME credit to participants. Finally, Dr. Jones is eager to prescribe medication X to her patients with NSCLC who have this other mutation, rather than the previously approved mutation. However, she is very concerned regarding her malpractice liability as well as the potential for FDA legal action against her for her speaking engagements.

Dr. Jones's speaking engagements can be considered off-label promotion and must be scrutinized closely. The FDA is mainly concerned with regulating off-label promotion by manufacturers. Therefore, her speaking engagements sponsored by the manufacturer will certainly be under the FDA's jurisdiction as off-label promotion. As discussed previously, such speech is considered to be commercial speech and is afforded some protection under the First Amendment. Although traditionally the FDA had a complete ban on such off-label promotion, in part as a result of recent court rulings, the FDA's stance has evolved to tolerate such activities as long as the statements during these events are truthful and non-misleading. Truthfulness is fairly easy to understand and establish; however, the threshold for what is considered non-misleading promotion has not been defined by regulators or the courts. Nonetheless, sharing the results of peer-reviewed publications is likely to be found truthful and non-misleading. Dr. Jones should carefully coordinate with the manufacturer's legal department to ensure that her statements during these engagements are not in violation of the FDA misbranding regulations, which can carry civil and criminal penalties for both her and the manufacturer.

On the other hand, her presentation at the state's medical society, which is independent of the manufacturer, would be considered outside of the FDA's jurisdiction and is unlikely to carry any significant liability. She would be wise to disclose her relationship with the clinical trial and the manufacturer and must follow any applicable accreditation rules and state laws.

Prescribing medication X, a previously approved medication, for an unapproved use outside of a clinical trial falls under off-label use and is considered to be part of the practice of medicine; therefore, it is outside of the FDA's jurisdiction. Nonetheless, the tort law malpractice liability associated with the practice of medicine still applies. Dr. Jones must weigh the risks of using a medication that does not appear to have been incorporated as a standard of practice for this particular mutation against the potential benefits her patient may gain. A thorough informed consent is of vital importance. Although courts seem to agree that off-label nature of the use on its own is not a material risk, this analysis may vary from state to state, and irrespective of its treatment in a given jurisdiction, it would be prudent that she disclose the off-label nature of the use to the patient.

In summary, as the American Academy of Pediatrics noted in their recent policy statement, "the off-label use of a drug should be done in good faith, in the best interest of the patient, and without fraudulent intent."[22] To secure more protection against potential malpractice claims associated with off-label use of medical products, physicians should (1) obtain a comprehensive informed consent including disclosure of off-label use; (2) ensure that the primary purpose for off-label use is to prevent, diagnose, or treat and the primary motivation is to benefit the patient for whom the drug or device is being used or, stated differently, that the needs of the patient are placed first; (3) ensure the use is based on sound clinical judgment; (4) ensure the use is supported by sound scientific evidence; and (5) ensure the use is generally supported by the opinions and practices of the medical community, especially local colleagues.[6]

On the topic of off-label promotion, although there may be other considerations, such as Accreditation Council for Continuing Medical Education (ACCME) rules on disclosures, clinicians participating in activities exempt from the FDA's regulations do not need to be concerned with any adverse FDA actions. Alternatively, if clinicians engage in activities involving off-label promotion that are not exempt from the FDA's jurisdiction, then it is recommended to coordinate with the sponsor's legal department to verify compliance with all relevant laws and regulations. Moreover, extra steps must be taken to ensure that the presented material is truthful and non-misleading.

PREAPPROVAL ACCESS

Preapproval access is an umbrella term that describes various legal schemes outside of a clinical trial for patients suffering from serious medical conditions who have exhausted all other approved modalities to gain access to medications and medical devices that have not been fully and formally approved (or cleared) by a country's regulatory system.[23] Of note, other commonly used terms to describe such access include, but are not limited to, *compassionate use*, *named patient programs*, and *managed access*. Outside of clinical trials, in the United States, the law provides for three distinct pathways for preapproval access: (1) Emergency Use Authorization (EUA), (2) expanded access programs (EAPs), and (3) the Right to Try (RTT) Act.[24] Unlike off-label use, discussed earlier in this chapter, these pathways can provide access to drugs and devices that have not yet been approved (or cleared) by the FDA for any purpose. Some authors do not include EUA, which is only available during a declared emergency, as a pathway within the construct of preapproval access. However, it does meet the criteria for inclusion under the broader definition used in this chapter. Of note, EUA and EAPs allow eligible patients to access both drugs and devices, whereas the RTT Act is only limited to drugs. All pathways only entitle patients to access the investigational product through a prescriber with the expressed agreement of the manufacturer; however, none entitles the patient or the prescriber to be provided with the desired product. In fact, in a case involving a terminally ill patient claiming a constitutional right to preapproval access to cetuximab, the US Court of Appeals for the District of Columbia, in *Abigail Alliance v von Eschenbach*, held that patients have no legal right to demand "a potentially toxic drug with no proven therapeutic benefit" and further that "there is no fundamental right . . . to experimental drugs for the terminally ill."[25] The Supreme Court declined to review the case.

Emergency use authorization

The EUA program was established in 2004 when the Project Bioshield Act amended section 564 of the FDCA to permit "the FDA Commissioner to authorize the use of an unapproved medical product or an unapproved use of an approved medical product during a declared emergency."[26] It is uncommon for a clinician to sponsor a product under an EUA, and therefore, the details of the process are not discussed in this chapter. More commonly, clinicians will find themselves with the option of administering or prescribing a medical product available under an approved EUA (hereafter referred to as EUA medical products). Therefore, the focus of this section will be on potential malpractice liability associated with EUA medical products. However, it is important to first understand the circumstances under which an EUA can be issued.

Before the FDA can issue an EUA, the HHS secretary must declare that circumstances exist justifying the authorization (i.e., EUA declaration). The requirements for the basis of such a declaration are detailed in the law and can be based on a domestic, military, or public health emergency.[27] The FDA commissioner, after appropriate consultations and in compliance with other statutory requirements, may then authorize the emergency use of an unapproved product or an unapproved use of an approved product. The EUA may subsequently be revoked by the FDA if it is determined that the required criteria are no longer met or such revocation is appropriate to protect public health or safety.[28] Furthermore, EUAs issued based on an EUA declaration will no longer be in effect upon termination of that EUA declaration.[29] Finally, unlike the other pathways discussed later, EUA does not require any additional documentation of individual informed consent beyond what is required in the regular course of the practice of medicine.[30]

Section 564 of the FDCA, which established the EUA program, does not provide any liability protection. However, Public Readiness and Emergency Preparedness Act (PREP Act) enacted in 2005 does provide a mechanism to limit tort liability associated with EUA medical products or, as referred to in the PREP Act, covered countermeasures. (Countermeasures may be qualified pandemic or epidemic products, security countermeasures, EUA medical products, any other approved medical products, or some other medical products under the direction of a government agency.[31]) Although the liability protection is not automatically attached to the EUA product, the PREP Act authorizes the HHS secretary to issue a separate declaration (this is a different declaration than the EUA declaration described earlier) immunizing individuals and entities from federal and state tort liability associated with any claim for losses caused by administration or use of a covered countermeasure. Such declaration will identify covered persons (covered persons are individuals and entities protected under immunity from liability; such protection is limited to those who are specified in the declaration, determined at the discretion of the HHS secretary, and may include manufacturers, distributors, program planners, qualified persons [including health care providers], officials, agents, and employees of the above and the United States[31]), countermeasures, category (or categories) of diseases, health conditions or threats to health, population, geographic area, any limitations on distribution, and the declaration's effective time period. Liability protection is fairly sweeping and generally preempts state law. Nonetheless, its protections only extend to losses arising from administration or use of covered countermeasures in accordance with the declaration (e.g., during the effective period of the declaration, for what has been specified in the declaration and for a patient who is in the population specified by the declaration). Furthermore, the immunity does not cover acts or omissions resulting in serious physical injury or death proximately caused by willful misconduct (willful misconduct requires that the covered person act [1] intentionally to achieve a wrongful purpose; [2] knowingly without legal or factual justification; and [3] in disregard of a known or obvious risk that is so great as to make it highly probable that the harm will outweigh the benefit[31]). The PREP Act specifically holds that, as a matter of law, acts consistent with applicable directions, guidelines, or recommendations of the HHS secretary are not to be considered "willful misconduct" so long as a federal, state, or local health authority is notified regarding the suffered loss associated with the administration or use of the covered countermeasure within seven days of actual discovery of such information.[31]

The law also provides a separate compensation mechanism for eligible individuals injured as a result of administration or use of a covered countermeasure through the Countermeasures Injury Compensation Program (CICP).[32]

Therefore, when deciding to administer or use an EUA medical product, clinicians should take extra precautions to ensure that there is a separate declaration by the HHS secretary providing immunity under the PREP Act, that clinicians are covered under such declaration (usually under covered persons), and that their administration or use of the EUA medical product is consistent with such declaration. In doing so, clinicians ensure protection against any associated potential tort liability. Failure to do so may increase clinicians' liability given the nature of EUA medical products and the circumstances in which they are typically used.

Expanded access program

Although since the 1970s the FDA has facilitated access to investigational drugs, the EAP was originally formalized in 1987 (drugs and biologics) and 1996 (devices). It was further codified in law in 1997 and underwent significant revision in 2009. The EAP provides a potential pathway for patients with an immediately life-threatening condition or serious disease or condition to gain access to an investigational medical product for treatment outside of clinical trials in absence of alternative options. Additionally, potential benefits for the patient must justify the potential risks of the treatment.[33-35]

An immediately life-threatening disease or condition is one for which there is a "reasonable likelihood that death will occur within a matter of months or in which premature death is likely without early treatment."[36] A serious disease or condition is one that it is associated with morbidity that has substantial impact on day-to-day functioning. The determination of whether a condition constitutes a serious disease or condition is based on clinical judgment, incorporating factors such as its impact on survival, functional status, and prospects of progression without treatment.[36]

Licensed physicians are authorized to become sponsors for requesting access to an investigational medical product under the EAP. The sponsor must then submit the required FDA forms, secure institutional review board (IRB) approval, and obtain informed consent from the patient(s). The medical product may be shipped and treatment may begin 30 days after the application is received by the FDA, unless otherwise advised by the FDA. Due to the nature of the EAP, there are provisions for emergency use. This is only available when there exists an emergency requiring the patient to be treated before a written submission can be made. In such instances, for drugs and biologics, the licensed physician can contact the FDA by telephone (or other rapid means of communication), whereas medical devices can be used without first contacting the FDA. Subsequently, the FDA must be notified and appropriate reports must be filled within a specified time period. There are additional reporting requirements for the sponsor and manufacturer as detailed in the regulations.

Liability

Unlike the other FDA programs that provide preapproval access to investigational drugs, the EAP does not provide any liability protection. Although some of the liability risk can be mitigated by obtaining a thorough informed consent, the involved physician will most likely be placed at a higher risk of liability than encountered in the typical course of clinical practice given the clinical situations in which EAP use is contemplated. Furthermore, medical product manufacturers may be reluctant to provide access to their investigational medical product given the increased liability risk. Nevertheless, a recent study specifically looking at product liability found no legal precedent for actions against pharmaceutical companies related to providing access to an investigational medical product under the EAP.[37] Finally, although theoretically possible, it is highly unlikely that there will be any additional liability for declining to become a sponsor under the EAP.

Project facilitate

To assist oncologists and regulatory professionals in navigating the complexities of the EAP, the FDA's Oncology Center of Excellence has implemented Project Facilitate. This is a pilot program that provides a single point of contact for the FDA's oncology staff to assist physicians and their team in the process of submitting an expanded access request for an individual patient with cancer. It would be prudent for physicians embarking on such a journey to use this resource to the fullest.[38]

The FDA has permitted the vast majority of the expanded access requests. Between 2010 and 2013, the FDA imposed clinical holds on only 2 of the 2472 individual requests.[39]

As discussed, securing access to investigational medical products through the EAP involves multiple steps requiring coordination among multiple stakeholders (e.g., patient, physician, manufacturer, IRB, and FDA), which can be time consuming. Based on a survey study, administrative burden associated with supporting an EAP application for an individual patient is estimated to be approximately 30 hours, inclusive of physician and staff time. Often, this time is not reimbursed by payers.[33] The associated administrative burden and potential cost must be fully considered by a physician prior to commencing on this path.

Right to try act

The RTT Act (also known as the Trickett Wendler, Frank Mongiello, Jordan McLinn, and Matthew Bellina Right to Try Act of 2017) was signed into law on May 30, 2018. The RTT Act allows an eligible patient access to eligible investigational drugs.[40]

An eligible patient is one who has been diagnosed with a life-threatening disease or condition, which, for the purposes of this act, is defined as a disease or condition that results in a high likelihood of death unless the course of disease is interrupted or for which there is a potentially fatal outcome.[41] Furthermore, the act requires such patients to have exhausted approved treatment options and be unable to participate in a clinical trial involving the eligible investigational drug; both conditions must be certified by a physician in good standing with his or her licensing organization or board and who is not being compensated directly by the manufacturer. Finally, the patient or a legally authorized representative of the patient must provide written informed consent regarding the eligible investigational drug to the treating physician.[40]

An eligible investigational drug is a drug that has completed phase I clinical trial but has not been approved or licensed by the FDA for any use. Additionally, the drug must have had an application filed with the FDA or must be under investigation in a clinical trial as part of establishing effectiveness in support of FDA approval and must be the subject of an active investigational new drug application submitted to the FDA. Lastly, the drug's active development or production must be ongoing, and it must not have been discontinued by the manufacturer or placed on clinical hold by the FDA. As opposed to the other pathways discussed earlier in this chapter, investigational medical devices are not eligible for preapproval access under the RTT Act.

Ultimately, if the previously listed criteria for patient eligibility and the investigational drug are satisfied, access to the investigational drug can be secured directly from the sponsor, typically through the treating physician, without any other regulatory requirements. Unlike the EAP, where the FDA plays a pivotal role in regulating access to an investigational medical product, under the RTT Act, the FDA does not review or approve requests. Its role is limited to receipt and posting of certain information as required by law. Patients may be charged by the manufacturer for the direct cost associated with providing the investigational drug.[40] Reporting requirements specifically for the RTT Act are limited to annual summaries submitted by the investigational drug's sponsor, although the act does not limit any other reporting requirements.

Finally, to further incentivize an investigational drug sponsor's willingness to participate, the RTT Act, with very narrow exceptions, exempts the use of any clinical outcome associated with the use of an investigational drug under the RTT Act to delay or adversely affect the review or approval of such drug.[40]

Liability

The RTT Act explicitly shields sponsors, manufacturers, prescribers, dispensers, and other individual entities from most tort liabilities in the absence of reckless or willful misconduct or gross negligence. Of note, the RTT Act does not provide any liability protection for causes of action arising from intentional torts under state law. Therefore, in jurisdictions that still construe absent or inadequate informed consent as battery, an intentional tort, clinicians may not be shielded from liability, although there does not appear to be any precedent for such cause of action involving the RTT Act. Consequently, obtaining a thorough informed consent (as previously discussed in this chapter) is vital, especially in such jurisdictions. However, malpractice suits brought under negligence theory (absent reckless or willful misconduct or gross negligence) are preempted by the act. Moreover, the RTT Act protects the previously listed entities against liability if they elect not to participate.[42] Table 19-1 compares the EAP to the RTT Act.

Overall, there is fairly limited case law surrounding liability issues in preapproval access. At the time of the this writing, there are very few publicly available decisions, mostly involving the PREP Act and relate to the H1N1 vaccine. One addresses the merits of the immunity defense under the PREP Act (see *Parker* case below). Nonetheless, it is anticipated that this number will dramatically increase in the coming years given the number of medical products that were widely used under an EUA and were a covered countermeasure under the PREP Act in relation to the coronavirus disease 2019 (COVID-19) pandemic.

Table 19-1. **Expanded Access Program versus Right to Try Act**

	Expanded Access Program	Right to Try Act
Eligible patients	Patients with immediately life-threatening condition or serious disease or condition	Patients with life-threatening disease or condition
Eligible patient population size	Individual, intermediate size, and widespread patient population	Individual patient only
Eligible drugs	Drugs and biologics that are used in a clinical investigation	Drugs that have completed phase I and have an application filed with the US Food and Drug Administration (FDA)
Eligible devices	Medical devices that are used in a clinical investigation	None
Physician's role	Clinically determine patient's eligibility, assess availability of alternative options, work with industry, and file necessary paperwork; physician responsible for patient care and reporting	Must certify patient's eligibility and work with industry; cannot be compensated directly by the manufacturer
Manufacturer's role	Provides access to the medical product; submits safety and annual reports; performs specific responsibilities as outlined by the FDA; may also act as a sponsor	Provides access to the drug; submits annual summary
FDA's role	Determines if patient eligibility criteria are met and if potential risks outweigh benefits; ensures the use will not interfere with the clinical investigation of the medical product	Limited to receipt and posting of certain information.
Institutional review board (IRB) role	IRB provides oversight	No role
Reporting requirements	Safety report, annual summary (if applicable), summary report, and amendments by the sponsor	Annual summary submitted by the sponsor
Liability	No statutory limitation	Statutory limitation against liability in absence of willful misconduct or gross negligence (not including intentional torts)

CASE LAW # 4

In *Parker v St Lawrence County Public Health Department*, the parents of a minor child brought suit against the public health department, which inoculated the child against H1N1 without the parents' informed consent. The New York State appellate court noted that the "breadth of the preemption clause together with the sweeping language of the statute's immunity" implies that Congress intended to preempt all state law tort claims against covered persons administering a covered countermeasure. Subsequently, the court found that the vaccine was a "covered countermeasure" and the public health department qualified as "covered persons" under the PREP Act declaration. Therefore, the court ruled that the lawsuit was preempted by the PREP Act and the case was dismissed.[43]

CASE LAW # 5

During the H1N1 influenza epidemic of 2009, Dr. Casabianca was a patient at Mount Sinai Medical Center, where he underwent small bowel transplant. After an extended hospital stay due to surgical complications, he was discharged home but was allegedly never immunized against H1N1 during his hospital stay. He subsequently contracted H1N1 influenza and died from its complications. In *Casabianca v Mount Sinai Medical Center, Inc.*, his estate brought a malpractice suit against the hospital and his physicians for allegedly failing to administer the H1N1 vaccine, a covered countermeasure under the PREP Act, during his hospital stay. The defendants filed a motion to dismiss the case raising preemption of state law and immunity under the PREP Act. However, the New York State court held that the preemption and immunity only apply when a covered countermeasure is administered by covered persons. Failure to administer a covered countermeasure, however, is not protected under the PREP Act, and the malpractice claim was allowed to proceed.[44]

CLINICAL VIGNETTE # 2

Jennifer, a 65-year-old woman, had previously been diagnosed with acute myeloid leukemia (AML) and underwent hematopoietic stem cell transplantation. She now presents to the hematology/oncology service with fever and respiratory symptoms concerning for COVID-19 infection and is admitted. Within a few days of admission, her condition worsens, and she is transferred to the medical intensive care unit for respiratory distress. Besides supportive care, there is no known effective treatment for her condition, and she is ineligible to enroll in any ongoing clinical trial. It is feared that death is imminent.

Medication A is undergoing clinical trials with promising results but has not yet been approved by the FDA. So far, there appears to be a clinically significant survival benefit in patients, especially immunocompromised patients. Medication B was previously approved by the FDA for treatment of an unrelated infection, but the manufacturer has been able to obtain a new indication of use for treatment of COVID-19 under an EUA. However, the FDA is strongly considering revoking the EUA based on reported side effects. There are currently no formal guidelines recommending the use of either of these medications in patients with COVID-19.

An emergency declaration has been issued under the PREP Act, which includes all EUA authorized drugs and devices as covered countermeasures and includes physicians under covered persons.

Jennifer's husband is demanding that both medication A and medication B be administered to the patient immediately. However, the attending physician is not convinced that either of these medications would be effective in treating Jennifer and is concerned regarding his liability if he administers these medications or decides not to do so.

Although both medications fall under preapproval access, as defined in this chapter, they need to be addressed separately.

Medication A has not yet been approved by the FDA for any use, and therefore, it is not available outside of a clinical trial. In this case, the patient is not a candidate for enrollment in a clinical trial. Therefore, the only means of obtaining medication A is through a preapproval access pathway. Based on this scenario, the manufacturer of medication A has not sought an EUA, and therefore, the medication can only be obtained through the EAP or the RTT Act. As discussed earlier, the EAP involves a process that must be initiated by the physician or the manufacturer and must go through appropriate channels at the FDA, whereas under the RTT Act, the access can be secured upon request from the physician and agreement by the manufacturer. Based on the case scenario, the patient has a life-threatening condition, there is no other effective treatment available, and she is not eligible for any clinical trial, thus meeting regulatory criteria for both programs. Under the RTT Act, there is statutory liability protection for both the manufacturer and the physician when deciding whether to administer or to withhold medication A. Although the EAP does not explicitly provide any liability protection, it is unlikely that either choosing to administer medication A under the EAP or choosing to withhold the medication would result in a successful malpractice claim against the physician or the manufacturer.

Medication B, on the other hand, has been previously approved and is available outside of preapproval access (i.e., off-label use). Nonetheless, the existence of an EUA and emergency declaration under the PREP Act changes the liability calculus. As long as the emergency declaration is in place and medication B has an active EUA, there is wide liability protection for its administration under the PREP Act, which preempts state tort law claims. Alternatively, if the physician decides not to administer medication B, then the immunities of the PREP Act no longer apply and the usual negligence cause of action analysis applies. However, in this scenario, it is unlikely to be found that administration of medication B is considered to be standard of care given the absence of clinical guidelines or any other information to suggest that community practice standards endorse its use. Therefore, withholding medication B is unlikely to be a deviation from standard of care, a required element of medical malpractice under the negligence theory. Finally, the scenario contemplates the FDA's potential revocation of the EUA for medication B. Once the EUA is revoked, the protections under the PREP Act will immediately cease to apply, and the administration of medication B will be treated as an off-label use.

CONCLUSION

Preapproval access provides an alternative pathway to accessing medical products that have not undergone full approval (or clearance) by the FDA. Outside of clinical trials, in the United States, the law provides for three distinct pathways for preapproval access: (1) EUA, (2) EAP, and (3) the

RTT Act.[24] Each pathway approaches tort liability differently, but generally, when there is adequate informed consent and in absence of gross negligence, the overall risk appears to be low. These observations will be challenged as case law in this area develops further with the expected litigation that will surely arise from widespread use of EUA medical products during the COVID-19 pandemic.

KEY POINTS:

- The FDA is not involved in regulating the practice of medicine.
- Off-label use of drugs and devices in the regular course of practice of medicine is outside of the FDA's jurisdiction, and the usual malpractice liability rules apply. Physicians should take extra steps, especially with regard to disclosure, in order to decrease liability risk associated with off-label use.
- Off-label promotion of medical products falls under the jurisdiction of the FDA. However, the FDA does not regulate activities (programs and materials) that are produced independently from the influence of companies marketing the products. When off-label promotion activities are by or on behalf of the company marketing the product, then extra care must be taken to ensure that, at minimum, the off-label promotion is supported by sound evidence in order to meet the truthful and non-misleading standard.
- Preapproval access is an umbrella term that describes various legal schemes outside of a clinical trial for patients suffering from serious medical conditions who have exhausted all other approved modalities to gain access to medications and medical devices that have not been fully and formally approved (or cleared) by a country's regulatory system.[23]
- EUA is only available during times of declared domestic, military, or public health emergencies. There can be liability protection for administration or use of EUA medical products, but this requires a separate declaration by the HHS secretary under the PREP Act, and such protection is limited in scope.
- The EAP allows physicians to become sponsors for patients to be able to access unapproved drugs and medical devices under the FDA's oversight but does not afford any liability protection.
- The RTT Act is an alternative pathway for accessing unapproved drugs but not medical devices. There is very limited FDA involvement in the process, and the act provides statutory limitation on liability.

References:

1. What does FDA do? US Food and Drug Administration. Updated March 28, 2018. https://www.fda.gov/about-fda/fda-basics/what-does-fda-do. Accessed August 2, 2020.
2. What is the difference between the Federal Food, Drug, and Cosmetic Act (FD&C Act), FDA regulations, and FDA guidance? US Food and Drug Administration. Updated March 28, 2018. https://www.fda.gov/about-fda/fda-basics/what-difference-between-federal-food-drug-and-cosmetic-act-fdc-act-fda-regulations-and-fda-guidance. Accessed August 2, 2020.
3. 21 CFR § 10.115.
4. Regulated products and facilities. US Food and Drug Administration. Updated October 2019. https://www.fda.gov/media/131874/download. Accessed August 2, 2020.
5. Johns M. Informed consent: requiring doctors to disclose off-label prescriptions and conflicts of interest. *Hastings Law J.* 2007;58(5):967–1024.

6. Riley JB Jr, Basilius PA. Physicians' liability for off-label prescriptions. *Nephrol News Issues*. 2007;21(7):43–47.

7. *Femrite v Abbott Northwestern Hospital*, 568 NW2d 535 (Minn App 1997).

8. Stafford RS. Regulating off-label drug use: rethinking the role of the FDA. *N Engl J Med*. 2008;358(14):1427–1429.

9. Dresser R, Frader J. Off-label prescribing: a call for heightened professional and government oversight. *J Law Med Ethics*. 2009;37(3):476–396.

10. *Klein v Biscup*, 673 NE2d 225 (Ohio Ct App 1996).

11. Edersheim JG, Stern TA. Liability associated with prescribing medications. *Prim Care Companion J Clin Psychiatry*. 2009;11(3):115–119.

12. *R.T. v Knobeloch*, 111 NE3d 588 (2018).

13. Mazer D, Curfman GD. FDA sanctions off-label drug promotion. *Health Affairs Blog*. Published July 19, 2016. https://www.healthaffairs.org/do/10.1377/hblog20160719.055881/full/. Accessed August 2, 2020.

14. Jacobson L. Don't fix what ain't broken—off-label marketing, the FDA's regulatory regime, and the First Amendment. *Emory Corp Gov Account Rev*. 2018;5:19-60.

15. Ventola CL. Off-label drug information: regulation, distribution, evaluation, and related controversies. *P T*. 2009; 34(8):428–440.

16. Industry supported scientific and educational activities. US Food and Drug Administration. Published November 1997. https://www.fda.gov/media/75334/download. Accessed August 16, 2021.

17. *Central Hudson Gas & Elec Corp v Public Serv Comm'n of NY*, 447 US 557 (1980).

18. *United States v Caronia*, 703 F3d 149 (2d Cir 2012).

19. *Central Hudson Gas & Electric Corp v Public Service Commission*, 447 US 557 (1980).

20. *Amarin Pharma v U.S. Food and Drug Administration*, No. 15-3588 (SDNY August 7, 2015).

21. Fleder JR, Gibbons DC. Amarin announces a proposed settlement of its First Amendment lawsuit against FDA: coming full circle in a new era of the regulation of off-label promotion. FDA Law Blog. Published March 2016. https://www.fdalawblog.net/2016/03/amarin-announces-a-proposed-settlement-of-its-first-amendment-law-suit-against-fda-coming-full-circle/. Accessed October 2020.

22. Frattarelli DA, Galinkin JL, Green TP, et al. Off-label use of drugs in children. *Pediatrics*. 2014;133(3):563-567.

23. Kimberly LL, Beuttler MM, Shen M, Caplan AL, Bateman-House A. Pre-approval access terminology: a cause for confusion and a danger to patients. *Ther Innov Regul Sci*. 2017;51(4):494–500.

24. Working Group on Compassionate Use and Preapproval Access, frequently asked questions. NYU Langone Health. https://med.nyu.edu/departments-institutes/population-health/divisions-sections-centers/medical-ethics/research/working-group-compassionate-use-preapproval-access/frequently-asked-questions#what-is-preapproval-access. Accessed August 2, 2020.

25. *Abigail Alliance v von Eschenbach*, 495 F3d 695 (2007).

26. Institute of Medicine Forum on Medical and Public Health Preparedness for Catastrophic Events. *Medical Countermeasures Dispensing: Emergency Use Authorization and the Postal Model, Workshop Summary*. Washington, DC: National Academies Press; 2010. Emergency Use Authorization. https://www.ncbi.nlm.nih.gov/books/NBK53122/. Accessed August 16, 2021.

27. FDCA § 564 (b).

28. FDCA § 564 (f), (g).

29. Emergency use authorization of medical products and related authorities. US Food and Drug Administration. Published January 2017. https://www.fda.gov/media/97321/download. Accessed August 2, 2020.

30. Van Norman GA. Expanding patient access to investigational new drugs: overview of intermediate and widespread treatment investigational new drugs, and emergency authorization in public health emergencies. *JACC Basic Transl Sci*. 2018;3(3):403–414.

31. 42 US Code § 247d-6d.

32. 42 CFR § 110.

33. Expanded access program. US Food and Drug Administration. Published May 2018. https://www.fda.gov/media/119971/download. Accessed August 2, 2020.

34. 21 CFR § 312 subpart I.
35. 21 CFR § 812.
36. 21 CFR § 312.300.
37. McKee AE, Markon AO, Chan-Tack KM, Lurie P. How often are drugs made available under the Food and Drug Administration's expanded access process approved? *J Clin Pharmacol*. 2017;57(suppl 10):S136–S142.
38. Project Facilitate. US Food and Drug Administration. https://www.fda.gov/about-fda/oncology-center-excellence/project-facilitate. Accessed August 2, 2020.
39. Darrow JJ, Sarpatwari A, Avorn J, Kesselheim AS. Practical, legal, and ethical issues in expanded access to investigational drugs. *N Engl J Med*. 2015;372(3):279–286.
40. Pub L No. 115–176.
41. 21 CFR § 312.81.
42. Pub L No. 115–176(b).
43. *Parker v St Lawrence County Public Health Department*, 102 AD3d 140 (NY App Div 2012).
44. *Casabianca v Mount Sinai Med Ctr, Inc.*, 2014 NY Slip Op 33583 (NY Sup Ct 2014).

CHAPTER 20

Clinical Trials

Aarthi B. Iyer, JD, MPH, Jessica Huening Poppenk, JD, and Michelle Francis, JD, MPH

INTRODUCTION

Medical malpractice lawsuits are a common domain among plaintiff's attorneys in clinical care. While human subjects research does contain some parallels to clinical care, litigation in clinical trials has stemmed from an array of legal claims including lack of informed consent, products liability, fraud, battery, infliction of emotional distress, breach of patients' rights protected by state law, violation of federal regulations, and violation of civil rights protected under the constitution.[1] Layering on top of the actual claims is the breadth of individuals and institutions against which lawsuits have been commenced. Cases have been brought against universities, academic medical centers, hospital systems, investigators, clinical trial sponsors, institutional review board (IRB) members, and bioethicists.[2,3]

Private sector funding associated with clinical trials has been growing at an astounding pace,[4] consequently growing in relevance to the careers of investigators. Legal challenges have also increasingly contoured the discourse surrounding research and clinical trial design, conduct, integrity, and safety. This chapter identifies context and considerations in conducting clinical trials with a focus on the role of the investigator and highlights areas in which lawsuits can arise.

The complex regulatory, ethical, professional, and scientific backdrop

Various regulations and practice standards apply to investigators and other stakeholders of clinical trials depending upon what is being investigated, who is funding the activity, and the populations being studied. Research supported by US federal funds, such as that funded by the National Institutes of Health (NIH), is generally subject to the "Common Rule." The Common Rule is a generic reference to a shared policy on human subject protections among several federal agencies.[5,6] US Food and Drug Administration (FDA) oversight is applicable when there is a clinical investigation of a test article (an investigational drug or device) or data regarding a product are intended for submission to the FDA.[7,8] Beyond regulatory provisions, FDA has adopted the Good Clinical Practice (GCP) transnational quality standards provided by the International Conference on Harmonization (ICH-GCP) as nonbinding guidance.[9,10]

Both federal regulations and ICH-GCP require protections be in place for any individual enrolling in a clinical trial. For example, federal regulations require that an ethics committee, referred to in the United States as an IRB, review all research involving human subjects against core research ethics tenants and regulation. This includes the obligation to obtain informed consent, a topic discussed later in this chapter.[11,12] Because many individuals enroll in oncology trials when other clinical alternatives have failed, the experimental drug is often viewed by the human subject (and sometimes the investigator) as another treatment option. Evaluation of this "therapeutic misconception" is part of the ethics review because, without appropriate safeguards, it may lead to individuals agreeing to take on greater risks than they would otherwise accept.

Investigators often carry both clinical care and research responsibilities, and it can be a challenge to balance time, effort, emotional capital, and, sometimes, conflicting duties. Clinical care providers measure success by delivering the best health care for their patients.[13] In contrast, investigators face professional demands to provide generalizable knowledge and large volumes of research data for sponsors; publish in peer-reviewed journals; obtain and grow their research funding portfolios; acquire academic appointments and promotions; advance innovation in the field; and earn respect from peers.[13,14] Further complicating matters, unlike standard training and licensure requirements to practice medicine, there is no mandated prerequisite for investigators to demonstrate qualification and expertise to conduct clinical trials.[15] Although institutional policy often identifies who can serve in research roles and required training, the lack of defined competencies can pose challenges in measuring, evaluating, and validating investigator capabilities.

Resting beneath and weaving within a researcher's ethical, professional, and regulatory obligations is the most fundamental guardrail—the scientific method. In oncology research, effective trial design is vital to build evidence of an experimental drug's safety and effectiveness. The gold standard for oncology studies is the randomized clinical trial, with the use of placebo where ethically appropriate.[16,17] Research design considerations include selecting an appropriate sample size and study population, establishing the experimental and control regimens, developing an interim analysis and toxicity monitoring plan, and analyzing and presenting final results.[16,17] Importantly, producing scientifically valid results depends on the faithfulness with which the investigator and research staff follow the research protocol and document their work. Thus, following ICH-GCP standards helps an investigator ensure integrity of the research data, which is necessary for protecting human subjects and for obtaining approval of experimental treatments by FDA or another relevant regulatory agency.

As investigators grow their research experience, they should be aware of some of the most common legal issues that can arise in the context of clinical trials, along with the associated claims and defenses. This chapter covers four common legal claims that human subject plaintiffs bring against investigators: lack of informed consent, conflicts of interest, research misconduct, and fraud.

INFORMED CONSENT

One of the cornerstones of western research ethics is the obligation to respect an individual's choice of whether to participate in a research study. The primary mechanism to give effect to this right is to obtain informed consent (i.e., to provide enough information about the research to individuals considering enrolling so that they can make a truly informed and voluntary choice about whether to enroll and whether to expose themselves to any potential risks or benefits that might ensue).

Government regulations and standards

In the United States, federal regulations require that informed consent be obtained and certain key information be presented to each potential human subject, usually in the form of an informed consent document (e.g., a description of the research procedures, time commitment, anticipated risks and benefits to the subject, privacy and confidentiality measures, ability of the subject to withdraw from the study without penalty).[18,19] Importantly, these federal regulations do not provide a private right of action (the right of a private individual, rather than the government or other public agency, to bring a lawsuit claiming injuries caused by another's violation of the regulation). Instead, the primary penalty is incurred by the institution conducting the research, in the form of loss of federal funding or suspension of the research and/or research program.[20,21]

Human subjects can, however, bring negligence claims if they believe they have received an injury as a result of participating in a clinical trial. Negligence is a type of civil claim involving a plaintiff seeking compensation for a harm caused by the defendant's failure to meet a duty of care owed to the plaintiff. One of the primary negligence claims in the area of oncology research is a lack of informed consent.

A typical claim might involve an individual who agreed to enroll in a clinical trial of an investigational cancer drug and suffers a serious toxic side effect from the study drug. The human subject might bring a negligence claim, arguing that the researcher had a duty to provide all relevant information about the study, including any potential risks, to prospective subjects but that they did not receive adequate information from the investigator about the potential side effects of the study drug. The human subject asserts that, had they known about the possibility of the serious side effect, they would not have agreed to enroll in the study and would not have suffered the injury. Key areas of dispute in such lawsuits usually involve establishing what kind of duty, if any, a researcher owes to a research subject and if there is a corresponding standard for informed consent that was not met.

Basis of a research negligence claim

In the medical malpractice context, a negligence claim for lack of informed consent to treatment must include the following elements: (1) a duty of care owed by the physician to the patient; (2) breach of that duty; (3) injury or harm to the patient; and (4) a causal link between the breach of duty and the patient's injury. Some courts have extended this framework to the research context if the plaintiff can establish a fiduciary relationship between the investigator and the human subjects that results in the investigator having a duty to the human subject to obtain informed consent before the subject agrees to enroll in a research study.

As an initial matter, the biggest challenge to extending the medical malpractice framework to the research context is establishing that a researcher owes a duty of care to a research subject. The goal of clinical care is to treat the patient, and so a physician's first duty is to their patient's well-being. In contrast, the goal of research is to contribute to generalizable knowledge, and therefore, the investigator's first duty is to science and not to the individual research subject. Historically, this distinction resulted in a lack of a legally recognized fiduciary relationship between the investigator and human subject and is often proposed as the reason the federal regulations offer no private right of action.[1,20–22]

Because most research negligence lawsuits settle before going to trial, there is little published case law and the legal landscape is still developing. Courts do, however, appear to be moving toward recognizing that a fiduciary relationship can exist between an investigator and a human subject such that some level of duty is owed to the human subject. For example, several courts have found that the informed consent document itself creates a quasi-contract with duties owed to the human subject.[21,23,24] Courts have also found a "special relationship" and duty of care when the investigator and human subject had a preexisting doctor-patient relationship or when a nontherapeutic study involved a particularly vulnerable population such as children.[20,23,25]

Although this chapter focuses on claims against an investigator, it is important to note that plaintiffs may also bring claims against the institution supporting the research, the study sponsor, university officials, the IRB, individual IRB members, and even the university bioethicist.[1,26] Similar to the analysis for individual investigators, courts will look to see whether a fiduciary relationship exists between the plaintiff and any named individual defendant.[27] A court may find the institution owes a duty of care to the human subject where the research is subject to federal regulations requiring informed consent and where the institution has established an IRB to review the research and to ensure legally effective informed consent is obtained.[27] Conversely, because study sponsors do not conduct the actual research procedures, courts have not found a direct legal relationship between the human subject and study sponsor that would support a negligence claim for lack of informed consent (although a sponsor could otherwise be liable to the human subject under a fraud or product liability claim).[28,29]

If a court agrees with the plaintiff that the researcher owes a duty of care, it must next determine whether the researcher met the standard of care. In the medical informed consent context, courts use two different tests to determine the relevant standard: the professional practice standard and the "reasonable person" standard. The professional practice standard requires expert testimony to determine the professional standard for disclosure, whereas the reasonable person standard is based on what kind of information a reasonable and prudent patient in similar circumstances would want to know before agreeing to the medical treatment. Courts considering a research informed consent negligence case have either adopted the professional practice standard and looked to the federal regulations or assessed whether a reasonably prudent person in a similar situation would not have consented to the research if the missing information had been disclosed.[21,30,31]

Plaintiffs have successfully made the argument that a researcher did not meet their duty to provide adequate information to the human subject where there was a failure to disclose a key aspect of the study, for example, where parents were not informed that the purpose of the study was to observe levels of blood lead contamination in their children or where a human subject was not told she would not be able to receive the planned dose of a study drug if she was unable to ingest the oral version.[23,31]

However, under the reasonable person standard, it can be very difficult to show that an individual would not have participated in a study if they had known of a specific risk or other missing information such as an investigator's potential financial conflict of interest.[20,32] In oncology research, enrolling in a clinical trial of an investigational drug is often an individual's final option after exhausting all other treatment possibilities, and therefore, the individual may be more willing to accept additional study risks. In one of the few research negligence cases that went to trial, the jury found that the plaintiffs did not prove that any missing information would have changed the plaintiffs' decision about whether to enroll in the research.[20,32] In fact, several jurors later indicated their belief that the human subjects would have been willing to take on extra risks for the chance at a cure.[33] Additionally, some jurisdictions recognize "assumption of risk" doctrines that allow for a defense that the human subject was aware of the study risks and agreed to assume those risks. In these jurisdictions, courts have sometimes limited recovery only to risks that were not described in the informed consent document.[30]

Under the professional practice standard, where the federal regulations act as the standard for informed consent, an investigator's defense is to demonstrate that they complied with the federal requirements, for example, that an IRB reviewed and approved the consent document used to enroll the plaintiff. While case law has not established clearly that compliance with the federal regulations acts as a complete defense to a negligence action, several courts have ruled for defendants who demonstrated compliance with the federal rules.[21]

Finally, to prevail on an informed consent negligence claim, the human subject must demonstrate that they suffered an injury that was caused by their participation in the research protocol. This can be particularly challenging in biomedical research, especially in the context of oncology research, where a human subject often has underlying medical conditions that make it difficult to demonstrate the injury is a result of the investigational drug, as opposed to the human subject's existing comorbidities.

Human subjects seeking to recover for their losses under a research informed consent negligence claim will usually seek to recover compensatory damages for physical, psychological, and emotional injury. Depending on the age and health of the human subject when the injury occurred and the seriousness or permanence of the injury, costs can easily add up to millions of dollars. Punitive damages may also be sought if an investigator, research institution, or other defendant acted with reckless disregard and there is a desire to deter future bad behavior.[34] Because most research negligence cases settle out of court, exact figures awarded by juries are scarce. However, many high-profile research cases have resulted in multimillion-dollar settlements.

CONFLICTS OF INTEREST

With upward of 70% of the money for clinical trials in the United States being provided by industry, the research enterprise has shifted from government-sponsored projects to an environment of increased commercialization of research, where there is more competition for research dollars, more potential for institutions to generate profits for their own academic ecosystems, and, notably, more instances of conflicts of interest.[14,35,36] For the purposes of this chapter, a conflict of interest is defined as an interest that is inconsistent with the official responsibilities of a person in a position of trust, where institutions and investigators who carry out research, for example, are persons in a position of trust.[36]

Investigator conflicts of interest

There are a variety of tangible and intangible individual conflicts of interest that investigators are constantly asked to traverse. Intangible conflicts can originate from career advancement pressures as well as the researcher's own bias and decreased objectivity in the clinical research environment. Examples of tangible incentives that can create conflicts of interest include bonus payments for boosting subject enrollment or meeting enrollment deadlines; gifts from sponsors, including discretionary funds, research equipment, and support for travel to professional meetings; equity interests; and consulting fees.[37] These conflicts of interest can influence how research questions are selected and positioned; an investigator's choice of trial design and technology utilized; recruitment and enrollment of human subjects; fidelity in reporting adverse events; and how data are collected, analyzed, interpreted, and ultimately published. Thus, if such conflicts of interest are unmitigated, they can result in questionable research data, injury and harm to study subjects, sanctions and punitive regulatory actions, and public scrutiny and skepticism.

Institutional conflicts of interest

A hospital or university's own financial investments, intellectual property, or intangible interests may just as significantly affect the conduct of clinical trials. Scenarios where institutional conflicts may arise include the following: (1) receiving significant royalty from the sale of a product covered by a patent when that product is proposed to be used in human subjects research projects at the institution; (2) holding significant equity interests in research sponsors, through its technology licensing activities or investments related to such activities; (3) receiving substantial gifts from a potential sponsor or a company that owns products being studied in human subjects research; and (4) leadership serving on the board of an entity that has a significant financial interest in human subjects research.[38] Whereas individual conflicts of interest for a majority of research activities are addressed via federal regulatory standards, there are no corresponding compliance frameworks for institutional conflicts. However, professional societies and associations have developed policies and a portfolio of topic-specific resources on conflicts of interest in order to provide structure and guidance to institutions around this complex, nuanced, and oft-hidden issue.[39-42]

IRB member conflicts of interest

Current regulations require that no IRB may have a member participate in the IRB's initial or continuing review of any project in which the member has a conflicting interest, except to provide information requested by the IRB.[43,44] However, these regulations feature an (inadvertent) blind spot, because academic IRBs often include department chairs, deans, senior administrators, and researchers.[35] Members may be perceptive to the value of research profits to the institution, and their judgments on IRB approval and oversight may be contoured by priorities around patent value, stock price, or related financial interests.[35] An ongoing government investigation highlighting the reality of these risks stems from an inquiry of the two largest, private-equity-owned IRBs (commercial IRBs), evaluating whether there is pressure to increase profits by approving as many studies as rapidly as possible and whether this leaves significant vulnerabilities in review of studies, leaving human subjects exposed to unnecessary risks.[45] Because commercial IRBs oversee approximately 70% of all drug and medical device trials in the United States,[45] this investigation has the potential to cause major shifts in and deeper scrutiny of IRB conflicts of interests across the research spectrum.

Government regulations and standards

Prior to 1980, the federal government retained the rights to the research inventions and discoveries of the investigators it funded, and industry was limited in its ability to obtain licenses to manufacture and market these discoveries. In order to unblock the transfer of technology from universities to the marketplace, Congress passed the Bayh-Dole Act, giving nonprofit entities rights to inventions developed under federally funded research activities and lead roles in patenting and licensing discoveries.[46] As universities now encourage their faculty to patent discoveries and benefit from shared royalties, experts warn of adverse impacts on academic freedoms and the prescribing patterns of investigator-clinicians owning drug patent rights.[14,47]

The increasing use of the research process to generate profits for institutions and investigators does not mean all conflicts of interest are inherently untrustworthy. However, it does illustrate that these entities must operate with an increased volume of disclosures and federal agencies must preserve integrity and objectivity in research.[36]

US federal agencies have thus promulgated conflicts of interest regulations and policies applicable to publicly funded research. The US Public Health Service (PHS), which includes the NIH, requires that institutions receiving funding establish standards and procedures that, among other aspects, require funded investigators to disclose aggregate financial interests of more than $5,000 to the institution.[48,49] Institutions must designate an official to review disclosures and manage conflicts of interest, including reporting to federal agencies if the official believes an investigator's financial interest could affect the research.[48]

The National Science Foundation has similar standards for its grantees, except that the significant financial interest disclosure threshold is $10,000.[50] Federal Acquisition Regulations prescribe responsibilities, general rules, and procedures for identifying, evaluating, and resolving organizational conflicts of interest for contracts with either for-profit or nonprofit organizations.[51] FDA's disclosure reporting requirements apply to an entity (sponsor) that has submitted a marketing application to the FDA, and investigators are obligated to provide the sponsor with sufficient financial information to enable the sponsor to meet its disclosure obligations.[35] FDA analyzes such disclosures and retains the right to conduct audits of the data from the questioned clinical investigator, request further analyses, request independent studies, and refuse to consider the data from the covered clinical study.[35]

Basis of a conflict of interest claim

In considering the overarching goals of oncology research, the investigator's professional interests, and the human subjects' expectations, there is a persuasive argument to be made that the investigator's motives and the human subject's best interests may not be in alignment, especially if there are apparent tangible conflicts of interest—ripe conditions for lawsuits.[1]

At the center of the conflicts of interest challenges, plaintiffs claimed that they were not informed of the investigators' and institutions' financial investments and that, had they been so informed, they would not have consented to enrollment in the trial.[35] In one case, the plaintiffs alleged an investigator had left the cancer center to start the company that would research and develop the investigational product, with the cancer center standing to gain considerable amounts in stocks and licensing fees, plus a percentage of the sales of the company.[52,53] In addition, as highlighted in Case Law # 1 in this chapter, the director of a university's gene therapy institute owned stock in a company standing to financially benefit from the outcome of a clinical trial where the university's agreement with the company gave the company rights to gene research discoveries at the institute in exchange for substantial financial support.[54,55]

As mentioned earlier, many research-related cases settle or are resolved in early stages of the legal process. As a consequence, the following questions related to legal liability remain unanswered: What are the circumstances under which an undisclosed conflict of interest would result in liability for the individual(s) and/or entities who are in the conflict position? Do other parties who know of the conflict or who ought reasonably to have known about the conflict and are in a position of authority have a legal obligation to intervene to prevent the research from proceeding on the basis of the conflict? Does the existence of an undisclosed conflict of interest give a plaintiff the legal basis to argue that the consent given was not truly informed?[26]

RESEARCH MISCONDUCT

The term research misconduct can mean different things depending on the context in which it is being used, but fundamentally, it reflects a failure to meet the responsibilities or requirements necessary to carry out research. Research misconduct can be a result of deliberate malfeasance or negligence, with resulting differences in liability. Thus, to minimize legal risk to investigators and institutions, it is important to understand the roles and responsibilities of key stakeholders in the research process.

Investigator responsibilities

FDA defines an investigator as the individual who conducts the clinical investigation and, if there is a study team, the responsible leader of the team.[56] Paramount among investigator responsibilities is ensuring the clinical trial is conducted in accordance with the study protocol and applicable rules; that human subjects' rights, safety, and welfare are protected; and that the drugs under investigation remain under the investigator's control.[57] FDA emphasizes that enrolled human subjects are not adequately protected if they failed to meet study criteria, particularly when those criteria are intended to exclude human subjects on the basis of risk. Failure to perform safety assessments within the protocol-specific time frames also inadequately protects human subjects in clinical trials.[57]

Investigators may delegate certain study-related tasks and responsibilities to employees, colleagues, or other parties not under their direct supervision. However, because the investigator is ultimately responsible for regulatory violations, procedures for adequate training and supervision must be in place and delegated tasks must be documented. Additionally, even if study activities are appropriately carried out, there is no way to effectively establish whether that is the case if those activities are not documented in the research record.

Sponsor-investigator responsibilities

A sponsor-investigator is an individual who both initiates and conducts an investigation, which is often referred to as investigator-initiated research. Sponsor-investigators are responsible for both the investigator and sponsor responsibilities under the applicable rules, regulations, and standards. Sponsors have unique responsibilities such as selecting qualified investigators, maintaining appropriate regulatory submissions, and ensuring the FDA and all participating investigators are promptly notified of significant new adverse effects or risks. In evaluating appropriate conduct, sponsor-investigators are held to a higher combined standard for maintaining responsibility for the overall study.

Negligence claims of research misconduct

Litigation related to negligent conduct and monitoring is on the rise.[58,59] Although no express cause of action is provided against investigators in the federal regulations, clinical trial subjects can bring negligence claims if they believe they have received an injury because of participating in a clinical trial due to research misconduct. Of note, it is fairly regular practice for institutions to negotiate clinical trial agreements where sponsors provide indemnification to cover the institution's and investigator's performance of a clinical trial, including expenses for defending claims of human subject injuries suffered in a clinical trial. While this is a viable protective practice, sponsors typically carve out indemnification coverage where the institution's or investigator's behavior is deemed negligent or resulting from willful misconduct.[60]

Suits involving claims of research misconduct are often settled before going to court and reflect varied examples of study misconduct beyond problems with informed consent. For example, as described in Case Law # 1 in this chapter, a case from Pennsylvania included claims that investigators failed to follow the study's eligibility rules and enrolled an individual who did not qualify; failed to obtain the required federal review of the research gene therapy procedures; and failed to properly store and control the investigational product.[2] In another action, the plaintiff's malpractice claims focused on the negligent conduct of the sponsor-investigator in a vaccine clinical trial that included errors in the regulatory submissions provided to FDA, enrolled more than three times the number of approved human subjects, lacked safety monitoring, and failed to control the investigational product.[3]

The FDA Bioresearch Monitoring (BIMO) Program reports that of the 1,402 inspections performed by BIMO in 2019, just over half of those inspections were of clinical investigators.[61] Frequently cited observations included (1) failure to follow the investigational plan or protocol deviations; (2) failure to comply with Form FDA 1572; (3) inadequate and/or inaccurate case history records or inadequate study records; (4) inadequate subject protection or informed consent issues; and (5) inadequate safety reporting or failure to report and/or record adverse events.[61]

Regulatory research misconduct

In addition to risk of litigation from human subject plaintiffs, investigators face risk of regulatory sanctions and consequences due to deliberate research malfeasance as addressed under government policy. PHS defines research misconduct as fabrication, falsification, or plagiarism in proposing, performing, or reviewing research, or in reporting research results, but does not include honest error or differences of opinion.[62] Examples of litigated findings of PHS violations, usually by researchers subject to imposed penalties, include falsification of data for grant funding,[63] plagiarism of others work as part of a grant application,[64] and fabricated conclusions, data, and images in publications.[65]

Per PHS requirements, institutions must have written policies and procedures for addressing allegations of research misconduct that facilitate an impartial and just review process, including procedures to ensure confidentiality of parties relevant to the research misconduct claim, a fair review process free from conflicts of interest, appropriate notice and opportunity to be heard, and appropriate practices to handle research records and evidence.[66] Institutions have the burden of proof in making a finding of research misconduct, and the respondent has the burden to establish affirmative defenses or any mitigating factors by a preponderance of the evidence standard.[67]

In order to find research misconduct under PHS policy, there must be a significant departure from accepted practices of the relevant research community, and the misconduct must be committed intentionally, knowingly, or recklessly.[68] The allegation must be proven by beyond a preponderance of the evidence standard.

Defenses to findings of research misconduct often consist of breach of employment contract claims by which the institution making a finding of research misconduct violated their own institutional policies. This may include arguments that the preponderance of the evidence standard was not satisfied in establishing the level of misconduct and, specifically, that the misconduct did not meet the PHS regulatory threshold of being conducted intentionally, knowingly, or recklessly and/or in absence of honest error.

Consequences of research misconduct

Penalties for research misconduct may include (1) termination of employment; (2) suspension or termination of a research grant; (3) enforcement actions and sanctions; and (4) suspension or debarment from receiving federal funds.[69,70] For example, in 2001, the Office of Human Research Protection (OHRP) concluded that an investigator and IRB at Johns Hopkins erred in the design,

Table 20-1. US Food and Drug Administration (FDA) Enforcement Actions and Sanctions

FDA Sanction	Description
Warning letter	Letter issued when there have been significant violations of FDA regulations. Letter advises of the noted violations and requests a response to establish steps that will be taken to correct the violations. Warning letters are publicly posted.[a]
Formal disqualification	FDA may disqualify investigators after repeated or deliberate failure to comply with FDA regulations or submission of false information to the sponsor or FDA. Disqualified investigators are not eligible to receive investigational products and are not eligible to conduct any clinical investigation that supports an application for a research or marketing permit for FDA-regulated products. Investigators subject to disqualification proceedings are made publicly available.[b]
Clinical hold	Order issued by FDA to the sponsor to delay or suspend an ongoing investigation. Grounds for imposing a clinical hold include if human subjects are or would be exposed to unreasonable and significant risk or injury or the clinical investigators are not qualified in scientific training and experience to conduct the investigation.[c]
Criminal prosecution	Individuals or firms can be criminally prosecuted for misdemeanor (fines and/or 1 year imprisonment) and felony (fines and/or up to three years imprisonment) convictions under Title 18 of the US Criminal Code as well as for violations of Section 301 of the Federal Food, Drug, and Cosmetic Act.

[a]Warning letters. Food and Drug Administration Compliance Actions and Activities. https://www.fda.gov/inspections-compliance-enforcement-and-criminal-investigations/compliance-actions-and-activities/warning-letters. Accessed February 1, 2021.

[b]Clinical investigators: Disqualification proceedings. Food and Drug Administration Compliance and Enforcement Regulatory Activities. https://www.accessdata.fda.gov/scripts/SDA/sdNavigation.cfm?sd=clinicalinvestigatorsdisqualificationproceedings&previewMode=true&displayAll=true. Accessed February 1, 2021.

[c]21 CFR § 312.42 (2020).

review, and implementation of an investigator-initiated clinical investigation that resulted in the death of a healthy control human subject. As a result, all federally funded research at Johns Hopkins was temporarily suspended.[71]

FDA enforcement actions and sanctions vary based on the nature of the violation, the public health concern, current policy, and history of other violations (Table 20-1).[72] FDA is particularly concerned with falsification of clinical trial data as it poses risks to human subjects and compromises the integrity of safety and effectiveness data.[71] In such cases, FDA can criminally prosecute investigators for fraud and conspiracy.[71]

FRAUD

All fraud by definition is misconduct, but not all misconduct is fraud.[73] Because fraud and misconduct are sometimes used interchangeably, this section will address aspects of human subjects research historically implicated by a common law claim of fraud (also referred to as fraudulent misrepresentation or intentional misrepresentation), which always contains intent, be it via misstatements or omissions, featuring an element of deliberate action.[74] Contrastingly, as illustrated in the research misconduct section of this chapter, misconduct covers a broader range of activities and need not be an intentional action, but rather an act of poor management or failure to follow established protocols where the failure results in unreasonable risk or harm to human subjects.[75] For the purposes of this section, an overarching definition of fraud, as used by federal courts, is "the knowing breach of the standard of good faith and fair dealing as understood in the community, involving deception or breach of trust, for money."[76]

The notion of fraud in clinical trials has widespread, far-reaching historical consequences ranging from questions regarding the validity of data and research results to impacts on human subjects' dignity, rights, welfare, and safety. Data from the Office of Research Integrity (ORI) show that it receives 265 reports of research fraud each year.[76] Some earlier research-related fraud has involved significant harm and abuse of human subjects, perhaps most notably the Tuskegee Syphilis Study, an endeavor designed to study the natural progression of untreated syphilis where human subjects were enrolled under the impression that they were receiving free health care from the government.[77] However, subjects were never told they had syphilis, nor were they offered penicillin, which was widely used as a curative treatment for syphilis during the time of the study.[77] Claims related to fraud have also impacted oncology research, such as a government-sponsored study where live cancer cells were injected into debilitated elderly patients at a hospital, without their knowledge or consent, and a case involving human subjects with a severe form of brain cancer who were subjected to experimental treatment, also allegedly without their knowledge or consent.[78,79]

In exploring motivations that may catalyze fraud, investigators' professional obligations and expectations, discussed earlier in this chapter, may serve as a cascade into performance pressures, eventually resulting in fraud. Other investigators may even believe they are correct in their deliberate actions, despite lack of supporting data and evidence.[76] Given these powerful underlying factors, investigators may intentionally continue to commit fraud despite the risks, perhaps thinking, or rather hoping, they will not be discovered.

Basis of a fraud claim

The definition of fraud centers on the defendant's state of mind—knowingly or intentionally engaging in the bad conduct. From there, the definition requires an assessment of community standards of good faith and fair dealing. As illustrated earlier, courts continue to work through understanding the standards related to clinical trials conduct. In the informed consent context, fraud claims raise issues of what human subjects were told by the researcher and, subsequently, what information each subject relied on when giving consent. Breach of trust may stem from "special relationships," as discussed earlier in this chapter, whereby certain duties or parallels to fiduciary obligations exist within a researcher–human subject relationship. Pivoting to injury and damages, depending on the substantive nature of the claim, direct harms may be related to money, including where there are alleged financial conflicts of interest, and courts have also allowed this definition to encompass loss arising from fiduciary or agent relationships.[76]

While the elements of fraud claims vary from state to state, one class action suit involving injuries to subjects in a melanoma vaccine trial put forth the following elements regarding allegations that investigators fraudulently misrepresented the purpose, risks, and benefits of the study: (1) defendants committed common law fraud in intentionally misrepresenting the risks of participating in the trial; the nature, scope, and legitimacy of the trial; and the reason for terminating the trial; (2) the misrepresentations were done with the knowledge that they were false when made; (3) plaintiff justifiably relied upon the misrepresentations in making the decision to participate and continue in the trial; and (4) as a direct and proximate result of defendants' intentional and material misrepresentations, plaintiff participated and continued in the trial to her detriment.

For a representation to be actionable, the subject of the misstatement or omission must be knowable as either true or false, such as the case where investigators committed fraud by not revealing that previous human subjects enrolled in a study had died.[2] Courts have even found sufficient basis for fraud claims where a plaintiff claimed that the sponsor, through the informed consent form provided (to the institutional investigator) for use in the study, materially misrepresented the severity of the side effects of the investigational drug and failed to provide sufficient warnings that the sponsor had knowledge of and had previously reported in its annual reports.[80] In order to be actionable, statements are ordinarily made as to past or existing facts, but predictions and opinions are rarely actionable as fraud.[81] As actions regarding deception revolve around making false representations or lies, if the alleged misstatement was determined to not be a lie but the truth, the claim would likely be dismissed since truth is a defense.[82]

Importantly, a defendant's actions are evaluated based on knowledge and intent at the time the misrepresentations are made. In the context of research, the knowledge gained during a study is constantly evolving, often incomplete in terms of statistical power and scope, and subject to downstream data validation of results. Thus, informed consent forms often state that not all risks are known at the time the research is being conducted, new information may be learned in the future, or there may be no benefit to an individual subject through participation.

Finally, the plaintiff must also actually rely on the false representation, showing that the misrepresentation affected the plaintiff's conduct to their detriment. Additionally, courts may evaluate whether the reliance was reasonable, where the standard is based on the particular plaintiff.

Because fraud claims raise questions of deception and breach of trust, these allegations can draw significant public attention, providing insight into how jurors may view the magnitude of damages and impacts to plaintiffs and how the public's trust in investigators may erode if there is a belief that research is being done for a researcher's personal and financial gain.[1] Lawsuits alleging fraud therefore stand to have large damage awards, especially for punitive damages, in order to make an example of fraudulent defendants and deter others from making the same missteps.

BEST PRACTICE RECOMMENDATIONS

Being aware of the competing demands, common major pitfalls, and the shifting research landscape in conducting clinical trials can help minimize risk to investigators and institutions overall. Indeed, clinical trials in oncology can present unique challenges in the management and care of trial subjects, as treatment with cancer drugs is often associated with significant risk from known toxicities and off-label therapy with cancer drugs is common practice.[83] With a spirit of mitigating or even altogether preventing the regulatory and legal dilemmas investigators may encounter when conducting clinical trials, we recommend the following proactive and protective strategies to implement in daily practice.

Adhere to institutional policies

Since so much of the legal analysis across all the issues discussed in this chapter hinges on whether an investigator met the standard of care, it is critically important that any investigator follow institutional policies and processes, be it regarding IRB review, conflicts of interest disclosures, clinical trial conduct, training and education, or recordkeeping. Additionally, institutional policies are sensitive to local contexts and standards and also provide guidance on how to operationalize regulatory commitments, something often lacking in the regulations themselves.

Engage experts and mentors in clinical trial design and execution

Prior to starting the clinical trial, if investigators are inexperienced or they are otherwise serving as a sponsor-investigator, it is beneficial for them to get in touch with the groups at their institution that provide quality assurance for FDA submissions and also support setting up study case report forms, regulatory binders, and other essential documents.[84] Because there are no formal educational requirements for becoming an investigator, it is vital for those choosing this pathway to gain hands-on knowledge and lessons learned from senior mentors. These experienced individuals can provide guidance on working through the operational, technical, and clinical trial implementation responsibilities that investigators are expected to meet and maintain.

Provide clear, concise, and constant communication with human subjects

Because many legal claims stem from issues with informed consent, it is crucial for investigators to prioritize engaging in genuine dialogue with human subjects throughout the phases of a clinical trial. When disclosures are being made directly to human subjects, communication should be in line with regulatory requirements around informed consent (e.g., concise and focused presentation of key information),[18] with diligence around providing meaningful and clear content about conflicts of interests and related risk considerations. These steps to create a more collaborative dynamic between investigator and human subject will also facilitate well-reasoned informed consent. With the rise in pragmatic clinical trials and real-world evidence, soliciting ongoing feedback from human subject voices can lend valuable insights into real-world practicalities related to clinical trials, including design, implementation, and, notably, perceptions on what is deemed material information from the perspective of a human subject.

Be vigilant about recordkeeping and monitoring

Should a legal claim arise, maintaining documentation of the investigator's compliance with the consent requirements (e.g., maintaining a regulatory file for each human subject, documenting that the steps of the informed consent process were followed, including notes taken on any discussions with the human subject) will help build a stronger defense both that the federal regulatory standards were met and that the human subject was, in fact, aware of all anticipated study risks.

In conducting the research, investigators must be diligent to adhere to protocol requirements and to report protocol deviations that occur, whether due to error or the need to eliminate immediate hazards to human subjects. If it is discovered that noncompliant conduct has occurred, it is important to immediately assess the situation, report it to necessary parties as applicable, and develop a corrective and preventative action plan to prevent future reoccurrence.

CASE LAW # 1

Jesse Gelsinger, an 18-year-old human subject, died while participating in a phase I gene therapy clinical trial conducted at the Institute for Human Gene Therapy (IHGT) of the University of Pennsylvania.[2] The trial's goal was to develop a liver-directed gene therapy pathway to target an inherited deficiency in ornithine transcarbamylase (OTC). On September 13, 1999, Gelsinger was given an infusion of the experimental drug, a corrective OTC gene encased in a dose of attenuated adenovirus, injected into his hepatic artery. Gelsinger experienced severe complications related to vector administration and died four days after receiving the infusion. A co-investigator on this clinical trial, who also served as the director of the IHGT, held patents on several gene therapy delivery techniques and was a founder of Genovo, Inc., a company involved in gene transfer research and development. The company had rights to market the investigator's discoveries related to gene transfer and also provided funding to support the activities of the IHGT. Along with the investigator, the University of Pennsylvania held equity interests in the company, and all three parties had financial interests in a successful outcome of the research involved in the clinical trial.

Gelsinger's family filed a lawsuit against an array of defendants including Genovo, Inc., the University of Pennsylvania, the Children's Hospital of Philadelphia, the lead researchers (the principal investigator and co-investigators), and the institution's bioethicist. Plaintiffs asserted that Gelsinger died as a direct result of the carelessness, negligence, recklessness, and wanton and willful conduct of the defendants, under a variety of claims, including, among others, lack of informed consent, financial conflicts of interest, and common law fraud. The complaint specifically highlighted that (1) the risks of the toxic effects of the injection of the adenovirus particles were understated and intentionally misrepresented; (2) no mention was made that monkeys injected with the virus had become ill and/or died; (3) no mention was made that patients who had previously participated in the trial suffered serious adverse effects; (4) the representation was made that IHGT had achieved certain efficacy with respect to the treatment of OTC; (5) the extent to which investigators and the University of Pennsylvania had a conflict of interest was not adequately disclosed; and (6) the ammonia level in Gelsinger's blood exceeded the limit in the protocol the day before he received the gene transfer. It was contended that the effects of such misrepresentations and nondisclosures were that Gelsinger and his family believed the risks of experimental intervention were minimal and the potential benefits of participation to the future treatment of OTC patients in the clinical trial were enormous and that, had they known these underlying issues existed, Gelsinger would not have enrolled in the clinical trial or suffered death as a result.

While the lawsuit was confidentially settled out of court in November 2000, these events catalyzed government investigations from various federal agencies including FDA, Office of Human Research Protections, and NIH, as well as congressional inquiries. The investigations raised questions about noncompliance in several aspects of clinical trial conduct, including documentation of findings, timeliness and accuracy of adverse event reports to the IRB and FDA, completeness of protocol-mandated tests, adherence to eligibility and stopping criteria, adequacy of clinical staff training, delivery and content of the consent process, completeness of subject monitoring following vector dosing, and timely notification to FDA of animal toxicity data acquired subsequent to initiation of the study.[84] While the government investigations were ultimately resolved without admission of wrongdoing by the University of Pennsylvania or the investigators, they triggered the delay and investigation of other gene therapy clinical trials on a national scale and the development of new regulatory as well as institutional review and monitoring processes for performance of gene therapy research.[84]

CLINICAL VIGNETTE # 1

The following clinical vignette describes a hypothetical lawsuit involving a research subject who died because of toxic side effects from an experimental chemotherapy regimen. The details are taken from several different real-world examples. As you read through the vignette, try to think about the legal rules discussed in this chapter and how you would apply them to this case.

Angela was a 62-year-old cancer patient who died from severe organ damage while enrolled in a breast cancer study at a prominent academic medical center. The study was designed to determine whether the maximum-tolerated dose of a standard chemotherapy regimen could be increased when used in an experimental combination with another drug XRS. Preliminary data showed that XRS might offer protection against the organ-damaging effects of the chemotherapy regimen in question. The primary research aim was to establish XRS's efficacy. The principal investigator owned patent rights in XRS and owned stock in the company sponsoring the study.

Angela had previously tried several different breast cancer treatment regimens, all of which had been unsuccessful, and she had consequently turned to considering experimental alternatives. Before Angela agreed to join the study, she and her daughter Briana met with Dr. Smith, the principal investigator, to go over the study details and the consent form. Dr. Smith told Angela and Briana that XRS would protect Angela from organ failure by blocking the toxic effects of the chemotherapy drugs. Angela had a history of being unable to tolerate oral drugs and was assured by Dr. Smith that an intravenous version of XRS would be available. Dr. Smith did not tell Angela that the supplier of XRS had announced six months before that it would no longer supply the intravenous form of the drug. Dr. Smith did not mention, nor did the consent form state, that she had financial interests in the study drug and in the study sponsor.

Angela agreed to enroll in the study. She became nauseous and vomited after almost every dose of oral XRS and died four months later from acute organ failure resulting from the chemotherapy regimen. Briana, acting as the personal representative of Angela's estate, files a lawsuit against Dr. Smith. Briana claims Dr. Smith was negligent in obtaining informed consent, was negligent in conducting the research, and committed fraud. (Note that this chapter limits the analysis to claims against the investigator. A plaintiff would likely also bring claims against the academic medical center and the IRB that reviewed the research consent form.) Does Briana have a cause of action to recover under theories of negligent informed consent, research misconduct, and fraud?

The theory of informed consent liability in Briana's case is that Dr. Smith owed a duty of care to Angela such that she was required to obtain her informed consent to participate in the research, but that this duty was breached and this breach directly caused Angela's death. In a negligence case, the human subject (or their representative) has the burden to prove the elements of the claim. While the case law is still unsettled and the application will vary from state to state, courts appear to be moving toward general acknowledgement that researchers owe some duty of care to their human subjects, particularly in oncology research, with informed consent being a primary duty. Thus, Briana will likely clear the hurdle of the duty element. Depending on the state, the standard for disclosure will vary slightly, but most jurisdictions will require the plaintiff to demonstrate that key information was not provided. Briana will therefore need to focus on the lack of disclosure related to the following facts: Dr. Smith's financial interest in the study sponsor; the positioning of XRS as "protective" when there was no proven efficacy; and the fact that only the oral form of the drug was available.

Whether or not the investigator's financial interests should have been disclosed will require Briana to provide evidence of the academic medical center's existing conflict of interest policies, including whether these policies were, in fact, followed. Expert testimony may even be called to explain the conflicts disclosure and management standards in the academic research community. However, even if Dr. Smith's financial interest was found to be a material fact, given the potential therapeutic outcomes in oncology research, it may be quite difficult for Briana to convince a jury that her mother would not have enrolled in the study if she had known of the financial ties.

The information most likely to be found dispositive under any standard of disclosure is the information that the effectiveness of XRS had not yet been proven and that only the oral version of the study drug was available. Briana's argument would be that, without the ability to absorb the specified dose of XRS, Angela was exposed to a higher dose of the chemotherapy regimen than accepted medical practice and that, if a reasonable person in the same circumstances had been told this and also been told that the effectiveness of XRS had not been yet proven, they would not have enrolled in the research and would not have experienced organ damage from the chemotherapy regimen. The consent document itself will be crucial, as the actual wording and whether it contained overpromising statements related to the drug's efficacy or indicated whether intravenous XRS was available will be objective evidence that informed consent was not obtained. If the consent document is not defective, the parties, in a battle of "who took the best notes," will produce any other evidence they have regarding the conversations to show whether or not Dr. Smith overstated XRS's efficacy or misrepresented the availability of intravenous XRS.

Finally, Briana will have to demonstrate that Angela's organ damage was a result of the chemotherapy regimen she was exposed to as part of the study and not a result of her underlying cancer, other comorbidities, or other prior medical interventions. Given the complexity of oncology treatment regimens, most jurisdictions will use expert testimony to establish the likelihood that the organ damage was caused by the study chemotherapy regimen. Given organ damage was a known side effect of the chemotherapy regimen used in the study, Briana will likely be able to show causation.

The question of whether Dr. Smith misrepresented the availability of intravenous XRS will also be key in the research misconduct claim. Similar to informed consent negligence, the theory of research misconduct liability in this case is that Dr. Smith owed a duty of care to Angela such that she was required to conduct the research in conformance with the research protocol and federal regulations, but that this duty was breached, and this breach directly caused Angela's death. A critical argument in Briana's claim should be that Dr. Smith was obligated to follow the study protocol's eligibility criteria and that Dr. Smith should have found Angela ineligible to participate because she knew Angela was unable to tolerate oral medications and knew intravenous XRS was not available. Thus, Dr. Smith violated her duty of care to Angela, which resulted in her exposure to the toxic side effects of the chemotherapy regimen that caused her organ damage.

As with the informed consent negligence, Briana will likely prevail in demonstrating that Dr. Smith owed a duty of care to Angela that required her to meet her regulatory-compelled investigator obligations, including complying with the protocol. The outcome for the research misconduct claim will be very fact specific and depend on the precise eligibility criteria laid out in the research protocol and whether the evidence shows that, by enrolling an individual who could not tolerate oral medications, Dr. Smith violated the study protocol and thus breached her duty of care. If a breach of duty is found, the analysis will require walking through the same causation considerations as in the informed consent negligence claim.

The alleged behavior of Dr. Smith in the research misconduct claim will bear some similarity to the fraud claim. However, in research misconduct negligence, Dr. Smith's actions are positioned as resulting from a lack of care or diligence. Conversely, intentionality is key in claims of fraud. Specifically, the theory of fraud in Briana's case is that Dr. Smith intentionally misrepresented to Angela the effectiveness of XRS and the availability of intravenous XRS; that Dr. Smith was aware she was deceiving Angela; that Angela justifiably relied upon Dr. Smith's misrepresentations when deciding to enroll in the research; and that as a direct and proximate result of Dr. Smith's misrepresentations Angela was exposed to levels of a chemotherapy drug that caused her to die from organ damage.

In order for Dr. Smith's misrepresentation to be actionable as fraud, Briana must show that the misstatements are knowable as true or false. In oncology research, this can be a difficult bar to meet if the alleged misstatements relate only to the investigator's opinions or predictions relating to a drug's potential efficacy. However, the study protocol can be used here to show that it was known that the effectiveness of XRS had not been established and that Dr. Smith, as the principal investigator, would have been aware of this. Briana will need to produce evidence that Dr. Smith made statements affirmatively asserting XRS would "protect" Angela from organ damage by "blocking" the toxic effects of chemotherapy. Dr. Smith's precise statements to Angela will be a key source of dispute between the parties, with Dr. Smith asserting that she only expressed her general opinions about the prospects of XRS's efficacy. Briana will also need to produce evidence both that (1) Dr. Smith knew intravenous XRS would not be available to Angela (e.g., communications from the XRS supplier to Dr. Smith that preceded the date of their conversation) and (2) Dr. Smith stated to Angela that intravenous XRS would be available (e.g., e-mail communications, meeting notes). If Briana can produce this evidence, she will have a stronger case that Dr. Smith knowingly made untrue statements to Angela.

Finally, Briana will need to demonstrate that Angela relied on Dr. Smith's statements and that this reliance caused Angela's death. Depending on the state, Briana may also need to argue that this reliance was reasonable. Given Angela's known intolerance to oral medication and the fact that she was seeking experimental options in the hopes of therapeutic value, Briana should be able to demonstrate that Angela would not have agreed to enroll in the research without first relying on Dr. Smith's statements. Demonstrating causation will follow a similar analysis as in the preceding negligence claims.

In jurisdictions where reasonable reliance is a factor, Dr. Smith will produce any evidence demonstrating that Angela's reliance was unreasonable (e.g., any study materials, including the consent document, that stated that XRS's effectiveness was unknown or that only oral XRS was available). However, given the trend toward courts finding the investigator sits in a fiduciary role to the human subject, Briana may still be successful in demonstrating that Angela's reliance on Dr. Smith's oral statements was reasonable, even if they contradicted the written study materials.

Based on the current trends in research-related litigation, as well as the facts in this vignette, it is likely that Briana has a valid cause of action that Angela did not provide informed consent, that Dr. Smith engaged in research misconduct, and that Dr. Smith engaged in fraudulent misrepresentation.

CONCLUSION

As illustrated in the legal actions discussed throughout this chapter, there is a diverse bases for claims made in the context of clinical trials. Additionally, courts continually grapple with applying established standards for clinical liability to the complex and constantly evolving human subjects' research landscape. Further obfuscating the analysis is the prevailing trend for clinical trial cases to settle before going to trial. Investigators and institutions are therefore often left to speculate on what may have occurred and how to successfully avoid adverse legal consequences. Despite this uncertainty, the existing case law reveals that legal risk can still be minimized if investigators and institutions avoid common major pitfalls, balance competing professional demands, and understand best practice recommendations.

KEY POINTS:

- Research and clinical care have different goals, which result in different relationships and duties between a physician and patient and a researcher and human subject.
- Cancer patients who have participated in a clinical trial may believe the experimental drug caused their condition to worsen.
- Human subjects can bring lawsuits against the investigator conducting the research claiming the investigator's negligent or fraudulent behavior caused their research-related injury.
- Potential defendants can also include the study sponsor, research institution, institution officials, and IRB members.
- The primary negligence claims in research lawsuits are lack of informed consent and research misconduct.
- Financial conflicts of interest and research fraud have also been the bases of several prominent research-related lawsuits.
- The elements of a research negligence claim are (1) a duty of care owed by the investigator to the human subject; (2) breach of that duty; (3) injury or harm to the research subject; and (4) a causal link between the breach of duty and the research subject's injury.
- Central to the research negligence analysis is determining whether the investigator owes a duty to the research subject and what is the relevant standard of care.
- The elements of a research fraud claim vary by state but generally require that (1) the investigator made an intentional misrepresentation of fact; (2) the misrepresentation was known to be false when made; (3) the research subject justifiably relied on the misrepresentation in making the decision to participate; and (4) a causal link between the misrepresentation and the research subject's injury.
- Careful planning and attention should be taken in the design and implementation of a study protocol, and investigators should make themselves aware of the regulatory requirements and institutional policies governing the conduct of their research.

References:

1. Mello MM, Studdert DM, Brennan TA. The rise of litigation in human subjects research. *Ann Intern Med*. 2003;139(1):40–45.
2. Complaint, *Gelsinger v Trustees of the University of Pennsylvania*, Phila County Ct Com Pl (September 18, 2000). http://www.sskrplaw.com/links/healthcare2.html. Accessed August 22, 20221.
3. Complaint, *Robertson v McGee*, N Dist of Okla (January 29, 2001), No. 01CV00G0H (M). http://www.sskrplaw.com/gene/robertson/complaint.html. Accessed August 22, 2021.
4. Morin K, Rakatansky H, Riddick FA Jr., et al. Managing conflicts of interest in the conduct of clinical trials. *JAMA*. 2002;287(1):78-84.
5. Federal Policy for the Protection of Human Subjects, 82 Fed Reg 7149 (January 19, 2017).
6. Revised Common Rule. Office of Human Research Protections. Published January 19, 2017. https://www.hhs.gov/ohrp/regulations-and-policy/regulations/finalized-revisions-common-rule/index.html. Accessed February 1, 2021.
7. 21 CFR §§ 50, 312, 812 (2020).
8. Chapter 48: Bioresearch monitoring (FDA Form 2438g). US Food and Drug Administration. https://www.fda.gov/media/75927/download. Accessed August 22, 2021.

9. ICH guidance documents. US Food and Drug Administration. Published March 29, 2018. https://www.fda.gov/science-research/guidance-documents-including-information-sheets-and-notices/ich-guidance-documents. Accessed February 1, 2021.

10. ICH harmonised guideline integrated addendum to ICHE6(R1): guideline for good clinical practice ICH E6(R2) ICH consensus guideline. Good Clinical Practice Network. https://ichgcp.net/. Accessed February 1, 2021.

11. 45 CFR §§ 46.107-111 (Subpart A) (2020).

12. 21 CFR § 56 (Subpart C) (2020).

13. Coleman CH. Duties to subjects in clinical research. *Vanderbilt L Rev*. 2005;58:387.

14. Bodenheimer T. Uneasy alliance: clinical investigators and the pharmaceutical industry. *N Engl J Med*. 2000;342(20):1539–1544.

15. Saleh M, Naik G. So you want to be a principal investigator. *J Oncol Pract*. 2018;14(6):e384–e392.

16. Glass KC, Waring D. Effective trial design need not conflict with good patient care. *Am J Bioeth*. 2002;2(2):25–26.

17. Hamilton EP, Peppercorn JM. Ethical issues in adult oncology randomized clinical trials. *Clin Invest*. 2011;1(5):629–636.

18. 45 CFR § 46.116 (Subpart A) (2020).

19. 21 CFR § 50.20 (Subpart B) (2020).

20. Koch VG. A private right of action for informed consent for research. *Seton Hall L Rev*. 2015;45:173.

21. Jansson RL. Researcher liability for negligence in human subjects research: informed consent and researcher malpractice actions. *Wash L Rev*. 2003;78:229.

22. Morreim EH. Litigation in clinical research: malpractice doctrines versus research realities. *J Law Med Ethics*. 2004;32(3):474–484.

23. *Grimes v Kennedy Krieger Institute*, 782 A2d 807 (Md 2001).

24. *Dahl v Hem Pharmaceuticals Corp*, 7 F3d 1399 (9th Cir 1993).

25. *Moore v Regents of the University of California*, 793 P2d 479 (Cal 1990).

26. Zlotnik Shaul R, Birenbaum S, Evans M. Legal liabilities in research: early lessons from North America. *BMC Med Ethics*. 2005;6:E4.

27. *Karen Lenahan v University of Chicago*, 348 Ill App3d 155 (1st Dist Ct 2004).

28. Mello MM, Joffe S. Compact versus contract: industry sponsors' obligations to their research subjects. *N Engl J Med*. 2007;356(26):2737–2743.

29. *Abney v Amgen, Inc.*, 443 F3d 540 (6th Cir 2006).

30. Henry LM, Larkin ME, Pike ER. Just compensation: a no-fault proposal for research-related injuries. *J Law Biosci*. 2015;2(3):645–668.

31. Order Granting Plaintiff's Motion for Partial Summary Judgement on Informed Consent Claim, *Berman v The Fred Hutchinson Cancer Research Center, et al.*, WD Wash, (August 2002), No. C01-0727L (BJR).

32. *Wright v Fred Hutchinson Cancer Center*, 269 FSupp2d 1286 (WD Wash 2002).

33. Davis WN. When clinical trials fail. *Am Bar Assoc J*. 2004;90:20.

34. Resnik DB. Compensation for research-related injuries. Ethical and legal issues. *J Leg Med*. 2006;27(3):263–287.

35. Barnes M, Florencio PS. Investigator, IRB and institutional financial conflicts in interest in human-subject research: past, present and future. *Seton Hall L Rev*. 2003;32:525.

36. Jordan KA. Financial conflicts of interest in human subjects research: proposals for a more effective regulatory scheme. *Wash Lee L Rev*. 2003;60:15.

37. Goldner J. Regulating conflicts of interest in research: the paper tiger needs real teeth. *St Louis L J*. 2009;53:1211.

38. Institutional conflicts of interest in human subjects research policy. University at Buffalo Research Integrity. Published October 25, 2018. http://www.buffalo.edu/news/key-issues/research-integrity.host.html/content/authoritative/policy/institutional-coi-human-subjects.detail.html. Accessed February 1, 2021.

39. Conflicts of interest and transparency initiatives. Association of American Medical Colleges Medical Research. https://www.aamc.org/what-we-do/mission-areas/medical-research/conflicts-of-interest. Accessed February 1, 2021.

40. Conflicts of interest. Association of American Universities Key Issues. https://www.aau.edu/issues/conflicts-interest. Accessed February 1, 2021.

41. Conflict of interest. Council on Governmental Relations. https://www.cogr.edu/ConflictofInterest. Accessed February 1, 2021.

42. Woo SL. Policy of the American Society of Gene Therapy on financial conflict of interest in clinical research. *Mol Ther*. 2000;1(5 Pt 1):383–384.

43. 45 CFR § 46.107(d) (2020).

44. 21 CFR § 56.107(e) (2020).

45. Senators Warren, Brown, and Sanders Call for the government watchdog to investigate for-profit institutional review boards (IRBs). Elizabeth Warren. Published June 18, 2020. https://www.warren.senate.gov/oversight/letters/senators-warren-brown-and-sanders-call-for-the-government-watchdog-to-investigate-for-profit-institutional-review-boards-irbs. Accessed February 1, 2021.

46. Bayh-Dole Act: landmark law helped universities lead the way. AUTM. Accessed February 1, 2021. https://autm.net/about-tech-transfer/advocacy/legislation/bayh-dole-act.

47. Engelberg AB, Kesselheim AS. Use the Bayh-Dole Act to lower drug prices for government healthcare programs. *Nat Med*. 2016;22(6):576.

48. 45 CFR § 94 (2020).

49. Resnik DB, Ariansen JL, Jamal J, Kissling GE. Institutional conflict of interest policies at U.S. academic research institutions. *Acad Med*. 2016;91(2):242–246.

50. National Science Foundation Office of Budget Finance and Award Management. National Science Foundation Grant Policy Manual NSF 05-131: Chapter V – grantee standards, 510 conflicts of interest policies. National Science Foundation. Published July 2005. https://www.nsf.gov/pubs/manuals/gpm05_131/gpm5.jsp#510. Accessed February 1, 2021.

51. 48 CFR § 9.5 (2020).

52. Complaint, *Berman v The Fred Hutchinson Cancer Research Center, et al*, WD Wash, (May 2001), No. C01-5217 RSL.

53. Price EA, Lemons JA. Clinical trials: protecting the subject, avoiding liability, and managing risk. *Health Law Digest*. 2002;30(1):3–13.

54. Goldner JA. Dealing with conflicts of interest in biomedical research: IRB oversight as the next best solution to the abolitionist approach. *J Law Med Ethics*. 2000;28(4):379–404.

55. Icenogle DL. IRBs, conflict and liability: will we see IRBs in court? Or is it when? *Clin Med Res*. 2003;1(1):63–68.

56. 21 CFR § 312.3(b) (2020).

57. Investigator responsibilities: protecting the rights, safety, and welfare of study subjects. US Food and Drug Administration. 2009. https://www.fda.gov/regulatory-information/search-fda-guidance-documents/investigator-responsibilities-protecting-rights-safety-and-welfare-study-subjects. Accessed August 22, 2021.

58. Dembner A. Lawsuits target medical research. *IRB*. 2002;24(4):14–15.

59. Rozovsky FA, Adams RK. *Clinical Trials and Human Research: A Practical Guide to Regulatory Compliance*. San Francisco, CA: Jossey-Bass; 2003.

60. BIMO inspection metrics: FY'19. US Food and Drug Administration. Published April 8, 2020. https://www.fda.gov/science-research/clinical-trials-and-human-subject-protection/bimo-inspection-metrics. Accessed February 1, 2021.

61. 42 CFR § 93.103 (2020).

62. *Fei Wang v Board of Trustees of University of Illinois*, No. 18-cv-07522 2020, WL 1503651 (ND Ill 2020).

63. *Helm v Ratterman*, No. 3:16-CV-00771-TBR, 2017 WL 2800865 (WD Ky 2017).

64. *Bois v United State Department of Health and Human Services*, No. 11-1563 (ABJ), 2012 WL 13042904 (DDC 2012).

65. 42 CFR § 93.304 (2020).

66. 42 CFR § 93.106 (2020).

67. 42 CFR § 93.104 (2020).

68. 42 CFR § 93.309 (2020).

69. 42 CFR § 93.318 (2020).
70. Woollen SW. Misconduct in research: innocent ignorance or malicious malfeasance? US Food and Drug Administration Media. https://www.fda.gov/media/75682/download. Accessed February 1, 2021.
71. Clinical investigations compliance and enforcement. US Food and Drug Administration Clinical Trials and Human Subject Protection. Published March 30, 2018. https://www.fda.gov/science-research/clinical-trials-and-human-subject-protection/clinical-investigations-compliance-enforcement. Accessed February 1, 2021.
72. Barrett J. Clinical research fraud. *Res Ethics*. 2006;2(4):136–139.
73. Gupta A. Fraud and misconduct in clinical research: a concern. *Perspect Clin Res*. 2013;4(2):144–147.
74. Jessen J, Robinson E, Bigaj S, Popiolek S, Goldfarb NM. Unreported clinical research fraud and misconduct. *J Clin Res Best Pract*. 2007;3(1):1–5.
75. Sheehan JG. Fraud, conflict of interest, and other enforcement issues in clinical research. *Cleve Clin J Med*. 2007;74(suppl 2):S63–S69.
76. Kim WO. Institutional review board (IRB) and ethical issues in clinical research. *Korean J Anesthesiol*. 2012;62(1):3–12.
77. *Hyman v Jewish Chronic Disease Hospital*, 251 NYS2d 818 (NYApp2 Dept. 1964); rev'd, *Hyman v Jewish Chronic Disease Hospital*, 206 NE2d 338 (NY 1965).
78. *Heinrich v Sweet*, 44 F8upp2d 408 (D Mass 1999) (Heinrich I); *Heinrich v Sweet*, 49 F8upp2d 27 (D Mass 1999) (Heinrich II); *Heinrich ex rel Heinrich v Sweet*, 62 FSupp2d 282 (D Mass 1999) (Heinrich III).
79. *Butler v Juno Therapeutics, Inc.*, No. H-18-898, 2019 WL 2568477 (SD Tex, June 21, 2019).
80. Fraud and deceit: what are they and how do you prove it. Law Offices of Stimmel, Stimmel & Roeser. https://www.stimmel-law.com/en/articles/fraud-and-deceit-what-are-they-and-how-do-you-prove-it. Accessed February 1, 2021.
81. *Franklin Theatre Corp v City of Minneapolis*, 198 NW2d 558, 560 (Minn 1972) (quoting *Rien v Cooper*, 1 NW2d 847, 851 [Minn 1942]).
82. IND exemptions for studies of lawfully marketed drug or biological products for the treatment of cancer. US Food and Drug Administration. 2004. https://www.fda.gov/regulatory-information/search-fda-guidance-documents/ind-exemptions-studies-lawfully-marketed-drug-or-biological-products-treatment-cancer. Accessed August 22, 2021.
83. National Center for Complementary and Integrative Health Clinical research toolbox. National Center for Complementary and Integrative Health Grants and Funding. https://www.nccih.nih.gov/grants/toolbox. Accessed February 1, 2021.
84. Wilson JM. Lessons learned from the gene therapy trial for ornithine transcarbamylase deficiency. *Mol Genet Metab*. 2009;96(4):151–157.

CHAPTER 21

Artificial Intelligence

Junying Zhao, PhD, PhD, MPH, MBBS and Glen Cheng, MD, JD, MPH

INTRODUCTION

Artificial intelligence (AI) tools in medicine are rapidly advancing in technical ability and are increasingly being relied on by physicians to guide clinical decisions. In this chapter, we provide an overview of AI tools in oncology, with several examples of state-of-the-art diagnostic and therapeutic tools. We follow this overview with a discussion of legal liability for both AI manufacturers and physicians when AI tools are used in the course of patient care. Next, we discuss ethical implications of AI algorithm design and use in clinical care. We end with a discussion of how AI tools promise to shift financial risk for various health care stakeholders.

ARTIFICIAL INTELLIGENCE IN ONCOLOGY

Oncology is a branch of medicine that focuses on the prevention, diagnosis, and treatment of tumors. Oncologists traditionally work with radiologists and pathologists and manually read images and clinical notes, a process that is susceptible to individual subjectivity resulting in delay and diagnostic irreproducibility. In contrast, AI takes advantage of big data, automates classification and prediction, and thus provides early detections that may be invisible to the human eye and treatment recommendations that incorporate the vast volume of medical literature and comply with up-to-date guidelines.

AI is the branch of computer science concerned with the automation of intelligent behavior. It refers to intelligent machines (computer algorithms and robots) that think or act rationally or human-like.[1] In fact, AI has evolved from being mathematical logic based during the 1960s to 1990s to statistical learning based (machine learning [ML]) since the 1990s and has advanced since 2012 with new methods such as deep learning (DL).[2,3]

The mechanism of AI is a function, mapping from an object to a class to which the object belongs. This process can be visualized as a machine whose input can be an image of an object (e.g., magnetic resonance imaging [MRI] scan of brain tumor) and whose output is the classification of that object (e.g., a predicted label of the tumor as cancerous or not). The machine works through three main steps: First, extract and refine features of the input. Second, select a classifier (e.g., decision tree, naive Bayes, maximum entropy, hidden Markov model) that analyzes those features and produces the class/label to which the input belongs. Third, evaluate the performance of the classifier.[4] Based on the one-layer mapping described earlier, DL adds additional layers of mapping—artificial neural networks (ANNs)—to achieve better performance.

Input consists of two types: (1) structured data in electronic health records (EHRs) that are entered into drop-down boxes and point-and-click fields, and (2) unstructured data in narrative forms in clinical notes such as written case reports taken from consultations.[5] Depending on the type of input, AI has different areas including, but not limited to, (1) image recognition that processes and classifies pictures, (2) natural language processing (NLP) that works on texts, and (3) speech recognition that classifies voices.

There are four significant types of ML models. In supervised learning, the true label of the training data is compared with the predicted label. One can count true positives (TPs), true negatives (TNs), false positives (FPs), and false negatives (FNs); using these measures, one can calculate various performance measures, such as accuracy [accuracy = (TP + TN)/(TP + TN + FP + FN)].[6] In contrast, in unsupervised learning, the training data provide no true labels, and the algorithm extracts features and recognizes patterns on its own. Semi-supervised learning takes a middle ground; the classification learned from a small amount of labeled data is extrapolated to a larger set of unlabeled data. Alternatively, reinforcement learning modifies an algorithm with a reward system, providing positive feedback when a classifier performs best in a particular situation.[7,8]

In medicine, in general, AI has been applied to expert systems for imaging and clinical decision support since the 1980s.[9] AI has also been quickly adopted in EHRs and mobile health technology (mHealth) with the help of the Internet since 1995 and smartphones since 2002. Both EHRs and mHealth have demonstrated great potential to collect and analyze personal health data for clinical medicine and public health.[10] By 2017, the health care AI industry had more than 100 startups, more than half of which raised funding from third-party investors.[5] In 2019, medical AI was defined by the US Food and Drug Administration (FDA) as a medical device and by the American Medical Association (AMA) as augmented intelligence.[11,12]

In oncology, in particular, AI has affected imaging processing and NLP. In the next two sections, we discuss how imaging recognition has been applied to perform cancer detection and characterization. We further address how image recognition and NLP have been employed in cancer drug development and treatment recommendations.

Diagnostic and screening tools

The main task in oncology is abnormality detection. Traditional conventions require radiologists and pathologists to manually read images, a process that is susceptible to individual subjectivity and delay. In contrast, AI automates the classification process and provides early and sensitive detection of cancer.

Detection refers to the localization of objects of interest in radiographs; computer-aided detection (CADe) can be used to reduce omission errors. Characterization consists of segmentation, diagnosis, and staging of tumors. Segmentation defines the extent of an abnormality. Because the subsequent diagnosis of a benign or malignant tumor can be susceptible to the subjective, qualitative experience of radiologists and oncologists, it can be enhanced by computer-aided diagnosis (CADx). Moreover, AI-based monitoring of tumor development promises to provide many features in addition to predefined metrics such as the longest diameter of a tumor.[13] Various types of input include texts and images (e.g., x-rays and ultrasound, MRI, and computed tomography [CT] scan images).

In addition to individual patients, AI can also be applied to the population for cancer screening. Peer-reviewed publications in this area soared from approximately 100 in 2005 to nearly 1000 in 2017, which signals that AI can be further leveraged as a powerful tool to detect cancer, improve diagnosis, and monitor treatment, thus improving prognosis and saving lives.

Specific AI applications to the detection and diagnosis of three types of tumors—breast cancer, lung cancer, and brain cancer—are discussed here.

AI has been recently used for screening mammography in communities in the United Kingdom and the United States to predict risks of breast cancer. The top three AI models have been identified and ranked in terms of accuracy: unsupervised homogeneous fuzzy logic inference applied to mammogram data obtained 99.73% accuracy[14]; support vector machines (SVMs) used on Wisconsin Breast Cancer data obtained 99.51% accuracy[15]; and supervised backpropagation neural network (BPNN) used on ultrasound images generated 99.28% accuracy.[16]

Lung cancer has a dramatically high death rate and is often advanced and widespread by the time it is diagnosed. Therefore, it is crucial for AI to improve its early detection and characterization by differentiating benign from malignant nodules. Ada[17] applied the supervised BPNN to CT scan images and achieved 96.04% accuracy. Similarly, using CT scan images, Tariq et al.[18] employed an unsupervised model, adaptive neuro fuzzy inference system (ANFIS), and obtained 95% accuracy.[18] Kanakatte et al.[19] applied SVM to positron emission tomography (PET) images and obtained 97% accuracy.

Brain tumors include gliomas and meningiomas, as well as metastatic brain tumors. Sapra et al. applied the supervised probabilistic neural network (PNN) to MRI images and produced 100% accuracy.[20] Similarly, Al-Naami et al. used another supervised learning model (nonlinear autoregressive with exogenous neural networks [NARXNNs]) on MRI images and generated 99.1% accuracy.[21] Sharma employed an unsupervised ANFIS gradient descent and backpropagation algorithm to MRI images and obtained 98.67% accuracy.[22]

Therapeutic tools

Both of the subfields of ML—image recognition and NLP—have been applied to cancer therapy development, prediction of response to therapy, and recommendation of treatment plans.[23,24] Take the IBM Watson Health as an example; it is an AI system commercialized in genomics, drug development, and oncology. It can read 800 million pages per second, drawing content from sources such as PubMed, the Sanger Institute's Catalogue of Somatic Mutations in Cancer database, the National Cancer Institute's Drug Dictionary, and studies registered on ClinicalTrials.gov.[5]

Image recognition AI models have been accelerating drug discovery and achieving drug synergy for cancer treatment using genomic and chemical data. First, AI can be used to train algorithms to achieve a desired three-dimensional molecular structure in weeks, much shorter than the traditional timelines of approximately one year.[25] For example, a study trained the generative tensorial reinforcement learning (GENTRL) algorithm using data of chemical structures that target the tyrosine kinase discoidin domain receptor 1 (DDR1), which is involved in various cancers. Algorithms then run simulations to predict lead compound and receptor binding, maximizing the targeting of DDR1 while minimizing the targeting of other tyrosine kinases receptors.[26] Second, a cancer patient often has a genomic profile, including multiple molecular aberrations. Thus, drug combination therapy can help address multiple drug targets, improving treatment efficacy. However, testing all possible drug combinations at multiple doses for each drug is impossible and may result in unforeseen toxicity. Thus, AI can be used to optimize combination design, simultaneously identifying the best drugs and doses for combination while minimizing toxicity.[25] For example, a study experimentally determined the cytotoxicity of antitumor drugs alone and in combination on cell lines.[27] The study then trained ANNs with backpropagation on these experimental results and predicted the cytotoxicity of 60 combinations of antitumor drugs, which markedly reduced the number of experiments needed to evaluate the cytotoxicity of all possible combinations in the range of chosen doses.[28]

Image recognition AI models can also help predict patients' responses to radiotherapy, chemotherapy, and immunotherapy. Based on significant features of images of patients with cancer, AI models have been developed to identify patients who will show a pathologic complete response at the end of treatment and those who will not respond to therapy at an early stage of the treatment. For example, a study examined 55 patients with locally advanced rectal cancer who underwent 3-tesla MRI, acquiring T2-weighted images before, during, and after neoadjuvant chemoradiotherapy. In the study, AI models were built by training a random forest classifier, and model performances were estimated using a receiver operating characteristic (ROC) curve and a decision curve analysis. The AI models showed good discrimination power with mean areas under the ROC curve (AUC) of 0.86 for the complete response classification and 0.83 for the no response classification. Decision curve analysis confirmed higher net patient benefit when using AI models.[29] Similarly, AI models applied to CT scans and circulating biomarkers were reported to predict patients' response to radiotherapy and immunotherapy.[30,31]

Furthermore, NLP AI models are applied to text data for clinical decision support systems, especially cancer treatment recommendations. For example, IBM Watson for Oncology was launched in 2012 and primarily uses NLP to learn both the structured and unstructured text (e.g., clinical notes) data in the EHR of cancer patients and search the databases of vast medical literature on cancer in order to provide cancer treatment options ranked in three categories: recommended, for consideration, and not recommended.[5] Specifically, key phrases about diagnosis, symptoms, and so on, extracted from the health records of a patient will be searched and matched with similar key phrases in databases of official clinical guidelines and the outcomes of published medical literature, which triggers the closely related treatment phrases in these databases and the probability of the relevance of each treatment, based on which the "evidence-based" treatment options are produced and ranked.[32]

As a therapeutic decision support system, Watson for Oncology is expected to feature strengths such as its storage of the vast up-to-date medical literature that is published every day and that is beyond human memory and its computing power, which examines hundreds of variables in these records (e.g., demographics, tumor characteristics, treatments, and outcomes) and discovers patterns invisible to or treatments not thought of by human physicians.

Studies have compared Watson for Oncology's treatment recommendations to those of human oncologists and have found mixed results. In these studies, the concordance percentages indicate how often the advice of Watson matches that of human oncologists. For example, a study at Memorial Sloan Kettering Cancer Center examined 362 total cancer cases consisting of 112 lung, 126 colon, and 124 rectal cancers and found Watson concordance in 96.4% of lung, 81.0% of colon, and 92.7% of rectal cancer cases.[33] Three independent studies in China, with more than 300 patients each, reported that the concordance rates were 77% for patients with breast cancer and 72.8% for those with cervical cancer.[34,35] A study in India evaluated Watson on 638 breast cancer patients and found a 73% concordance rate.[36] Another study in South Korea found Watson's top recommendations for 656 colon cancer patients matched those of the experts only 49% of the time.[36] Factors that affect concordance rates include, but are not limited to, tumor stage, metastatic status, patient age, surgical preference, absence of neoadjuvant/adjuvant chemotherapy, reimbursement plan of an antitumor drug, and substitution of a particular drug for another.[35]

Moreover, Watson for Oncology performs poorly when the data are time dependent (e.g., therapy timelines) or written down ambiguously (e.g., acronyms). One study at the University of Texas M.D. Anderson Cancer Center applied Watson to approximately 1000 patient EHRs and a Medline database of more than 23 million published abstracts. In the study, NLP was trained to summarize patients' cancer history, based on which NLP recommended approved therapy in the medical literature and screened for eligible clinical trials on ClinicalTrials.gov. Although NLP did well in extracting static terms (e.g., diagnosis) from patient history documents with F1 scores of 90% to 96%, it performed poorly for time-dependent concepts (e.g., therapy history timeline) with F1 scores of only 63% to 65%, which did not succeed in constructing dynamic patient profiles.[37] In another pilot study for leukemia at M.D. Anderson, Watson could not interpret certain words or acronyms that have alternative meanings in different contexts. For instance, *ALL* is often the shorthand for *allergy* but is also the acronym for *acute lymphoblastic leukemia*. To correctly interpret *ALL* in a clinical scene requires the Watson NLP to take in additional words in the contextual environment of the target word *ALL*. If the neighboring context includes high white blood cell counts or bone marrow, *ALL* more likely means leukemia rather than an allergy.

To date, studies have examined whether therapeutic AI tools can perform as well as human oncologists. However, few studies on cancer decision support tools have demonstrated sufficient value in improving outcomes or saving costs, based on which a hospital can justify the financial investment.

LIABILITY

Physician liability when using AI tools for diagnosis or treatment

AI tools that assist in diagnosis or treatment recommendations have been heralded as the stethoscope of the 21st century, helping human physicians to achieve optimal health outcomes for patients. Indeed, AI can serve many roles in the course of medical care, from patient education to medical management. Here, AI used to assist in patient diagnosis or treatment is discussed and the following question is addressed: Who is liable when an AI diagnostic or treatment recommendation leads to patient harm? A brief discussion regarding the conceptualization of the AI system and its implications for manufacturer liability is in order, followed by a treatment on liability for the treating physician.

The role of the AI system and implications for product liability

Several analogies have been made to conceptualize the relationship between a physician, a patient, and a consulted AI system. AI can be viewed as a product or, alternatively, as a consultant, yet neither analogy fits perfectly. The AI-as-product analogy downplays the significant analysis and recommendations that the AI tool provides to the treating physician. For example, a chest x-ray CADe algorithm can provide significant guidance to the physician regarding a number of cardiovascular and pulmonary conditions, and in this sense, it is not simply relaying data but rather highlighting likely clinical diagnoses much in the way a physician consultant would. On the other hand, the AI-as-consultant analogy risks anthropomorphizing inert preprogrammed algorithms, virtually all of which disclaim liability for rendering medical judgment on diagnoses or treatments. Given the difficulties in conforming AI manufacturer liability to traditional legal theories of negligence or product liability, some scholars have proposed legislation creating so-called "enterprise liability" for AI systems, wherein both the provider and the manufacturer bear joint and several liability as a group for the damages resulting from medical errors.[1] These yet-unsettled theories have different liability implications for both AI manufacturers and treating physician using AI tools.

If the AI tool is a product, then product liability would attach to the AI manufacturer on a showing that the product is defective. Please refer to Chapter 27 on product liability for full discussion of manufacturer liability for defective products. If the manufacturer were found liable for designing a defective AI product, this finding could reduce the treating physician's liability because the AI manufacturer would be at least jointly or severally liable for the harm to the patient. However, depending on the level of AI automation,[2] the physician would still be liable for any negligence in using the AI product or failing to substitute medical judgment for an erroneous AI recommendation.

Alternatively, the AI tool could be viewed as a consultant, taking the role of a physician consulted for advice on diagnosis or treatment by the treating physician. This theory potentially avoids a product liability cause of action and exposes the physician to greater liability, since the AI tool would merely supplement rather than replace the physician's judgment. When consulting an AI tool for medical information, the treating physician would retain responsibility for the care of the patient and all diagnostic and therapeutic decisions. Moreover, the conceptualization

---

[1] See David C. Vladeck, Machines without Principles: Liability Rules and Artificial Intelligence, 89 WASH. L. REV. 117, 150 (2014)
[2] See discussion in the following section on financial risk.

of AI as a consultant potentially reduces the AI manufacturer's liability under a tort theory of negligence. This is because negligence requires the plaintiff to demonstrate a physician-patient relationship with a consulted physician, and in the absence of that relationship, the consulted physician does not owe a duty of care to the patient.[38] Courts have in some cases declined to find that a physician-patient relationship exists where the consulted physician did not see the patient.[39,40] In the case of an AI system consulted by the treating physician, there is no direct physician-patient relationship between the AI and the patient. Thus, plaintiffs may be left to pursue negligence claims solely against the treating physician.

AI tools and liability for the treating physician

Independent of whether a plaintiff sues an AI manufacturer on a product liability theory, the plaintiff may choose to pursue a medical malpractice negligence claim against the treating physician. To prevail in a medical malpractice case, the plaintiff needs to establish each element of the negligence claim: duty, breach of duty, causation, and harm.

Regarding duty, a plaintiff in a medical malpractice action must first establish the existence of a provider-patient relationship.[38,41] If this relationship exists, the health care provider then owes a duty of care to the patient.

To demonstrate breach of duty, the plaintiff must show that a medical provider breached the standard of medical care by failing to act as a reasonably prudent physician.[35] To establish that a physician consulting an AI system breached his or her duty of care, a key question is whether consulting and following the recommendation of an AI system fall within the standard of medical care. A review of the case law performed for this chapter (as of July 2020) did not reveal any published judicial opinions involving medical malpractice claims where AI tools were consulted in diagnosis or treatment. Given this uncertainty, physicians can reduce their liability exposure by obtaining patients' informed consent to consult an AI system for assistance in medical care, including diagnosis and treatment. Legal commentators have also noted that the medical malpractice standard promotes conservative care, because providing care that deviates from the standard of care renders a physician vulnerable to liability. The medical malpractice negligence standard thus incentivizes physicians to ignore AI recommendations when those recommendations conflict with the existing standard of care, even if such AI recommendations would provide an improvement in patient outcomes over the existing standard of care. To protect themselves from medical malpractice suits, therefore, physicians should carefully evaluate AI diagnostic or treatment recommendations when those recommendations conflict with the current standard of care. AI systems capable of both identifying the current standard of care and explaining why a proposed course of treatment conforms to or deviates from that standard of care thus provide a clear benefit to the physician.

To establish causation, a plaintiff must demonstrate that the physician caused the claimed injury. Causation becomes more complicated when a treating physician consults an AI system and adopts the AI recommendation for treatment. In such cases, the patient or physician may make a claim for product liability against the AI developer, which could bring a third party into the lawsuit. The AI manufacturer could then be liable for a portion of the damages resulting from the harm to the patient. Note that physicians are generally protected from product liability suits, because physicians are providing a service using the AI system rather than selling the AI system. The physician is, however, responsible for exercising due care in broader patient management and care decisions. Thus, it is important that physicians recognize when AI recommendations deviate from the standard of care because physicians retain responsibility for managing patients' care.

To demonstrate harm, the plaintiff must show that they suffered a different or worse outcome than they would have had the standard of care not been breached. Accordingly, if a physician is convinced that an AI diagnostic or treatment recommendation will result in an improvement in an optimal patient outcome, the physician should follow the AI recommendation. However, following a course of action recommended by an AI system might result in a different harm than would result under the standard of care. For example, an AI recommendation for chemotherapy could result in chemotherapy side effects (despite overall improved survival), whereas a standard of care wait-and-see approach could result in avoidance of chemotherapy side effects albeit with a lower survival rate. Therefore, clinicians should fully disclose all benefits and risks when recommending courses of action to patients.

Best practices for physicians using AI tools

This discussion brings us back to a foundational principle of good medical practice—autonomy, which involves patients in their own care. Informed consent enables patient autonomy by informing patients of the different options available, including the risks and benefits of each option.[42] Studies have shown that patients who are informed and who choose their own course of action experience better outcomes than patients who are told which course of action to follow. By involving patients in each step of the treatment journey, physicians allow patients to weigh their own values and choose the course of action in line with their desired outcomes. This approach is especially important in oncology because outcomes are often uncertain and involve considerable risk. Facilitating patient autonomy in treatment decisions in turn reduces physician liability.

Treating physicians may find it difficult to decide whether to follow an AI recommendation when the two negligence claim elements of breach of duty and harm are in tension. On the one hand, following an AI recommendation that results in an optimal patient outcome could result in an improved patient outcome and avoid harm to the patient. On the other hand, disregarding AI recommendations that conflict with current standards of care protects physicians from claims that the duty of care has been breached. Physicians will inevitably feel more comfortable following AI recommendations, and can more readily explain the course of action to patients, when physicians understand the rationale behind the AI recommendation. Therefore, we recommend that AI developers build explanations into their tools regarding how the AI recommendation comports with the current standard of care and, if the AI recommendation conflicts with the current standard of care, why the AI recommendation is expected to result in a more optimal outcome compared to the current standard of care.

Ultimately, the decision whether to use an AI system as an aid in diagnosis or treatment is an individual professional choice, much as it is a driver's decision regarding whether to use self-driving tools when operating a vehicle. AI systems that guide physicians to the current standard of care will have high value, particularly if they explain how their recommendation conforms with the current standard of care. Physicians are, however, potentially exposed to greater liability when relying on AI recommendations that deviate from the standard of care, especially when physicians unilaterally pursue novel treatment regimens without close patient involvement. Finally, because diagnostic or treatment-recommending AI tools may eventually become standard of care, practitioners would do well to begin familiarizing themselves with such tools sooner rather than later.

Oncology case examples

In this section, two previously litigated oncology malpractice cases, based on failure to diagnose and failure to treat, are discussed. These actual cases are followed by a hypothetical case examining physician liability when choosing whether to follow an AI treatment recommendation that deviates from the current standard of care.

CASE LAW # 1

Decedent's wife brought a medical malpractice action on behalf of her deceased husband, Robert Salazar, alleging negligent failure to diagnose lung cancer based on chest x-rays, resulting in a 10-month delay in diagnosis.[43] The court decided for the plaintiff, finding that the patient likely had stage I lung cancer at the time of the initial x-ray scan and that the physician negligently failed to diagnose the cancer. Testimony at trial revealed that the decedent "was in pretty good shape . . . for a 75-year old man." The court credited expert witness testimony that the patient's survival rate was 48% at the time of the initial scan and that he would have "had a reasonable chance of cure." The court held that the 10-month delay in diagnosing the patient's lung cancer was "a substantial factor" in causing the patient's death and that, absent the delay, the patient "would have had a chance at a better outcome."[43]

CASE LAW # 2

Decedent's son brought a medical malpractice action on behalf of his mother, Lula Rowsey, who was falsely diagnosed and treated for terminal lung cancer that she did not have. The patient died three years later from a heart attack.[44] A pathologist diagnosed the patient with squamous cell lung cancer based on cytology, and an oncologist-initiated chemotherapy. The court found neither the pathologist nor the oncologist liable for medical malpractice. The court, however, held that the patient's family physician breached the standard of care by failing to reevaluate and correct the improper diagnosis after the family physician took over care from the oncologist. The family physician considered the patient to have terminal squamous cell lung cancer, changed the chemotherapeutic agent, failed to consult with any oncologist during the course of the patient's treatment, and failed to reevaluate the diagnosis of lung cancer with serial chest x-rays every two months. The family physician continued chemotherapy for three years, at which point the patient died of a heart attack. An autopsy found no sign of cancer. The court found that the diagnosis of terminal squamous cell lung cancer could have been corrected at the six-month mark because most patients would have been expected to live six months to one year and chemotherapy is not expected to be curative for terminal lung cancer.

CLINICAL VIGNETTE # 1

S am is a 53-year-old woman who presents to her physician with burning and a feeling of heaviness in her right breast, accompanied by fatigue and a 10-lb weight loss in the past three months. Physical exam reveals a 1.5-cm round mass in her right breast and tenderness of the nipple. Mammogram reveals a 1.5 × 1 cm mass in her right breast, and biopsy confirms the diagnosis of invasive ductal carcinoma that is estrogen and progesterone receptor negative and HER2/neu positive. Sam's physician consults AI software to determine the risk of systemic recurrence for breast cancer and to obtain a treatment recommendation (see, e.g., Oncotype Dx, https://www.oncotypeiq.com/en-US/breast-cancer/healthcare-professionals/oncotype-dx-breast-recurrence-score/about-the-test). The AI software classifies the invasive ductal carcinoma as moderate risk and, based on a recent randomized controlled trial, recommends trastuzumab (Herceptin)–based chemotherapy and avoidance of surgery and radiation therapy if Sam has a complete clinical and imaging response to chemotherapy. Sam's physician is surprised by this recommendation for chemotherapy alone since the standard of care treatment would be chemotherapy along with breast-conserving surgery and adjuvant radiation therapy. However, the AI predicts that, given Sam's specific patient profile, chemotherapy alone will result in reduced side effects, reduced likelihood of disability, and equivalent five-year survival rate compared to the standard of care.

What liability is Sam's physician exposed to if he follows the AI's treatment recommendation for chemotherapy alone versus if he follows the standard of care and recommends breast-conserving surgery along with chemotherapy and adjuvant radiation therapy?

Medical malpractice liability hinges on whether a physician breaches the duty of care owed to his or her patient. Here, the AI recommends an avant-garde treatment regimen that deviates from the current standard of care but promises to provide an improved outcome, namely, reduced side effects and reduced likelihood of disability, and an equivalent five-year survival rate. The AI prediction for an improved patient outcome is based on precision personalized oncology algorithms that run sto-chastic modeling, taking account of Sam's individual patient characteristics in light of large popula-tion data sets.

A safe route would be for Sam's physician to follow the standard of care, rejecting the contrary AI recommendation. This course of action is safe because Sam's physician is not a guarantor of patient outcomes. Instead, Sam's physician is only legally required to exercise his duty of care owed to the patient, which Sam's physician satisfies by providing medical care consistent with the standard of care. While this route is arguably safe for the time being, it is subject to change if consulting and relying on AI recommendations become standard of care.

If Sam's physician follows the AI recommendation to provide chemotherapy only, rather than the standard of care chemotherapy plus local surgery and adjuvant radiation, three outcomes are gen-erally possible. If Sam takes chemotherapy only, she could fare better than, the same as, or worse than the outcome she would have had under the standard of care. It is only this last possibility—if Sam suffers a worse outcome under the AI recommendation to deviate from standard of care—that could lead Sam's physician to face liability. This is because if Sam faces a better outcome or the same outcome under the AI recommendation, Sam will not be able to demonstrate that she suffered harm relative to the standard of care.

If Sam suffers a worse outcome under the AI recommendation for chemotherapy only, Sam could potentially sue the AI manufacturer under a product liability theory. This could be accomplished if either Sam or Sam's physician joined the AI manufacturer as a party to the medical negligence suit. Such a maneuver could potentially reduce Sam's physician's liability if a portion of the damages were assigned to the AI manufacturer. However, for the AI manufacturer to be liable in such a case, the plaintiff or co-defendant would need to show that the AI system was defective under product liability law.

A reductionistic discussion of legal liability would be incomplete if it failed to account for the patient's preferences. Indeed, a patient may be more likely to sue if she feels denied the opportunity for agency and self-determination, even if the treatment she received resulted in an improved out-come relative to what she would have chosen. Here, Sam's physician would do well to present Sam with the different treatment options, detailing the risks and benefits of each approach, and to allow Sam to select the treatment she wishes to receive.

FINANCIAL RISK

To err is human, but machines make mistakes, too. AI application to medicine in general, and to oncology in particular, is currently at the early stages of research and development. There has been neither a hospital incidence report nor an insurance claim or lawsuit for the commercial implementation of AI in medicine.

However, there have been AI-related injuries in other industries such as the automotive industry. There are five levels of automated driving, of which levels four to five do not require the passenger's attention and thus are considered autonomous driving. A level three conditionally automated car needs a driver who is not required to monitor the environment but is ready to take control of the vehicle at all times with notice. A level two partially automated car requires a driver to engage in driving tasks and monitor the environment at all times.[45] As of 2019, there have been five confirmed level two fatalities, of which four driver fatalities involved Tesla Autopilot and one pedestrian fatality involved an Uber experimental robotaxi. The crash rate of level two automated cars is estimated to be 5% of the crash rate of traditional human-controlled vehicles.[46] Car crashes kill more than 30,000 people per year in the United States, and 94% of these crashes are caused by human errors.[47]

Once lower-level automated cars are advanced to higher-level autonomous cars and networked on public roads, the finance industry estimates that there will be at least an 80% reduction in crash rate and a 60% decrease in cash flow of the auto insurance premium. Cheap car insurance may be offered by car manufacturers at the time of purchase. Real-time dynamic insurance may also be possible once the stream data of networked autonomous cars become available.[46]

Implications of medical AI for insurance

Similar to the autonomous car, AI in medicine faces safety issues, legal uncertainties, and financial risks. Admittedly, an autonomous car is a product for individual customers/drivers, whereas medical AI can be a product for not only individual consumers (e.g., who buy skin cancer detection on their smartphones) but also health care service providers (e.g., IBM Watson for oncologists) at the individual level (e.g., a visit to an oncologist) and at the aggregate level (e.g., Memorial Sloan Kettering Cancer Center). Therefore, financial responsibilities will vary accordingly.

When individual consumers use medical AI for consultation without human physicians, the liability pertains solely to the product. For example, an app falsely predicts that a consumer's mole is not a melanoma, which delays the diagnosis and treatment, causing extended absenteeism from work and hospital stay and thus greater loss of income and higher costs of health care. In such a situation, compensation should be covered by software developers under the product liability law.

When medical AI is used by health care service providers, compensation for patient injuries will be determined by the proportion of the doctor's liability and product's liability. It is more complex to distinguish between the two types of liability. Here, we propose levels of automation of medical AI from the perspective of health care service providers, similar to the levels of the autonomous car.[48]

In addition to private liability insurance, public insurance may be designed in the future. For autonomous cars, some legal theorists recommend creating a national insurance fund to pay for all damages resulting from accidents.[49] Similarly, in medicine, a typical public insurance is the state-run vaccination fund. However, both products—autonomous cars and vaccines—justify public insurance because the utilization of both has externalities. In contrast, applying AI to individual diseases (with the exception of some conditions such as infectious diseases) does not typically have externalities and thus may not have a strong justification for public liability insurance.

Level 1: physician assistance—AI acts as a physician assistant. Human physicians make conclusions regarding tumor detection, diagnosis, and treatment. AI may offer some predictions as suggestions when consulted.

Level 2: partial automation—Automatic functions are combined with physicians' practice (eg, all medical images or clinical notes are automatically read and classified by AI). Physicians remain engaged in detecting, diagnosing, and treating cancer patients; checking concordance with AI predictions; and monitoring the AI system's overall workflow at all times. Human physicians make all ultimate professional decisions.

Level 3: conditional automation—Human physicians need to be present but are not required to check the concordance of AI predictions all the time; they remain available to intervene in tasks of detecting, diagnosing, and treating patients if necessary.

Level 4: high automation—AI performs all tasks of detecting, diagnosing, and treating patients under certain conditions.

Level 5: full automation—AI is capable of performing all tasks under all conditions.

In extreme scenarios like levels four and five, for any harm done to patients, such as the sudden death of a patient during surgical removal of tumor caused by failure to predict venous thrombosis, liability should be assumed by software developers. If the patient died as a result of a surgical robot's broken components, then the liability should be assumed by hardware manufacturers under product liability insurance.

However, product liability insurance has specific issues when applied to medical AI: (1) Should the product liability insurance be compulsory for manufacturers and/or developers? (2) Does the product liability insurance cover poor maintenance of the AI (e.g., failure to upgrade) by the health care service providers? (3) Does the product liability insurance include causes external to the AI?

In scenarios regarding levels one and two, physicians are the ultimate decision makers and gatekeepers of AI, so if harm is done to patients, it is more likely to be covered by medical professional liability insurance.

However, recall that traditional medical liability insurance faced excessive numbers of claims and costly judgments during the 1970s when juries were sympathetic to injured patients. Many medical liability insurance companies went bankrupt to the extent that no insurers remained in some states. If this occurred again, since people tend to have higher expectations for technology than for humans to prevent errors and juries are sympathetic to injured victims, the number of claims and the amount of compensation per claim will likely rise. Thus, professional liability premiums could increase, which would offset the costs saved by a reduction in the number of injuries. The degree of offset is an empirical question depending on the availability of data. This uncertainty motivates physicians and medical centers to mitigate AI-related errors for patient safety, health care quality, and cost containment.

The middle level of medical AI, level three, is the most complicated. When human physicians and AI systems work together, how would fault be partitioned if AI made diagnostic or therapeutic errors but human physicians were inattentive?

For example, if a surgical robot performing intersphincteric resection for a very low rectal cancer accidentally cuts the external anal sphincter, how much should the algorithm of the surgical robot expect the human surgeon to recognize the error and take control? Would it be reasonable for the robot to continue the error? After surgery, if the patient experiences anal incontinence, what proportion of product liability and malpractice liability should the robot and the human surgeon assume, respectively? If one liability insurance covers the injury, should the other liability insurance compensation be automatically waived in order to achieve tort goals of cost containment or deterrence?

Given so many foreseeable legal and financial issues of medical AI at various levels, the US FDA proposed a regulatory framework for medical AI as a medical device.[50] Nevertheless, state legislatures have not addressed medical AI issues to date. Furthermore, the AMA defines AI as augmented intelligence, emphasizing its assistive role to human physicians at level 1.[11]

Legislation and regulation are needed to (1) initially distinguish between levels of automation of medical AI, (2) clarify legal relationships among multiple parties (e.g., AI software developers, hardware manufacturers, EHR vendors, individual consumer/patients, individual health care providers, health care organizations, product liability insurers, and medical professional liability insurers), and (3) identify how liability shifts from one party to another in subrogation claims. Finally, plaintiff personal injury attorneys and medical experts who give testimony in court will need additional skill sets and knowledge regarding the kinds of software defects in automated medical AI systems that cause harm.

ETHICAL IMPLICATIONS

Conflict of principles

AI in medicine imposes ethical and technical challenges in data security, nondiscrimination, consumer privacy, and data interoperability. These problems in health informatics correspond to principles in medical ethics. Data security pertains to digital information safety and *harm* prevention. Unfair predictions from biased input data violate the *justice* principle. Consumer (e.g., patient) privacy and data interoperability fall into the realm of the *autonomy* principle. When conflicting with one another, the principles cause ethical dilemmas.

Consider the following hypothetical case. A patient requests her bypass surgery costs paid by her insurer (e.g., Anthem) and postsurgical electrocardiogram data to be transmitted from her care provider (e.g., Petaluma Health Center in Sonoma County, California) via the EHR patient portal managed by the vendor (e.g., eClinicalWorks) and stored by the cloud computing company (e.g., Amazon) to mHealth apps (e.g., Apple Watch ECG) on the patient's smartphone developed by the software designers (e.g., Apple). In this case, the *autonomy* principle guides clinicians to respond to the patient's request and share her data. The care provider, however, also knows that the payer Anthem was fined $16 million for exposure of patient health information (PHI) of 79 million people after a series of cyberattacks51 and that the vendor eClinicalWorks was fined $132,500 for failure of data breach notification.[52,53] Both may *harm* the current patient's *privacy* and even finance. To share or not to share is the dilemma.

Avoidance of bias

A major goal in medical AI development is to avoid designing systems that perpetuate systemic bias, such as racism, sexism, or ageism, in health care. Although current AI systems do not consciously choose to perpetuate bias, neither are they exceptional. Indeed, AI systems are susceptible of perpetuating precisely because they are designed and trained by humans. AI systems are limited by the data sets on which they are trained.[22] For example, if an AI system is trained on a specific hospital's data set, but that hospital had a history of providing life-sustaining care to White versus Black patients, the AI system could integrate that racial bias into its treatment algorithm for end-of-life care. This bias bears an even greater danger of being perpetuated if the AI system does not explain the rationale behind its recommendations but instead practices "black box" medicine.

One of the highest values that a clinician can offer to a patient is empathy, which includes compassion, patient-centeredness, equity, and trust. Clinicians, who are empowered to protect and promote their patients' health, would do well to be aware of potential biases in AI systems and avoid overreliance on systems that implicitly or explicitly promote bias.

To sum up, the application of AI to medicine, and to oncology in particular, faces technical challenges and also imposes legal, ethical, and financial risks that will require legislation, regulation, and mitigation measures to achieve efficiency, safety, and quality.

CONCLUSION

AI tools show immense promise in improving patient care and, indeed, in eventually becoming standard of care for medical practice. These powerful tools, however, are not without significant risks. The careful clinician will consider the limitations of AI tools and their attendant liability in using these tools to supplement clinical judgment. In addition, wise clinicians will be cognizant of ethical considerations in the design of AI tools and will be aware of limitations when using tools that were trained only on specific patient populations. Finally, health care stakeholders, ranging from hospitals to physician practice groups, payors, medical device companies, and biopharmaceutical companies, will pay close attention as AI tools have the potential to shift financial risk across the large health care ecosystem. While many trends in health care AI have yet to run their course, one thing is clear: AI in health care has come of age and will make its impact known.

KEY POINTS:

- AI takes advantage of big data, automates classification and prediction processes, and hence provides early detection and treatment of cancer that may be invisible to the human eye.
- AI has excelled in cancer diagnosis and screening in the areas of image recognition and processing of structured data. However, AI faces challenges in treatment recommendations in the area of natural language processing of unstructured clinical data.

- Physician liability in using AI diagnostic or therapeutic tools is uncharted territory. There are currently no decided court cases involving medical malpractice claims where AI tools were consulted in diagnosis or treatment.
- Physicians remain ultimately responsible for exercising due care in broader patient management and care decisions, regardless of whether AI tools are consulted.
- To limit medical malpractice liability, physicians should:
  - Carefully evaluate AI diagnostic or treatment recommendations, particularly when those recommendations conflict with the current standard of care.
  - Obtain informed consent from patients when consulting AI tools for recommendations on diagnosis or treatment.
  - Fully disclose all benefits and risks regarding different diagnostic or treatment options.
- By involving patients in each step of the treatment journey, physicians allow patients to select an optimal course of action based on their own values and goals.
- AI developers should build explanations into their tools regarding (1) how the AI recommendation comports with the current standard of care and (2) if the AI recommendation conflicts with the current standard of care, why the AI recommendation will likely result in a more optimal outcome compared to the current standard of care.
- Legal, medical, ethical, and financial implications of medical AI for manufacturers, developers, and insurers need further exploration among stakeholders, patients, medical experts, legal experts, lawmakers, and policymakers.

References:

1. Russel P, Norvig SJ. *Artificial Intelligence: A Modern Approach*. 3rd ed. Upper Saddle River, NJ: Prentice Hall; 2009.
2. Luger GF, Stubblefield WA. AI *Algorithms, Data Structures, and Idioms in Prolog, Lisp, and Java*. 6th ed. Albuquerque, NM: University of New Mexico Press; 2006.
3. Arel I, Rose DC, Karnowski TP. Deep machine learning: a new frontier in artificial intelligence research. *IEEE Comput Intell Mag*. 2010;5(4):13–18.
4. Manning CD, Schütze H. *Foundations of Statistical Natural Language Processing*. Cambridge, MA: MIT Press; 1999.
5. Schmidt C. M.D. Anderson breaks with IBM Watson, raising questions about artificial intelligence in oncology. *J Natl Cancer Inst*. 2014;109(5):4–5.
6. Bishop CM. *Pattern Recognition and Machine Learning*. New York, NY: Springer; 2006.
7. Hastie T, Tibshirani R, Friedman J. *The Elements of Statistical Learning Data Mining, Inference, and Prediction*. 2nd ed. New York, NY: Springer; 2016.
8. Bramer M, Petridis M. *Research and Development in Intelligent Systems XXXIII: Incorporating Applications and Innovations in Intelligent Systems XXIV*. New York, NY: Springer; 2016.
9. Buch VH, Ahmed I, Maruthappu M. Artificial intelligence in medicine: current trends and future possibilities. *Br J Gen Pract*. 2018;68(668):143–144.
10. Zheng K, Zhao J. Public health informatics. In: Boulton ML, ed. *Maxcy-Rosenau-Last Public Health and Preventive Medicine*. 16th ed. New York, NY: McGraw-Hill Professional Publishing; 2019.
11. Augmented intelligence in medicine. American Medical Association. 2019. https://www.ama-assn.org/amaone/augmented-intelligence-ai. Accessed August 30, 2021.
12. Crigger E, Khoury C. Making policy on augmented intelligence in health care. *AMA J Ethics*. 2019;21(2):e188–e191.
13. Bi WL, Hosny A, Schabath MB, et al. Artificial intelligence in cancer imaging: clinical challenges and applications. *CA Cancer J Clin*. 2019;69(2):127–157.

14. Jain R, Abraham A. A comparative study of fuzzy classification methods on breast cancer data. *Australas Phys Eng Sci Med.* 2004;27:213–218.

15. Ubaidilah SHSA, Sallehuddin R, Ali NA. Cancer detection using artificial neural network and support vector machine: a comparative study. *Jurnal Teknologi.* 2013;65:173–181.

16. Swathi S, Rizwana S, Babu GA, et al. Classification of neural network structures for breast cancer diagnosis. *Int J Comput Sci Appl.* 2012;3(1):227–231.

17. Ada RK. Early detection and prediction of lung cancer survival using neural network classifier. *Int J Innov Technol Manag.* 2013;2:6.

18. Tariq A, Akram MU, Javed MY. Lung nodule detection in CT images using neuro-fuzzy classifier. Paper presented at the Computational Intelligence in Medical Imaging, 2013 IEEE Fourth International Workshop. https://ieeexplore.ieee.org/document/6583857. Accessed August 30, 2021.

19. Kanakatte A, Mani N, Srinivasan B, et al. Pulmonary tumor volume detection from positron emission tomography images. Paper presented at the BioMedical Engineering and Informatics 2008. https://ieeexplore.ieee.org/document/4549165. Accessed August 30, 2021.

20. Sapra P, Singh R, Khurana S. Brain tumor detection using neural network. *IJISME.* 2013 Aug:2319–6386.

21. Al-Naami B, Bashir A, Amasha H, Al-Nabulsi J, Almalty AM. Statistical approach for brain cancer classification using a region growing threshold. *J Med Syst.* 2011 Aug;35(4):463–471.

22. Sharma K, Kaur A, Gujral S. Brain tumor detection based on machine learning algorithms. *Int J Comput Appl.* 2014 Oct;103(1):7–11.

23. Shortliffe EH, Sepúlveda MJ. Clinical decision support in the era of artificial intelligence. *JAMA.* 2018; 320(21):2199–2200.

24. Liang G, Fan W, Luo H, et al. The emerging roles of artificial intelligence in cancer drug development and precision therapy. *Biomed Pharmacother.* 2020;128:1–5.

25. Ho D. Artificial intelligence in cancer therapy. *Science.* 2020;367(6481):982–983.

26. Zhavoronkov A, Ivanenkov YA, Aliper A, et al. Deep learning enables rapid identification of potent DDR1 kinase inhibitors. *Nat Biotechnol.* 2019;37:1038–1040.

27. Pivetta T, Isaia F, Trudu F, et al. Development and validation of a general approach to predict and quantify the synergism of anticancer drugs using experimental design and artificial neural networks. *Talanta.* 2013;115:84–93.

28. Tsigelny IF. Artificial intelligence in drug combination therapy. *Brief Bioinform.* 2019;20(4):1434–1448.

29. Ferrari R, Mancini-Terracciano C, Voena C, et al. MR-based artificial intelligence model to assess response to therapy in locally advanced rectal cancer. *Eur J Radiol.* 2019;118:1–9.

30. Tran WT, Jerzak K, Lu FI, et al. Personalized breast cancer treatments using artificial intelligence in radiomics and pathomics. *J Med Imaging Radiat Sci.* 2019;50(4):S32–S41.

31. Benzekry S. Artificial intelligence and mechanistic modeling for clinical decision making in oncology. *Clin Pharmacol Ther.* 2020;108(3):471–486.

32. Malin JL. Envisioning Watson as a rapid-learning system for oncology. *J Oncol Pract.* 2013;9(3):155–157.

33. Somashekhar SP, Sepúlveda MJ, Norden AD, et al. Early experience with IBM Watson for Oncology (WFO) cognitive computing system for lung and colorectal cancer treatment. *J Clin Oncol.* 2017;35(15):8527.

34. Zhao C, Zhang Y, Ma X, et al. Concordance between treatment recommendations provided by IBM Watson for Oncology and a multidisciplinary tumor board for breast cancer in China. *Jpn J Clin Oncol.* 2020;50(8):852–858.

35. Zou FW, Tang YF, Liu CY, et al. Concordance study between IBM Watson for Oncology and real clinical practice for cervical cancer patients in China: a retrospective analysis. *Front Genet.* 2020;11:200.

36. Strickland E. IBM Watson, heal thyself: how IBM overpromised and underdelivered on AI health care. *IEEE Spectrum.* 2019;56(4):24–31.

37. Simon G, DiNardo CD, Takahashi K, et al. 2019 Applying artificial intelligence to address the knowledge gaps in cancer care. *Oncologist.* 2019;24(6):772–782.

38. Moore TA. *Medical Malpractice: Discovery and Trial.* 7th ed. New York, NY: Practising Law Institute; 2004.

39. *Hill v Kokosky*, 463 NW2d 265.266 (Mich BT App 1990).

40. *Ellis v Wallsend District Hospital*, 17 NSW, R 553 (1989).

41. *Kuznar v Raksha Corp*, 750 NW2d 121, 128 (Mich 2008).

42. *Matthies v Mastromonaco, DO*, 733 A2d 456, 460 (NJ 1999).

43. *Gonzalez v United States*, No 17CIV3645GBDOTW, 2020 WL 1548067 (SDNY Mar 31, 2020).

44. *Rowsey v Jones*, 26,823, 655 So 2d 560 (La App 2 Cir 1995).

45. Preliminary report: highway HWY19FH008. National Transportation Safety Board, 2019. https://www.ntsb.gov/investigations/AccidentReports/Reports/HWY19FH008-preliminary.pdf. Accessed July 15, 2020.

46. Naylor M. *Insurance Transformed: Technological Disruption*. New York, NY: Palgrave Macmillan; 2017.

47. Ball G. *En garde*: a civil law approach to autonomous vehicle liability under Louisiana law. *Tulane Law Rev*. 2019;94(1):155–182.

48. Automated vehicles for safety. National Highway Traffic Safety Administration, US Department of Transportation. https://www.nhtsa.gov/technology-innovation/automated-vehicles-safety. Accessed July 15, 2020.

49. Schroll C. Splitting the bill: creating a national car insurance fund to pay for accidents in autonomous vehicles. *Northwest Univ Law Rev*. 2015;109(3):803–833.

50. Proposed regulatory framework for modifications to artificial intelligence. US Food and Drug Administration. 2019. https://www.fda.gov/medical-devices/software-medical-device-samd/artificial-intelligence-and-machine-learning-software-medical-device. Accessed August 30, 2021.

51. Stipulated penalties and exclusion for material breach. US Department of Health and Human Services, Office of Inspector General. 2018. https://oig.hhs.gov/fraud/enforcement/ciae/stipulated-penalties.asp. Accessed August 30, 2021.

52. Phishing. US Department of Health and Human Services, Office for Civil Rights. 2018. https://www.hhs.gov/sites/default/files/cybersecurity-newsletter-february-2018.pdf. Accessed August 30, 2021.

53. Vanderpool D. HIPAA compliance: a common sense approach. *Innov Clin Neurosci*. 2019;16(1–2):38–41.

CHAPTER 22

Telemedicine

Cindy Jacobs, RN, JD

INTRODUCTION

There is no single or universal definition of telemedicine, but in general, it means the practice of medicine by electronic communication or other similar means by a health care professional in one location whose patient is in another location, with or without an intervening health care professional.

The primary legal and regulatory issues surrounding telemedicine from the physician's perspective include the following:

- Is telemedicine a treatment?
- Does it have a separate standard of care?
- Can a patient-provider relationship be established via telemedicine?
- Are there prescribing limitations related to telemedicine?
- Is consent required for telemedicine?
- Cross-state licensing issues: When is an out-of-state license needed?
  - Consultation exemptions
  - Reciprocity and compacts

STANDARD OF CARE ISSUES IN A TELEMEDICINE CONTEXT

Because telemedicine is not a treatment per se, but rather a treatment delivery mode or method, it does not really have a separate standard of care. For example, the Washington Medical Commission has stated in its telemedicine guidelines that its "practitioners using Telemedicine will be held to the same standard of care as practitioners engaging in more traditional in-person care delivery, including the requirement to meet all technical, clinical, confidentiality and ethical standards required by law."[1]

Elements of professional negligence claim

A medical malpractice claim is simply a professional negligence claim brought against a health care provider. The structure of a malpractice claim may vary slightly from state to state, but the basic elements of such a claim, of which establishing a failure to meet the standard of care is one and all of which the plaintiff/patient has the burden of proving, are as follows[2]:

- The health care provider and the patient had established a patient-provider relationship.
- The health care provider failed to meet the standard of care (usually defined as the degree of care and skill expected of a "reasonably prudent" health care provider acting in the same or similar circumstances).
- The health care provider's failure to meet the standard of care "proximately caused" the patient's injury and/or related damages.

Establishing a patient-provider relationship

As noted earlier, a threshold element in a medical malpractice claim that must be established by the plaintiff is the presence of a patient-provider relationship. Most state medical boards have taken the position that a patient-physician relationship *must* be established for telemedicine practice (presumably meaning that establishing this element would be relatively easy for a plaintiff in a telemedicine medical malpractice case). Until not that long ago, however, some states did not allow this relationship to be established via telemedicine. The requirement to establish the relationship in person is no longer present in any state (except in some prescribing circumstances; see next section). A common admonishment in state medical board telemedicine policies and/or regulations is that using a questionnaire to establish the relationship and basing a plan of care (including prescriptions) solely on the questionnaire are not appropriate.

Scope of practice and prescription requirements

In theory, a physician's scope of practice would not be affected by telemedicine, except that as a practical matter, telemedicine imposes technical limitations on a physician's ability to perform some activities that are within the full scope of practice. This makes any "telemedicine scope of practice" regulation by a state medical board redundant. Many state boards have either recognized this affirmatively or remained silent about any limitations on the scope of telemedicine practice.

Prescribing, however, is one area where some state boards have articulated varying restrictions on telemedicine scope of practice. For example, some states prohibit telemedicine prescribing of any controlled substance (Schedule II drugs, which include many pain, anxiety, and sleep medications), at least without an in-person evaluation. These prohibitions are generally consistent with the federal law restrictions that have long been in place under the Ryan Haight Act,[3] which was intended to curb indiscriminate Internet prescribing that was perceived as a serious problem in the 1990s.

Essentially, the Ryan Haight Act prohibits telemedicine prescribing of Schedule II drugs unless the physician has conducted at least one in-person exam of the patient or meets an exception to the act's in-person exam requirement. Most of these exceptions involve what the act defines as "the practice of telemedicine," but that definition is extremely narrow.

Oncologists, of course, would find themselves needing to prescribe Schedule II drugs, so they should be aware of any telemedicine prescribing restrictions in their state as well as the Ryan Haight Act restrictions. As a practical matter, however, the restrictions have a more significant effect on behavioral health telemedicine; in the oncology setting, any telemedicine prescribing presumably would take place during follow-up/monitoring visits after at least one in-person exam has taken place.

CONSENT ISSUES IN A TELEMEDICINE CONTEXT

State medical boards have not historically regulated in the area of informed consent requirements for health care professionals, as these requirements generally are found either in court opinions (case law) or separate statutes passed by the legislature that are not related to licensing requirements. However, in recent years, many state boards have set forth informed consent criteria specific to telemedicine, although sometimes referencing established informed consent principles.

Most of these state board requirements involve some type of mandated informed consent for telemedicine. This is somewhat confusing because clinical informed consent principles are targeted at treatment and care; as noted, telemedicine is not in and of itself treatment and care, but rather a delivery method for treatment and care. Some state boards have clarified that the physician should conduct and document normal and customary informed consent discussions with telemedicine patients but should also include appropriate discussion of how the telemedicine setting might affect the treatment and care, including technology capabilities and limitations.

Despite the fact that some states have articulated a specific informed consent requirement for telemedicine, the core of those requirements is still embedded in general informed consent principles. Accordingly, the best overall approach to take is to conduct (and document) a normal informed consent process for whatever treatment scenario is underlying the telemedicine visit, while considering and including relevant telemedicine information that would be considered a "material fact" about which the "reasonably prudent patient" would want to be aware before making an overall decision about whether to consent to the proposed treatment itself. This would include, for example, explaining and discussing limitations of the telemedicine process (e.g., no ability to assess the patient in person).

The following are the basic elements of informed consent (these are from Washington State, but informed consent elements are fairly universal across the United States):

- The health care provider has a duty to secure the patient's informed consent for treatment by informing the patient of material facts related to the treatment.
- A fact is defined as or considered to be a material fact if a reasonably prudent person in the position of the patient or his or her representative would attach significance to it deciding whether or not to submit to the proposed treatment.
- Material facts include:
  - The nature and character of the treatment proposed and administered;
  - The anticipated results of the treatment proposed and administered;
  - The recognized possible alternative forms of treatment; or
  - The recognized serious possible risks, complications, and anticipated benefits involved in the treatment administered and in the recognized possible alternative forms of treatment, including nontreatment.[4]

Applicable facts about the telemedicine process might materially relate to the nature and character as well as to the serious possible risks, complications, and anticipated benefits of the treatment.

CROSS-STATE LICENSING ISSUES IN TELEMEDICINE

Requirements for licensure

The Federation of State Medical Boards (FSMB), which is a professional organization and not itself a licensing board (membership comprises the US state and territorial medical licensing boards), has stated in its model telemedicine policy[5] that the practice of medicine occurs at the "location" of the patient. The policy does not specify whether "location" means "residence" (as opposed to a patient who is temporarily in the state, e.g., traveling).

The risks of running afoul of the medical licensing board in the patient's state for engaging in telemedicine activities without a license include the following:

1. The unlicensed practice of medicine is a crime in most states.
2. Unlicensed practice constitutes professional misconduct, and once a patient's state takes action on this issue, the physician's home/licensing state will be notified and also may take action.

Most state medical licensing laws define the practice of medicine very broadly. For example, Washington State's definition provides as follows:

A person is practicing medicine if he or she . . . offers or undertakes to diagnose, cure, advise, or prescribe for any human disease, ailment, injury, infirmity, deformity, pain or other condition, physical or mental, real or imaginary, by any means or instrumentality.[6]

Overall, then, a physician engaged in telemedicine practice with a patient either must be licensed in or must qualify for a licensing exemption in the patient's state (see further discussion in the following section).

Consultation exemptions and other licensing exemptions

The specifics of various state schemes vary, but overall, the presumption should be that a physician needs full licensure in the patient's state in order to engage in the practice of medicine with that patient via telemedicine, unless an exemption or "special license" is expressly provided under the state's licensing law.

The most common exemption applicable to telemedicine is the consultation exemption. The details differ from state to state, but the consultation exemption basically provides that no license is needed under the following circumstances:

- The physician must be duly licensed in their home state.
- The total number of consultations by the physician must not exceed the state's threshold (some states identify a specific number, which is usually 10-12 per year; others limit the number to "occasional" or "infrequent," without a specific number).
- Most states require the consultation to be at the request of the patient's treating physician who is licensed in the state. Some states, such as Nevada and Montana, require requesting physicians to report or register these consultations by out-of-state physicians to or with their medical board.

- Some states require that the consultation must be intraspecialty to qualify for the exemption.
- Some states require that the consultation be at no charge to qualify for the exemption.

Most states (47) have some type of consultation exemption (Alabama, Alaska, Arizona, Arkansas, California, Colorado, Connecticut, Delaware, District of Columbia, Florida, Georgia, Hawaii, Idaho, Illinois, Indiana, Iowa, Kansas, Kentucky, Louisiana, Maine, Maryland, Massachusetts, Michigan, Minnesota, Mississippi, Missouri, Montana, Nebraska, Nevada, New Hampshire, New Jersey, New Mexico, New York, North Carolina, North Dakota, Ohio, Oklahoma, Oregon, Pennsylvania, Rhode Island, South Carolina, South Dakota, Tennessee, Texas, Utah, Vermont, Virginia, Washington, West Virginia, Wisconsin, and Wyoming).

So far, only Washington State has specifically articulated a licensing exemption for situations where a patient residing in one state has previously been treated in a different state by a physician licensed in that state and is having a brief follow-up related to the prior treatment through telemedicine with that physician after returning home to the patient's home state.[7]

In addition, some states have a special or limited telemedicine license or certificate available, although that trend actually has reversed itself in recent years with states that have discontinued those licenses in favor of requiring full licensure or adopting the interstate licensing compact (see discussion in the next section). The seven remaining states with telemedicine special purpose licenses or certificates are Alabama, Georgia, Oklahoma, Louisiana, Nevada, New Mexico, and Tennessee (osteopaths only). In addition, Alaska has a separate, mandatory "Telemedicine Business Registry"; however, the requirement to register does not apply to individual health care providers.

Still other medical boards make allowances for practice (not necessarily limited to telemedicine) in contiguous states (e.g., the Washington, DC, Maryland, and Virginia medical boards) or in certain situations where a temporary license might be issued provided the specific board's licensing conditions are met.

Reciprocity and compacts

Twenty-nine states, the District of Columbia, and Guam have adopted the FSMB's Interstate Medical Licensure Compact (referred to as IMLC or the Compact). Compact adoption allows for the national Interstate Commission's expedited licensure process to be used for licensed physicians to apply for licenses in other states. Participation is entirely voluntary for states, which adopt the Compact by passing its language as legislation. The Compact creates an expedited pathway for a state's home-licensed physicians to obtain a license in another Compact state; it does not otherwise change a state's existing medical practice laws. Regulatory authority remains with each participating state medical board, not with national Compact staff. Medical boards in participating states must share complaint or investigative information with each other.

A Compact license process originates through the physician's home state of licensure. As an example, both Wyoming and Washington have adopted the IMLC. If a Wyoming-licensed physician wants to practice telemedicine in Washington, the process would work as follows:

1. The physician would apply and pay $700 to the national Compact office, of which $400 would go to their home license state of Wyoming and $300 would go to the Compact general fund.
2. Wyoming would issue a licensing approval letter to Washington (where the physician is seeking licensure).

3. The physician would then pay the full normal Washington licensing fee to the Washington Medical Commission, which would issue a Washington license based on Wyoming's approval letter.
4. The physician also could pay the Compact $100 each for the release of additional letters to additional states but still would pay the full licensing fee to each new state.

CASE LAW QUANDARY

There is very little case law (law created through court decisions) in the telemedicine arena that relates to physician practice. There is some case law concerning physician licensing requirements in a telemedicine context, but the case is primarily related to antitrust allegations against the Texas Medical Board. One of the few cases involved a medical malpractice action where the defendant physician was not licensed in the patient's state—and the diagnosis at issue was a cancer diagnosis.[8]

CASE LAW #1

In August 2007, the physician was working as a pathologist in Washington State. She reviewed the plaintiff's pathology slide, which had been collected in and sent from Idaho, and interpreted it as showing a benign skin lesion. A biopsy later revealed malignant melanoma. The plaintiff alleged negligence by the physician for failure to diagnose, with damages related to decreased chances of survival based on the early, curable stage reflected by the original pathology slide. As part of the court proceedings, the plaintiff requested a declaration that the physician had violated the Idaho Medical Practices Act by rendering a medical diagnosis for an Idaho resident without holding a license to practice medicine in Idaho.

The Idaho law at issue prohibited the practice of medicine "in this state" without a license, and the defendant physician argued that this applied only to the practice of medicine when the *physician* was within Idaho borders. The court disagreed, noting that the Idaho Board of Medicine had specifically noted in August 2006, based on a policy set forth by the College of American Pathologists, that "pathologists who review tissue samples taken from Idaho patients and who render diagnoses from those samples for inclusion in an Idaho patient's chart are practicing medicine in the state of Idaho, regardless of where they are physically located."[8] Note that this approach also is consistent with the FSMB policy discussed earlier.

Consistent with the overall lack of physician practice-related case law, there is essentially no evidence of "telemedicine malpractice" in reported information about medical malpractice settlements, verdicts, and judgments. For example, an April 2019 research letter in the *Journal of the American Medical Association* noted that a review of 551 reported malpractice cases between October 1, 2018 and November 1, 2018, revealed none that involved claims targeting telemedicine services. [9]

This lack of specific "telemedicine malpractice" cases is consistent with the previously-discussed principle that telemedicine does not have a separate or unique standard of care. Accordingly, the usual accepted oncology standards of care would apply in a telemedicine setting. Two primary recommendations in this regard are to be aware of (1) what types of malpractice claims have the highest frequency and severity in oncology practice, as discussed more fully below; and (2) where a telemedicine setting may be unduly likely to limit the provider's ability to adhere to the "reasonably prudent oncologist" standard of care, particularly in high-claim categories such as those described below.

1. Oncology Malpractice Closed Claims Study[10]

The following data analysis is from a Doctors Company review of 101 medical and two surgical oncology claims—which were excluded from the reported study data—and lawsuits among its 500+ insureds that closed between 2012 and 2018.

- Only 26% of the closed claims resulted in a payment to the patient or their family, half of which were less than $100,000.
- 68% of the claims comprised three primary case types, 29% diagnosis-related, 24% treatment management-related, and 15% medication management-related.
- Diagnosis-related claims were highlighted by either "failure to reconcile relevant signs, symptoms, and test results, or a narrow diagnostic focus where it was presumed that the patient's chronic condition was the cause of current symptoms." Contributing factors included patient behavior (52%), inadequate patient assessment (38%), communication among providers (21%), and communication between the patient/family (or family members) and providers, including language barriers (17%).
- The other prevalent claim types (treatment and medication-management related claims) also were associated with the same or similar factors.

Reducing risk of a malpractice claim in the telemedicine arena, then, is more likely if the provider pays attention to how the contributing factors described above might be exacerbated by a telemedicine setting for care episodes.

CLINICAL VIGNETTE # 1

Dr. Faraway works at the Memorial Hospital where she has privileges, and the hospital is trying to increase its use of telemedicine. They have asked Dr. Faraway to obtain patient informed consent for upcoming procedures, including, e.g., chemotherapy port placement, via a telemedicine visit instead of in person. Is this okay? What are the conditions and limitations, if any?

In general, there is no designated "scope" for what may or may not be undertaken during a telemedicine visit versus in person from a regulatory perspective, with the exception of prescribing limitations as noted and a few states that require an in-person exam to establish a patient-physician relationship (the ability of those states to enforce that restriction is questionable due to the fact that the existence of that relationship is construed from the perspective of the patient, not the physician).

Limits on what may or may not be done during a telemedicine visit come from the medical malpractice concept of standard of care (i.e., Would the reasonably prudent provider in like or similar circumstances do XYZ via telemedicine?). Informed consent, however, has its own set of statutory elements that are separate from medical malpractice elements. Informed consent is not based on a provider standard of care the way medical malpractice is; rather, the consent process must meet certain criteria in order to constitute informed consent, and whether the process met those criteria is determined by asking whether the "reasonable *patient*" would believe they had provided informed consent. The customary elements for informed consent can all be easily met via telemedicine.

As with in-person informed consent, make sure of the following:

- Whoever provides the educational portion of the consent process (which may be delegated in general, e.g., to a nurse educator) needs to cover all of the elements (e.g., description, risks, benefits, alternatives).
- If the health care provider performing the procedure did not provide the educational portion, he or she should make sure the patient understands the procedure and consent and answer any remaining questions the patient has.
- On the day of the in-person procedure, the provider performing the procedure should reconfirm whether the patient has questions and answer them accordingly (and document). A signed consent form is not generally required by law, but with appropriate content, it can serve as *prima facie* evidence of informed consent. An electronic signature process can be used for this in telemedicine settings.

CLINICAL VIGNETTE # 2

Dr. Jones has an outpatient clinic in the state of Oregon, which is close to the Washington-Oregon border. She often treats patients who come to her practice from Washington, and sometimes she admits them to the Oregon hospital where she has privileges. Can she have follow-up telemedicine visits with these patients after they return to their Washington homes without being licensed in Washington?

As discussed earlier, Washington is actually the only state that had specifically addressed this issue prior to the COVID-19 pandemic, when most states relaxed licensing requirements for purposes of addressing the public health emergency. If the provider is licensed in, for example, Oregon, Montana, or Idaho and is treating patients from Washington at their Oregon, Montana, or Idaho location, they are expressly permitted to do a brief follow-up related to the prior treatment through telemedicine without obtaining a Washington license. This suggests that even Washington would require a license for telemedicine visits associated with an *ongoing* course of care.

If the provider will be treating any out-of-state patient for an ongoing course of care and they would like to do telemedicine visits with them while they are in their home, they have the options listed below. Note that options generally will be broader in states that have not returned to their tighter pre-COVID licensing requirements; some states may make those relaxed requirements permanent, with Idaho being farthest along on that path.

1. If the patient is from a bordering state, from which the provider presumably has other patients, the most efficient and lowest risk option is to obtain a license there. This is easier and quicker to do if their state and the bordering state are both IMLC states.
2. In the case of a patient who has traveled to their provider's practice or hospital from a state whose residents they rarely see, they may be able to follow the patient via telemedicine once the patient is back home through a consultation exemption—if the state has one that is applicable (discussed earlier)—by working with the patient's primary care provider. As noted, in many states, they would need to be careful not to exceed the maximum number of telemedicine visits they perform under a consultation exemption.

CLINICAL VIGNETTE # 3

Dr. Baker is conducting a routine follow-up visit via video telemedicine with his established pancreatic cancer patient. The patient informs him that she has had some intermittent cramping abdominal pain for the past few days. What are the liability risk issues associated with seeing this type of patient through video? What if the patient signs a liability waiver before the telemedicine visits?

The liability risks in this situation are actually standard of care considerations. That is, can the provider safely evaluate their patient via video telemedicine, or do they need to redirect the patient so that they or another health care professional (e.g., in an emergency department) can conduct a hands-on exam or have the patient undergo other in-person evaluation? In this setting, a liability waiver is essentially useless. A court would not uphold a waiver beyond knowing the assumption of risks that a patient is affirmatively taking related to their own behavior, which would never extend to a waiver their negligence under medical malpractice principles (see earlier discussion in "Elements of Professional Negligence Claim").

CONCLUSION

Telemedicine can greatly improve access to care, especially for patients in rural settings or who otherwise have access limitations. It can also make physician practice settings more efficient and streamlined. To optimize the potential benefits of telemedicine while minimizing the clinical risk for patients and the legal/regulatory risks for providers, health care professionals should be aware of and comply with applicable standard of care and consent principles and state licensing requirements, as discussed in this chapter.

KEY POINTS:
- -

- It is acceptable in most situations to establish a new patient-provider relationship via telemedicine; however, it must involve actual interaction with the patient and not rely on a questionnaire or form. One exception is in the case of patients for whom providers will be prescribing Schedule II drugs, which requires an initial in-person evaluation under federal law.
- It is important to always obtain a patient's informed consent for any treatment or treatment plan, whether that plan is proceeding entirely in person or partially via telemedicine.
- For treatment visits that are proceeding via telemedicine, providers should ensure that the informed consent elements are or have been met for the treatment plan itself, as well as include information about any material facts related to how telemedicine limitations might affect the visit or the overall plan.
- When providers are conducting patient care visits via telemedicine, the appropriate standard of care does not differ from in-person patient care (i.e., target goals should be the same). They should use their clinical judgment to determine whether their goal for a visit can safely be accomplished without putting hands on the patient. If not, they should move that patient to an in-person visit as quickly as indicated by the circumstances.
- If providers regularly treat out-of-state patients via telemedicine who are in their homes (or any originating site in their home state, such as their primary care provider's office), they should be licensed in those states unless there is an applicable licensing exemption, such as a consultation exemption. Care must be taken to observe any limitations on licensing exemptions (e.g., maximum annual frequency for consultations).

References:

1. Appropriate use of telemedicine. Washington Medical Commission. 2014. https://wmc.wa.gov/sites/default/files/public/Telemedicine%20Guideline.pdf. Accessed August 25, 2021.
2. See RCW 7.70.040.
3. 21 USC §§802(50)-(56), 829(e), 841(h).
4. See RCW 7.70.050.
5. Model policy for the appropriate use of telemedicine technologies in the practice of medicine. Federation of State Medical Boards. 2014. https://www.fsmb.org/siteassets/advocacy/policies/fsmb_telemedicine_policy.pdf. Accessed August 25, 2021.
6. RCW 18.71.011.
7. Telemedicine and continuity of care. Washington Medical Commission Policy Statement. POL2018-01. Washington Medical Commission. March 2, 2018. https://wmc.wa.gov/sites/default/files/public/documents/TelemedicineAndContinuityOfCarePOL2018-01.pdf. Accessed August 25, 2021.
8. *Smith v Laboratory Corporation of America, Inc*, Case No. C09-1662 (WD Wash February 3, 2011).
9. Fogel AL, Kvedar JC. Reported cases of medical malpractice in direct-to-consumer telemedicine. *JAMA*. 2019;321(13):1309–1310.
10. "Oncology Closed Claims Study," Doctors Company (https://www.thedoctors.com/articles/oncology-closed-claims-study/)

CHAPTER 23

Liability Involving Midlevel Practitioners

Eric E. Shore, DO, JD, MBA, FCLM

INTRODUCTION

Midlevel practitioners (MLPs) are increasingly becoming an important fixture in American health care, and although their use provides great opportunities to improve the provision of health care around the country, the novelty of their increasing scope of practice in a burgeoning number of jurisdictions presents their supervisors, and them, with the possibility of increased legal liability. It is important, therefore, to define who they are, what they do, and how best to protect them and their supervising physicians and institutions from liability. First, any reference to "physicians" or "doctors" in this chapter refers to graduates of accredited medical schools with the degrees of MD or DO. For our purposes, an MLP is a practitioner who is performing a function that has traditionally been thought of as being within the purview of medicine but who is not a physician. While there may be other providers that fit some portion of this category, for practical purposes, our discussion is limited to nurse practitioners (NPs), including those who have a doctorate in nursing practice (DNP), and physician assistants (PAs). Moreover, although these practitioners dislike being referred to as MLPs, that designation was placed on them more as a billing standard by the Centers for Medicare and Medicaid Services (CMS) than by physicians. MLPs came into existence for a reason, they persist for a reason, and when properly utilized, they can provide significant contributions to patient care and the efficiency of the health care system. It is only when their practice overreaches their education, training, and experience or they practice in a manner for which their training has not prepared them that difficulty begins. First, therefore, some background is provided.

The first program to produce an MLP was at Duke University in 1965 and was founded by Eugene A. Stead, Jr., MD, then chairman of Duke's Department of Medicine. It was proposed in partial answer to an impending primary care physician shortage in the United States, and because it occurred during the Vietnam War, it was reasoned that if military medics entered the program, they would already have a significant amount of clinical experience, especially with trauma, and could supplement physicians working in their offices, hospitals, and clinics. It was a two-year program meant to fill the gap between physicians and nurses, and graduates were referred to as PAs.[1]

Perhaps wanting to protect the place of nurses in health care, the first program to graduate NPs was founded at the same time at the University of Colorado by Loretta Ford, RN, and

Henry Silver, MD. The goal was to "increase the supply of primary care providers, especially in underserved urban and rural areas by training Registered Nurses ("RN") in clinical care so they could . . . free up physicians for those patients who really needed their attention."[2]

Early on, PAs and NPs worked in physicians' offices, clinics, or rural health settings, in many cases making house calls or seeing patients who did not need a higher level of care. For example, it was not unusual for an MLP to see a patient with an upper respiratory infection in the physician's office, so that the physician could spend more time caring for difficult patients with pathology such as heart failure, uncontrolled hypertension, or a complicated urinary tract infection. In the beginning, when MLPs finished seeing a patient (and depending on their arrangements with the physician), they would approach the physician to sign a prescription for treatment and then give it to the patient. Later, as they became more trusted, they were sometimes given a book of presigned prescriptions so they would not have to bother the physician to sign a prescription for each patient. It was expected, though, that if MLPs ran into anything they were unsure about, they would consult with the physician before acting.

Much of this has now changed, and we must now separate PAs from NPs. PAs are licensed by the board or medicine in each jurisdiction, whereas NPs are generally licensed by the board of nursing. This is a critical distinction because, for practical purposes, physicians have little control in many, if not most, jurisdictions over what an NP is allowed to do, this being the responsibility of the board of nursing and the state legislature. Not surprisingly, therefore, there has been a push by NPs and boards of nursing to extend practice authority to allow NPs to practice independently of physician oversight, counting on them to know their limitations and refer to physicians when needed. Additionally, a similar push for independent practice has begun among PAs as well. Despite a backlash from physicians, NP lobbying efforts have succeeded in convincing at least 22 states and the District of Columbia to allow independent practice of NPs, while 16 states have opted for reduced practice (must have a contractual arrangement with a physician to review a percentage of their charts and be available for consultation), and the remainder allow only restricted practice (must work directly under a physician).[3] This situation remains fluid and will undoubtedly change over time. Definition and scope of practice also vary by state as well. For example, some states may choose to limit practice in one area of practice while allowing it, independently, in another. These practice limitations change over time as well, so the scope of an NP's permitted practice will depend on the state and the date of the care in question.

How, then, do these restrictions apply to oncology, and what difference does it make? The answers are complex and cannot be presented in an exhaustive manner here, but the basic difference can be discussed. It is extremely unlikely that NPs or PAs will be the practitioners to ultimately diagnose and prescribe treatment for cancer. They may, however, care for comorbid conditions and, undoubtedly, will often be the first health care provider to see a patient with signs of cancer. Therefore, it is incumbent upon them to recognize these signs and differentiate them from signs of more mundane illnesses; whether for NPs or physicians, this is always a matter of training. Moreover, if properly trained, there are specific procedures that MLPs can perform such as injections and intravenous chemotherapy, even when the oncologist is not physically present. Still, even "simple" issues may be complex in the context of the oncologic patient. If a cancer patient has a simple urinary tract infection, then the person prescribing treatment must be cognizant of the fact that the patient may be immunosuppressed and may require both a different interpretation of their symptoms and lab studies as well as different treatment and testing than a nonimmunosuppressed patient. Other issues include whether an NP is able and trained to evaluate a patient's progress if the patient lives in a rural area without immediate access to the oncologic service. This raises the important issue of training.

TRAINING

The average family physician, when they complete their residency, will have had more than 15,000 hours of clinical training and experience, whereas the average NP may have as little as 500 hours or as much as 1500 hours.[4,5] Many NPs also have substantial experience caring for patients before entering training to become an NP. Moreover, some who work in areas such as anesthesia and psychiatry do have additional training in those areas. Unfortunately, although this was the original premise of their education, there are nurses with little experience who become NPs. Additionally, because there is no enforceable national accreditation policy for NPs, the quality of NP graduates may vary greatly, which places them in the same position as MDs in the early part of the 20th century when Dr. Flexner published his report on the state of medical education at the time. The results of that report would end the diploma mills that had sprung up granting MD degrees to poorly educated and trained students.[6] Some NP programs are excellent and require strict minimums for entrance and program completion, whereas others have few requirements for entrance and minimal standard requirements for completing their programs. In addition, the relatively new designation of doctor of nursing practice (DNP) has been created. This is a *terminal* degree (the highest degree in the field) that is largely meant to prepare NPs for administrative duties and is frequently available to be earned mostly (if not entirely) online. Because of its implications for legal issues, it will be discussed in greater detail later. For now, it is only necessary to know it exists.

Finally, perhaps the most important concept that will bear on legal issues is the independent practice of NPs. With anywhere from 3% to 10% of the training and experience of even the shortest physician residency programs, few would argue that NPs have the same education as physicians. Perhaps a more important question is whether they will be held to the same standard of care as physicians and who can testify to that standard of care. In most jurisdictions, the standard of care is the same.[7] However, who may testify at trial about the standard of care can vary widely. Additionally, one of the first things any physician learns as they gain medical knowledge is how little they know about something and to call for help as soon and as often as needed. While this seems self-evident, studies by Dr. Dunning and Dr. Kruger have shown that it is not only not self-evident but, in fact, the reality is clearly counterintuitive. People who have less knowledge appear to be more confident in their abilities than those with more knowledge, leading to more incorrect decisions. This is known as the Dunning-Kruger effect[8]:

The Dunning-Kruger effect represents a bias in estimating our own ability that stems from our limited perspective. When we have a poor or nonexistent grasp on a topic, we literally know too little of it to understand how little we know. Those who do possess the knowledge or skills, however, have a much better idea of where they sit. But they also think that if a task is clear and simple to them, it must be so for everyone else as well.[9]

In a situation where a judgement is required as to whether one's own knowledge is sufficient to make a diagnosis and/or prescribe treatment or needs to be supplemented by that of a physician, the very existence of lesser education and training is what may cause a critical error by the MLP and potential disaster for the patient, leading to many of the issues that follow. Clearly, it is in the best interest of both the MLP and supervising physician to closely supervise the MLP until the MLP becomes more comfortable with their level of knowledge and experience and are thus enabled to do more with less supervision. This is especially true in oncology, where recognition of malignancy is important, diagnosis is difficult, and treatment can change on a frequent basis—aspects that cause even nononcologic physicians to find the field intimidating. The most important way to make MLPs more valuable and better able to increasingly manage patient care, at least partially on their own, is education, which, as in a medical residency, is the responsibility of the oncologist. Not only does education improve patient care and decrease the probability of untoward effects and liability, but ultimately, it makes the MLP that much more valuable to the oncologic practice since more responsibilities can be given to them with less concern for error.

LIABILITY

Having briefly reviewed the basis of the discussion, it is now time to discuss liability for NPs or PAs, their employers, and any physicians providing oversight. This must begin with the caveat that, although MLPs have certainly been involved in many lawsuits, both as primary and secondary defendants, there has been limited litigation so far defining their standard of care compared with that of physicians or delineating who may testify in such cases, with many cases being cases of "first impression," wherein the court must determine who may testify to that standard. Therefore, in many cases, what is expressed here may change as new information and statutory and case law become available. It is not the intent here to define each of these issues, as they are relatively jurisdictional and need to be researched on a case-by-case basis. Moreover, some of what follows applies to any agent (i.e., anyone who stands in the place of or represents another) of a physician, group, or corporation, and only a few cases are selectively applicable to MLPs or NPs.

NEGLIGENCE

The first issue to face any practitioner in health care is always *negligence*. Briefly, negligence can be defend as a breach in the standard of care. (When negligence exists but no damage is caused, it is frequently referred to as "negligence in the air.") Most jurisdictions have rules stating that the expert testifying at trial must be someone in the same or similar specialty, in clinical practice for a specific number of years, and/or demonstrably familiar with the issue being addressed. Each of these requirements, however, can be waived by a court as circumstances require. What happens when apples are compared with oranges, such as when the standard of care of MLPs is equated to that of physicians?

Suppose the person on trial for negligence is an NP, Mr. Y, who is accused of failure to diagnose a severe illness because he failed to perform a particular test. Along comes Dr. X who opines that Mr. Y breached the standard of care by not performing the test. Mr. Y may counter that Dr. X is not entitled to testify because Dr. X is not a nurse and is not *legally* capable of defining the standard of care for Mr. Y. What about the reverse? Can Mr. Y testify that Dr. X breached the standard of care since he is not a physician? There is no clear answer to these questions, and various courts and jurisdictions have wrestled with the problem. Examples might begin with Pennsylvania Statute Title 40, which states, in relevant part:

> An expert testifying on a medical matter, including the standard of care, risks and alternatives, causation and the nature and extent of the injury, must meet the following qualifications:
>
> 1. Possess an unrestricted physician's license to practice medicine in any state or the District of Columbia.
> 2. Be engaged in or retired within the previous five years from active clinical practice or teaching.[11]

The statute then goes on to add:

> Provided, however, the court may waive the requirements of this subsection for an expert on a matter other than the standard of care if the court determines that the expert is otherwise competent to testify about medical or scientific issues by virtue of education, training or experience.[10]

In other circumstances, courts have attempted to deal with this issue but appear to be evolving in their decisions. In 2010, the Indiana appeals court ruled that an NP's testimony was inadmissible, stating:

> Although the Medical Malpractice Act allows health care providers, such as registered nurses, to serve on medical review panels and provides that the panel's opinion is admissible in court, we conclude that Indiana Evidence Rule 702, which trumps any statute, may prohibit such non-physician health care providers' opinions as to medical causation from being admitted in court to create a genuine issue of material fact in a summary judgment proceeding or to serve as substantive evidence at trial. This is because the health care providers may not be qualified by knowledge, skill, experience, training, or education to give opinions as to medical causation.[11]

By 2017, however, the same Indiana appeals court appears to have revised its opinion, ruling:

> [W]e are not prepared to declare a blanket rule that nurses cannot qualify as expert witnesses under Indiana Evidence Rule 702 and testify as to whether a healthcare provider breached a standard of care or whether an alleged breach caused an injury. Indiana Evidence Rule 702(a) provides "a witness qualified as an expert by knowledge, skill, experience, training, or education, may testify thereto in the form of an opinion or otherwise." Just as the Rule states, we hold a nurse could qualify as an expert regarding medical standards of care and causation in some circumstances. The determinative

question is whether the nurse has sufficient expertise, as provided in Rule 702(a), with the factual circumstances giving rise to the claim and the patient's injuries.[12]

In 2012, a Kentucky court appears to have extended this further, holding that a nurse can be an expert witness against a doctor, but only through an exception based on the knowledge and experience of the individual, not on the individual's degree:

It may be possible that a nurse could obtain the "knowledge, skill, experience, training, or education" required to qualify as an expert on the standard of care required of a doctor treating a patient with [name of patient]'s symptoms. Fed.R.Evid. 702. One can imagine a nurse who specializes in a field (for example cardiology), reads the relevant literature, and works closely with doctors to treat patients on a regular basis. Over time, the nurse might become as qualified to opine on the standard of care her supervising physician must meet as that physician himself . . . But [name of expert] is not that nurse.[13]

These rules can be confusing because there is no national standard for standard of care testimony requirements, and many jurisdictions are dealing with this issue as a matter of first impression.

An additional issue with potential legal liability for MLPs is the doctrine of *respondeat superior*. In short, this is a legal doctrine, commonly used in tort, that holds an employer or principal legally responsible for the wrongful acts of an employee or agent, *if such acts occur within the scope of the employment or agency*. Typically, when *respondeat superior* is invoked, a plaintiff will look to hold both the employer and the employee liable. As such, a court will generally look to the doctrine of joint and several liability (if available) when assigning damages. (Joint and several liability is the doctrine that each defendant is liable for the entire amount of damages so that, if one defendant is unable to pay their share, the remaining defendant[s] must shoulder the burden.) This is similar to, but broader than, the old "captain of the ship" rule (which has fallen out of favor), making the operating surgeon responsible for anything that happens in the operating room regardless of who caused it. However, when the "agent" is not directly employed by the "superior," other causes of action such as negligent supervision or negligent oversight, by which a professional corporation or even a hospital may be added to the list of defendants, are frequently seen. Thus, it is possible that a physician who has agreed to provide oversight to an NP by reviewing 20% of the NP's medical records may be sued in a case where the NP breached the standard of care, even if the physician never saw or even know of the patient and did not approve the diagnostic process or treatment.

It is important to mention that even if there is no agreement to supervise NPs or PAs, liability may still attach. Like most clinicians, oncologists often informally consult with their colleagues both by asking questions and seeking suggestions for care of their patients (i.e., "hallway" consults), which usually benefits both the physicians and the patients they serve. However, some jurisdictions permit negligence claims arising from informal consults. For example, in April 2019, in *Warren v Dinter*,[14] the Minnesota Supreme Court ruled that a clinician can be liable for medical malpractice, even when there is no established patient-physician relationship, when negligent advice is given and it is reasonably foreseeable that a patient could be injured by that advice.

CASE LAW # 1

In *Warren v Dinter*,[14] an NP in an outpatient clinic felt that a patient needed to be admitted to the hospital, but the nearest hospital was a distance away and part of another health care system. She called the hospitalist at that system and presented the case. Based solely on the NP's description of the clinical situation, the hospitalist did not recommend hospitalization. The NP accepted this recommendation and sent the patient home, where the patient died three days later. The physician provided answers based solely on the NP's presentation, never saw or even spoke with the patient, did not bill, and had no supervisory responsibility for the NP, yet was held liable. Those who work around NPs or PAs, even if they have no supervisory agreements with the MLPs, and who base their answers to questions upon wrong or inadequate information provided by the MLPs may still be liable.

INFORMED CONSENT

For practical purposes, the right of privacy, granted pursuant to the liberty guarantee of the US Constitution, gives all Americans authority over their own bodies and what can be done to them.[15] It is a basic tenet of American law, however, that any such consent to treat must be *informed*.[16] Perhaps the clearest example of this was the Pennsylvania Supreme Court's holding in *Shinal v Toms*, stating that "a physician's duty to provide information to a patient sufficient to obtain her informed consent is non-delegable."[17] In that case, the consent for the procedure was obtained by a resident whom the surgeon had asked to obtain it. The court explained that the resident was in training and therefore not as knowledgeable as the surgeon; thus, only the surgeon could be expected to present a coherent picture of what was to be done and answer all of the patient's questions adequately. This would certainly apply to consent obtained by an NP as well. This case raises the question of whether an NP or PA can legally obtain informed consent for a procedure to be performed by a physician. Further, is any consent to treat informed if obtained by an NP prior to treating a patient on his or her own if the patient has not been informed of the difference in education and experience between a physician and an NP? This comes down to the question of whether the patient would have granted their consent if they *had* known. Moreover, this becomes even more important when the NP holds a DNP degree and introduces themselves to the patient as "Dr." Jones.

MISREPRESENTATION

Misrepresentation is, essentially, causing or allowing someone to believe something that is not true, with that person relying on that information to their detriment. Put more simply, the elements of misrepresentation are as follows:

1. The defendant made a material misrepresentation.
2. The defendant had knowledge of the misrepresentation or acted with gross neglect.
3. The defendant intended for the plaintiff to rely on the misrepresentation.

4. There was actual and justifiable reliance on the part of the plaintiff.

5. There were damages sustained by the plaintiff.

In addition, a fraudulent concealment of material facts may also be considered misrepresentation.[18]

CLINICAL VIGNETTE # 1

Imagine a patient lying on a gurney outside of an operating room waiting for emergency surgery. A physician walks up to the patient and introduces himself, stating that he is about to operate on the patient and explaining what he is going to do. The patient signs the consent form, goes into surgery, and suffers an untoward consequence. Later, it is determined that the doctor was, in fact, not really a surgeon at all, but a surgical assistant who was taking the case because the surgeon with whom he worked had not yet shown up. Although the doctor never actually said, "I am a surgeon," a *reasonable person* in the patient's position would have assumed that to be the case. The patient, who was injured by the surgery, sues the physician and hospital because, among other things, the doctor, by omission, represented himself to the patient as a qualified surgeon and thus obtained the patient's consent and confidence before surgery.

CLINICAL VIGNETTE # 2

An NP, Dr. Jones, is assigned to a patient as a primary care provider by the patient's insurance company, largely for financial reasons. Dr. Jones is listed on her website as a DNP, but this is not something the patient has seen and the sign outside of the office only reads, "Dr A. Jones, Family Medicine." After waiting in the examination room for a while, a young lady walks into the room wearing a long white coat with the name "Dr A. Jones" embroidered on the coat and a stethoscope around her neck. The patient signs the consent forms, and Dr. Jones proceeds to take a history, examine the patient, and prescribe treatment. Only when things go awry, however, does the patient find out that Dr. Jones is a DNP, not an MD or DO. At no time did Dr. Jones explain this to the patient, nor did she inform the patient that she was not a physician (although there are some NPs who now insist upon calling themselves "cathopathic physicians"). A lawsuit ensues, and the usual issue of *negligence* is claimed but is then followed by *misrepresentation* and *lack of informed consent*.

It is important to note that many NPs will advertise themselves as specialists, even when no such nursing specialty exists. In this case, NPs may call themselves oncologic NPs, and a patient who relies upon that designation to their detriment has been misled as surely as any other. Unlike physicians, however, there is no control exercised in many jurisdictions over the use of these terms, so NPs are legally permitted to use them despite their misleading implication of additional training.

FRAUD

Perhaps the easiest way to think of fraud is that it is the *intentional* use of deceit, trick, or other dishonest means to deprive another person of their money, property, or a legal right. More formally, fraud requires showing by clear and convincing evidence an intentional and knowing misrepresentation of material fact made with intent to mislead and relied upon by another to his or her detriment.[19] In the case of oncology, the most likely place for this to occur is in billing. An attorney defending a client against fraud charges will most frequently use the "intentional" and "knowing" part of the definition (what is known as *mens rea* in criminal law) to have the charges (in a criminal proceeding) or lawsuit dropped, alleging that there was no *intent*, only *error*. This works best in criminal proceedings but can work in civil proceedings as well. What happens, though, when the evidence shows something else, and why does it matter to our discussion here? It matters because, as pointed out later in this section, the physician is rarely the one who actually transmits the invoice.

There are two possibilities in medical practice: self-employment (or employment by your professional corporation) or employment by a health care system or hospital (which could also contract with your professional corporation). As with physicians, MLPs may be sole proprietors, may work for a corporation, or may work under a corporate structure that contracts with others and therefore falls within the penumbra of the issue of sending invoices to payers. It is unusual, therefore, for a physician to closely monitor the invoices sent for an MLP's services. Even if one is in solo practice (perhaps *especially* in solo practice), most doctors assume that they have checked the right box or that their billing clerk, computer, or electronic medical record will enter the right code. If a billing service is used, there is even another step removing the physician from the actual invoice transmitted for payment. Now, to be clear, errors happen, and people rarely get into trouble if a few errors are made and then corrected. What happens, though, if errors become pervasive, and how might that occur? Many oncologists as well as MLPs work for themselves or are in a group practice, whereas many others work for a hospital, health care system, or similar entity. When they are presented with billing forms to sign, physicians do not always examine every form critically or spend valuable time on what many consider to be a trivial pursuit. If the "system" routinely sends a bill for a *physician's* services that the NP actually performed, it may be considered fraud, and even if there was no *intent* on the part of the physician, it could lead to civil or even criminal litigation against the physician or group. How this mistake happens is simple and not easy to prevent: if a physician employs an MLP or the MLP is employed by an entity the physician works for or contracts with and the physician signs the chart after the fact as part of the physician's oversight function, the system may interpret this as the physician's provision of the service and bill it as such. Perhaps more important are the more nefarious and intentional occurrences of this type of fraud.

Health care systems throughout the United States have been charged with fraud, and there is a difference in reimbursement between a service provided by an MLP and one provided by a physician.[20] The reason for that difference is obvious, but for some corporations (as well as unscrupulous independent physicians), it seems worth the risk to receive millions of dollars in additional compensation. Moreover, if one is on salary, they may not even know that their name, education, and license are being used for this purpose. It is important, therefore, that invoices are periodically examined to avoid this issue. Even if another person has committed the fraud, in many cases, the physician may also be held liable for damages.

How does this relate to oncology? A good example is given us by the court in *Kelly Woodruff, MD, and Hawaii Children's Blood and Cancer Group v Hawaii Pacific Health et al*. Here, a hematology/oncology group was sending in bills for procedures performed by an NP, including (1) "Chemotherapy into CNS [Central Nervous System]"; (2) "Bone Marrow Aspiration"; (3) "Bone Marrow Biopsy"; and (4) "Lumbar Puncture, Diagnostic."[21] In this case, the facility was already under a compliance agreement with the federal government, and despite this appeal, the court held the oncology group liable for the illegal billing.

Finally, another example that may be applicable, especially in the field of oncology, is billing an NP's services as *incident to* those of a physician. Generally speaking, if a visit is billed under the MLP's own billing personal identification number, the service will be paid at about 85% of the amount paid for a physician. If billed as *incident to* a physician visit, it will be paid at 100% of the physician's fee amount. The rules for this can be found on the CMS website, but for practical purposes, *incident to* services are defined as "those services that are furnished incident to physician professional services in the physician's office (whether located in a separate office suite or within an institution) or in a patient's home."[22] While this sounds simple enough, there are specific criteria that must be met before such billing can legally occur. For example, for an *incident to* bill to be legitimate, the physician must be physically present in the office and remain "actively involved" before such services can be billed. In addition. The services provided by the NP must be:

- An integral part of the patient's treatment course
- Commonly rendered without charge (included in the physician's bills)
- Of a type commonly furnished in a physician's office or clinic (not in an institutional setting)
- An expense to the physician[22]

Importantly, the NP cannot be treating a new condition, only one that already exists. Unfortunately, much confusion surrounds this type of billing. For example, if an NP is employed by an oncologist and is completing the patient visit after the patient was briefly seen by the physician and the patient raises a new problem that was not previously discussed, is appropriately treated by the NP, and leaves the office, was that visit still *incident to* the physician visit? If the NP treated a new problem, possibly not, but it is obvious how these types of bills can get sent out as *incident to* the visit when they do not meet the criteria. If this happens a few times, it is unlikely to be picked up by the system, let alone prosecuted, but if a practice makes it a habit to bill this way, it will eventually raise red flags.

PREVENTION

Perhaps the most important question to ask in this chapter is as follows: What can be done to prevent these issues from adversely affecting physicians and/or their institutions?

The first and most important action that can be taken to prevent issues is simple *identification*. All employees should wear name badges that identify their medical degrees. There should be no lab coats and scrubs that read, for example, "Dr John Jones," but rather, they should read "John Jones, MD" or "Jane Jones, DO." That means that an MLP should wear a tag reading, for example, "Mary Doe, NP" or "John Doe, PA." A nurse with a DNP should not wear a tag that says "Dr," but rather, "Mary Jones, DNP."

Second, an information brochure should be made available to all patients, and perhaps available on the website as well, listing the academic credentials and education of all practitioners in the group. *There is no lack of informed consent if the patient is informed.*

Third, the work of an NP or PA should be reviewed, or if in a collaborative agreement, physicians should ensure they are indemnified by *their* insurance or their own employer's insurance for patients who are seen and treated without their knowledge (e.g., the 80% of charts they never got to review). Additionally, whenever possible, physicians should take a minute to see (even via telemedicine) their patient before the patient leaves the office and make sure the patient is aware that their approval of the patient's case was dependent on the MLP's presentation. While this may not represent part of the standard of care, it will go a long way toward making patients comfortable with the care they receive and reassure them that, when necessary, their care is being appropriately overseen.

Fourth, it is important to keep as nearly perfect records as possible of the relationship and interactions with an MLP involved in patient care. It does not take long for a physician to dictate one or two sentences each time the physician offers an opinion that the MLP may or may not follow regarding patient care, but such brief notes have the potential to keep the physician out of the defendant's chair. Moreover, the same goes for the MLP. If an MLP discusses a patient with a physician, the MLP should be sure to note that discussion in the medical record. It may be the MLP's best defense in court.

Finally, the physician should provide as much oversight of the MLP as possible. Remember this one immutable fact, especially in oncology: patients are already emotionally traumatized by their diagnoses and the treatments involved. They are afraid and, in many cases, facing death. They may not remember what the physician told them, even when the explanation was perfect, so the better the record keeping and relationship with the patient, the better the legal outcome.

CONCLUSION

MLPs (or advanced level practitioners as they prefer to be called) are a growing and valuable addition to the panoply of health care providers in the United States, and when properly utilized in appropriate venues and situations, they tend to make health care more affordable and available to many who would otherwise either have a long wait or go without. Unfortunately, like all good things, there are caveats and liabilities that follow. The first issue is their education, which is appropriate to their place in health care but not well understood by the general public. Unfortunately, the education of MLPs is not well overseen by credentialing bodies, as was the case in medicine prior to the Flexner report. Moreover, in addition to longer and more formal training, additional licensing and board examinations should perhaps be added to educational minimums for MLPs before achieving any degree of autonomy in practice, especially in a field as complex as oncology. Perhaps MLPs could then justifiably claim to be oncologic NPs because of their additional training and certification. MLP practice is also fraught with the liability issues all practitioners face, such as negligence and informed consent, in addition to issues that less frequently touch physicians, such as misrepresentation. In addition, although many practitioners in health care face issues such as fraud, there are additional landmines to be avoided when billing for services provided by MLPs. Finally, there are legal issues involved with MLP practice, especially autonomous practice, such as setting and testifying to the standard of care to be applied in each situation. Until these issues are surmounted and the answers clarified by the courts, there will continue to be uncertain liability for physicians and others who employ, work with, supervise, or are even in professional contact with MLPs in clinical practice.

KEY POINTS:

- MLPs are becoming increasingly important members of the health care team in the United States.
- An increasing number of jurisdictions are allowing independent practice of NPs and PAs.
- Differences in education between physicians and MLPs mandate that the supervising physician or facility, as well as the MLPs themselves, be careful that the medical practice of MLPs does not overreach their education, training, and experience.
- Just as with physicians and health care facilities, there are both the usual liability issues with MLPs and some that are specific to them.
- The best solution is prevention, and there is no better means of prevention than education of the patient and clear identification of the person providing care.

References:

1. Duke physician assistant program: the birthplace of the physician assistant profession. Duke University and Duke University Health System. https://fmch.duke.edu/duke-physician-assistant-program/news-and-events/duke-physician-assistant-program-birthplace. Accessed August 30, 2021.
2. Kohler S. The development of the nurse practitioner and physician assistant professions. The Commonwealth Fund, Robert Wood Johnson Foundation, and Carnegie Corporation of New York, 1965. https://cspcs.sanford.duke.edu/sites/default/files/descriptive/nurse_practitioners_and_physician_assistants.pdf. Accessed August 30, 2021.
3. State practice environment. American Association of Nurse Practitioners. May 2020. https://www.aanp.org/advocacy/state/state-practice-environment. Accessed August 30, 2021.
4. Family Nurse Practitioner Program information. Vanderbilt University https://nursing.vanderbilt.edu/msn/fnp/index.php. Accessed August 30, 2021.
5. Primary health care professionals: a comparison. American Academy of Family Physicians.
6. Flexner A. *Medical Education in the United States and Canada: A Report to the Carnegie Foundation for the Advancement of Teaching.* New York, NY: Hardpress Publishing; 1910.
7. See *Harvey v Kindred Healthcare Operating, Inc.*, 578 SW3d 638, 648 (Tex App 2019); *Thompson v Center for Pediatric & Adolescent Medicine, LLC*, 244 So 3d 441 (La App 1 Cir, 2018).

8. Kruger J, Dunning D. Unskilled and unaware of it: how difficulties in recognizing one's own incompetence lead to inflated self-assessments. *J Pers Soc Psychol*. 1999;77(6):1121–1134.

9. Micu A. The Dunning-Kruger effect, or why the ignorant think they're experts. Feature Post, Psychology Science. February 13, 2020. https://www.zmescience.com/science/the-dunning-kruger-effect-feature/. Accessed August 30, 2021.

10. Pa Stat Tit 40, § 1303.512.

11. *Nasser v St Vincent Hospital and Health Services*, 926 NE2d 43 (2010).

12. *Aillones v Minton*, 77 NE3d 196 (2017).

13. *Hamilton v Pike County, Kentucky et al.,* No. 7:2011cv00099, Document 61 (ED Ky 2012).

14. *Warren v Dinter*, 926 NW2d 370 (Minn 2019).

15. See *Roe v Wade*, 410 US 113, 93 S Ct 705; 35 L Ed 2d 147 (1973 US LEXIS 159).

16. See *Canterbury v Spence*, 464 F2d 772 (US App DC 1972).

17. *Shinal v Toms*, 162 A3d 429 (2017).

18. See, for example, *Hart v Browne*, 103 Cal App 3d 947 (1980), and *Metric Investment, Inc. v Patterson*, 244 A2d 311 (NJ 1968).

19. See generally *Flippo v CSC Assocs. III, LLC*, 262 Va 48, 547 SE2d 216).

20. See *Shanti v Allstate Insurance Company*, 356 SW3d (Tex App, Houston [14 Dist] 2011), in which, *inter alia*, the physicians and facility were held to be liable for services provided by a nurse practitioner but billed as though provided by a physician.

21. *Kelly Woodruff, MD, and Hawaii Children's Blood and Cancer Group v Hawaii Pacific Health et al.*, No. 29447 (Haw Ct App January 14, 2014).

22. MLN Matters. Centers for Medicare and Medicaid Services. https://www.cms.gov/outreach-and-education/medicare-learning-network-mln/mlnmattersarticles/downloads/se0441.pdf. Accessed August 30, 2021.

CHAPTER 24

Quality Improvement

William J. Pao, MD, JD, FACR

INTRODUCTION

Oncologists can run afoul of the law when conducting quality improvement projects in three different scenarios. The first is in the setting of a quality review related to patient care. Many states have enacted immunity statutes for quality improvement review, and Congress has enacted the Health Care Quality Improvement Act, where most of the litigation in this subject has been focused. The second is if a quality improvement study becomes a research project, encroaching on a patient's self-determination and well-being. Finally, the third is in the context of payment for quality improvement, where the quality improvement study is linked to increased payment for clinical services.

Taguchi and Clausing[1] state that "quality is being on target with minimal variation." The idea of quality improvement began with guild craftsmen in 13th century Europe.[2] However, quality concepts did not influence the practice of medicine until the 20th century. Health care quality is often associated with the reduction of medical errors, a concept credited to Dr. Ernest Codman, a founder of the American College of Surgeons (ACOS). Codman noted that most medical journals only touted good results. He stated that real improvements would be made when clinicians wrote about their errors and how to reduce them.[3] By the 1980s, with the rise of health care technology (and profits), the corporatization of health care led to industrial methods to achieve quality improvement. Deming, Juran, Berwick, Donabedian, and others pioneered quality concepts in health care.[4] Oncologists usually get involved in quality management by serving on hospital committees, including credentialing and cancer committees. The American Society of Clinical Oncology (ASCO) has implemented their Quality Training Programs in the United States and abroad. Quality improvement literature in oncology has increased ten-fold in the past decade.

A widely quoted definition of quality in health care is from the Institute of Medicine (IOM), the predecessor of the National Academy of Medicine, and states that "quality of care is the degree to which health services for individuals and populations increase the likelihood of desired health outcomes and are consistent with current professional knowledge."[5] Today, many organizations in health care evaluate methods, metrics, compliance, and outcomes. Table 24-1 lists a sampling of the larger organizations. At the heart of quality improvement is the collection of data.[6] The goal of quality improvement is improved patient outcomes, which are often achieved by reduction of medical errors by following clinical pathways or guidelines. Because much of

Table 24-1. Health Care Quality Improvement Organizations

Organization	Notes
Centers for Medicare and Medicaid Services (cms.gov) QIO-Like Entity	Designated under § 1903(a)(3)(C) of the Social Security Act
Agency for Healthcare Research and Quality (ahrq.gov)	Provides funding for health-related quality improvement projects
The Joint Commission (thejointcommission.org)	Accrediting agency evaluates quality process and outcomes
National Academy of Medicine (Former Institute of Medicine) (nam.edu)	Created by Congress in 1863 Advises government on health care policy
National Committee for Quality Assurance (ncqa.org)	HEDIS data set measures health data on 190 million Americans
National Quality Forum (nqf.org)	"Driving measurable health improvements"
Robert Wood Johnson Foundation (rwjf.org)	Funding health care and health equality initiatives
Kaiser Family Foundation (kff.org)	Studies the effects of diseases and health policy on communities
Institute for Healthcare Improvement (ihi.org)	Optimize health system performance Population and individual health Per capita cost of health care

Abbreviations: HEDIS, Healthcare Effectiveness Data and Information Set; QIO, quality improvement organization.

medical practice (including oncology) is not always grounded on level I or level II scientific evidence,[7,8] which data points to be measured in a quality improvement study can be subject to debate. Another reason quality improvement is important to oncology practices is that, by reducing error, adverse events are decreased, which in turn lowers the risk of medical malpractice lawsuits. Finally, many health care payment contracts are tied to quality metrics (adherence to clinical practice guidelines), which, when achieved, lead to higher payments for clinical services.

CLINICAL PRACTICE GUIDELINES

The IOM's definition of quality ends with the phrase "consistent with current professional knowledge," which is embodied in clinical practice guidelines (CPGs) in the practice of oncology. CPGs are used to promote quality care in oncology, and they are developed by various oncology organizations. CPGs have the following limitations: (1) They may be developed using other factors outside of scientific evidence (e.g., access and cost). (2) Guidelines apply to the "perfect patient" and may not apply to every individual. (3) Guidelines often become outdated.[9] (4) Guidelines from oncology societies often has a disclaimer. For example, a guideline from ASCO, the American Society of Therapeutic Radiology and Oncology (ASTRO), and the Society of Surgical Oncology (SSO) states that "the information is not intended to substitute for the independent professional judgment of the treating physician, as the information does not account for individual variation among patients."[10]

CPGs have no intrinsic legal significance. Several states (Maine, Florida, Kentucky, and Minnesota) tried to incorporate CPGs as standards of care in the 1990s, but most have been repealed.[11]

Courts have neither equated deviation from CPGs as negligence nor equated adherence to CPGs as release from liability. Most courts will admit CPGs as evidence depending on their reliability and relevance to a particular case.[12] In *Ellis v Eng*, the appeals court in New York considered ASCO guidelines in exculpating the liability of the defendant physician.[13] Although legal scholars predicted decades ago that CPGs would carry more weight as evidence,[14] the progress has been glacial. CPGs are more often included as one of the determinative factors, but not the sole element, in the standard of care.[15]

LEGAL LIABILITY IN QUALITY REVIEW

Quality improvement in oncology

Cancer programs, similar to many other health care organizations, participate in quality initiatives at local, regional, and national levels. For many hospitals and clinics, morbidity and mortality (sentinel event) reviews (M&M) focus on near misses and adverse patient outcomes, usually within a specific specialty. Several courts have held that M&M reviews do fall under quality peer review confidentiality,[16] as discussed in the next section.

In health care, quality improvement is often tied to peer review. In many health care organizations, adverse events occur, which in turn lead to quality management reviews. Because adverse events are often tied to mistakes attributed to the actions of health care providers, peer review of those actions becomes a part of that quality improvement review. Medical organizations participate in the ACOS Commission on Cancer (CoC) Quality Improvement Projects, and the topics often focus on the six attributes of quality health care as defined by the IOM (Table 24-2).[17] The CoC Rapid Quality Reporting System (RQRS) looks at monthly updates to oncology metrics such as postlumpectomy radiation therapy rates, endocrine therapy for estrogen receptor–positive breast cancer, and 12 regional nodes removed during colon cancer surgery. On a national level, ASTRO sponsors the Radiation Oncology Incident Learning Service (ROILS), which allows its 500 participant institutions to send internal incidents, near misses, and unsafe conditions to a federally listed patient safety organization. The data are blinded, and reports are updated at least on a monthly basis, with the aim to achieve correct administration of radiation treatments.

Table 24-2. Elements of Quality Health Care

1. **Safety:** Freedom from accidental injury of patients and health care workers from care intended to help patients.
2. **Effectiveness:** Care based on scientific evidence. Includes prevention, diagnosis and treatment that produces better outcomes than other alternatives, including the alternative of doing nothing.
3. **Patient-Centeredness:** Care tailored to meet the physical and psychological needs of the specific patient, including the ability to make informed decisions about their own care.
4. **Timeliness:** Delivery of care without excessive delay.
5. **Efficiency:** Reduction of waste and reduction of administrative or production costs.
6. **Equity:** Equal access to health care and equity in caregiving.

The healthcare quality improvement act

The most common cause of legal action in quality improvement occurs in the context of health care provider decision making within a health care organization committee. Quality review in this context is distinguished from peer review in a research context (e.g., peer review of a scientific paper) or peer review of a physician's conduct (e.g., harassment of coworkers, absenteeism). Quality improvement review in this setting is primarily connected with patient-centered metrics, such as timeliness of care, patient safety, and clinical outcomes.

Quality review committees were the outgrowth of two unrelated concepts: hospital liability and Medicare payments. Prior to 1950, hospitals were not liable for their patients' medical mishaps. However, by the 1970s, hospitals were often found guilty of medical malpractice under the legal concepts of *respondeat superior* (liability through the actions of their employees and physicians)[18] and corporate negligence (the corporate practice of medicine).[19] By 1965, in order to receive Medicare and Medicaid funding, a hospital had to receive accreditation by The Joint Commission, and one part of the accreditation process involved the establishment of a hospital quality improvement committee. Quality review committee members were subject to litigation by physicians who lost hospital privileges and by injured patients seeking information on the defendant-physicians subjected to peer review. As hospitals also became defendants in these legal actions, medical and hospital associations lobbied their state legislatures and the US Congress to enact legislation to immunize peer review proceedings from discovery in litigation[20] to a allow fair and honest evaluations in the peer review process. As a result, many states have enacted their own version of health care quality improvement statutes (Table 24-3).

The tipping point for enacting a federal law occurred in the case of *Patrick v Burget*. Dr. Timothy Patrick, a solo practice surgeon, sued the Astoria Clinic and its physicians under the Sherman Antitrust Act for antitrust and sham quality review resulting in loss of hospital privileges and income. The case was appealed to the 9th Circuit Court of Appeals, which ruled in Patrick's favor, awarding him $2.3 million and disbanding the Astoria Clinic.[21] This case was discussed in the *New England Journal of Medicine*[22] and caused many physicians to avoid participating in peer review committees fearing future litigation. As one step in turning the tide of increased medical malpractice litigation, Representative Ron Wyden introduced the Healthcare Quality Improvement Act (HCQIA), which was signed into law by President Ronald Regan in 1986.[23]

Peer review immunity

The HCQIA (42 USC 11101) was enacted in two parts. The first part provides immunity, and the second part requires reporting of the findings to a national data bank. The first part of the HCQIA provides immunity for quality review committee physicians and witnesses from liability in damages "regarding the professional conduct of a physician . . . under any law of the United States or of any State."[24] To be eligible for this immunity, the peer review must satisfy the following four requirements under the HCQIA:

1. in the reasonable belief that the action was in the furtherance of quality of medical care,
2. after a reasonable effort to obtain the facts of the matter,

Table 24-3. **Healthcare Quality Improvement Statutes and Case Law by State**

State	Statute	Case Law
Alabama	§6–5–333	*Lindsay v Baptist Health Sys, Inc.*, 154 So3d 90 (Ala 2014)
Arizona	36-45.02(B)	*Goodman v Samaritan Health System*, 990 P2d 1061 (Ariz App 1999)
California	BPC 11-809	*Fahlen v Sutter Center Valley Hosp*, 318 P3d 833 (Cal 2014)
Colorado	§12-36.5-101	*Nicholas v North Colorado Med Ctr*, 12 P3d 280 (Colo App 1999)
Connecticut	§19a-17b	*Grenier v Stamford Hosp*, 3:14-cv-0970 (VLB) (D Conn 2016)
Delaware	24 Del C §1768	*Lipson v Anesthesia Services, PA*, 790 A2d 1261 (Del Super 2001)
Florida	766.101, Fl Stat	*Fullerton v Florida Medical Ass'n, Inc.*, 973 So2d 1144 (Fla App 2006)
Hawaii	Ch 671D	
Illinois	735 ILCS 5/8-2101	*Valfer v Evanston Nw Healthcare*, 31 NE3d 883 (Ill App 2015)
Indiana	§34-30-15-19	*Mann v Johnson Memorial Hosp*, 611 NE2d 676 (Ind App 1993)
Kansas	65-442	*Hildyard v Citizens Med Ctr, Non-Profit Corp*, 286 P3d 239 (Kan App 2012)
Kentucky		*Univ of Ky v Bunnell*, 532 SW3d 658 (Ky Ct App 2017)
Louisiana		*Tebault v E Jefferson Gen Hosp*, No. 18-C-539 (La App 2019)
Maine	Tit 32 Ch 48 §3293	
Maryland		*Cornfeld v Board of Physicians*, 921 A2d 893 (Md App 2007)
Massachusetts		*Gargiulo v Baystate Health, Inc.*, 826 F Supp 2d 323 (D Mass 2011)
Michigan	331.531(3) and (4)	*El-Khalil v Oakwood Health Inc.*, 934 NW2d 665 (Mich 2016)
Minnesota	§§145.63-145.64	*Larson v Wasemiller*, 738 NW2d 300 (Minn 2007)
Mississippi	§41-63-1	*Som v Natchez Reg'l Med Ctr*, 98 So3d 500 (Miss App 2012)
Missouri		*Johnson v SSM Healthcare Sys*, 988 F Supp 2d 1080 (ED Mo 2013)
Montana	§37-2-201	
Nevada	§49.117	*Clark v Columbia/HCA Info Servs*, 25 P3d 215 (Nev 2001)
New Hampshire	§329:13-b	
New Jersey	§2A:84A–22.10	*Hurwitz v AHS Hosp Corp*, 103 A3d 285 (NJ Super App Div 2014)
New Mexico	§41–9–1 to –7	*Tanner v McMurray*, 405 F Supp 3d 1115 (D NM 2019)
New York	Art.131 – 6527	*Morshed v St Barnabas Hosp*, 16 Civ 2862 (LGS) (SD NY 2017)
North Carolina	§131E–95	*Estate of Ray v Forgy*, 783 SE2d 1 (NC App 2016)
North Dakota	23-12-12; 23-31-01	
Ohio		*Wilson v Barnesville Hosp*, 783 NE2d 554 (Ohio App 2002)
Oklahoma	Tit 63 §1-1709	*Cohlmia v St. John Med Ctr*, 906 F Supp 2d 1188 (ND Okla 2012)
Oregon	Tit 4 §41.675	
Pennsylvania	63 PRPA §425	*Estate of Krappa v Lyons*, 211 A3d 869 (Pa Super Ct 2019)
South Carolina	§40-71-10	

(Continued)

Table 24-3. Healthcare Quality Improvement Statutes and Case Law by State (*Continued*)

State	Statute	Case Law
South Dakota	§36-4-25	*Miller v Huron Reg'l Med Ctr*, 145 F Supp 3d 873 (D S Dakota)
Tennessee	§63-6-219	*Pinkard v HCA Health Serv of Tenn, Inc.*, 545 SW3d 443 (2017)
Texas	§160.001	*Batra v Covenant Health Sys*, 562 SW3d 696 (Tex App 2018)
Utah	§58-13-4	*Levitt v Iasis Healthcare Holdings, Inc.*, 442 P3d 1211 (Utah App 2019)
Vermont	26 VSA §1445-8	
Virginia	§8.01-581.13	
Washington	RCW 70.41.200	*Lowy v PeaceHealth*, 280 P3d 1078 (Wash 2012)
West Virginia	§§30-3C-1—5	*Earhart v Elder*, 5:18-CV-01000 (SD WVa 2019)
Wisconsin	§146.37	*Rechsteiner v Hazelden*, 753 NW2d 496 (Wis 2008)
Wyoming	§35-2-910	

3. after adequate notice and hearing procedures are afforded to the physician involved after such other procedures are fair to the physician under the circumstances, and
4. in the reasonable belief that the action was warranted by the facts known.[24]

In addition, the findings need to be reported to the national data bank, and if there is non-compliance, the immunity privilege will not apply. Finally, the HCQIA allows the quality review committee to recuperate attorneys' fees and costs in the defense of the lawsuit if the claim was "frivolous, unreasonable, without foundation or in bad faith."[25]

The national practitioner data bank

The second part of the HCQIA creates a data bank that requires the quality review committee to report an action that "revokes or suspends (or otherwise restricts) a physician's license or censures, reprimands, or places on probation a physician" or "to which a physician's license is surrendered."[26] Any actions are required to be reported to the Board of Medical Examiners, and such reports must be updated on a monthly basis.[27] In addition, all hospitals are required to query the data bank when a new physician applies for medical privileges.[28] The Department of Health and Human Services (HHS) developed the data bank, called the National Practitioner Data Bank (NPDB), in 1988, and it began operation in 1990. The major purpose of the NPDB was to legally mandate communication among states regarding disciplined physicians. This was to prevent physicians disciplined by one medical board from relocating to another state to practice substandard medical care. Today, the NPDB covers all licensed professionals involved in health care, from physicians to cytologists and athletic trainers and even insurance brokers.[29] The second part of HCQIA also provides for confidentiality of the information to the NPDB—the information in the peer review is confidential except for a future peer review process or medical malpractice actions.[30]

The HCQIA and quality peer review statutes as applied in the courts

For a physician or committee performing a quality review to acquire immunity, the following four requirements of the HCQIA must be satisfied:

1. The review must be performed for purposes of quality health care, which is often tied to patient care. Courts have given wide latitude to the peer review process for many aspects of patient care, including being nonresponsive to patients, lack of documentation,[31] poor clinical judgment, and high postsurgical infection rates.[32] Some courts have extended the cause for peer review based on the "totality of circumstances" and not on individual patient cases.[33] In *Robinson v Reg'l Hematology and Oncology*, the court extended the peer review privilege in a medical malpractice case, preventing the plaintiff from accessing the quality review records.[34] Personal conduct outside the hospital can also be justified in a peer review process. In *Moore v Williamsburg Regional Hospital*,[35] where a general surgeon who treated both adults and children was found guilty of sexually abusing his daughter and lost his hospital privileges, the court ruled that the hospital (the defendant) could use the HCQIA immunity privilege for its peer review members, as long as the hospital used a fair and reasonable process for its determination. Even consumption of alcohol while on call can be grounds for a quality review process protected by the HCQIA.[36]

2. The review is reasonable and fact based. The HCQIA does not provide guidelines as to the review process. Factors considered by courts as to the reasonableness of the inquiry include (1) whether the information is factual and unbiased; (2) whether the physician investigated was interviewed and allowed to rebut the evidence[37]; and (3) whether witnesses were interviewed.[38] In *Brandner v Bateman*,[39] the court explained that the HCQIA does not require a hospital to "carry out its investigation in any particular manner; it is only required to conduct a factual investigation that is reasonable under the circumstances." Moreover, the HCQIA only requires a reasonable inquiry and not a perfect investigation.[40] There is no requirement that any of the reviewers be of the same specialty as the physician being reviewed.[41]

3. The physician being reviewed must be given fair notice. This is the due process clause of the HCQIA. There are no definitive rules to determine the fairness of the process, but it is apparent that physicians cannot be abruptly summoned to the review committee and then stripped of their privileges.[42] The HCQIA states that (1) the physician can choose to be represented by another person or an attorney; (2) the physician is notified of specific cases to be reviewed and the witnesses to be present; (3) the physician can testify, cross-examine the witnesses, and bring their own expert witnesses; and (4) a written recommendation is presented to the investigated physician.[24,43]

4. The action taken by the review committee is based on the known facts. The HCQIA gives the benefit of the doubt to the quality review committee, it is presumed that the facts and conclusions of the quality review committee are correct and justify its actions, and it is up to the investigated physician to present evidence to overcome the conclusions.[44] Members of the quality committee should not be in direct economic competition with the investigated physician.[45] However, the conclusions of the quality committee have to be based on a "reasonable belief."[24] Courts have held that reasonable belief is an objective standard that is upheld "if the reviewers, with the information available to them at the time of the professional review action, would reasonably have concluded that their actions would restrict incompetent behavior or would protect patients."[46] In other words, the facts have to support the conclusions.

CASE LAW # 1

In *Peyton v Johnson City Medical Center*, a radiation oncologist was removed from the medical staff after the quality committee found five wrongful radiation treatment incidents in a single year, including 30 treatments to the left kidney for a right-sided renal tumor, placing a radioactive source in the wrong site in two separate patients, and unduly exposing the public with improper storage of radioactive material after a brachytherapy procedure.[47] In *Drabnick v Sebelius*, a quality committee found that a medical oncologist's incorrect calculation led to an overdose 5-flourouracil, causing the death of a cancer patient and leading to a report in the NPDB.[48] When properly applied, the HCQIA immunizes quality review committees in lawsuits by physicians dismissed or reported for improper practice.

Piercing the veil of the HCQIA

Even when the previously listed four requirements are satisfied, there are instances in which the HCQIA would fail to provide immunity for the quality review committee members. One explicit exception occurs when the suit involves a civil rights matter (e.g., discrimination). This is explicitly stated in the HCQIA.[49] That provision has been upheld in federal court when plaintiffs have alleged the quality review committee violated their civil rights, whether based on gender and disability,[50] race,[51] or a Health Insurance Portability and Accountability Act violation.[52]

A second exception occurs if the physician is not a member of the organization that performed the quality review on that physician; HCQIA immunity only applies to members within the peer review organization. In *Austin v American Association of Neurological Surgeons*,[53] a neurosurgeon was suspended from membership in the American Association of Neurological Surgeons, and he filed an action for damages and injunctive relief against the association, alleging that the suspension was in retaliation for his having testified as an expert witness for the plaintiff in a medical malpractice action brought against another neurosurgeon, who was also a member of the association. The 7th Circuit Court affirmed the trial court's entry of summary judgment against the neurosurgeon. However, in *Fullerton v Florida Medical Association* (FMA),[54] the FMA issued a statement that the plaintiff's (Dr. Fullerton) testimony in a medical malpractice trial fell below medical standards. Dr. Fullerton sued the FMA, alleging defamation and tortious interference. The FMA used the HCQIA's immunity statute for defense. The court of appeals ruled that the immunity privilege applied only to a physician in the same organization being reviewed by a quality assurance committee and not medical testimony. Because Fullerton was not a member of the FMA, the HCQIA immunity privilege did not apply.

A third exception occurs during credentialing of physicians to join a medical staff. In *Jacksonian v Temple University Health System*,[55] the plaintiff in a malpractice suit successfully compelled the hospital's credentials committee to reveal whether it had queried the NPDB before admitting the defendant physician into its medical staff. The HCQIA does not grant immunity in the quality review of admitting new physicians into the medical staff. However, under state law in certain jurisdictions, immunity is granted to the peer review process in credentialing potential hires.

Finally, some states have opted out of the HCQIA. Prior to the HCQIA, several states enacted their own peer review immunity statutes, most notably in California and Maryland (both opted out of many HCQIA provisions with their own peer review statutes). However, all states are still required to report sanctioned physicians to the NPDB. The quality review immunity privilege continues despite much litigation regarding its validity in varied facts and circumstances.

The patient safety and quality improvement act

A major role of quality improvement is the reduction of medical errors. In response to the IOM's report of widespread medial errors in US health care,[56] Congress enacted the Patient Safety and Quality Improvement Act (PSQIA) in 2005. The PSQIA (Pub L 109-41) was intended to create patient safety organizations (PSOs) and immunizes "patient safety work product" from discovery or subpoenas.[57] The PSQIA is administered under the Agency for Healthcare Research and Quality (AHRQ). Courts have ruled that "work product from patient safety reviews" is privileged in malpractice cases,[58] although civil rights litigation voids that privilege.[59] The PSQIA also indemnifies whistleblowers and does not allow "adverse employment actions" against an employee who submits a report if "the individual in good faith reported information." The protections are only afforded to the whistleblower if the PSO is federally certified. In *Bulhoff v Hospital of University of Pennsylvania*, an employee was not afforded protection for termination after she reported the misadministration of oncology medication in an outpatient clinic; the court ruled that the University of Pennsylvania's Safety Net reporting system was not a federally certified PSO.[60]

PSQIA immunity has been challenged in several states. For example, Florida passed Amendment 7 in 2003 (adding Section 25 to Title X of the Florida Constitution), which allows patients access to "any records made or received in the course of business by a health care facility or provider relating to any adverse medical incident." In *S Baptist Hospital of Florida, Inc, v Charles*, the Florida Supreme Court ruled that the Florida Constitution allows discovery of "safety evaluation report" proceedings in a medical malpractice case.[61] The Federal District Court in Florida also weighed in on this matter in *Florida Health Sciences Center v Azar*, holding that the PSQIA does preempt Florida's Amendment 7.[62] In Kentucky, the state supreme court narrowly interpreted the PSQIA immunity privilege in *Tibbs v Bunnell*,[63] ruling that an incident report was not privileged under the PSQIA. The above litigation continues to challenge the confidentiality of information reported to PSOs, such as ASTRO's ROILS.

The HCQIA and PSQIA persist today to immunize the quality review committee but continue to be challenged in the courts. Moreover, as more physicians and health care providers are employed by hospital systems, their termination (often for providing substandard care) may no longer go through a formal quality review process. In fact, risk managers (who are not immunized by the HCQIA) who mine the data from electronic medical records can analyze practice patterns among the health care staff. The termination may be via contractual language, and the event will not be recorded in the NPDB. By bypassing the formal quality review process, potentially more substandard practitioners can evade detection by credentialing committees. The HCQIA and PSAQIA may need further modernization to adapt to current health care practices.[64]

QUALITY IMPROVEMENT VERSUS HUMAN RESEARCH

Oncologists can violate the law and biomedical ethics when the quality improvement projects they perform become research. The Common Rule was established in 1981 by the HHS to regulate biomedical research in the United States via the institutional review board (IRB). The first revision was in 1991 (Title 45 CFR 46), and the second revision was in 2017. Quality improvement, at its core, collects and analyzes data on patients to improve a health care interaction. Research requires that a patient knowingly consents (without enticement or coercion) to one of several alternate interventions to obtain a less certain outcome (e.g., treatment or placebo). Table 24-4 compares the differences between quality improvement and research studies. A major difference is that research usually requires a patient's informed consent, but quality improvement projects usually do not. Many IRBs have checklists that help clinicians differentiate between the two. Although rare, large disease databases created for quality studies have been alleged to be converted to human research projects in order to acquire government funds. In a case involving the Roswell Park Cancer Institute, a senior researcher unsuccessfully sued the institution for converting a prostate cancer database to clinical research without IRB approval.[65] In today's world of electronic medical records and artificial intelligence in health care systems, the line between quality improvement and research is increasingly blurred.

Table 24-4. **Quality Improvement versus Research**

	Quality Improvement	Research
Knowledge	Implement current knowledge	Designed to develop new knowledge
Routine care	Part of routine care	Independent of routine care
Scope	Local or regional implementation	Generalizable practice
Duration	Short (months)	Long (years)
Purpose	Integrate standard of care into routine health care delivery	Seeks new knowledge and new standards of care
Design	Flexible, adaptive; rapid feedback	Rigid, minimal changes; results not known until data analysis later
Benefits	Directly benefits a process or program; intends to benefit patient care	May or may not benefit the research subjects; intends to benefit science
Risks	None or minimal risk to patients; possible loss of data privacy	Can place research subjects at risk of harm
Awareness	Subjects unaware as part of clinical process	Subjects required to be informed
Obligation	Participation as part of the care process	No obligation to participate
Consent	No consent required; not possible to obtain consent	Informed consent often required

Violation of the Common Rule can lead to loss of present and future institutional funding by the government and sanctions against performing research for both the institutions and individuals involved. Department of Defense (DOD) military personnel can be sanctioned under the Military Code of Justice, and civilian employees of the DOD can be terminated. Some states have stricter standards for the conduct of human research, but only California allows for sanctions for failure to obtain informed consent. The California Safety Code (Vol 40B § 24176, 1995) authorizes monetary sanctions for failure to obtain informed consent ($1000), for willful conduct (up to $5000), and if a person is exposed to "a known substantial risk of serious injury, either bodily harm or psychological harm" (incarceration of up to one year and fines up to $10,000).

The latest revision of the Common Rule (45 CFR 690) was finalized in 2017, and ASCO published its summary of the changes in April of 2018. The revised Common Rule did not address the differences between quality improvement and research but did allow for "public health surveillance activities." In July of 2020, the Office of Human Research Protection issued guidance on its website on elimination of IRB review of (selected) research applications and proposals.[66] This implies that the regulation of data mining, including quality improvement studies, may face less regulatory scrutiny in the coming decade. Commentators have noted that the revised Common Rule is already outdated because companies such as 23andMe and Facebook can gather large amounts of health care information on individuals and sell that information for enormous profits.[67]

QUALITY IMPROVEMENT AND FINANCIAL INCENTIVES

Although rare, oncologists can run afoul of the law when quality improvement data are tied to financial incentives. Quality metrics used to be completely separated from medical payments in the past. Prior to the mid-1990s, payment was fee-for-service from insurance and Medicare; claims were submitted by health care providers without specific metrics for the quality of care delivered. As a result of the increasing cost of Medicare, the Centers for Medicare and Medicaid Services (CMS) began exploring alternate payment models (APMs) for medical services. Moreover, in the Medicare Modernization Act of 2003, Congress directed the CMS to explore performance aligned with payment.[68] One effort was the enactment of the Health Information Technology for Economic and Clinical Health Act (HITECH) in 2009, which incentivized physicians and health care organizations to adopt electronic health records (EHRs). The Patient Protection and Affordable Care Act (ACA), signed into law by President Barack Obama in 2010, created the Medicare Shared Savings Program (MSSP), which in turn created accountable care organizations (ACOs); in ACOs, the CMS provides approval for a group of physicians to provide care for a defined population, and any savings that accrue are shared with the physicians. ACOs in oncology had to meet certain quality metrics in order to receive additional payments from CMS; an analysis performed in 2018 showed that 58% of analyzed oncology ACOs met their targets for health care savings.[69] Other such programs are tied to the Hospital Value-Based Purchasing Program for Medicare and include metrics such as readmission rates, drug procurement, and hospital-acquired conditions rates.[70] In 2015, the Center for Medicare and Medicaid

Innovation (CMMI) started the Oncology Care Model (OCM), which determined value-based payments for oncologist. One such initiative held participating medical oncologists accountable for controlling the costs of oncology drugs, which have risen exponentially. An analysis in 2019 showed that over 30% of oncologists had not met their targets mainly due to the administration of immunotherapy drugs.[71]

Tied to all these electronic and alternate payment models are quality metrics that determine payments for services. Beginning in the late 1990s, the federal government began using the False Claims Act (FCA; 31 USC § 3279), a Civil War era statute, to prosecute fraudulent claims by federal contractors, including physicians. To successfully prosecute an FCA claim, the government must prove that (1) the defendant made a statement or representation in an application for payment under a federal program, (2) the statement was false, and (3) the defendant knowingly and willfully made the statement.[72] Many of the FCA prosecutions came from whistleblower (*qui tam*) legal actions. The Department of Justice website (www.justice.gov) is replete with successful prosecutions and settlements of oncology entities convicted of fraudulent practices. For example, in 2017, 21st Century Oncology, Inc., was fined $26 million for FCA violations due to their EHR program under the HITECH Act.[73] Submitting claims under quality incentives to the government requires increased accuracy and scrutiny in order to avoid criminal and civil penalties.

CLINICAL VIGNETTE #1

Dr. Kirk is the newly hired chair of medical oncology at Springfield Memorial Hospital. The department participates in clinical research studies and has been enrolled in the CMS OCM since 2018. While performing an audit of the OCM data, Dr. Kirk notes that Dr. Lee, a staff medical oncologist, has a high oncology pharmacy utilization volume. In addition, as part of the Cancer Committee quality improvement reports, Dr. Kirk notes that Dr. Lee has a much higher rate of chemotherapy delivery within four weeks of a patient's date of death—one of the quality metrics in the oncology department. When approached by Dr. Kirk, Dr. Lee notes that he has generated quality improvement data in the use of chronomodulated endocrine immunotherapy in the treatment of metastatic cancer. Although the agents used are approved by the US Food and Drug Administration for the disease, the timing and combination do not comport with CPGs. While discussing his practice patterns, Dr. Lee notes that he "wanted always to do the best for his patients and never give up." Dr. Kirk is concerned that Dr. Lee's clinical performance may constitute a research issue and a patient safety issue (over treatment of disease) and could jeopardize the OCM reimbursements.

In this particular scenario, the following medicolegal issues need to be considered:

1. Should Dr. Lee be subject to a formal quality review to examine his practice patterns in administering chemotherapy?

2. Is Dr. Lee doing clinical research without IRB approval and patient consent?
3. Will overutilization of oncology pharmaceuticals decrease or void the CMS OCM payments?

To address the first question, conducting a formal peer review should not be taken lightly, as the consequences of an adverse review can lead to loss of clinical privileges. Dr. Lee should be given notice that he will be subjected to a formal review; the date and time should be mutually agreed upon, and he can opt for legal representation and present his own witnesses. To overcome the findings of the quality committee, Dr. Lee has to rebut the presumption of the findings of the committee by a preponderance of the evidence. After review is conducted, the review committee sends the written recommendations to the health care authority in charge of credentialing.

To address the second question, the quality committee also needs to determine whether administering chronomodulated immunotherapy is actually clinical research without IRB approval or patient consent. If this treatment regimen is novel (i.e., untried in the published scientific literature), then it is more likely to be research. Documentation review is performed to ascertain whether patients were informed of this novel regimen versus other therapeutic alternatives or no treatment.

Finally, to address the third question, a utilization committee needs to determine if Dr. Lee overprescribed oncology pharmaceuticals compared to other oncologists in the same practice or region and compared to national benchmarks.

An adverse outcome can lead to Dr. Lee losing his clinical appointment and being reported to the NPDB. By following procedures, the quality committee can acquire immunity from the HCQIA. If Dr. Lee is found to be conducting research without consent and IRB approval, Springfield Memorial Hospital could lose federal funding for research and be sanctioned against performing research temporarily or permanently. Finally, if it is determined that there is overutilization of oncology pharmaceuticals, the institution can have its OCM reimbursement decreased; in egregious cases, the case may be referred to the Department of Justice for investigation for abuse in clinical practice.

CONCLUSION

Quality management is woven into the fabric of clinical oncology. Collection of data, (pertaining to structure, process, and outcomes) are now integrated into oncology practice. The HCQIA and PSQIA codify protections for those who measure quality improvement, and penalties for those who violate the standards of quality in healthcare; the legal standards continue to be modified in legislatures and the courts. Research and quality management are becoming more intertwined. Healthcare payments are increasingly linked to quality metrics, as oncologists seek outcomes to be on target with minimal variation.

KEY POINTS:

- Physicians are often asked to serve on quality review committees.
- Quality committees often review the performance of the organization's health care providers.
- In order to acquire immunity from litigation in the performance of a quality peer review, members of the quality committee must adhere to the 4 requirements of the HCQIA:
  - The review must be related to quality improvement (tied to patient care).
  - The review must be fact based.
  - The reviewed physician must be given fair notice.
  - The conclusion must be based on the facts.
- In an adverse finding by the quality committee, the findings must be report in a timely manner to the NPDB.
- Beware of inadvertently conducting human research while performing quality studies.
- When quality metrics are tied to payment incentives from the government, ensure that proper documentation and procedures are followed. The penalties for committing Medicare or Medicaid fraud can be severe.

References:

1. Taguchi G, Clausing D. Robust quality. *Harvard Business Rev*. 1990;68:65–75.
2. Wolek F. The lesson of guild history: variance reduction must be balanced with innovation. *Qual Manage J*. 2004;11(2):33–41.
3. Neuhauser D. Ernest Amory Codman. *Qual Saf Health Care*. 2002;11(1):104–105.
4. Blumenthal D. Part I: quality of healthcare—what is it? *N Engl J Med*. 1996;335(12):891–894.
5. Lohr KN, ed. Volume II: sources and methods—defining quality of care. In: *A Strategy for Quality Assurance. Medicare: Institute of Medicine (US) Committee to Design a Strategy for Quality Review and Assurance in Medicare*. Washington, DC: National Academies Press; 1990:5. https://www.ncbi.nlm.nih.gov/books/NBK235476/. Accessed August 30, 2021.
6. Brook R, McGlynn E, Cleary P. Part II: quality of healthcare—what is it? *N Engl J Med*. 1996;335(13):966–970.
7. Poonacha T, Go R. Level of scientific evidence underlying recommendations arising from the national comprehensive cancer network guidelines. *J Clin Oncol*. 2011;29(2):186–191.
8. Fervers B, Burgers J, Haugh M, et al. Predictors of high quality clinical practice guidelines: examples in oncology. *Int J Qual Health Care*. 2005;17(2):123–132.
9. Samanta A, Samanta J, Gun M. Legal considerations of clinical guidelines: will NICE make a difference? *J R Soc Med*. 2003;96:133–138.
10. Tung N, Boughey J, Pierce L, et al. Management of hereditary breast cancer: American Society of clinical Oncology, American Society of Radiation Oncology, and Society of Surgical Oncology Guideline. *J Clin Oncol*. 2020;38(18):2080–2106.
11. LeCraw L. Use of clinical practice guidelines in medical malpractice litigation. *J Oncol Pract*. 2007;3:254.
12. *Conn v United States*, 880 F Supp 2d 741 (SD Miss 2012).
13. *Ellis v Eng*, 2010 NY Slip Op 1453 (NY App Div 2010).
14. Mello M. Of swords and shields: the role of clinical practice guidelines in medical malpractice litigation. *U Pa L Rev*. 2001;149:645.
15. Taylor C. The use of clinical practice guidelines in determining standard of care. *J Leg Med*. 2014;35(2):273–290.
16. *Weekoty v US*, 30 F Supp 2d 1343 (D NM 1998). See also *Tanner v McMurray*, 405 F Supp 3d 1115 (D NM 2019).

17. Institute of Medicine. *Crossing the Quality Chasm: A New Health System for the 21st Century*. Washington, DC: The National Academies Press; 2001.
18. *Bing v Thunig*, 1 AD2d 887 (NYS 1956).
19. *Darling v Charleston Memorial Hospital*, 211 NE 2d 253 (Il 1965).
20. Rowland JM. Enforcing hospital responsibility through self-evaluation and review committee confidentiality. *J Leg Med*. 1988;9(3):377–419.
21. *Patrick v Burget*, 800 F2d 1498 (9th Cir 1986).
22. Dolin L. Antitrust law versus peer review. *N Engl J Med*. 1985;313(18):1156–1157.
23. Leedy L. Health care quality improvement act and physician peer review: ingredients for effective dispute resolution. *Ohio State J Dispute Res*. 1990;5(2):401–419.
24. 42 USC 11111 § 412.
25. 42 USC 11111 § 413.
26. 42 USC 11111 § 422.
27. 42 USC 11134.
28. 42 USC 11135.
29. Code lists. National Practitioner Data Bank. 2019. https://www.npdb.hrsa.gov/software/CodeLists.pdf. Accessed August 30, 2021.
30. 42 USC 11135 § 427.
31. See *Dekalb Med Ctr V Ob*ekpa, 728 SE2d 265 (Ga App. 2012).
32. *Eyring v Fort Sanders Parkwest Medical Center*, 991 SW2d (Tenn 1999).
33. *Burros v Northside Hospital et al*, 671 SE2d 176 (Ga App 2008).
34. *Robinson v Reg'l Hematology and Oncology, PA, CA*, No. N16C-06-077 (Del Super 2018).
35. *Moore v Williamsburg Regional Hospital*, 560 F3d 166 (4th Cir 2009).
36. *Murphy v Goss*, 103 F Supp 3d 1234 (D Or 2015).
37. *Obey v Frisco Medical Center*, No. 4:2013cv00656, Document 91 (ED Tex 2015).
38. *Smigaj v Yakima Valley Memorial Hospital Association*, 269 P3d 323 (Wash App 2012).
39. *Brandner v Bateman*, 349 P3d 1068 (Alaska 2015).
40. *Berg v Shapiro*, 36 P3d 109 (Colo App 2001).
41. *Pfenninger v Exempla Inc.*, 116 F Supp 2d 1184 (D Colo 2000).
42. *Peper v St Mary's Medical Center*, 207 P3d 881 (Colo App 2008).
43. *Hurwitz v AHS Hospital Corp*, 102 P3d 285 (NJ Sup Div App 2014).
44. *Wahl v Charleston Area Medical Center*, 562 P3d 599 (4th Cir 2009).
45. 42 USC 11112(b)(3). See *Smith v Ricks*, 798 F Supp 605 (ND Cal 1992).
46. *Pamintuan v Nanticoke Memorial Hospital*, 192 F3d 378 (3rd Cir 1999).
47. *Peyton v Johnson City Medical Center*, 101 SW3d76 (Tenn App 2002).
48. *Drabnick v Sebelius*, No. 1:10-CV-1841 (MD Pa 2012).
49. 42 USC 11111(a)(1)(D).
50. See *Gargiulo v Baystate Health, Inc*, 826 F Supp 2d 323 (D Mass 2011).
51. *Virmani v Novant Health Incorp*, 259 F.3d 284 (4th Cir 2001).
52. *Ciox Healthy LLC v Azar*, No. 18-cv-0040 (DDC 2020). https://ecf.dcd.uscourts.gov/cgi-bin/show_public_doc?2018cv0040-51. Accessed August 31, 2021.
53. *Austin v American Association of Neurological Surgeons*, 253 F3d 967 (7th Cir 2001).
54. *Fullerton v Florida Medical Ass'n, Inc.*, 973 So2d 1144 (Fla App 2006).
55. *Jacksonian v Temple University Health System*, 862 A2d 1275 (Pa Sup Ct 2004).
56. Kohn L, Corrigan J, Donaldson M. *To Err Is Human: Building a Safer Health System*. Washington, DC: The National Academies Press; 2000.
57. Riley W, Liang B, Rutherford W, et al. The Patient Safety and Quality Improvement Act of 2005: developing and error reporting system to improve patient safety. *J Patient Saf*. 2008;4(1):13.

58. *Quimby v Community Health Systems Professional Services Corporation*, 222 F Supp 3d 1038 (D NM 2018).
59. *Morshed v St Barnabas Hospital*, 16 Civ 2862 (LGS) (SD NY 2017).
60. *Bulhoff v Hospital of University of Pennsylvania*, Civil Action No. 18-4532 (ED Pa 2019).
61. *S Baptist Hospital of Florida, Inc v Charles*, 209 So3d 1199 (Fla 2017).
62. *Florida Health Sciences Center Inc v Azar*, 420 Supp 3d 1300 (MD Fla 2019).
63. *Tibbs v Bunnell*, 2012-Ca-000603-MR (Ky 2014).
64. Matzka K. It's time to rewrite the Healthcare Quality Improvement Act of 1986. *Physician Leadersh J.* 2017;4(1):52–55.
65. *Underwood v Roswell Park Cancer Institute*, Case No. 15-CV-684-FPG (WD NY 2017) (where the plaintiff alleged the defendant physician "had acquired funding grants based upon representations that the Prostate Database would be used in clinical research, even though the Prostate Database had only been approved for internal quality control and had not been approved by the Institutional Review Board . . . for use in clinical research.").
66. OHRP guidance on elimination of IRB review of research applications and proposals. Office for Human Research Protections, Department of Health and Human Resources. https://www.hhs.gov/ohrp/regulations-and-policy/guidance/elimination-of-irb-review-of-research-applications-and-proposals. Accessed August 31, 2021.
67. Yuan A. Blurred lines: the collapse of the research/clinical care divide and the need to for context-based research categories in the revised common rule. *Food Drug L J.* 2019;74(1):46–79.
68. Pub L No 108-173, 117 Stat 2066 § 238.
69. Aviki E, Schleicher S, Mullagni S, et al. Alternate payment and care-delivery models in oncology: a systematic review. *Cancer.* 2018;124:3293–3306.
70. Value-based programs. Centers for Medicare and Medicaid Services. https://www.cms.gov/Medicare/Quality-Initiatives-Patient-Assessment-Instruments/Value-Based-Programs/Value-Based-Programs. Accessed August 31, 2021.
71. Lyss A, Supalla S, Schleicher S. The oncology care model—why it works and why it could work better. *JAMA Oncol.* 2020;6(8):1161–1162.
72. Favre D, Bodaken A, Freyets V, et al. Health care fraud 2020. *Am Crim L Rev.* 2020;57(3):895.
73. 21st Century Oncology to pay $26 million to settle false claims act allegations. US Department of Justice. https://www.justice.gov/opa/pr/21st-century-oncology-pay-26-million-settle-false-claims-act-allegations. Accessed August 31, 2021.

CHAPTER 25

Medicolegal Ethics and Professionalism

Cody Miller Pyke, MD, JD, LLM, MSBe

INTRODUCTION

The practices of medicine and law are both full of complex ethical and philosophical questions. Oncology further complicates the ethics landscape by introducing a plethora of nuanced variables—vulnerable patient populations, end-of-life decisions, experimental treatments, and high costs of care, to name a few. The question is not *if* but *when* oncology clinicians will encounter legal and ethical dilemmas. When such a dilemma arises, oncology clinicians and legal professionals can adopt a systematic approach based in applied medicolegal ethics.

It should be noted that this chapter is intended as a primer on medicolegal ethics and professionalism. A complete exploration of legal and ethical issues in oncology would merit volumes of discussion. Therefore, the scope of this chapter is limited to an accessible analytical framework for approaching these issues.

Before analysis of an ethical issue can occur, professionals must familiarize themselves with the foundational bases of medicolegal ethics. Once a foundation is established, a medicolegal ethics analysis can be applied to a variety of dilemmas, including conflicts of interest, oncologic research, and experimental treatments.

FOUNDATIONS OF MEDICOLEGAL ETHICS

To create a solid starting point for a medicolegal ethics analysis, professionals in legal oncology should consider collectively (1) the organizing principles of biomedical ethics, (2) the fiduciary-beneficiary relationship, and (3) models of professional responsibility.

Biomedical ethics principles

Biomedical ethics analysis relies on a framework of four moral principles to guide professionals to a normative (i.e., based in common morality) conclusion. These principles are nonhierarchical—each principle is considered to be obligatory (*prima facie*) "unless it conflicts on a particular occasion with an equal or stronger obligation," like another principle.[1]

The four principles of biomedical ethics are (1) respect for autonomy, (2) nonmaleficence, (3) beneficence, and (4) justice.

Respect for autonomy

The principle of respect for autonomy requires clinicians and other professionals to respect the rights of persons to make informed choices. Applied to oncology, this principle requires that respect must be given to the intentional choices made by patients. The principle further requires that patients be empowered to make intentional choices by being provided the information necessary to do so with understanding and that they are able to make such choices without undue external influences controlling their actions.

In oncology, as with virtually all forms of medical care, the question of *paternalism* will often arise. By definition, paternalism occurs when a clinician acts in what they believe is the best interest of the patient but against the patient's autonomous choice or preference. Paternalism in medicine is to some extent unavoidable but should always be considered carefully. The principle of respect for autonomy also forms the bedrock of the doctrine of informed consent in health care. Regardless of whether a paternalistic action slightly or seriously diverges from a patient's wishes, the patient (or the patient's surrogate decision maker) is entitled to honesty and transparency from the care team.

Nonmaleficence

The next principle of nonmaleficence requires that one not harm another. Although often equated with the medical maxim of antiquity, *primum non nocere* ("First, do no harm"), it should be noted that nonmaleficence is not prioritized above other biomedical ethics principles. Additionally, nonmaleficence does not require intent on the part of the actor, and even unintentional harms are prohibited by this ethical principle. Thus, when evaluating an action through a bioethics framework, both known and potential unintended harms must be considered and weighed.

Nonmaleficence is ever present in oncology. Whether a patient's course of treatment includes surgery, radiation, chemotherapy, or a combination of these, harm will come to the patient in some form. Nonmaleficence is also notably implicated in end-of-life issues, particularly in the subtle distinctions between withholding and withdrawing lifesaving treatment and between actively "killing" and passively "letting die." These subtleties should be kept in mind when evaluating an ethical dilemma in oncology practice.

As with all the biomedical ethics principles, nonmaleficence cannot be absolutely enforced. Existence simply does not allow for a perfect prevention of harm. Ethicists and theologians have addressed this truth through the *doctrine of double effect*. The doctrine broadly states that an otherwise impermissibly harmful action or bad effect may be morally justified if it is done to bring about a sufficiently good effect. It is not an "ends justifying means" doctrine, however, as the bad effect must not create the good outcome itself. Rather, the bad effect must be a side effect of a morally good or neutral action that itself produces the good effect. One formulation of the doctrine involves four requirements[2]:

For an action that has a good effect and a bad effect:

1. The action done must itself be morally good or at least indifferent;
2. The good effect, and not the bad effect, must be intended;

3. The effect must not be the result of the bad effect; and
4. The good effect must be desirable enough to outweigh allowing the bad effect.

For an example of the doctrine of double effect in clinical practice, see Clinical Vignette # 1, later in this chapter.

Beneficence

Along a spectrum of actions, there is not a clear point where minimizing harm to a patient (nonmaleficence) transforms into seeking to increase benefit to that patient (beneficence). The key distinction between these two principles lies in the extent of obligation. Where nonmaleficence may simply require an avoidance of harm, beneficence may require action by a health care provider to affirmatively provide benefits to a patient. Additionally, health care providers are required to avoid harm impartially, regardless of their biases, whereas the extent to which health care providers engage in acts of kindness or charity is more subject to their partial preferences. Said another way, where nonmaleficence is a perfect negative prohibition of action, beneficence is an imperfect positive requirement for action.

In oncology, the principle of beneficence is bolstered by the fiduciary obligation of the physician to act in the best interest of the patient. This obligation is explored further in the "Fiduciary Relationships" section.

Justice

The final principle of justice is perhaps the most difficult to strictly define. What one defines as just and fair is the product of a multitude of sociocultural factors and personal beliefs. For example, theories of justice may be egalitarian or utilitarian, retributive or rehabilitative, or sacred or secular.

In biomedical ethics, a focus is often brought to the concept of *distributive justice*. A theory of distributive justice requires an equitable and fair distribution of rights and responsibilities across members of society. Distributive justice may be applied to an array of issues in oncology, including but not limited to financial barriers to care, distribution and availability of clinicians, research, and the development of novel drugs.

CLINICAL VIGNETTE # 1

Harper is a 62-year-old, African American female patient with a significant history of cigarette smoking. She was recently hospitalized for a broken leg after an automotive accident, where emergency department physicians incidentally discovered suspicious opacities on her chest x-ray. After an uncomplicated recovery from her accident, she presents to Dr. Lee, an oncologist, for treatment.

Dr. Lee diagnoses Harper with small-cell lung cancer and determines that she would benefit from chemotherapeutic treatment with cisplatin. Cisplatin is known to be highly nephrotoxic. Harper's kidney function tests show her kidney function is within guidelines for cisplatin treatment but only by a small margin. Dr. Lee is concerned about potential damage to her kidneys.

To make matters worse, Harper does not have health insurance. Although she works two part-time jobs, neither provides health benefits, and her combined income makes her ineligible for federal assistance. Between the cost of her care and the lost income from missing hours at work in order to receive her chemotherapy treatments, the total cost of her initial treatment is estimated to be around $10,000. When Dr. Lee tells Harper the cost estimate, she bursts into tears, saying, "Doctor, I just can't imagine ever being able to afford that."

Assuming no other therapeutic options are available for Harper, how can Dr. Lee proceed with cisplatin treatment while upholding the principles of biomedical ethics?

We can address Dr. Lee's situation by considering each of the four principles of biomedical ethics. First, under the principle of respect for autonomy, Dr. Lee is required to discuss all the risks and benefits of cisplatin treatment with Harper. Providing Harper with the information she needs—in a nondirective way—not only satisfies the legal requirement of informed consent to medical treatment but also empowers her to make her own autonomous choices without undue outside influence.

Second, we analyze Dr. Lee's responsibility to minimize harm to Harper under the principle of nonmaleficence. Before starting treatment, Dr. Lee must balance the risk of harm to Harper's kidneys (and the other harms associated with chemotherapy) against the expected benefits of therapy. In this case, Dr. Lee is medically permitted to start cisplatin therapy as long as he closely monitors Harper's kidney function and makes appropriate adjustments in her treatment plan to minimize harm as much as possible. Morally, Dr. Lee's actions are permissible under the doctrine of double effect. The act of providing medical treatment (by prescribing a medicine, cisplatin) to a patient is an inherently good or morally indifferent act. The cisplatin itself causes the reduction of cancerous cells and increases the likelihood of Harper having a longer and healthier life, a desirable good effect. The cisplatin also may cause damage to Harper's kidneys, a bad effect. However, because the kidney damage does not itself give rise to the benefit of treating the cancer and because treating the cancer is presumably sufficiently desirable to justify the risk of kidney damage, the act is justified by the doctrine.

Third, the principle of beneficence requires that Dr. Lee act in the best interests of the patient. There is an obvious requirement that Dr. Lee try to effectively treat Harper's cancer and promote her well-being. Less obvious, however, is an arguable duty based in both beneficence and the fourth principle of justice. Because Harper is a member of the society in which both she and Dr. Lee live, distributive justice is putatively violated when she cannot reasonably access treatment for her health needs. Dr. Lee, under the principle of beneficence, may be compelled to take some degree of action to help Harper access care, rather than abandon Harper to her own devices. Dr. Lee might achieve this by helping Harper find a prescription discount coupon for her chemotherapy, coordinating her care with an infusion clinic that is open when she is not working to minimize lost wages, and considering a payment plan or write-off to assist her with expenses. This is not to say Dr. Lee's duties to Harper supplant legitimate interests in keeping the clinic financially solvent and operational. Rather, the principle of beneficence simply calls on Dr. Lee to reasonably pursue opportunities to address the justice issues affecting Harper.

If all the principles of biomedical ethics are adhered to (or, if not adhered to, as long as any nonadherence is justified through a balancing of legitimate interests), then Dr. Lee can proceed with cisplatin treatment upon receiving Harper's informed consent.

FIDUCIARY RELATIONSHIPS

A fiduciary relationship is a relationship between someone who is legally and morally required to act (the fiduciary) in a manner according to the best interests of another (the beneficiary). The fiduciary-beneficiary relationship is centrally important in both medicine and law but is not necessarily only applicable to providers and attorneys.

Provider-patient

Physicians, nurses, midwives, pharmacists, and other health care professionals all have a fiduciary duty to the patients under their care.[3] They must be honest and transparent with their patients and must act according to the best interests of patients. Respect for provider-patient relationships is essential to an effective health care system, as patients need to be able to trust their providers with sensitive personal information and to trust the provider to put patient needs first and foremost.

The power of the provider-patient relationship is not limitless, however. Mandatory reporting laws, subpoenas, and other legal avenues may often require a provider to violate their fiduciary duty in order to serve another purpose for society. Because limits and exceptions to the provider-patient relationship vary by jurisdiction, providers should be as intimately familiar with medical fiduciary and privacy laws in their jurisdiction as they are with federal privacy protections such as the Health Insurance Portability and Accountability Act (HIPAA).

Attorney-client

The relationship between an attorney and their client is an archetypal example of a fiduciary relationship. Attorneys arguably have one of the strongest fiduciary obligations because they are agents of their clients in legal proceedings—acting as if they *are* the clients in legal proceedings. Attorneys owe their clients duties of candor, loyalty, care, and confidentiality.[4]

The duties of candor and confidentiality are fairly self-explanatory. Attorneys must be honest and forthcoming with their clients, and they must keep their clients' information private unless disclosure is required by law. Next, under the duty of loyalty, attorneys must advocate for their clients' interests, even potentially above their own in some circumstances.[4] This is especially important to keep in mind when attorneys represent organizations or public entities, rather than individual people, as clients. Finally, the duty of care owed by attorneys to their clients can loosely be summarized as exercising due diligence and maintaining professional behavior in the course of representing a client.[4] Examples of things covered by the duty of care include working cases in good faith, properly researching the relevant law, communicating material updates effectively with the client, following client instructions, and acting appropriately within the scope of the attorney's authority.[4]

Researcher-subject

Although the obligations of research ethics are distinct from those found in clinical biomedical ethics, patients with cancer diagnoses are often case studies of the blurred boundary between these two worlds. When a cancer patient has not responded to traditional treatment, enrollment in a clinical trial of a novel therapy may be the patient's best chance at increased duration or quality of life. There are strong arguments for regarding these "patient-participants" as patients for the purposes of determining the presence of a fiduciary provider-patient relationship, with the strongest arguments focusing on later stages of clinical trials (e.g., phase III or IV trials).[5]

Enrollment in experimental treatment trials and its implications on biomedical ethics principles are discussed in more detail later in the "Experimental Treatments and 'Right to Try'" section.

Other fiduciary-like relationships

As a final point on fiduciary relationships, it should be noted that there will be cases where a patient lacks either capacity or competency. *Capacity* is a medical determination of decision-making ability, and it may be changed at any time by clinicians based on their professional judgment. A patient who "lacks capacity" or "is incapacitated" does not have the ability to express their autonomous choice and thus cannot make informed decisions. *Competency*, although similar to capacity, is a legal status determined by a court. If a patient has been declared "incompetent" or "lacking competency" by a court of law, a judicial decision is necessary to reinstate that patient's legal ability to make informed decisions.

When a patient lacks capacity or competency, their autonomy rights pass to their surrogate decision maker, who in turn makes informed choices for the patient. Jurisdictions vary on the hierarchical order of potential surrogate decision makers for incapacitated patients. In determining who is the patient's surrogate decision maker, if an individual has a medical power of attorney (MPOA) over the patient, then that individual's legal authority ordinarily supersedes the surrogacy presumed by personal or familial relationships.

All surrogate decision makers, whether determined through an MPOA or relationship to the patient, are required to act in good faith in accordance with what they believe the patient would have decided if they had the capacity to make their own choices. Though not per se a fiduciary relationship in the legal sense, surrogate decision makers nonetheless have a normative ethics obligation to take on a "fiduciary-like" role bound by the same fiduciary principles.[6]

PROFESSIONAL RESPONSIBILITY

It is well known that physicians and attorneys have explicit fiduciary duties to their patients and clients. However, these professionals also have other obligations, which exist outside of a specific fiduciary-beneficiary relationship. These broader duties, termed *professional responsibilities*, may overlap with patient care or client service but do not require a specific preexisting fiduciary-beneficiary relationship. Examples may include a professional's interactions with other professionals, business dealings, or relationship with society.

Physicians

Following a rich historical tradition of codified ethical codes in medicine, the American Medical Association (AMA) first adopted a professional code of ethics in 1847. Last revised in 2001, the AMA Code of Medical Ethics provides 9 guiding principles[7]:

1. A physician shall be dedicated to providing competent medical care, with compassion and respect for human dignity and rights.
2. A physician shall uphold the standards of professionalism, be honest in all professional interactions, and strive to report physicians deficient in character or competence, or engaging in fraud or deception, to appropriate entities.
3. A physician shall respect the law and also recognize a responsibility to seek changes in those requirements which are contrary to the best interests of the patient.
4. A physician shall respect the rights of patients, colleagues, and other health professionals, and shall safeguard patient confidences and privacy within the constraints of the law.
5. A physician shall continue to study, apply, and advance scientific knowledge, maintain a commitment to medical education, make relevant information available to patients, colleagues, and the public, obtain consultation, and use the talents of other health professionals when indicated.
6. A physician shall, in the provision of appropriate patient care, except in emergencies, be free to choose whom to serve, with whom to associate, and the environment in which to provide medical care.
7. A physician shall recognize a responsibility to participate in activities contributing to the improvement of the community and the betterment of public health.
8. A physician shall, while caring for a patient, regard responsibility to the patient as paramount.
9. A physician shall support access to medical care for all people.

We can loosely group the AMA code's nine principles into three groups. First, principles 1, 3, 4, and 8 establish the fiduciary and legal relationship between physician and patient. These principles also establish the physician's duty to advocate for their patients, even outside of the clinic, by promoting human rights and advocating for changes in law that benefit patients' best interests.

Second, principles 2 and 5 hold physicians to a professional standard that requires they not only maintain their own qualifications and knowledge (also implicated in principle 1—the dedication to providing *competent* care) but also to participate in the betterment and growth of the field of medicine as a whole. Principle 2 specifically requires physicians both be honest in all their work and participate in the monitoring and reporting of their colleagues.

Finally, the third grouping of principles 6, 7, and 9 guides the physician's relationship with society at large. Principle 6 creates rights for the physician couched in a duty to treat anyone in an emergency situation, and principles 7 and 9 both deal with the physician's role as an advocate for promoting the general health and welfare of the public.

Attorneys

Attorneys are governed by strict rules of decorum and professionalism. Every state in the United States has adopted some version of the American Bar Association *Model Rules of Professional Conduct*.[4] Failure to adhere to the rules can lead to public or private discipline of attorneys, censure, and temporary or permanent suspension of legal license (disbarment). Breaches of the rules may also be considered as evidence in civil malpractice suits.

Other professionals

The professional responsibility model is not exclusive to physicians and attorneys, nor are these the only professions with codes of professional ethics. Individual professional organizations often develop codes of ethics and model rules of conduct for their members, such as seen with the American Nurses Association and the American Psychological Association.[8,9] The codes and rules developed by professional organizations often more specifically explore issues common to their members' practices. Nonetheless, these codes and rules should be interpreted, to the extent possible, in such a way to maintain harmony with general principles of medical and legal ethics.

PROMINENT ISSUES IN LEGAL ONCOLOGY

As stated earlier, this chapter is only intended as a primer on medicolegal ethics in oncology. A complete exploration of the metaphysical and philosophical debates present in oncology exceeds the scope and purpose of this book. Therefore, the chapter concludes by briefly considering a few frequent ethics issues that arise in oncology and two legal case examples.

Conflicts of interest—research

A conflict of interest arises when two legitimate interests are at odds with one another. In oncology, this may arise in clinical research. For example, consider a treating physician who has a financial interest in the clinical trials of a new chemotherapeutic drug. The physician also has a professional interest in continuing to improve the field of oncology. The physician's patient is eligible for the clinical trial but is unsure of whether to enroll.

Under a normative ethics analysis, the physician cannot unduly persuade the patient to enroll in the trial. Respect for autonomy requires both that the physician is nondirective in the counseling given to the patient and that the physician disclose all financial stakes they have in the trial to the patient. It is also essential that the patient be informed of the experimental nature of the drug in addition to normal disclosure of potential risks and benefits. Finally, the physician must carefully evaluate whether recommending the new treatment is truly benefitting the patient. Nonmaleficence requires minimization of harm, and if the expected benefit of the drug is speculative, a patient may be better off transitioning to comfort care rather than furthering clinical research (note, though, that some patients may *wish* to participate in purely research-oriented treatment as a form of altruism in line with their values, but this decision should be informed and voluntary rather than coerced).

CASE LAW # 1

John Moore was diagnosed with hairy cell leukemia in 1976 by Dr. David Golde at the University of California at Los Angeles (UCLA) Medical Center. At Golde's recommendation, Moore consented to and underwent a splenectomy to slow the progress of his illness. Prior to the operation, Golde and a researcher employed by UCLA, Ms. Shirley Quan, made arrangements to obtain portions of Moore's spleen for research purposes. Neither Golde nor Quan informed Moore of their research plans, nor did they ask his permission. Moore's spleen was removed, and he shortly thereafter moved to Seattle, Washington.

Over the next seven years, Moore returned from Seattle to Los Angeles several times at Golde's instruction. Each time, Golde collected samples of blood, serum, skin, bone marrow, and semen. Moore believed—based on Golde's representations—that these trips to Los Angeles were necessary and that proper treatment of his illness could not be accessed close to his home. In actuality, Golde and Quan had discovered that Moore's blood and tissues were useful for generating a line of cells for cancer research, which they patented and dubbed "Mo."

Investigation further revealed that Moore could have easily continued his treatment in Seattle and that Golde and Quan were not only engaging in unnecessary procedures and tissue sampling but also actively concealing their research activities from Moore. By the time Moore became aware of the commercialization of his cells, UCLA Medical Center, Golde, and Quan had profited hundreds of thousands of dollars from the patented licensing of the Mo cell line.

This case represents a clear conflict between the patient's right to autonomous decision making, which requires fully informed consent, and the physicians' and researchers' business interests (and, potentially, the altruistic societal interest in cancer research—it is impossible to know the exact motives of Golde and his associates). Moore brought his suit against UCLA, Golde, Quan, and two other parties. After a convoluted legal battle, the case was finally decided by the Supreme Court of California in 1990.[10] In its decision, the court held that although Moore had a cause of action for "breach of fiduciary duty and lack of informed consent," he did not have a property interest in his cells and thus was not entitled to any share in the profits generated from the unethically acquired Mo cell line.

In 1990, the estimated value of the Mo cell line was $3 billion,[11] and in 2021, sample cultures of the cells sell for upward of $600 each. Moore was never compensated, receiving only a small settlement to cover his legal fees. While his cancer was in remission from 1976 to 1996, Moore ultimately died from a recurrence of his illness in 2001.[12]

Conflicts of interest—end of life

A conflict of interest may also arise when a patient reaches a point where end-of-life discussions need to be had. End-of-life care may create conflicts of interest between physicians and their patients, between physicians and patient families acting as surrogates, or even between groups of treating physicians. The circumstances are often as unique as the individual patients.

A guiding principle when dealing with end-of-life conflicts of interest is to recenter discussions around the dying patient. The patient's wishes and best interests must be, foremost, subject to the limitations of medical futility and other applicable law.

Medical futility and living wills

While the details in the law vary across jurisdictions, physicians are ordinarily under no legal or ethical obligation to provide futile medical care. The issue of medical futility overlaps with a conflict of interest, because the physician's fiduciary obligation to the patient may be at odds with best practices and responsibilities to society. Even when a patient insists that they want to "try everything and anything" in an effort to overcome an illness or condition, if further treatment is definitively futile, then the physician's duty to society to refrain from providing superfluous care (thereby avoiding using up resources that could be equitably distributed elsewhere) is controlling. This also avoids putting unnecessary costs onto patients themselves.

Contrastingly, there may be situations where an incapacitated patient would likely benefit from a particular treatment but has provided an advance directive to physicians (i.e., a living will) expressly refusing that treatment. Here, again, the strictness and specifics of the laws governing advance directives differ by jurisdiction. However, regardless of law, a physician should avoid paternalistically and unilaterally invalidating an advance directive by assuming it is invalid or legally unenforceable. Doing so undermines the public trust in the medical profession and opens the door to potential litigation. Medical treatment without informed consent can easily constitute battery and malpractice. Whenever possible and barring an emergency, physicians should give credence to advance directives unless they are shown to be inapplicable. This is true even if the physician is certain a patient could significantly benefit from treatment.

CASE LAW # 2

One of the most famous cases dealing with the issue of medical futility and withdrawal of life-sustaining treatment was the case of Nancy Beth Cruzan.[13] In January 1983, 25-year-old Cruzan was driving near Carthage, Missouri, when she lost control of her vehicle, was ejected from the vehicle, and landed face down in a water-filled ditch. She was resuscitated by paramedics but ultimately entered a persistent vegetative state (PVS). As part of her long-term care, a feeding tube was placed by her providers.

Five years later, Cruzan's parents requested the removal of their daughter's feeding tube. However, because removing the tube would lead to Cruzan's death, the Missouri hospital providing her care refused to do so without a court order. From 1988 to 1990, Cruzan's parents were subject to a painful and intense legal battle and sensationalized media exposure. The legal question at issue was the constitutionality of Missouri's law requiring "clear and convincing evidence" from Cruzan's parents that she would want life-sustaining treatment to be withdrawn. Cruzan did not have a living will or other advance directive.

In 1990, the Supreme Court of the United States held that (1) the US Constitution did not forbid Missouri from requiring clear and convincing evidence of an incompetent's wishes regarding the withdrawal of life-sustaining treatment; (2) the state supreme court did not commit constitutional error in concluding that evidence adduced at trial did not amount to clear and convincing evidence of the patient's desire to cease hydration and nutrition; and (3) due process did not require the state to accept substituted judgment of close family members absent substantial proof that their views reflected those of the patient. The case was an important precedent in that it established (1) that the right to die was not a right guaranteed by the US Constitution and (2) that states may each determine their own right-to-die laws and standards.

Following the Supreme Court's decision, Nancy Cruzan's parents amassed more evidence to support their claim that she would want her life support terminated. Having already won the larger constitutional debate, the State of Missouri withdrew its case and allowed the Cruzans to remove their daughter's feeding tube. Nancy died on December 26, 1990, nearly eight years after her initial car accident.

Experimental treatments and "right to try"

The "right to try," or the right of a patient to access experimental treatments not yet approved for a patient's condition, is another hotly debated topic in legal oncology. Terminally ill patients vary widely in their reasons for wanting to try experimental treatments, from hoping for a last-ditch cure to finding peace through an altruistic act at the end of their life. Proponents of the right to try feel patients have a right to access these treatments in the interest of distributive justice and the greater good of advancing medical science. Critics, on the other hand, worry that experimental treatments often do not actually benefit patients and that terminally ill patients are a vulnerable population being taken advantage of by the clinical research industry.

Regardless of one's views on the right to try, it is likely to come up at some point in the practice of oncology. Jurisdictions apply widely different approaches to the issue, with several states having no right to try law at all.[14] Although a federal right to try law was passed in 2018, its preemptive power over state law is not well established.[15] Providers and representing attorneys should still make sure they are familiar with applicable laws in their jurisdiction.

CLINICAL VIGNETTE # 2

Charles Brown is an 89-year-old patient who presents to his radiation oncologist, Dr. Bloom, with diffuse metastatic bone lesions from his prostate cancer, with tenderness to palpation over his T11 vertebra. On clinical assessment, he appears to have moderate dementia. The MPOA is listed in his medical records as his daughter, Charlotte, whom he has not seen in over 30 years. Accompanying Charles at his appointment is his girlfriend of the past ten years, Lucille. Dr. Bloom determines that Charles is a potential candidate for radiation treatment, but his exact prognosis is unclear.

While Dr. Bloom presents the treatment options, Charles shouts, "I'm sick of all this medicine. Just let me die, already!" Lucille follows, saying, "He's just cranky this morning, Doctor. I'm sure he wants you to do everything you can to help him get better." When Dr. Bloom calls the contact information listed for Charlotte and describes her father's condition, she responds, "Dad and I never really talked about this kind of stuff, but I'm pretty sure he wouldn't want to take extravagant measures. He always was a very proud man."

Should Dr. Bloom proceed with Charles Brown's radiation treatment? Why or why not? What sort of ethical issues are present in this case?

Given Charles's advanced metastatic disease, the first and foremost ethical issue to be resolved is how aggressive his treatment, if any, should be. On the one hand, as a patient with diffuse disease, Charles may be a candidate for treatment with radium-223, but this comes with significant side effects. On the other hand, targeted beam therapy of his T11 vertebra may relieve some of his pain and improve quality of life with minimum side effects but would leave other lesions untreated. Dr. Bloom should weigh the options carefully and make sure that no treatments are being given without considering the ramifications for Charles's quality of life.

The next issue to consider is that of Charles's moderate dementia. As discussed in more detail in Chapter 2, there is a distinct difference between "consent" and "assent." Considering his mental state, Charles is able to assent to care but not able to provide informed consent. Here, however, neither is present, and Charles is ostensibly refusing care. Dr. Bloom should make an effort to speak with Charles directly and investigate his concerns. While a surrogate decision maker can provide the legal consent required for treatment, it is nonetheless best practice to attempt to acquire assent from incapacitated patients whenever possible.

Lack of capacity functions bidirectionally—that is, it cuts both ways. It would be deeply unethical to take Charles's assent to treatment as tantamount to informed consent. Said another way, physicians must not selectively recognize when patients lack capacity. If a patient lacks the capacity to refuse treatment, the patient also lacks the capacity to accept it. Thus, regardless of whether assent can be acquired from Charles, Dr. Bloom must still consult with a surrogate decision maker.

There are two options for a potential surrogate here: Charlotte (Charles's estranged daughter) or Lucille (Charles's girlfriend). Assuming the MPOA held by Charlotte is durable (i.e., did not have any sort of provisions that render it presently invalid), then Charlotte is legally the surrogate to whom Dr. Bloom should defer. However, the estrangement from her father makes Charlotte a less than ideal surrogate, and Lucille's more recent closeness to Charles may make her more familiar with his wishes. Dr. Bloom's best option would be to call a family meeting, potentially also involving a consult of the clinical ethics team (if available). The goal of such a meeting would be to clearly explore what Charles's expressed wishes reflected prior to him losing capacity, ideally ending with a consensus among all parties. Ultimately, if no resolution can be agreed upon, Dr. Bloom must defer to the legally binding authority of the MPOA.

As a final note, the potential conflict of interest experienced by Lucille in this scenario should be considered. Lucille, as Charles's girlfriend, has a legitimate interest in wanting her partner to continue living. Her "do everything" statement reflects such an interest. However, Lucille's interest may be at odds with several other interests, namely the patient's wishes (Charles's objection to treatment), Charlotte's stance as the MPOA (no "extravagant measures"), or potential medical futility issues at future appointments Dr. Bloom must compassionately navigate discussions with Lucille by recognizing the validity of her interests and emotions, but also reminding her that decisions must be in Charles's best interest—expressing Charles's own autonomy wherever possible and opting for palliation over aggressive treatment when appropriate.

CONCLUSION

This chapter has but scraped the surface of the complex ethical dilemmas that arise in the practice of oncology. Providers should maintain their knowledge of the relevant laws and policies in their jurisdictions that govern them as much as they maintain their expertise for taking care of cancer patients. There is no one perfect system for addressing all conflicts. However, with an analytic framework based in normative ethics and professionalism, even the toughest situations can come to an amicable and patient-centered resolution.

KEY POINTS:

- Legal oncology invariably raises complex legal and ethical questions.
- Oncology clinicians and legal professionals should build a strong foundational understanding of medicolegal ethics in order to address these dilemmas.
- A medicolegal ethics analysis uses a framework based on (1) the four principles of biomedical ethics (respect for autonomy, nonmaleficence, beneficence, and justice), (2) the fiduciary-beneficiary relationship, and (3) models of professional responsibility.
- The doctrine of double effect and the balancing test of risk versus benefit are tools used to evaluate the appropriateness of a given action or treatment decision.
- The fiduciary-beneficiary relationship is both morally and legally required between physicians and their patients and between attorneys and their clients.
- Complex ethical dilemmas, such as end-of-life issues and the right to try experimental therapies, are often affected by local and state law. Providers and attorneys should make sure they know which laws apply in their jurisdiction.

References:

1. Beauchamp TL, Childress JF. *Principles of Biomedical Ethics*. 5th ed. Oxford, United Kingdom: Oxford University Press; 2001.
2. McIntyre A. Doctrine of double effect. *The Stanford Encyclopedia of Philosophy*. March 21, 2019. https://plato .stanford.edu/archives/spr2019/entries/double-effect/. Accessed August 30, 2021.

3. McCullough LB. John Gregory (1724–1773) and the invention of professional medical ethics and the profession of medicine. *J Clin Ethics*. 1997;8(1):11–21.

4. American Bar Association. *Model Rules of Professional Conduct*. 2020. https://www.americanbar.org/groups/professional_responsibility/publications/model_rules_of_professional_conduct/. Accessed August 30, 2021.

5. Bernabe RD, van Thiel GJ, Raaijmakers JA, van Delden JJ. The fiduciary obligation of the physician-researcher in phase IV trials. *BMC Med Ethics*. 2014;15:11.

6. Kohn NA. Fiduciary principles in surrogate decision making. In: *The Oxford Handbook of Fiduciary Law*. May 2019. https://www.oxfordhandbooks.com/view/10.1093/oxfordhb/9780190634100.001.0001/oxfordhb-9780190634100-e-12#oxfordhb-9780190634100-e-12-div1-99. Accessed August 30, 2021.

7. American Medical Association. AMA Principles of Medical Ethics. AMA Code of Medical Ethics. 2016. https://www.ama-assn.org/about/publications-newsletters/ama-principles-medical-ethics. Accessed August 30, 2021.

8. American Nurses Association. *Code of Ethics for Nurses with Interpretive Statements*. Silver Spring, MD: American Nurses Association; 2015.

9. Ethical principles of psychologists and code of conduct. American Psychological Association. 2017. https://www.apa.org/ethics/code/. Accessed August 30, 2021.

10. *Moore v Regents of University of California*, 51 Cal 3d 120 (1990).

11. Ferrell JE. Who owns John Moore's spleen? *Chicago Tribune*. February 18, 1990. https://www.chicagotribune.com/news/ct-xpm-1990-02-18-9001140537-story.html. Accessed August 30, 2021.

12. McLellan D. John Moore, 56; sued to share profits from his cells. *Los Angeles Times*. October 13, 2001. https://www.latimes.com/archives/la-xpm-2001-oct-13-me-56770-story.html. Accessed August 30, 2021.

13. *Cruzan by Cruzan v Dir., Missouri Department of Health*, 497 US 261 (1990).

14. DelGrosso D. Fighting for your life in America: a study of "right to try" laws throughout the country. *St John's Law Rev*. 2017;91:743–766.

15. 21 USC § 360bbb–0 et seq.

CHAPTER 26

End-of-Life Care

Ana E. Dvoredsky, MD, MJ

INTRODUCTION

In cancer care, despite the many and significant advances in science, the matter of death and dying has not become trivial. Legal issues often arise throughout diagnosis and treatment and also as a complication of unresolved emotional or psychiatric complications of the events surrounding the end of life.

The study of the process of dying has been a late development in medicine. In the past, death was considered to be a familiar, fairly irreversible process, mostly held in the privacy of family and those who best knew the patient. It was generally supported by spiritual care, which has had centuries of experience in finding purpose in the passage as well as consolation of patients, family members, significant others, and caretakers who have become attached to those who are dying. In the 20th century, the process of dying and grieving began to be studied as a biological activity.[1-3] As therapies were discovered and previously invincible forces such as infection and trauma became easily vanquished, dying became the enemy of health care workers, and hospitals turned into combat zones. The patient's loved ones were not allowed to interfere with these heroic efforts, and the last moments of life became a lonely fight seen only by the patient and some strangers the patient hardly knew.

Modern research with people near the end of life is complex and unpredictable, requires methodologic flexibility, and is very difficult to negotiate in the constraints of a preapproved ethical regulatory framework. Therefore, it is difficult to define "best practices."[4] It is important to keep in mind that the process of dying and the moment of death will be as unique to each patient as their life was. The care of the patient does not end when the efforts to prolong survival have ended; it needs to continue as long as the patient is alive and even afterward, as will be discussed later in this chapter.

For the sake of clarification of legal issues, the discussion will be separated into (1) the process of dying and (2) the moment of death.

THE PROCESS OF DYING

Dying is defined as "approaching death" or "gradually ceasing to be."[5] There is no legal definition for this process. Legal professionals, including attorneys and courts, will fully rely upon health care professionals to define the onset, existence, and termination of the process of dying in the performance of their own duties such as preparation of deeds or wills, execution of estates, and dying confessions or other statements that may relate to civil or criminal procedures. Physicians must be ready to assist in these processes by fulfilling the patient's needs within the confines of the law.

Overall, the dying process is considered to be the period of time when the body begins to deteriorate in such a way that the probability of recovery or maintenance of a steady state is unlikely, until it ceases to function. The psychological effects of the dying process upon the patient, family, and health care staff are extremely important and not always stressed in the study of oncology. However, they are discussed only very briefly in this chapter because they are beyond the scope of this book. Their influence will be reviewed only as they affect legal issues. Resources are provided at the end of the chapter for the reader to learn about the psychological effects and support organizations.

Autonomy through the dying process

The most significant advances in clinical practice with respect to end-of-life care have been reached through concerns for the rights of the patient, especially that of autonomy. It used to be fairly common that patients who were diagnosed with cancer and other terminal diseases were treated like children: early on, decisions were made by family members, and later, patients' fate was taken over by the medical staff, who could force patients to receive therapies if the treatment team thought it was in the patients' best interest. Late in the 20th century, a significant movement arose to return the patient's autonomy in all areas of care, and this also included the area of oncology. Patients began to make their own choices regarding treatment, including the choice to stop therapy if that is what they desired. This was not an easy road to travel for the health care staff or family members, but it was gradually accepted because it provides significant support to patients who gain a modicum of control over their own bodies at a time of overwhelming uncertainty.

CLINICAL VIGNETTE # 1

Maude is a 60-year-old woman who has been diagnosed with breast cancer. She has had an excellent relationship with her primary care physician (PCP) for many years and is very unhappy at the thought of having to receive care in a different setting, with different people, after her diagnosis has been made. The PCP has a long conversation with Maude and finds out that she is worried about having new staff every time she goes for cancer care. Consistency seems to be an issue for Maude, and the choice of care must reflect her needs. The PCP refers Maude to a cancer care facility where the staff will not vary (rather than a university setting with rotating trainees), and the PCP will continue providing primary care.

Competency and capacity: making decisions during the dying process

When patients have a terminal diagnosis, they will need to make decisions as soon as they are ready to do so, and it will be necessary to confirm that their mental status is such that they show the competency to ensure that their decisions are legally valid.

Competency is a legal term referring to individuals "having sufficient ability . . . possessing the requisite natural or legal qualifications" to engage in a given endeavor.[6] As it appears, the definition will serve quite a broad scope of actions, including many legal activities, such as preparing a will, accepting or refusing a medical treatment, signing a contract, and others. It becomes essential to clarify the issue in question because the requirements will vary to determine competency. Simply put, competency refers to the mental ability and cognitive capabilities required to execute a legally recognized act rationally,[7] and each act has different requirements. For instance, competency to make decisions regarding medical treatment requires that the patient know the diagnosis, the proposed treatment as well as other management options, the natural course of the disease without treatment, and the complications of treatment. Legally, patients do not need to know the name of their grandchildren to make that decision. However, competency to make a will requires that patients know who their natural legal heirs are but does not require patients to know what the red pill they take is for. The ability to make a decision, legally, is called *capacity*. Capacity, then, is "the ability to do the job." When examining a patient for competency, it is essential to know which type of competency one is called to examine.

A physician should be involved in the determination of medical decisions as the physician will be uniquely prepared to verify that the understanding of the patient fits reality. For other types of competency that may be required during the dying period, such as writing a will or writing instructions on how to manage the patient's own death, it is suggested that an attorney be consulted.

CLINICAL VIGNETTE # 2

Matthew is 25 years old and loves his motorcycle to the chagrin of his parents. While riding the motorcycle one day, he runs into a truck. He is alert and conscious but suffers from multiple life-threatening wounds and is currently being seen in the emergency room. He knows his parents are in shock and angry at him. Matthew wants to donate all organs that can be used after his death. Desperate and anguished, he calls the physician to make this happen. What should the physician do? How would the physician make Matthew's wish become a reality? Does the physician know the procedure in the hospital? Who is the physician going to call?

Although assessing the patient's competency status is important in the decision-making process, it is imperative to be familiar with the hospital's policy and procedures. Policies may vary depending on the hospital and depending on the state and jurisdiction.

The right to die

Over the past 50 years, medicine has been faced with a significant ethical and legal problem as therapeutic techniques have become able to stave off death but not quite reverse the damages caused by disease or injury. Nowadays, patients may be saved from a critical episode only to remain severely functionally restricted or in coma for the rest of their lives. This situation has caused significant conflict for the public, health care providers, and ethicists who must grapple with the question of actively allowing or deferring the natural death of patients.

Simultaneously, this period of time has also seen the end of the paternalistic model, where physicians and healthy relatives made decisions for dying patients. A strong movement for patients' rights and autonomy in all areas of care, including a patient's own final days, has come to the forefront. These forces have changed how people perceive the care of the dying patient and have involved the courts in significant and public ways as they have been called to make the final decisions.

CASE LAW # 1

In 1976, Karen Ann Quinlan[8] ingested an unknown amount of sedatives and alcohol and, at the age of 22, was in a persistent vegetative state for months. The parents, as guardians, asked the physician to remove external life support, which the doctor refused to do. The Quinlans sued for their daughter's right to die. An appeals court recognized for the first time the concept of the *right to die*. The respirator was disconnected, but she continued to be fed. She died at age 31.

CASE LAW # 2

Terri Schindler Schiavo, at age 26, suffered a heart attack in Florida. Emergency medical technicians (EMTs) restored her heartbeat, but Terri ended up in a long-term care facility in a persistent vegetative state. Her husband, as guardian, asked to have supportive measures removed. Her parents went to court, arguing that she might recover, and a 15-year court battle ensued, with the parents and husband fighting over Terri's life support.[9] Terri never gained consciousness, and she died 13 days after the courts allowed her husband to remove life support. An autopsy confirmed that her vegetative state was irrecoverable.

This is and will always be a familiar quandary for a young physician: technical tools are developed faster than the wisdom to use them. Our medical world has created amazing techniques to keep individuals alive. The availability of such a plethora of therapeutic agents and techniques often makes a physician feel obligated to use them. Once the health care professional has installed the treatment method (e.g., in both cited cases, EMTs resuscitated patients who had been without a heartbeat for an unknown period of time), there is an obligation to continue with the consequences.

Society is quite torn regarding the idea of individually deciding whether to provide or abstain from providing life-prolonging measures. This is a decision that will always haunt a health professional and must be made with the patient's benefit in mind. Fortunately, the movement for patient rights and autonomy has determined that this choice must be left up to the patient whenever possible. Ultimately, it is the patient's right to die.

Caring for dying patients: advance directives

A directive is an instruction or a specific order. As the name indicates, an advance directive is an instruction provided by an individual before the situation occurs that requires the instruction to be used. In law, advance directives are a special type of document that the law accepts as valid to represent an individual's wishes even if the person cannot provide his or her opinion in person at the time because he or she is incompetent or dead. These documents were created around decisions that related to health care and were affirmed in the Uniform Health Care Decisions Act of 1993. They are effective as long as patients are unable to make decisions about their care and become void as soon as patients regain competency. The judicial system is supporting the citizen and the health care professional in ensuring that the patient's rights and autonomy are served always and that the patient's care follows his or her wishes even when the patient cannot clearly state them.

There are several tools patients can use to ensure that their wishes are followed regardless of their medical circumstances; these are (1) a living will, (2) a do-not-resuscitate (DNR) order, (3) health care proxy, and (4) organ donation instructions.

Living will

A living will is a legal document that provides specific instructions to the health care team regarding treatment conditions at the end of life. It may be specially written by a patient or consist of a form filled out by the patient. Forms can be obtained in health care facilities, through attorneys, and from other sources. Although all states accept living wills, there may be some variations in requirements, and the patient will need the living will appropriate for the state in which he or she is receiving care. Physicians should encourage patients to complete their living wills regardless of their health status.

Living wills include the patient's choice regarding when care should be terminated (e.g., coma, dementia), the level of survival to maintain (e.g., feeding, no intravenous line), heroic measures to use (e.g., dialysis, nothing), alternative treatments (e.g., music in the room), religious support (yes or no), autopsy (yes or no), and organ donation (yes or no; if yes, which organs). The living will allows for special requests to fit the patient's beliefs and wishes.

CASE LAW # 3

Nancy Cruzan lost control of her car and crashed in a ditch. EMTs resuscitated her, but she ended up in a persistent vegetative state. After four years without improvement, her parents requested to have life support removed. A long legal battle ensued in the Missouri courts, reaching the US Supreme Court,[10] where the right to refuse treatment was affirmed. Three friends testified to the fact that Nancy would not have wanted to live in a vegetative state, and the feeding tube was removed nine years after her accident. This is a case about the right to die, but it also shows how the patient's stated wishes to friends finally determined her fate.

Do-not-resuscitate order

Most patients are allowed to determine whether they wish to be resuscitated when they are admitted to a hospital. However, most individuals do not talk about this procedure outside of the hospital, for example, in case of a cardiac arrest at home or car accident. Oncology presents a more dire situation because crises may arise when the patient has been discharged home. Nonetheless, it is suggested that physicians talk about DNR orders with their patients in all circumstances, as was illustrated in the previous case law examples. To exert control over their own body, people's relatives should know what their choices would be in case of loss of function.

Durable power of attorney

Any person is entitled to allow another person to do something in their place. A document that allows another to do something in one's place is called a power of attorney (POA). A young man may want to give a POA to his dad to pick up his new car in his place while he is away at school, for example. It exists for that purpose while the young man is competent.

A durable POA is special in that it takes effect and retains its power only when a person loses legal capacity. It is often signed by patients who are very sick or old and have decided to trust a certain individual to make decisions for them. The person who takes control of the decisions is called the *agent*.

When dealing with a very ill patient, which is not rare in oncology, a physician should know whether the patient has signed a durable POA and identify the person who will be making decisions. Some treatment modalities cause the patient to become disoriented, unconscious, or simply so frail that the patient does not wish to make any decisions. In that case, it is important to learn who will be making decisions for the patient.

Decisions by surrogates: health care power of attorney

A specific subset of durable POA is the health care POA, where the power is delegated only to areas that concern health care. The patient may choose a relative or a friend to make decisions for the patient regarding health care, and this person is sometimes called the health care proxy or agent.

A health care POA is as important as a living will, and it should be encouraged. Patients sometimes have an emotional reaction to determining a living will or a health agent because they think that having that conversation means that they are about to die. Creating these documents should be raised as a normal part of health care because illnesses and treatments may cause periods of time when patients are not alert and the health care team needs to know to whom to direct any questions. However, as patients work through their end-of-life compromises, the creation of these documents will become continuously easier.

Organ donation

As transplantation technology has improved, transplantation procedures have multiplied. However, the public has not become as comfortable with the idea of donation. Options for organ donation are usually included in the living will, following the intensive efforts of the legislature through the national Organ Donation and Recovery Improvement Act (1984) and the creation of the United Network for Organ Sharing. This topic can be conflicting for oncology patients because they often feel the wish to donate part of themselves to others as a way to continue living, but the seeding of organs with cancerous cells or the damage produced by oncotherapies can make their organs of little use for transplantation. As an alternative, the possibility of donation to research facilities to further advances in the knowledge of pathologies might be raised.

Physician-assisted suicide and euthanasia

The term *euthanasia* (from the Greek meaning "a good death") has been defined as "directly or indirectly bringing about another person's death for that person's benefit." Its premise is the idea that contributing to someone else's death is a benefit because it saves that person from a larger evil, such as a terrifying or painful death.[11]

This concept represents a long battle fought by health care professionals, family members, and legal professionals who have been in the field, watching patients live their last days in a painful and degrading manner or simply linger in a semi-conscious or unconscious state while family members suffer through the remaining days of what may have been an otherwise happy life. These sad and extreme situations, which may extend over decades, as illustrated in the landmark cases previously cited, merit thoughtful assessment by physicians, families, and patients themselves prior to illness. However, the law is careful to protect citizens whose end of life might be accelerated by relatives who are interested in estates or new beginnings, guarding against rapid termination to lives that could still hold significant purpose. Both extremes are vividly possible in the practice of oncology.

The concept of a health care professional, who has sworn to fight illness and death as part of his or her profession, struggling with the idea of allowing death or even inducing death has been a very difficult topic to discuss and is frequently avoided in medical training and in patient consultations. However, avoidance does not make the issue disappear. It remains as a deeply concerning and always difficult topic fraught with legal and ethical issues.

To assist a new physician with this unavoidable situation, a couple of distinctions and definitions have been provided by the American Medical Association (AMA). One is the difference between *passive* euthanasia (letting someone die) and *active* euthanasia (creating the means of death and, therefore, killing). For many physicians, this distinction is helpful both ethically and legally. Active euthanasia is illegal, and it is ethically sanctioned. Passive euthanasia, involving the withholding of life-sustaining measures, is accepted within the medical and ethical communities and has been legally supported, as seen in the landmark cases previously quoted. However, not all cases can be clearly separated through the active/passive dichotomy. Other ethicists prefer to view these cases as either voluntary (where a patient has expressed the desire to end life or has selected a surrogate through a POA, who has chosen means to end the patient's life) or involuntary (where neither the patient nor a representative has given consent). Ethical and legal support is offered to all situations where the physician can show that the patient has, at one point, voluntarily selected a particular manner to induce, accelerate, or permit his or her own death. Nonvoluntary methods may be used when dealing with infants, where parents or health care professionals are making the decision; another situation is seen among demented patients who have previously selected agents to make health decisions in general without specifying a manner of death. Most of these events occur in a hospital or institutional setting.

An additional variation to this concept is called *physician-assisted suicide* (PAS), where a patient takes his or her own life in a setting of the patient's choice (usually at home) with the help of a physician (through medications prescribed by the physician or through the act itself). The AMA has provided a code of ethics for this practice.[12] In addition, a number of states have passed legislation that permits this type of death, and physicians should be familiar with the particular statutes in the states in which they practice, including the evaluations, conditions, and certifications required to provide a patient with PAS. (Physician-assisted death, also known as medical aid in dying, is legal in ten jurisdictions: California, Colorado, District of Columbia, Hawaii, Montana, Maine [as of January 1, 2020], New Jersey, Oregon, Vermont, and Washington.) Not all physicians are emotionally equipped to assist patients in dying, but oncologists should become familiar with this practice and find those who make it available if their patients request it. Practitioners interested in the long judicial road followed by those supporting PAS are referred to the book, *Physician-Assisted Suicide: The Anatomy of a Constitutional Law Issue.*[13]

CLINICAL VIGNETTE # 3

Ellen Marple is in her 80s. She is a keen, detail-oriented person. As she approaches her 90s, the issue of advance directives is raised by her physician, Dr. Jones. She has created a living will, signed a DNR order, and set limits on life-prolonging measures. Her nephew Harold is her health care proxy. She brings a copy of these papers to Dr. Jones's office to have in her file. Since all documents will be observed in hospitals and institutional settings, Dr. Jones suggests that Ellen have a visible document at home so EMTs know of her wishes prior to commencing resuscitation efforts.

Grief management through illness

Dr. Elizabeth Kubler-Ross provided a great understanding of the different phases people go through in the management of grief. Grief is the most common reaction to a significant loss. Kubler-Ross was able to distinguish several stages of grief: (1) denial and isolation, (2) anger, (3) bargaining, (4) depression, and (5) acceptance. Further information on these stages and grief can be found in the books *On Death and Dying*, by Kubler-Ross, and *On Grief and Grieving*, by Kubler-Ross and Kessler.

On a practical note, the stages defined by Dr. Kubler-Ross do not always occur in a smooth progression. A patient may move forward to a later stage, only to retreat for a short time to an earlier stage and then move forward again. In addition, a patient may not be uniformly at the same stage regarding all issues. For example, a patient may have accepted the diagnosis but still be in the bargaining stage regarding treatment choice. The clinician's patience is needed as patients travel through the stages of grief. Clinicians should also be mindful of the toll a close relationship with oncology patients can take and ensure self-care.

The moment of death

Death has been defined as the permanent cessation of all biological functions that sustain a living organism. This apparently simple definition has undergone significant changes, as medical advances have permitted the sustained function of some organs coexisting with the cessation of function of other organs equally important to a person's well-being. As a result of the complex situations created by semi-survival and the associated legal struggles, the definition of death in the United States was expanded in 1968 to include neurologic criteria, determining that the most important factor to consider is brain death.[14]

Legal death is the recognition under the law of a particular jurisdiction that a person is no longer alive. However, the law itself does not have any particular procedure to determine death. It requires a physician to declare a patient dead or a corpse to be identified. Only then can further medicolegal procedures, such as organ donation, be commenced. Therefore, it is extremely important that a physician assist in the legal process of determining the end of life.

There are a number of psychological and ethical issues regarding the determination of the moment of death. For the oncologist who has been caring for a patient and fighting for survival, this is the final moment of surrender, which needs to be accepted jointly with the patient and family. However, few issues are as striking as the legal implications of the moment of death.

As long as the patient was alive, the physician had a relationship with the patient and was likely attempting to fulfill the patient's wishes and maintain the patient's comfort at all times. The patient's intention determined the physician's conduct at all times, or at least this should have been the case. It is difficult to comprehend, but immediately after death, the patient becomes "a thing," with no will of its own, now the property of its heirs. It is incumbent upon the heirs or the executor of the will to decide what needs to be done with the body. Physicians may get caught up in disputes between what they heard their patient's intentions to be done after death and the patient's family members' plans for the remains. It is always a good idea to encourage patients to leave clear instructions in writing, including the determination of an agent to carry out those instructions, especially in time-dependent procedures such as organ donation.

Care of the patient after death

The patient does not cease to be attached to the physician after death. Many oncologists choose to attend the funeral of patients they have cared for through many years, and others remain friendly with the families. Legally, physicians need to talk with their patients about their duty to have a conversation with family members regarding any inherited disorders and how to prevent, screen, and care for them. This is a service a patient and a physician can provide even after the patient is dead.

CONCLUSION

Just as patient care is complex and rewarding in life, so it is throughout the dying process. Physicians can be of significant support to patients and family members not only by providing medical care but also by supporting patients at the end of life and reminding patients of the legal implications in all stages of their care.

KEY POINTS:

- The physician is an important actor throughout the stages of dying and later during death and postdeath care. It is valuable to be present and not to refer all care out during these stages.
- The dying phase of care begins when irreversible damage occurs.
- Although not all patients are alike, a significant number of dying patients prefer to have some degree of control over their decisions regarding death and dying.
- Physicians may be called upon to make decisions of legal competency and capacity of their patients. They are the best qualified people to perform this task and need to know how to perform it.
- All oncology patients should be able to discuss with their physician the significant legal documents that reflect their autonomy in the late stages of life, including (1) advance directives, (2) living will, (3) durable POA, (4) health care POA, (5) organ donation, and (6) physician-assisted suicide. Physicians need to become comfortable discussing these subjects with their patients and not delegate them to other health care providers.
- The right to die movement has gained validity in many states. To assist their patients, physicians needs to know the following: (1) the law in their area of residence, (2) the bylaws in their health care system, (3) the proper methods to use, and (4) the proper procedures to use. Physicians should also try to become comfortable discussing these issues with their patients who are nearing death.
- At the moment of death, the patient ceases to be a legal entity and becomes property owned by the heirs. It is important to have created a relationship with the family member who will make decisions in order to provide postdeath care (e.g., organ donation, inherited disorders).
- Dying is part of life. As the physician, do not avoid the patient or the family. The physician will be their mainstay. In addition, the physician will be the main source of data for all legal documents. If the physician is lucky and listens, patients and families will teach them more about medicine than any book.

References:

1. Kubler-Ross E. *On Death and Dying*. New York, NY: Simon & Schuster/Touchstone; 1969.
2. Kubler-Ross E, Kessler D. *On Grief and Grieving: Finding the Meaning of Grief Through the Five Stages of Loss*. New York, NY: Scribner; 2005.
3. Glaser BG, Strauss AL. Temporal aspects of dying as a non-scheduled status passage. *Am J Sociol*. 1965;71:48–59.
4. Borgstrom E, Ellis J. Introduction: researching death, dying and bereavement. *Mortality*. 2017;22:93–104.
5. Dying. Merriam-Webster. Merriam-Webster.com/dictionary/dying. Accessed September 3, 2021.
6. Garner B, ed. *Black's Law Dictionary*. 10th ed. New York, NY: Thomas Reuters; 2014.
7. Bisbing SB. Competency and capacity: a primer. In: Sanbar SS, Gibofsky A, Firestone MH, et al., eds. *Legal Medicine*. 4th ed. St Louis, MO: Mosby; 1998:32–43.
8. In the matter of Karen Quinlan, an Alleged Incompetent 70 NJ 10 (1976).
9. *Theresa Marie Schindler Schiavo, incapacitated ex rel, Robert Schindler and Mary Schindler, her parents and next friends, Plaintiffs-Appellants, v Michael Schiavo, as guardian of the person of Theresa Marie Schindler Schiavo, incapacitated, Judge George W. Greer, The Hospice of the Florida Suncoast, Inc., Defendants-Appellees*, 403 F3d 1261 (2005).
10. *Nancy Beth Cruzan, By Her Parents and Co-Guardians, Lester L. Cruzan, Et Ux, Petitioners v Director, Missouri Department of Health, et al.*, 110 S Ct 2841 (1990).
11. Vaughn L. *Bioethics*. 3rd ed. Oxford, United Kingdom: Oxford University Press; 2017:626.
12. Physician-assisted suicide. American Medical Association. https://www.ama-assn.org/delivering-care/ethics/physician-assisted-suicide. Accessed September 3, 2021.
13. Behuniak S, Svenson A. *Physician-Assisted Suicide: The Anatomy of a Constitutional Law Issue*. New York, NY: Rowman and Littlefield; 2003.
14. Bernat JL. A conceptual justification for brain death. *Hastings Cent Rep*. 2018;48(suppl 4):S19–S21.

ADDITIONAL SOURCES

Institute of Medicine and National Research Council. 2001. *Improving Palliative Care for Cancer*. Washington, DC: The National Academies Press; 2001. (https://www.nap.edu/catalog/10149/improving-palliative-care-for-cancer) (Free PDF available for download.)

Compassion and Choices (www.compassionandchoices.org)

Partnership for Caring (www.partnershipforcaring.com)

Oregon Department of Human Services. Death with Dignity Act. Oregon, March 2007 (https://www.oregon.gov/oha/ph/providerpartnerresources/evaluationresearch/deathwithdignityact/pages/index.aspx)

CHAPTER 27

Cancer Causation and Product Liability

Tony S. Quang, MD, JD, FCLM, Michelle S. Taft, JD, and Michael Vinluan, MD, JD, FCLM

INTRODUCTION

Exposure to cancer-causing agents can raise a variety of medical and legal issues for patients. Exposure to carcinogens usually changes patients' lives for the worse. Often, such exposures can lead to increased screenings and medical monitoring, including diagnostic testing such as x-rays and computed tomography (CT) scans that can increase the risk of cancer. Even if all test results come back negative, it is still stressful. It can disrupt patients' daily routines and affect their ability to work. If patients are diagnosed with cancer, they may have to undergo cancer treatments and follow-up. They may no longer be able to work or care for their families or themselves. Cancer and its exhausting treatments can be devastating physically, emotionally, and financially.

Patients often seek answers from their doctors to determine if their cancers were caused by exposure to various agents. Many feel they should be compensated for harm and injury caused by the company who made the agent, and they may file suit to seek justice and financial compensation. Along with the product manufacturer, distributors and retailers are often named as codefendants. Physicians who prescribed medications or surgeons who used medical devices at issue may also be named as codefendants.

If patients believe that a chemical agent they were exposed to caused their cancer and its resulting harms and injuries, they can turn to the field of product liability law to seek redress from the company that manufactured the agent. Product liability is the area of law dealing with claims of personal injury arising from the design, manufacture, distribution, or sale of a product.[1] In product liability lawsuits, the issue of cancer causation is critical when it comes to determining whether use or exposure to a certain product can cause cancer.

ELEMENTS OF A PATIENT'S CLAIM

Within the field of product liability law, there are three traditional causes of action (the legal basis or theories) upon which a patient can file a lawsuit: negligence, breach of warranty, and strict liability. Negligence occurs when a company fails to exercise reasonable prudence. Usually, the patient alleges that the company acted negligently in the design or manufacture of the product or in creating the warning, labels, and instructions that should accompany a product and inform the patient of the safe use of the product. Breach of warranty claims arise from a contractual relationship between the company and the patient. The basis of these claims is that the company made a false statement about the product and the patient reasonably relied on the false statement to their detriment; the understanding that the product being sold is suitable for ordinary purposes for which such goods are used; and the patient's reliance on the seller's skill or judgment to select the item for a special purpose. Finally, the theory of strict liability provides that if a company sells a product in a defective condition that is unreasonably dangerous to the patient, then the company is liable even if the company exercised all possible care and even if the patient did not enter into a contractual relationship with the company. Unlike negligence, under the theory of strict liability, patients need not prove fault on the part of the manufacturer to recover damages so long as the product is defective.

These three causes of action hinge on the concept of *product defect*—meaning that the design, manufacturing, or warnings and instructions accompanying the product were defective. However, defining the relevant product defect can be subjective, and courts have developed a variety of legal tests and standards to help them determine whether a product defect exists. The most commonly used legal standard is the *patient's expectations test*.[2,3] Under this test, a product is deemed unreasonably dangerous and, therefore, defective if it is dangerous to an extent beyond which would be contemplated by the ordinary patient. Other tests courts have used include the *risk-utility balancing test* and the *presumed knowledge test*.[4,5] When design defect is in question, the chosen design is considered defective if a safer feasible alternative design exists, the alternative design would have reduced or eliminated the risk of patient's injury, and not using the alternative design made the product unsafe.

An unusual product liability theory called medical monitoring is invoked when patients claim they were exposed to a hazardous or toxic product because of the company's negligence and therefore have become significantly more likely to develop cancer in the future.[6] In these scenarios, the patient's alleged injury is the cost of undergoing medical surveillance procedures during the time period between the present-day exposure and any future disease manifestation to detect the disease at its earliest stage and maximize the chances of a cure, rather than merely the increased risk of getting the disease in the future. A classic example of this legal theory in action is cigarette smoking. In 2020, the National Comprehensive Cancer Network and other medical societies recommend annual low-dose CT scan screening for high-risk individuals ages 55 to 74 years who have a 30-pack-year history of smoking, who are current smokers, or who have quit within the past 14 years.[7,8] This screening is costly—a detailed analysis of low-dose cancer screening showed that the cost of adding One good year to a person's life through CT screening is around $80,000—but tests or procedures that cost less than $100,000 per year added are considered cost effective.[9] Nevertheless, most states do not recognize medical monitoring claims because the patient's physical injury has not manifested. However, when medical monitoring may not be a cause of action by itself, some states may allow medical monitoring as part of the damages.

Related to but distinct from product liability claims, sometimes third-party payors, such as unions, insurers, and health funds that pay for part of the medical care or prescriptions of patients, have brought claims against manufacturers.[10] For example, an insurer may argue that the company misrepresented the efficacy or risks of a particular medical product and that physicians paid by that insurance would not have prescribed it had they known the facts. Even though patients may not have been necessarily harmed, if in fact these third-party payors over-paid, these third-party payors would feel they were economically harmed and should be compensated. However, these cases suffer from challenging legal questions such as standing (whether the third-party payor is the correct plaintiff to bring the lawsuit), causation (whether the company caused the payor's alleged harms), and injury (whether the payor suffered a loss for which the law can or should provide a remedy). For instance, New York's highest court ruled that an insurance company's claims for the costs of treating subscribers' smoking-related health costs are too remote for the insurer to raise.[11]

There are other potential causes of action related to product defects such as racketeering laws, consumer fraud statutes, conspiracy, public nuisance, securities law, and innovator liability, but they have been less applied in product liability related to cancer.

ISSUES RELATED TO CAUSATION

Central to any claim of product liability, no matter which theory or cause of action it is based on, is the legal element known as *causation*. Did the product defect cause the patient's cancer? In this context, a product defect means that a court will ask whether there was something wrong with the product that caused the patient to develop cancer as a function of the product's use, the patient's exposure to it, or the patient being uninformed of the product's dangers. Under virtually all product-based causes of action, there must be sufficient causal connection between the patient's injury and the product defect (or the seller's conduct related to that defect).

Courts have traditionally required patients to show evidence that the product was the *cause-in-fact* of the patients' harm, meaning that the court will ask "but for the product defect, would the patient not have been injured?" or, put another way, "was the defect a substantial factor in bringing about the patient's harm?" To make matters more complicated, causation can be divided into *general* and *specific* causation. General causation asks whether the substance or chemical at issue *is capable of causing* a particular injury or condition. For instance, can smoking cause cancer?[12] By contrast, specific causation relates to whether the substance or chemical *in fact caused* the patient's medical condition. For instance, did the patient's years of smoking actually cause the patient's lung cancer?[13] These types of cases often involve complex expert testimony on causation from experts in disciplines such as medicine, oncology, toxicology, and epidemiology. Not uncommon is a "battle of the experts" where different experts testifying for the patient and the company hold differing opinions on causation.

In some jurisdictions, a patient must show not only that they were injured by the product but that they were injured by a specific product of the company. This concept is often termed *product identification* because patients have to identify which specific product caused their harm. However, this can be complicated and difficult for patients to do because, over time, a patient may have used several brands of the same product. Historically, a minority of courts eased the patient's legal burden by allowing for a rule called *market share liability*, where a company is assigned fault based on its relevant market share. Courts that previously adopted this rule have considered the following factors: the generic nature of the product, the long latency period before manifestation of harm, the patients' practical inability to discover which company's product caused the harm, and the availability of sufficient market share data to support a reasonable apportionment of liability. The best-known example of market share liability comes from the diethylstilbestrol (DES) litigation.[14] The US Food and Drug Administration (FDA) had approved DES to be taken by expectant mothers to prevent miscarriages, but children of those mothers developed vaginal adenocarcinoma and adenosis. Courts concluded that companies that produced DES could be held liable for such harms in proportion to their share of the DES market, given the presence of all the factors described earlier.

Companies routinely offer a variety of defenses concerning their liability. These defense theories focus on whether patients misused the product, altered the product before using it, contributed in some way to their own injury, or cannot establish a causal chain between the product and their injury because of a third party's involvement. Another possible defense is the passage of time, where the company claims that the product was the best out there or was the state of the art at the time the product was sold and that it should not be judged with the benefit of hindsight many years later.

Another common defense is the statute of limitation defense, where a patient is barred from filing suit past a certain number of years following the injury or when the injury was or should have been discovered. In some states, another defense is the statute of repose, which bars a lawsuit a certain number of years, typically around ten years, after the product was sold to its first purchaser.

If patients can successfully show that a company's product caused their injury, patients normally seek to recover all their damages, past, present, and future. Recoverable compensatory damages include compensation for physical, psychological, and emotional injury. More specifically, patients can be compensated for permanent disability, pain and suffering, disfigurement, impairment of earning capacity, lost wages or profits, medical costs, out-of-pocket expenses, and loss of consortium or companionship if a partner is injured or deceased. These injuries are then translated into monetary figures. Less frequently, punitive damages are sought if a company was reckless and the patient brought the case out of a desire to deter the company from continuing this behavior.

PROMINENT CANCER CASES

Although there may be many cancer-causing agents, cigarettes, agent orange, DES, and asbestos cases have been the most prominent examples. Cases involving such carcinogens have been, for the most part, resolved on a large scale in complex litigation where cancer causation has been established and compensation has been awarded through various settlement agreements, either paying victims directly or paying states to cover medical costs. For instance, in the 1998 Tobacco Master Settlement Agreement between the four largest US tobacco companies (Philip Morris, Inc., R. J. Reynolds, Brown & Williamson, and Lorillard) and the attorneys general of 46 states, the tobacco companies agreed to pay a minimum of $206 billion over the first 25 years of the agreement. The states settled their Medicaid lawsuits against the tobacco industry for recovery of their tobacco-related health care costs. In exchange, the companies agreed to curtail or cease certain tobacco marketing practices, as well as to pay, in perpetuity, various annual payments to the states to compensate them for some of the medical costs of caring for persons with smoking-related illnesses. Although the Tobacco Master Settlement Agreement did not derive from traditional product liability causes of action, but instead from the violations of various state laws such as consumer protection laws and antitrust laws, it nevertheless shows the impact of large-scale litigations in shifting public policy and opinion about tobacco use.

While cancer causation cases like the famous ones listed earlier are relatively well settled, the Roundup scenario that follows is an example that has been more recently litigated. Roundup has become a frontrunner in the patient's arena in terms of presently litigated cancer-causing agents with large verdicts and settlements. The example that follows illustrates how lawyers might analyze such a claim and how it has evolved through the courts. The same type of analysis can be expected of other potential carcinogenic agents that are currently being litigated.

The following case scenario will help you think through the steps of analysis a lawyer would consider when evaluating a patient's potential claim. Lawyers begin by researching previous court cases to learn about the tests and standards courts have used in the past. As you read the legal case examples that follow, try to identify any legal rules or concepts that were used in each case. At the end of the case examples is a clinical vignette that describes a new patient's situation, and you will be able to practice evaluating how the legal rules from previous cases might apply if that new patient files a lawsuit.

Roundup is the brand name of a systemic, broad-spectrum, glyphosate-based herbicide originally produced by Monsanto and later acquired by Bayer in 2018.[15] Glyphosate is the most widely used herbicide in the United States. Monsanto developed and patented the glyphosate molecule in the 1970s and marketed it as Roundup from 1973. It retained exclusive rights to glyphosate in the United States until its US patent expired in September 2000. The Roundup trademark is registered with the US Patent Office. However, glyphosate is no longer under patent, so similar products use it as an active ingredient.[16] The main active ingredient of Roundup is the isopropylamine salt of glyphosate. Another ingredient of Roundup is the surfactant polyethoxylated tallow amine (POEA).

The toxicities of Roundup have been debated in the scientific literature with mixed reviews. The consensus among national pesticide regulatory agencies and scientific organizations is that labeled uses of glyphosate have demonstrated no evidence of human carcinogenicity.[17,18] The Environmental Protection Agency (EPA) has evaluated the carcinogenic potential of glyphosate multiple times since 1986. It initially ascertained glyphosate to be carcinogenic to humans. Then it switched position to say that it was not as likely to be carcinogenic to humans in 2017.[19-21] The International Agency for Research on Cancer classified glyphosate as probably carcinogenic to humans in 2015.[22] After this classification, over 300 federal lawsuits have been filed that were consolidated into a multidistrict litigation called In re: Roundup Products Liability Litigation.[23] The most recent and largest international pooled meta-analysis from the AGRICOH consortium in 2019 showed moderately increased risk for non-Hodgkin lymphoma from glyphosate.[24] As of

October 30, 2019, there were 42,700 plaintiffs who said that glyphosate herbicides caused their cancer.[25]

CASE LAW # 1

Dewayne Johnson brought a product liability action against Monsanto alleging he developed mycosis fungoides, a type of non-Hodgkin lymphoma, as a result of his exposure to glyphosate, which is contained in Monsanto's herbicides such as Roundup.[26] On August 10, 2018, he was awarded $289 million in damages (later cut to $78 million on appeal) after a jury in San Francisco found that Monsanto had failed to adequately warn consumers of cancer risks posed by the herbicide. Johnson had routinely used two different glyphosate formulations in his work as a groundskeeper, Roundup and another Monsanto product called Ranger Pro. The jury's verdict addressed the question of whether Monsanto knowingly failed to warn consumers that Roundup could be harmful, but the jury did not reach the question of whether Roundup causes cancer. Court documents from the case show the company's efforts to influence scientific research via ghostwriting.

CASE LAW # 2

On March 2019, Edwin Hardeman testified that he sprayed Roundup on poison oak and weeds on properties in Mendocino and Sonoma counties for 26 years.[27] He was awarded $80 million in a lawsuit claiming that Roundup was a substantial factor in causing his non-Hodgkin lymphoma. In July 2019, US District Judge Vince Chhabria reduced the settlement to $26 million. Chhabria stated that a punitive award was appropriate because the evidence "easily supported a conclusion that Monsanto was more concerned with tamping down safety inquiries and manipulating public opinion than it was with ensuring its product is safe." Chhabria also stated that there was evidence on both sides as to whether glyphosate causes cancer and that the behavior of Monsanto showed "a lack of concern about the risk that its product might be carcinogenic."[27]

CASE LAW # 3

Alva and Alberta Pilliod began using Roundup weed killer on their properties in the 1970s.[28] Alva and Alberta both developed non-Hodgkin lymphoma in 2011 and 2015, respectively. In May 2019, they sued Monsanto, alleging that it knew that its Roundup products were defective and were inherently dangerous and unsafe. They specifically stated that Roundup's active ingredient, glyphosate, could result in cancer. A jury in California ordered Monsanto's successor company, Bayer, to pay the couple $2 billion in damages after finding that the company had failed to adequately inform consumers of the possible carcinogenicity of Roundup. On July 26, 2019, an Alameda County judge cut the settlement to $86.7 million, stating that the judgement by the jury exceeded legal precedent.

CLINICAL VIGNETTE # 1

Jim is a 16-year-old male who presents to the primary care doctor for a swollen left neck mass. He endorses drenching night sweats and mild fever but no weight loss. He is a junior in high school and plays on the varsity basketball team. Past medical history is significant for spending five summers using Roundup to kill weeds in his neighbor's backyard. Workup includes a CT neck, which reveals a 3 × 5 cm lesion. Ultrasound-guided core biopsy is done. Pathology reveals diffuse large B-cell non-Hodgkin lymphoma. Jim is seen at Pink Acre Children's Hospital. His case is presented at an interdisciplinary tumor board and determined to be stage IB. He receives R-CHOP chemotherapy (rituximab, cyclophosphamide, doxorubicin, vincristine, and prednisolone) for six cycles followed by 30 Gy of consolidative radiation therapy. Posttreatment CT/positron emission tomography shows complete response. Jim is relieved. However, his quality of life has changed. He is now tired, and his energy level has decreased by 60%. He no longer has the stamina to play sports. He is worried that he may not be able to father children because of toxicity from the chemotherapy.

Did exposure to Roundup increase Jim's chance of getting non-Hodgkin lymphoma, and does he have a cause of action to recover damages?

The theory of liability in Jim's case is that glyphosate is a carcinogen and Monsanto failed in its duty to warn patients, thereby causing some exposed persons to develop cancer for which they will need to undergo chemotherapy and radiation therapy treatments. While not dispositive, there is a body of scientific literature to suggest that glyphosate causes cancer, especially non-Hodgkin lymphoma like Jim developed. In a legal context, Jim does not have to prove that glyphosate irrefutably causes cancer. Instead, he must simply show a probability of causation—that it is more likely true than not that glyphosate is carcinogenic. This concept can be a bit challenging for young clinicians because causation is often thought of in binary terms in medicine. Clinicians tend to understand cancer causation from the standpoint of deterministic effect: Was there a threshold in the use or exposure to a product that caused the cancer? Once that threshold is reached, then cancer results. Clinicians have a harder time grasping stochastic effect (i.e., the idea that there is no threshold of use or exposure to a product wherein cancer develops). Rather, in the legal context, the probability of carcinogenesis increases as a function of increasing use or exposure to a product. To establish legal causation, the standard of proof is simply a preponderance of evidence, or "more likely than not." More likely than not means more than 50% probability. The probability of carcinogenesis as a function of use or exposure to glyphosate does not have to be 55%, 65%, 75%, 85%, or 95%. It just needs to be more than 50%. Glyphosate fits the bill.

In a products liability case, the burden rests on the patient to establish legal causation—that the company's conduct, such as a failure to adequately warn, was a proximate cause of the patient's injuries. In other words, but for the alleged failure to warn, the defective design, or the manufacturing defect of the drug or device at issue, the patient's injuries would not occur. While the specific elements of a products liability claim and the evidentiary requirements thereof vary somewhat by state, most jurisdictions require that where a causal link is beyond the knowledge or expertise of a lay jury, expert testimony is required to establish causation. Due to the complex nature of medical causation in products liability cases, patients must typically call medical experts to explain the causal link between the drug or device and the patient's injury. These experts may rely on their own training, knowledge, and experience, as well as medical literature accepted within the relevant medical community. Companies often try to undermine patient experts' opinions on causation by citing purported inadequacy of studies, even if those studies were peer reviewed.[26] During trial, courts consider whether a particular expert opinion is reliable and whether a certain study has gained general acceptance in the scientific community. If admitted as evidence, the limitations of peer review studies go to the weight of the evidence, which is admissible for consideration by the jury. Undermining the basis of the opinions of a patient's expert is just one way in which a company can attempt to convince a jury that a patient has failed to meet the "more probable than not" threshold. Causation and expert testimony are discussed in more detail in those respective chapters.

Another argument that the companies may make is that epidemiology does not establish an unequivocal causal relationship. While this may be true, epidemiology does not need to confirm an unequivocal causal relationship; it only needs to establish that there is a more likely than not probability of a causal relationship despite confounding factors. Other arguments companies may use include erroneous extrapolation of in vitro data and the latency period being too short for the development of cancers.

CONCLUSION

Based on the compendium of scientific and medical literature, it is reasonable to say that glyphosate is more likely than not to cause cancer. Therefore, companies like Monsanto have the duty to warn and to mitigate any potential harm to patients like Jim. Failure to do so puts the company at risk of liability for harm and damages, as is evidenced by recent verdicts and settlements in favor of patients in glyphosate cases like the Johnson, Hardeman, and Pilliod patient cases described earlier.

KEY POINTS:

- Patients often seek answers from their doctors to determine if their cancers were caused by exposure to various agents.
- Product liability is the area of law dealing with claims of personal injury arising from the design, manufacture, distribution, or sale of a product.
- The three traditional causes of action in product liability lawsuits are negligence, breach of contract, and strict liability.
- These three causes of action hinge on the concept of product defect—meaning that the design or manufacturing of the product or warnings and instructions accompanying the product were defective.
- Central to any claim of product liability is causation. Did the product defect cause the cancer? The issue of cancer causation is critical when it comes to determining if a company is legally responsible for the patient's harm.
- In cancer causation cases (i.e., those regarding cigarette smoke or weed killer), patients use the concept of product defect to assert a legal claim.
- Not uncommon is a battle of the experts where the parties' different experts hold differing opinions on causation.
- The unusual theory of medical monitoring is invoked when patients claim that exposure to a hazardous or toxic product because of the company's negligence has made them significantly more likely to develop cancer in the future and that they are now burdened with obligations of monitoring and testing.
- In some jurisdictions, patients have to show not only that were they injured by a product in general but also that they were injured by a specific product of the company.
- Glyphosate more likely than not causes cancer, and that probability of causation can form the basis for patients' lawsuits.

References:

1. Wajert SP. *Product Liability Claims, Defenses and Remedies*. Washington, DC: Shook, Hardy & Bacon LLP; 2016:1–30.
2. *Southwest Pet Products, Inc. v Koch Industries, Inc.*, 273 FSupp2d 1041 (2003).
3. *Saller v Crown Cork & Seal Co*, 187 Cal App 4th 1220, 1234-37 (Cal Ct App 2nd Dist 2010).
4. *Sperry-New Holland v Prestage*, 617 So2d 248 (Miss 1993).
5. *Kent v Gulf States Utility Co*, 418 So2d 493, 497 (La 1982).
6. *Donovan v Philip Morris USA, Inc.*, 268 FRD 1, 13-17 (D Mass 2010).
7. Lung cancer screening. National Comprehensive Cancer Network. 2020. https://www.nccn.org/patients/guidelines/content/PDF/lung_screening-patient.pdf. Accessed September 3, 2021.
8. Guidelines for lung cancer screening. UpToDate. https://www.uptodate.com/contents/image?imageKey=PULM%2F64078. Accessed September 3, 2021.
9. Black WC, Gareen IF, Soneji SS, et al. Cost-effectiveness of CT screening in the national lung screening trial. *N Engl J Med*. 2014;371(19):1793-1802.
10. *Empire Healthchoice, Inc. v Philip Morris USA, Inc.*, 393 F3d 312 (2d Cir 2004).
11. 2D Cir. Reverses Insurer's Win Over Tobacco Companies Empire HealthChoice v. Philip Morris USA, ANTILR20 No. 9, *Andrews Tobacco Industry Litigation Reporter* 4.
12. *Parker v Mobil Oil Corp*, 824 NYS2d 584, 590 (N.Y. 2006).
13. *Milward v Rust-Oleum Corp*, 820 F3d 469, 471 (1st Cir. 2016).
14. *Hymowitz v Eli Lilly & Co*, 541 NYS2d 941 (NY 1989).

15. Monsanto no more: agri-chemical giant's name dropped in Bayer acquisition. NPR. June 4, 2018. https://www.npr.org/sections/thetwo-way/2018/06/04/616772911/monsanto-no-ore-agri-chemical-giants-name-dropped-in-bayer-acquisition. Accessed September 3, 2021.

16. California product/label database application. California Department of Pesticide Regulation. http://www.cdpr.ca.gov/docs/label/labelque.htm#regprods. Accessed September 3, 2021.

17. Tarazona JV, Court-Marques D, Tiramani M, et al. Glyphosate toxicity and carcinogenicity: a review of the scientific basis of the European Union assessment and its differences with IARC. *Arch Toxicol*. 2017;91(8):2723-2743.

18. Ludlow K. Australian Pesticides and Veterinary Medicines Authority. Sage. http://sk.sagepub.com/reference/nanoscience/n22.xml. Accessed September 3, 2021.

19. Revised glyphosate issue paper: evaluation of carcinogenic potential. Epa-Hq-Opp-2009-0361-0073. 2017. https://www.regulations.gov/document/EPA-HQ-OPP-2009-0361-0073. Accessed September 3, 2021.

20. EPA releases draft risk assessments for glyphosate. Environmental Protection Agency. December 18, 2017. https://www.epa.gov/pesticides/epa-releases-draft-risk-assessments-glyphosate. Accessed September 3, 2021.

21. BfR-contribution to the EU-approval process of glyphosate is finalised. Federal Institute for Risk Assessment. April 2, 2015. https://www.bfr.bund.de/cm/349/bfr-contribution-to-the-eu-approval-process-of-glyphosate-is-finalised.pdf. Accessed September 3, 2021.

22. International Agency for Research on Cancer. Glyphosate evaluation. *IARC Monogr*. 2015;112:321-412, https://www.iarc.who.int/featured-news/media-centre-iarc-news-glyphosate/. Accessed September 3, 2021.

23. In re: Roundup Products Liability Litigation (MDL No. 2741). US District Court Northern District of California. https://www.cand.uscourts.gov/judges/chhabria-vince-vc/in-re-roundup-products-liability-litigation-mdl-no-2741/. Accessed September 3, 2021.

24. Leon ME, Schinasi LH, Lebailly P, et al. Pesticide use and risk of non-Hodgkin lymphoid malignancies in agricultural cohorts from France, Norway and the USA: a pooled analysis from the AGRICOH consortium. *Int J Epidemiol*. 2019;48(5):1519-1535.

25. Bayer's roundup headache grows as plaintiffs pile into court. Bloomberg. October 30, 2019. https://www.bloomberg.com/news/articles/2019-10-30/bayer-is-now-facing-42-700-plaintiffs-in-roundup-litigation. Accessed September 3, 2021.

26. *Johnson v Monsanto Co*, No. CGC-16-550128, 2018 WL 2324413, at *1 (Cal Super May 17, 2018).

27. *Hardeman v Monsanto Co*, 216 FSupp3d 1037 (ND Cal 2016).

28. *Alva Pilliod and Alberta Pilliod v Monsanto Company*, 19 NW P I Lit Rpts 234.

CHAPTER 28

The Corporate Practice of Medicine

Sarah Diekman, MD, JD, MS, FCLM

I believe in corporations. They are indispensable instruments of our modern civilization. But I believe they should be so regulated that they shall act for the interests of the community as a whole.

—*Theodore Roosevelt*[1]

INTRODUCTION

This chapter covers the various types of legal restrictions governing the corporate practice of medicine. The core of these restrictions is that the physician and patient relationship cannot be interfered with by nonphysicians. In particular, it cannot be interfered with by nonphysicians who stand to make more money by controlling the diagnosis and treatment given to the patient by the physician. These laws arose to protect patient safety and create trust in the medical profession. In the current environment, there is evidence of room for improvement in both of these aims. This chapter explores the powers and limitations of corporate practice of medicine legislation. It ends with evidence from social science that addresses the root cause of many problems that the corporate practice of medicine laws seek to remedy. The balance of legal restrictions and social science (alternative to legal restrictions) can blend to create the win-win scenario where patients receive excellent and safe care, physicians feel they are actuating excellent care in a long and fulfilling career, and administrators are able to balance budgets and keep hospitals financially viable into perpetuity.

Understanding the history and origin of corporate practice of medicine law is important because it still guides how courts will interpret the law and gives information regarding social and legislative trends of the past, which, as with much of history, portends the future. The concept of the medical corporate practice and its bans arose from a series of reforms endorsed and originated by the American Medical Association (AMA). Of note, the historical portion of this chapter focuses on the AMA, which could imply that the history of MDs is the history of physicians. This implication should not be read into this text. It is only because the recorded reports of the legislative history of corporate practice of medicine law specifically credit the AMA that it is the focus of the historical part of this chapter. The history of physicians extends far beyond that of the AMA and MDs. Additionally, this chapter does not address the discriminatory application and pretextual purpose of many regulations and legislative efforts. The history section of this chapter is focused on the historical context that the courts will apply to current law by way of legislative intent interpretation.

HISTORY

The origins of the corporate practice of medicine started with the earliest actions of the AMA. Before there could be concerns of interference within the physician-patient relationship, there first was the issue of defining physician and patient. About 150 years ago, the newly formed AMA had concerns about the landscape of medicine. It was an open market that ranged from untrained dangerous fraudsters to experienced and science-based physicians. The AMA sought to bring standards and accountability to the profession of medicine.[2]

It was during the end of the 19th century that the AMA and its physician membership began a campaign to establish themselves as the professionals of medicine. They sought to protect the public from untrained people promising miracle cures to the public. Physicians sought to distinguish their profession as competent, regulated, and accountable for the care they provided. This meant that physicians would be registered, unlike the salesman of the time who would ride into town in a buggy, promising miracles from a secret potion. Physicians would be registered so that if they harmed someone they could be found. This path to accountability would lead to trust in the profession as a whole.[3]

The direct administration of unknown chemicals to patients, with unknown consequences, was something the AMA sought to stop. The majority of drug regulation would eventually happen on the federal level, with the first food and drug act signed by Roosevelt in 1906. Although the AMA did not seek direct regulation over drugs and medications, they did seek a common standard for physicians to follow when giving a substance to treat an illness. They wanted their profession to administer science-based treatments, not to take advantage of people's fears and desperation. The trustworthiness of medications played a role in this because, like the origins of trademark law, there was value seen in knowing you can trust what something is and where it came from. The AMA sought to have physicians be the gatekeepers that ensured trustworthy treatments were being used. Collectively, they would gain the public's trust by not overpromising cures, by not keeping secrets about medications for personal commercial value, and by holding the members of their profession accountable when they failed to live up to these standards.[4]

The AMA sought to achieve these goals through licensing standards for physicians. The AMA set out on an aggressive legislative campaign to pass restrictions on the practice of medicine in all states. To do this, they had to go state by state because, constitutionally, a restriction on health and safety cannot be passed via federal legislation. This is because, constitutionally, health and safety fall under the purview of the 10th and 11th Amendments, which leave these powers to the sovereignty of the states. In other words, the practice of medicine is defined state by state. An organization such as the AMA has to lobby each state to adopt a particular set of laws that adhere to their organization's set of ethics and values. Historically, this led to the establishment of medical societies in all states and the adoption of a medical practice act that makes it a criminal offense for anyone to practice medicine without a license. The practice of medicine is defined by a combination of statutory state medical practice acts, enumerated law, and common law, which defined who is a physician and who is a patient. When considering state laws, it is important to understand that this is a compromise between what the AMA as a lobbying group wanted and what the state legislators and politicians and the public wanted. The AMA has its own ethical guidelines that may or may not be adopted by state law.[5]

The AMA developed an internal ethical code for the first time in 1912. It outlined the established best practices for medical licensing. This included high-quality education requirements and raised the standards of medical education: a diploma from a licensed medical institution (additionally reformed and standardized), passing a state examination, training in a residency, and demonstrating bodily and intellectual soundness.[2] Although on its face, having standards and regulation creates certainty and trust, many of these regulations were discriminatory. Importantly, it is known that there was intentional malice behind critical pieces of these regulations, including the Flexner Report. The laws and restrictions served as pretext, used to effectuate racism and discrimination. This is a deep ethical problem that continues to this day. The medical education system has not adequately remedied it.[2]

Returning to restrictions on profit in medicine, there was a prohibition against physicians advertising. This actually runs afoul of the First Amendment, and such prohibitions are not enforceable. The 1912 code set out the basics of what is now the corporate practice of medicine doctrine. The guidelines severely restricted any consultation or skilled relationships between trained physicians and nonphysicians offering medical services. The AMA again sought to distinguish itself from secret potions and untraceable people. The AMA knew that, as a private organization, its code of ethics could only be enforced upon its members in their capacity as AMA members. If there were other concerns about maintaining high standards of patient safety, in order to stop corporations from controlling medicine and ruining the reputation of physicians through undue influence, state law would need to legislate to protect physicians' decisions from the invisible hand of corporate control via another legislative campaign.[6]

This legislative campaign began at the turn of the 20th century, after the success of the AMA medical licensing campaign. The increased regulations and requirements to practice medicine had led to more public trust in physicians. Physicians became valued and respected. As the public increasingly sought medical care exclusively from licensed physicians because they were experiencing quality care, the value of physician work hours increased. This led to increased corporate interest in controlling physicians and turning the public trust into a commodity. The AMA believed that this focus on money would compromise patient care and safety. The subsequent corporate practice of medicine guidelines and lobbying campaign sought to place a barrier between corporate power and the medical judgement of the physician. At its heart, these laws are supposed to protect the physician from being told what treatment to give a patient. This is to protect the patient from receiving expensive treatments that the physician does not believe will benefit the patient. These laws were not quick to take hold, and as the 20th century progressed, there was an upward thrust of massive corporations.[6]

Corporations were growing bigger and more powerful. Physicians who wished to care for patients, and not run a business, were agreeable to engaging with a corporation. In exchange, the physician could focus on medicine, not paperwork, overhead costs, billing, and regulations.

This led to less physician control over how patients were cared for. Corporations had more influence on the materials used in the practice, how patient charts were kept, and how patient care was administered. Individual physicians may have found that being employed by a corporation, rather than self-employed, benefited them as an individual. Collectively, when considering the effect of all these individual physicians' choices, the AMA was concerned that the net effect would be a public erosion of trust in physicians.[2]

Like the lobbying campaign to establish licensing requirements to practice medicine in all states, the AMA set out on a campaign to prohibit the corporate practice of medicine in all states. Unlike the previous campaign, this one did not establish a universal baseline across states. A small number of states did pass legislation that explicitly prohibited the corporate practice of medicine. More commonly, the courts implied prohibitions against the corporate practice of medicine when examining the legislative intent of the aforementioned licensing requirements to practice medicine.[4]

LEGAL DOCTRINE

The specific definitions and prohibitions on the corporate practice of medicine vary significantly from state to state. However, there are patterns for corporate practice of medicine restrictions, and knowing these principles can help one to examine and understand the meaning of the law in their state of interest. In broad terms, this legislation prohibits nonmedical professionals from the formation of business corporations in the medical field.

Across states, there is an exception to the prohibition against nonmedical professionals from the formation of business corporations, and that exception is nonprofit hospitals. This is a huge exception! It continues to become more significant as legislation has created more incentives for hospitals and put prohibitions on physicians owning hospitals. Nearly every state allows for the creation of professional corporations, which are corporations organized for the specific purpose of rendering a professional service. This includes allowance for the employment of physicians by certain entities. Each state varies in their exceptions; some explicitly permit hospitals to employ physicians, whereas others rely on court rulings based on implied law and public policy. No matter what the legal basis, the norm is that nonprofit hospitals are allowed to employ physicians. These exceptions carve out that hospitals are specifically prohibited from interfering with the independent medical judgment of the physician.[3]

The underlying rationale of corporate practice of medicine law is to prevent nonmedical factors from interfering with a physician's independent medical judgment, particularly when those factors are commercial. This is the intent that will be read into most corporate practice of medicine law. This commonly manifests within the law in 4 main ways: prohibiting business entities from employing physicians to provide medical care; requiring entities that provide medical services be owned and operated by licensed medical doctors; prohibiting professional fee splitting between licensed medical professionals and nonlicensed individuals or business entities; and setting the management fees stated within management services agreements at fair market value.[4]

The states with corporate practice of medicine laws require physician-controlled groups to obey certain boundaries when off-loading administrative tasks via management services agreements. Typically, a managed service agreement is the engagement of an outside company to perform the management services of the corporation. This is desirable to physicians who often prefer to spend their time caring for patients and wish to outsource issues of payroll, bookkeeping, budgeting, taxes, and insurance payments. Depending on the state's corporate practice of medicine law, this arrangement can be a violation. In the strictest states, in order to comport with the corporate practice of medicine laws, it is essential that management fees are at fair market value. The concern is for the improper incentives that arise if fees are too low, as this provides an inequitable income to the corporation, which allows for the management company to exert influence over the manner in which the physicians provide medical care. As such, this would be a violation of most states' explicit corporate practice of medicine laws.[4]

CLINICAL VIGNETTE # 1

Dr. Caring is a 45-year-old oncologist. For the past five years, she has been employed by a non-profit hospital, the Healing Hospital. Dr. Caring has found out recently that her salary is much lower than that of her male peers, and the Healing Hospital refuses to raise it. Not wanting to engage in an equal pay suit, Dr. Caring seeks to terminate her employment at the Healing Hospital and start employment at Our Lady of Equal Pay Hospital, which is across the state. The lawyers at the Healing Hospital inform Dr. Caring that she is bound by an employment contract with a noncompete clause. The lawyer further explains that Our Lady of Equal Pay Hospital is within the boundaries of the non-compete clause. Dr. Caring seeks legal advice. She explains to the lawyer that she does not want to bring an equal pay suit because she fears stigma and blacklisting from the medical community. She wants to explore legal options that are not based on a civil rights theory. Her lawyer suggests they explore the corporate practice of medicine laws of the state.

Under the corporate practice of medicine law of the state in question, is a contract between a hospital and a physician enforceable? The following case law explores whether a contract is void because of illegality if enforcing the contract would constitute the corporate practice of medicine. The outcome will vary by state law.

Many states have controlling case law that is 80+ years old. Depending on the amount of modern litigation, it can be unclear whether these cases are still good law, because medicine has changed so much that it is hard to compare the factual nexus. The modern cases tend to affirm a series of cases that were litigated in the early to mid-20th century.

CASE LAW # 1

In 1936, the Illinois Supreme Court issued its first ruling regarding the corporate practice of medicine in *People v United Medical Service*.[7] The attorney general of Illinois brought an action against United Medical Service, Inc., a domestic corporation. The attorney general demanded that United Medical Service produce proof of its "warrant ... to practice medicine or any of its branches or any system of treating human ailments."[7] At that time United Medical Service was a for-profit corporation with an issuance of 400 shares of common stock. The company was operating as a fixed-fee, low-cost medical service. It offered a variety of medical services including diagnosis, treatment, and minor surgeries. "[A]ll medical and surgical services which the respondent offers are rendered solely by physicians and surgeons licensed and registered by the State of Illinois."[7] The corporation published advertisements that depicted the nature of the business, including that it was *not* a charity, but rather was a for-profit enterprise. The court found that this structure was the corporate practice of medicine and was prohibited by the Illinois Medical Practice Act (Ill Rev Stat 1935, ch 91, par 1 et seq). "The corporation itself has never applied for or received a license to practice medicine in Illinois."[7] Thus, the court prohibited employment contracts from a for-profit corporation and a physician to engage in the practice of medicine.[7]

CASE LAW # 2

After the United Medical Service case, the courts of Illinois did not make any significant rulings until 1997 in *Berlin v Sarah Bush Lincoln Health Center*.[8] In this case, the Supreme Court of Illinois narrowed its reading of corporate practice of medicine, carving out an exception to the prohibition against the corporate practice of medicine to allow for enforcement of an employment contract between a hospital and physician. In this case, a physician sought to void an employment contract via a declaratory judgement from the court. The physician's position was that contracts between hospitals and physicians are not enforceable because they violate the corporate practice of medicine doctrine. The physician cited *People v United Medical Service* (see Case Law # 1) as binding precedent. The hospital contended that Illinois had no statutory prohibition against the corporate practice of medicine and that nonprofit hospital contracts with physicians are exempt from corporate practice of medicine doctrine as a matter of public policy.[8]

The court held that nonprofit hospitals are outside of the scope of any corporate practice of medicine doctrine that the state had adopted. Finding that the modern health care landscape necessitated contracts between physicians and nonprofit hospitals, the court stated, "We decline to apply the corporate practice of medicine doctrine to licensed hospitals. The instant cause is distinguishable from [past Illinois cases]. None of those cases specifically involved the employment of physicians by a hospital. More important, none of those cases involved a corporation licensed to provide health care services to the general public."[8] Based on this reasoning, the court enforced the contract between the hospital and the physician.

CASE LAW # 3

In *Gupta v Eastern Idaho Tumor Institute, Inc.*, there was a dispute about a contract between a radiation oncologist and a corporation. The radiation oncologist, Dr. Gupta, did not want the contract to be enforced. His case to the court was that the contract was illegal and therefore not enforceable. His basis for illegality was that the contract agreement was the corporate practice of medicine in violation of the Texas Medical Practice Act.[9]

Of note, this case contains references to California and Idaho. The ties to these states was not dispositive of the case and will not be addressed in this analysis. This case was litigated under Texas law where the clinic was physically located. The corporation in this case is Eastern Idaho Tumor Institute, Inc. This corporation was a consolidation of two corporations relevant to this case (the Ltd. and Gamma). The first of the two corporations, Northwest Radiation Medical Group, Ltd. (the Ltd.), was created in California in 1991 by four doctors practicing and licensed in Texas and two doctors practicing and licensed in California. The Ltd. was formed to open a radiation oncology clinic in Houston, Texas. After the purchase of the land, equipment, and construction of a specialized building, the Texas doctors had to part with their shares because they planned to refer to the Ltd. Without divesting their interest, the referrals would be a violation of federal law, which limits certain physician referrals (42 USCA § 1395). The four Texas doctors sold their interest in the Ltd. to the two California doctors, with the plan that the Texas doctors would refer patients to the clinic.[9]

The clinic operated for two years, from 1992 to 1994. Then the Ltd. sought to sell the clinic or find another doctor to operate it. In 1995, Dr. Gupta entered into a joint venture with the Ltd. Dr. Gupta would practice radiation oncology in the furnished building owned by the Ltd. Dr. Gupta would "provide, and be solely responsible for the payment of ... all necessary professional, medical, and administrative staffing necessary for the successful operation of the Joint Venture," and the Ltd. would "contribute all necessary equipment, office space, and machinery required for the successful operation of the Joint Venture."[9] The gross revenue would be divided equally.[9]

Now, the second corporation enters into the facts. Gamma Management, Inc. (Gamma), which was controlled by the Ltd., entered into an agreement with Dr. Gupta to manage the billings, collections, and accounts payable. Gamma and the Ltd. were consolidated into the single corporation, which was a party in this case, the Eastern Idaho Tumor Institute, Inc. (EITI). After the consolidation, EITI took over the billing, collections, and accounts payable on behalf of Gamma.[9]

Problems in the arrangement began in mid-1996 when Dr. Gupta ceased the sharing of billing information with EITI and instead performed more of the work himself. Dr. Gupta did not split the gross revenue with EITI for the remainder of the one-year joint venture. Near the end of 1996, the agreement expired, and the two parties negotiated without success to reach a new agreement. During the negotiation period, Dr. Gupta did not pay rent for the property or equipment and did not send EITI any portion of the gross revenue. Dr. Gupta defended his nonpayment to EITI because, as part of an oral agreement, EITI had agreed to have the four Texas doctors (the ones who divested their shares of the first corporation) refer patients to Dr. Gupta's clinic; however, Dr. Gupta contended that they were not referring patients to the clinic, and thus, he withheld payments to EITI.[9]

EITI attempted to evict Dr. Gupta several times, but because he was actively treating patients with courses of radiation and a closure of Dr. Gupta's practice would cause a lapse in care for patients at a critical time, medical ethics prohibited the eviction. Eventually, Dr. Gupta agreed to not take any new patients and vacate once all the existing patients had completed the IR radiation therapy, a process that took nearly one year.[9]

EITI filed suit against Dr. Gupta to recover damages for the time that Dr. Gupta was not paying rent on the building and equipment that EITI owned and not sharing a portion of the gross proceeds. A jury found in favor of EITI. Dr. Gupta appealed the finding on the basis that EITI was engaged in the corporate practice of medicine. He contended that this was a violation of the Texas Medical Practice Act and, thus, any contract between Dr. Gupta and EITI was void. Therefore, Dr. Gupta asserted that he should not have to pay damages for breaching a void contract.[9]

On appeal, the court held that this was a joint venture and EITI did not exert enough control over Dr. Gupta to be considered the corporate practice of medicine under the Texas Medical Practice Act. Specifically, the act, which was passed in 1993 (73rd Leg, RS, ch 862, § 17, 1993 Tex Gen Laws 3374, 3388; repealed and recodified 1999), defines practice of medicine. The act does not specify a definition for the corporate practice of medicine; it is inferred from this act. Under the act, a person is practicing medicine when they "[p]ublicly profess to be a physician or surgeon and ... diagnose, treat, or offer to treat any disease or disorder, mental or physical, or any physical deformity or injury by any system or method or to effect cures thereof; or [d]iagnose, treat, or offer to treat any disease or disorder, mental or physical, or any physical deformity or injury by any system or method and to effect cures thereof and charge therefor, directly or indirectly, money or other compensation."[9]

The court reasoned that Dr. Gupta was completely independent of EITI in regard to diagnosis, treatment, and any actions governed by the Texas Medical Practice Act. EITI did not have control over the work in a manner that would legally define it as Dr. Gupta's employer. The relationship was that of an independent contractor and therefore not the corporate practice of medicine as a violation of the Texas Medical Practice Act. Therefore, the underlying contract was found to be legal, and the judgment against Dr. Gupta was upheld.[9]

THE QUALITY CHASM

Despite the legal command that a physician's medical judgement must not be interfered with, there is an increasing feeling among physicians that third parties are dictating patient care. This means there is a large chasm between what the law is telling physicians and what physicians are perceiving as their reality. The reason for this could be the numerous exceptions to the laws, or it could represent a multitude of forces that combine to create pressures that interfere with patient care. Is the only solution to pass increasingly restrictive laws that narrow the exceptions to the prohibitions against the corporate practice of medicine? Would this even help physicians feel they can fully advocate for their patients? How can the leaders of current corporations manage health care systems in a way that allows physicians to fully advocate for their patients?

Patient safety and industrial organizational psychology research has shown that health care worker morale increases with patient safety. These fundamental stakeholders of medicine are not in opposition; they are in synergy. Therefore, the leaders of any corporation within medicine must look to the science of patient safety and health care worker health if they wish to be trustworthy in the eyes of the public. The alternative is to continue down a path that has led medical errors to increase from the eighth to the third leading cause of death in the United States. This is a system that the public has shown it will not tolerate. The literature on patient safety is clear. The literature on workplace burnout is clear. The implementation and execution of organizational leadership are needed for such leadership to maintain or re-earn legitimacy. The silver lining is that there are opportunities to achieve a system that is a win for everyone involved. Health care is not a zero-sum game.[11]

The public's reaction to adverse events in hospitals has been to increasingly legislate restrictions on health care corporations in an attempt to achieve *patient safety*. There is a common thread among the varying stakeholders of medicine, and it is *patient safety*. The heart of public trust is *patient safety*. The heart of corporate practice of medicine legislation is *patient safety*. The heart of health care worker morale is *patient safety*. How then does hospital management achieve this singular goal?

Patient safety benefits the financial bottom line of hospitals and the morale of health care workers, and most importantly, it realizes the purpose of medicine. Corporate culture has a strong influence on patient safety. This is an opportunity for corporate leadership to increase the morale of employees and patients. This change in perception is probably necessary if corporate healthcare systems do not want to be legislated out of existence.[12] History has shown that the public will rebel against corporate behavior that takes advantage of the current laws, especially when it affects their loved ones' health care, an issue that has polled as highly important to voters in recent years. Improving the safety and quality of care in hospitals is a path to public confidence.

SAFETY SCIENCE

Safety science is a science of its own. Competence in one field, such as medicine or finance, does not convey competence in safety science. As such, safety science deserves the focused attention and respect conveyed to the other aspects of health care. Safety science has been developed to understand the cause of adverse events so that they can best be avoided. Historical corporate management styles across fields have focused on punishing individuals for errors in an effort to avoid error. This is arguably a bad psychological motivator across industries, and specifically, safety science has shown it to be antithetical to safety.[11]

Over the past 30 years, social scientists have looked beyond the obvious when investigating error prevention. It is easy to do, but unhelpful to the future, to look at an accident such as an airplane crash and say, "The pilot ignored a warning light. He should not have done that. This is his fault. He was bad. We need to not hire bad people. If he was alive, we would fire him." This type of response to accidents is the "shame and blame" method. It focuses on individuals and holds them fully accountable for everything that happened. It also relies on hiring perfect human beings in order to prevent accidents. Safety science has explored these philosophies and found them to be flawed. First, does it make sense to place all of the responsibility for an accident onto one person? Certainly, the end user may have ignored the safety light, but did he control the fact that the safety lights routinely go off five times per flight and have always been false alarms? Did he control the corporate culture that led to the termination of three pilots who complained about the danger of routine false alarms? Safety science has found that organizational and corporate behaviors often have a lot more control over the accident than the end user. Is it fair or logical to say that a pilot had control of the situation when he ignored the light because, in the previous 1000 times he had seen it, it was a false alarm and his boss had told him to "stop complaining or find a new job"? Such a situation is what psychologists call a "double bind."[11]

A double bind is a situation where both options are flawed and distressing. Here, there can be no perfect employee because any choice the employee would make would lead to a bad outcome. Therefore, a system that relies on "shame and blame" is destined to have accidents and failures. Even more devastating is that those accidents and failures will be repeated over and over.

Safety science has sought to remedy this by looking at the system to see where errors were, in fact, predictable. The hope was and has been shown to be the reality: what can be predicted can be controlled. Systems failures can be uncovered, safety failures can be predicted, and tragedies can be avoided. This leads to the best outcome for all involved. Health care workers are able to care for patients as they dreamed of when they entered the field, and patients receive that care.[11]

This safety philosophy is formally described in two approaches: the person approach and the system approach. The person approach is the blame and shame approach. Individuals are sought out and given the responsibility of the error. In health care, this approach relies on the premise that there are good and bad health care workers and blames personal flaws, such as carelessness, intelligence, and lack of effort, for medical errors. This traditional approach has addressed hospital errors with the plan that if the "bad health care workers" can be found and culled from the herd, then the system will be free from errors. However, history has shown us that hardworking, careful, and intelligent individuals are involved with errors.[11]

The system approach concentrates on the conditions, routines, and policies surrounding the errors. This puts individuals in a role where the system is responsible for supporting their optimal performance. This has the advantage of system design, which can be resilient against human fatigue, human variability, and human interpretation. Humans cannot be separated from these intrinsic traits. This is the basic concept in human factors engineering. The premise is that the machine or system should not be designed for the perfect operator. Instead, the engineering should be designed with the realities of human beings in mind. This has been the approach of high-reliability organizations (demanding industries with low incident rates and an almost complete absence of catastrophic failures over several years), and the results are stellar records in safety despite the high potential for catastrophic errors. As Reason[11] stated, "Perhaps the most important distinguishing feature of high-reliability organizations is their collective preoccupation with the possibility of failure. They expect to make errors and train their workforce to recognize and recover from them. They continually rehearse familiar scenarios of failure and strive hard to imagine novel ones. Instead of isolating failures, they generalize them. Instead of making local repairs, they look for system reforms." In other words, if one person makes an error, the organization assumes others will make the same error and design a system to catch the error.[14]

COSTS

All industries have some form of liability risk. The physical safety of workers and the local environment factor into the management of all organizations. This cost factors into risk benefits analysis, as well as profit and loss considerations. Health care is arguably unique in that safety *is* the product. If patients are not safe, what is the purpose of health care? In addition to the costs of patient safety, health care has the usual cost of worker safety.

The most cynical and financially motivated managers should consider that patient safety is of huge financial interest to the organization. In terms of the general public and what might motivate the passage of increasingly restrictive legislation, the Institute of Medicine has estimated that preventable adverse events cost the nation $17 billion to $29 billion per year.[13]

Elastic costs associated with patient safety are the obvious hospital losses from legal judgments regarding injuries. There are large fluctuations in medical malpractice tort judgements and hospital-wide malpractice insurance based on performance. Another elastic loss is the unproductive costs of extra medical services for which the hospital cannot obtain payment because the extra hospitalization was due to poor care. The *inelastic* costs of medical errors are costs such as the operational cost of the risk-management office. However, if patient safety problems overwhelm the current personnel, they will become elastic because you have to hire new personnel to deal with the additional problems. The hospital may have to bring in consultants to fix problems such as regaining accreditation or hire public relations firms to fix a tarnished image.[13]

William Weeks and James Bagian[14] argued that two types of patient safety elements have indirect costs or benefits to the financial bottom line of the organization. First, the reputation of the hospital can be affected by word of mouth or more formal platforms such as the Leapfrog Group's publicly available safety information. Second, patient choice in the US free market system is a significant financial consideration, especially when a single incident can garner negative attention for years to come.[14]

MOTIVATION

Looking to the future of medicine, there is a need to increase the amount of attention and resources invested into the wellness of health care workers. In recent years, corporate leaders have realized that health care worker wellness has a very real relationship to retention of hospital staff and that such retention significantly affects a hospital's balance sheet. Both researchers and hospital leaders are realizing that health care worker burnout comes at a high price for the safety of patients and the financial bottom line of the hospital.

The issue of physician burnout has gotten the attention and respect of hospital chief executive officers (CEOs) in recent years. In 2016, a group of 10 CEOs of leading US health care organizations met with the AMA to address the issue of physician burnout. The result was an unequivocal statement that burnout is bad for business and the time has come to take it seriously. They issued a formal statement that said (among other things), "[we] unanimously concluded that physician burnout is a pressing issue of national importance."[17]

The financial cost of physician burnout has been taken more seriously in recent years. This has resulted in more research and estimates of the financial repercussions of physician burnout in the United States. The estimated cost to the health care industry is $4.6 billion a year. Studies have shown there is a financial link between physician burnout and the cost of patient safety failures. There are very real financial repercussions to a hospital with high physician burnout rates. The magnitude of the problem of health care worker burnout cannot be overstated. Studies performed prior to the COVID-19 pandemic estimated that at least half of physicians were feeling at least one of the symptoms of burnout, including emotional exhaustion, a feeling of detachment, or a diminished sense of personal accomplishment. This is twice the rate of the general public.[16]

Looking into the morphology of occupational burnout, there are theories that categorize it as a syndrome with three key dimensions: emotional exhaustion, feelings of cynicism and detachment from work, and a sense of low personal accomplishment. The downstream consequences of burnout have been shown to be negative clinical outcomes, decreased productivity, and increased absentee rates. Beyond the financial impact to a hospital based on those costs, physicians with burnout are more likely to reduce their work hours or leave the profession altogether. Specifically, studies have shown that for every one-point increase in burnout score, there is a 43% increase in the likelihood that a physician will be reducing their clinical effort during the following 24 months.[17]

The financial cost of burnout is interlinked with two component costs from physician turnover: the cost of physician replacement and the lost income from empty physician positions. Replacing a physician contains several loss components known as labor market friction costs: search costs, hiring costs, and physician orientation costs. Experts have quantified the cost of replacing a physician (resigns, retires early, changes careers, or dies) as between $500,000 and $1 million. This cost includes recruiting cost, lost revenue, and costs of training/onboarding new employee. These cost estimates do not account for any perpetually increased cost created by employee turnover increasing the likelihood of other employee turnover.[17]

At the 2016 summit mentioned earlier, the CEOs' collective statement defined burnout as an experience of emotional exhaustion, depersonalization, and feelings of low achievement and decreased effectiveness. They concluded that physician burnout is a pressing issue of national importance for patients and the health care delivery system. The statement was clear in stressing that the problem is not "physician shortcomings." Citing the rigorous selection process of physician training and pointing out that misapplying blame to work ethics of physicians detracts from actual problem solving and further contributes to burnout, the report stated:

> The spike in reported burnout is directly attributable to loss of control over work, increased performance measurement (quality, cost, patient experience), the increasing complexity of medical care, the implementation of electronic health records (EHRs), and profound inefficiencies in the practice environment, all of which have altered workflows and patient interactions. The result is that many previously well-adjusted and engaged physicians have been stressed to the point of burnout, prompting them to retire early, reduce the time they devote to clinical work, or leave the profession altogether.[17]

These comments speak to a level of control that is supposed to be prohibited by the corporate practice of medicine legislation. However, through various loopholes and exceptions, a great deal of control is exerted upon physicians. The corporate practice of medicine laws are not restraining this control. The nonlegislative solutions are garnering more respect.

The CEOs at the 2016 summit identified burnout as a warning sign of system-wide dysfunction. They cite high-quality patient care as a main driver of physician satisfaction. When physicians cannot deliver what they believe to be high-quality care to patients, they become burnt out.[17] Health care workers are the metaphorical "canary in the coal mine" of patient safety because health care worker dissatisfaction is driven by factors that impede patient care.

Barriers that will simultaneously decrease health care worker job satisfaction and patient safety include ineffective administrative and regulatory burdens, limitations of current technology, an inefficient practice environment, excessive clerical work, and conflicting payer requirements.[17]

The longevity and productivity of physicians are dependent on the reduction and prevention of burnout. The CEOs at the 2016 summit did more than identify that there is a problem; they set forth recommendations to their fellow health care CEOs: "Leaders of health care delivery organizations must embrace physician well-being as a critical factor in the long-term clinical and financial success of our organizations. There is a need for frameworks that prevent burnout and restore the joy of a career in medicine. Boards should hold CEOs accountable to implement these approaches to address physician burnout."[17]

MORAL INJURY

Beyond the concept of burnout, moral injury has been introduced as a theory of mental health problems in health care workers having a cause-and-effect relationship with patient safety. Historically, the theory or concept of moral injury was introduced alongside posttraumatic stress disorder (PTSD) as a result of the Vietnam War. Part of the injury that accompanied or caused PTSD was different than the mortal fear of one's death. Service members were suffering from something distinct from a survival instinct stressor; they were having an identity crisis in regard to their own moral compass. The acts they participated in during the war were incongruent with their previous identity of self and self-definition of a moral being. The war had forced them to act contrary to what their beliefs dictated was right. Researchers and clinicians observed this as a different category of psychological injury from the fear for life injuries. They also found that different treatments were required.[15]

With time, a term and definition arose. The term is *moral injury*. It is defined as the injury that occurs when an actor perpetrates, bears witness to, or fails to prevent an act that "transgresses our deeply held moral beliefs."[15] This type of injury has been implicated in health care and is logically consistent with the burnout evidence that links patient safety to health care worker burnout.[15]

In health care, the moral injury comes into play when the deeply held belief that time caring for the patient is paramount comes into conflict with the demands of third parties. The current hospital landscape is full of these double binds. While patients ask for health care workers' time and attention, health care workers are forced to dedicate their attention and mental resources to the electronic medical records, the insurers, the hospital, and other demands that feel like barriers to patient care. With each transaction where third parties get their needs met and patients do not, health care workers suffer the "sting of moral injustice." "Over time, these repetitive insults amass into moral injury ... Moral injury describes the challenge of simultaneously knowing what care patients need but being unable to provide it due to constraints that are beyond our control."[15]

There should be only one answer to the following question: Which do we take care of first: our patient, the hospital, the insurer, the electronic medical records, the health care system, or our productivity metrics? The current health care business framework of medicine creates multiple answers depending on the level of pressure from each stakeholder, thus distracting health care workers and leaving them with a feeling of divided loyalty. When health care workers set out on their mission of patient care, the answer is clearly that the care of the patient is always first. The dark reality is that, with time, the years of pressure tear at the seams of health care workers' moral compass, leaving them injured and without a path to return to their deepest ideals and motivations. Moral injury locates the source of distress in a broken system, and the solutions reside in creating a health care environment that finally acknowledges the value of the time clinicians and patients spend together developing the trust, understanding, and compassion that accompany a true relationship. The long-term solutions to moral injury include a health care system that prioritizes healing and allows health care workers to always put their patients' best interests first.[15]

Most health care workers enter into the profession to help patients, and the thought of a patient experiencing harm under their care is unthinkable. Yet, errors are so prevalent that it is the norm that a health care worker will be involved in one during their career. This takes a mental toll on the collective workforce. This issue deserves its own time and attention to mitigate the harmful effects.[15]

Studies have shown that being involved in an error increases the job-related stress of physicians. One study demonstrated the impact of errors on health care workers' well-being. After an error, health care workers reported increased anxiety about future errors (61%), loss of confidence (44%), sleeping difficulties (42%), reduced job satisfaction (42%), and harm to their reputation (13%). The impact of job-related stress was shown for *both* serious errors and near misses, demonstrating that events that may not even be recorded are having a negative impact on the mental health of health care workers.[18]

PREVENTING MEDICAL ERROR

Over the past 20 years, the problems of medical error and subsequent patient harm have gained the attention of major institutions. These authoritative and research bodies have established a body of knowledge that has shaped public policy and led to reforms in major institutions. In 1999 and 2001, the Institute of Medicine published two landmark reports that form the basis of modern patient safety philosophy. The reports revealed that the state of health care in the United States was one of quality failures and in urgent need of a redesign in order to achieve its most important aim of patient safety. This movement brought into existence practices that are so successful that recent trainees cannot imagine a system without them. One such example is the implementation of rapid response systems in hospitals across the country.[22]

HIGH-RELIABILITY ORGANIZATIONS

The science of safety has largely studied what is known as high-reliability organizations (HROs). The HROs "had carried out demanding activities with low incident rates and an almost complete absence of catastrophic failures over several years." HROs include nuclear aircraft carriers, air traffic control systems, and nuclear power plants. The organizations are certainly not medical or health care related, yet they share the relevant characteristics related to safety. Each of these fields, including health care, is complex, internally dynamic, and intermittently, intensely interactive. They have the potential for catastrophic failure. They performed exacting tasks under considerable time pressure and require maintaining the capacity for meeting periods of very high peak demand.[11]

HROs gained their name because they can be relied upon, and as such, patient safety experts have looked to them for practices that can be replicated and incorporated into medicine. A prominent feature of these successful organizations is that they recognize that "human variability" is part of a system and that good systems utilize this as a resource for "compensation and adaption to change" and to create safeguards when human variability may be a liability.[11]

In any organization or corporation, it is easy to look at the lack of adverse events at any given time and say that nothing bad is happening and that, therefore, the current state of affairs should continue. However, the inquiry into HROs has demonstrated that reliability is not static but is in fact a dynamic nonevent. James Reason[11] explains, "It is dynamic because safety is preserved by timely human adjustments; it is a non-event because successful outcomes rarely call attention to themselves." In other words, the situation is changing day to day and the people are changing day to day, and yet within that change, they are achieving the same outcome day to day: reliability. Therefore, it is paramount to look below the surface of "nonevents." Under the surface of daily nonevents, a plethora of situations can be unfolding. There could be daily near misses with health care workers who are highly aware that it is just a matter of time before a bad outcome occurs, or there could be an active system that is working to create nonevents each moment of the day. It is important to look below the surface and to carefully define what success is. Systems that punish reporting or warnings can have paradoxical effects on safety. An example is the common system that rewards "zero accidents" for so many days. Such a system rewards covering up accidents or subthreshold events. Reporting systems need to be evidence based to ensure that they are promoting behaviors that increase safety in a way that aligns with human nature. There is much to learn from the studies that have been done on HROs' success.[11]

THE CURRENT SYSTEMS MODEL

All models are wrong, but some are useful.

—George Box[19]

The safety onion systems model

Patient safety has been described as an onion, with all the pieces of the organization or corporation coming together toward a single "product." The product is patient safety. As Woodward et al.[20] state, "The systems approach of patient safety recognizes that most errors and adverse events arise from the fallibility of humans working within poorly designed care systems." This approach views patient safety as a function of the corporate operations. To fully realize the potential of maximum safety, the corporation must address all of the layers of patient safety and not quickly blame an individual when something goes wrong. Blaming individuals means that the problem will reoccur.[20]

The onion system approach starts with the layer of the "onion" that is the closest to the patient. The patient is the center of the metaphorical onion. This innermost layer includes behaviors and systems that are immediately involved in patient care, such as hand washing. The next layer are those measures that are less direct but still have an immediate effect on patient care, such as educational programs to reduce prescribing errors. Management decisions, such as nurse-to-patient ratios, might be made in rooms far away from patients. Even further from the center of the onion is the development of a bonus structure for health care workers and the development of checklists. At the edge of the onion, toward the metaphorical onion skin, are national patient safety measures. At different levels, a variety of actions may be effective. For some challenges, a checklist may be the most appropriate measure, whereas in other situations, a hard stop or education may be the right choice.[20]

The Swiss cheese model of system accidents

The most well-known systems model of medical error is the Swiss cheese model. In this model, a bad outcome results when multiple layers of defense fail in such a way that the strengths of each layer are not able to identify and compensate for the errors in a different layer. The imaginary visual model is that of several slices of Swiss cheese stacked on top of each other. The cheese represents the functioning portion of the system. The holes represent the specific failure on each level. A patient harm will occur when the events initiating the harm pass through each layer of health care (the cheese) and are undetected as a threat to the patient. This is akin to the holes of the cheese lining up, such that a finger (the danger) or the like could pass through. If even a single slice of cheese does not have the whole in the same place as the others, then the finger (the danger) cannot pass through. This block is equivalent to a health care system catching an error.

The modern system employs various safeguards to block patient harm by reducing the number of holes in the cheese. The less holes there are, the less likely it is that they will align.[11]

These defenses include engineered safeguards, the training of people, and administrative controls. Ideally, these would be completely effective and leave no holes and thus no opportunity for patient harm. "In reality, however, they are more like slices of Swiss cheese, having many holes—though unlike in the cheese, these holes are continually opening, shutting, and shifting their location."[11]

THE RELATIONSHIP BETWEEN MANAGEMENT AND HEALTH CARE WORKERS

One strategy that health care organizations have implemented in order to improve patient safety and relationships between health care workers and executives and managers is the implementation of executive walk rounds (EWRs). This method also reduces communication barriers that might lead to the corporate practice of medicine as administration creates policies with no feedback from the front lines. The execution of EWRs varies from institution to institution, but they share some general principles: hospital executives visit workers engaged in clinical care in the physical location of the patient care and discuss patient safety. The idea is to break down the communication barriers between executives or managers and the frontline health care workers. It also has the potential to dispel assumptions that those whose expertise is in other fields (e.g., finance, informatics) might have about the realities of patient care. During EWRs, "the executive may ask providers to discuss specific events or general processes that could put patients at risk for harm, they ask for suggestions to improve safety, and verbalize their commitment to improving safety. Discussions are documented and lead to action which is followed by feedback to participants."[21]

Ideally, this strategy identifies opportunities for improvement in patient care by maximizing the wisdom, experience, and expertise of health care workers. Further, this structure is designed to demonstrate leadership's commitment to patient safety and move away from a "shame and blame" culture that focuses on individual error. The goal is to create a culture that encourages error reporting and response. EWRs were investigated in a 2005 study. This study estimated that, at that time, at least 200 hospitals had used EWRs. These identified institutions were participating in a collaboration with the Institute for Healthcare Improvement. The study found that nurses who participated in EWRs had higher safety climate scores than nonparticipants. The study also found that only those who participated directly in the EWRs showed improved ratings, underscoring the importance of investment in full faculty participation.[21]

MEASURES OF SAFETY CULTURE

Not all scores of safety are accurate, and some measures can actually work against safety. Systems that reward cover-ups instead of acknowledging shortcomings will achieve a result that is counter to their aim. Many institutions have implemented systems to measure the safety of the institution. Some tie safety culture survey scores to the bonuses of managers. The effectiveness of such measures depends on multiple factors. To truly design an effective inventory tool and response, research is needed. Without identifying which of these characteristics is in play, the wrong things may be rewarded and punished. Safety culture is such that the wrong incentives can dramatically increase the wrong outcome. Just like other instruments in medicine, the instruments that measure safety culture must be valid and reliable. In other words, they must measure what you are trying to measure, and they should produce similar results with repetition. Studies have investigated safety measurement tools such as the Safety Climate Tool Survey. This survey was studied and validated in Canadian health care institutions. The long version of the Safety Climate Tool Survey overall (22 items) and the 13-item scale "had construct validity and sufficient reliability."[22] A shorter seven-item version was studied but was found to lack sufficient validity. Another survey, the Safety Attitudes Questionnaire (rather than just safety climate), is in use at the Johns Hopkins Hospital, where it is continually evaluated for validity and reliability. The findings have been that when one's unit engages in the measure and feedback process, other units express the desire to follow suit. Currently in the health care industry, the Safety Attitudes Questionnaire is the most widely used cultural assessment tool. To improve culture once it is assessed, the Comprehensive Unit-Based Safety Program (CUSP) has been shown to produce results. It provides a practical framework with a focus on improving patient safety. CUSP uses the mantra "culturally, clinically, and operationally" to describe the framework that is applied unit by unit. This piece-by-piece evaluation and response are important because culture is local and the hospital units are the functional units that combine to make the hospital as a whole.[22]

HEALTH CARE CULTURE PSYCHOLOGY

The health and wellness of health care workers are essential to the success of a hospital and patient safety. It is not breaking news that sleep deprivation is a problem in medicine. In 1971, Friedman et al. "demonstrated that interns made more errors reading ECGs at the end of shift."[20] This and subsequent studies have confirmed what common sense tells us—that the length of shifts are tied to patient safety. All high-reliability industries identify sleep deprivation as a risk to safety and utilize frameworks that eliminate it. Studies continue to show that medical workers suffer from fatigue, unsafe staffing levels, and inappropriate handovers. All of these factors increase the chance of error and affect the financial bottom line of the hospital. It is the choice of the leadership as to whether the money will be spent on an up-front investment in time and resources for workers or be paid through lawsuits after patients get hurt. Even further, the organization will pay with increased administrative burden as the public loses trust in the corporate hospitals and responds with increased corporate practice of medicine regulation.[23]

Although it may seem that medical and aviation workers have very little in common, aviation has been used as a model for medical safety. In fact, medicine and aviation have a great deal in common. They are both expected to function without error. The aviation industry has invested time and attention to issues of perceptions of fatigue, stress, and error. Medicine has attempted to follow suit. However, there is still a lot of work to be done before medicine can be said to have effectively tackled these issues. "Much progress has been made to create a culture in aviation that deals effectively with error, whereas in medicine substantial pressures still exist to cover up mistakes, thereby overlooking opportunities for improvement."[23]

Historically, aviation had safety in the public eye, almost from its inception. It is the nature of airplane accidents that they are public and receive a great deal of attention. This means that there is a strong external pressure on the aviation industry to have a perfect performance record or the industry will perish. In the 1950s, after the introduction of jet transport, there were very few accidents caused by mechanical failures. The research community, the National Aeronautics and Space Administration, and regulatory agencies revealed that the majority of accidents were caused by "breakdowns in crew coordination, communication, and decision making."[23] These organizations improved safety by shifting the culture within the aviation industry to a more open one that accommodated questioning and recognized human limitations.[23]

Through the years, the aviation industry has used survey tools to inventory pilot attitudes about safety and interpersonal interactions. This has allowed leaders and researchers to diagnose the strengths and weaknesses of the industry's culture and subsequently develop interventions. Somewhat surprising and definitely encouraging is their finding that individuals' attitudes are malleable and responsive to training interventions. Of note, the psychological concept of attitude (which is malleable) is distinct from the psychological concept of personality, which is persistent across time and situation.[23]

One example of a training intervention is known as crew resource management training. It uses surveys to inventory and then address the attitudes of the cockpit crew. These dynamics within hierarchies have been shown to be very important for safety. Several examples exist in aviation where junior crew pointed out errors that were ignored because of their junior status. The result was complete loss of life on the airplane. The attitudes survey has been shown to address specific attitudes, change related behavior, and improve performance of the cockpit crew. To translate these inventories from aviation to medicine, only slight changes in language are required, with no underlying changes in the principle of team dynamics. In aviation, the junior *cockpit crew* members should be able to question the decisions made by senior cockpit crew members, and in medicine, junior *team* members should be able to question the decisions made by senior team members. Researchers have proposed that these same survey measures can be implemented in medicine. They hypothesize that attitudes about errors, teamwork, and the effect of stress and fatigue are good subjects for survey studies. This can be done internally for the benefit of the corporation or as part of a study to publish. The advantage of surveys is that they are inexpensive. For a survey to be effective, it should tap into the attitudes toward stress, hierarchy, teamwork, and error. A good deal of evidence has shown that surveys that reach these issues are relevant to understanding error, predictive of performance, and sensitive to training interventions.[23]

INDUSTRIAL AND ORGANIZATIONAL PSYCHOLOGY

The specialty of industrial and organizational psychology (I/O psychology) is the field that specializes in studying human behavior in organizations and the workplace. "The specialty focuses on deriving principles of individual, group and organizational behavior and applying this knowledge to the solution of problems at work."[24] I/O psychology focuses on many issues that plague health care corporations, including issues of recruitment, selection and placement, training and development, performance measurement, workplace motivation and reward systems, quality of work life, structure of work and human factors, organizational development, and consumer behavior. Therefore, there is great potential to utilize the expertise of this field to make real change in health care corporations.[24]

I/O psychology has investigated the phenomenon of health care worker burnout and identified factors that need to be addressed and strategies to do so. The research has investigated the organizational stressors that lead to burnout and the modifiable workplace characteristics. A key finding is the moderation effect of job control on the relationship between workload and exhaustion. Studies have shown that workload predicts employee exhaustion (a positive association exists between workload and exhaustion). This correlation is strongest when job control is lower. In other words, the less control workers feel they have over the workplace, the more exhausted they will feel in proportion to the hours worked. In contrast, if workers feel they have control over the workplace, they will feel less exhausted even if they are working more hours. Both workload and job control play pivotal roles in healthy working condition.[25]

The literature on burnout shows that exhaustion comes before burnout. Therefore, it can be used as a warning sign for the need for organizational intervention. If CEOs wish to reduce the turnover in their organization, the literature shows that exhaustion needs to be taken seriously and intervened upon. Simply telling employees to "suck it up" or that their colleagues are able to handle the schedule is a recipe for burnout and turnover. The consequence of ignoring exhaustion is predictable and financially costly. Ignoring the problem may yield short-term gains, but in the long run, it erodes the vitality of the institution, and it may take decades to undo the damage. Time off for employees is an investment in long-term employee performance. I/O psychologists have found significant psychological impact from days off during work cycles. Specifically, Sonnentag and Fritz state:

> For most people, weekends—or other periods of one to three full days off work— provide more free time than workday evenings and therefore offer more opportunities for psychological detachment. Even when an employee does not fully detach during evening hours throughout the workweek, he or she might detach from work during one or more days off. This increased opportunity for detachment might be partly due to the larger amount of time that is available to unwind and recover. In addition, during off-work days, many people pursue other activities than during weekday evenings which by themselves may foster psychological detachment. Thus, in an optimal situation, an employee will detach from work during the nonwork days so that physiological strain levels and negative affective states are reduced and well-being increases. The more an employee detaches from work during the nonwork days, the more likely it is that job stressors experienced during the workweek lose their impact on employees' strain levels.[26]

The cumulative effect of chronic overwork is a maladaptive psychological compensation because there is no substitute for time off work. In health care training, there is a sense of "breaking in" of students—a belief that the human needs of sleep, eating, and relationships can be overcome by training. But are they really overcome by training, or are we experiencing large-scale maladaptive psychological compensation with the downstream effects of large-scale burnout, health care worker shortages, and suicides? The mind likely adapts to the absence of life necessities during health care training, by culturally devaluing those necessities, with the consequence of shortened careers. Sonnentag and Fritz describe the effect of continued depravation of time off work:

> If an employee tends not to detach from work over several weekday evenings or a few days off, this tendency of not detaching may develop into a habit (Ouellette & Wood, 1998) and may become the employee's usual way of spending evenings and weekends. This employee's overall level of psychological detachment will differ from that of an employee who successfully detaches from work during evenings or days off and who has developed leisure routines that help in detaching. Encountering job stressors day after day will reduce the likelihood of detachment so that over time, the lack of detachment turns into a chronic state. As a result, strain levels will remain chronically elevated. If this person, however, succeeds in detaching from work during evenings and off-work days despite high levels of stressors, strain levels will be relatively low and will not increase substantially over time.[26]

Researchers have laid out a framework for reducing the risk of burnout, exhaustion, or cynicism and increasing a sense of efficacy. The framework focuses on six key areas that need to be seriously addressed by leadership and managers. These areas are manageable workload, job control, reward, community, fairness, and values. This again reiterates the importance of control over work. In the current climate, the data clearly show that health care workers do not feel a sense of control over their work. In fact, they feel a devastating loss of control over their work.[25]

Among I/O experts, there is widespread agreement that "preventing burnout is a better strategy than waiting to treat it after it becomes a problem."[25] Further enforcing this concept is evidence that burnout is, so to speak, "contagious." Formally, this is known as a cross-over effect. The more burnt-out health care workers in an environment, the more likely others will become burnt out. This is proposed to be because the underlying cause of burnout is affecting both parties; in addition, downstream workers are affected by an environment that is full of burnt-out workers, which is an additional stressor.[25]

No doubt leaders and managers face challenges when trying to implement long-term strategies. There is always a balance that must be struck between the pressures for short-term gain and the delayed gratification of long-term benefit. For example, running a hospital with a minimal workforce and maximal patient load might yield short-term financial gains by lowering overhead and increasing revenue. However, month after month, this pace will put patients in danger and create burnout among the health care workers. The increase turnover and difficulty recruiting to an institution with a bad reputation among health care workers will, in the long run, outstrip any short-term gains that were made by running the hospital short staffed. Input from the health care workers as to the appropriate staffing levels of the unit will improve the workers' sense of control and provide valuable feedback about the realities of the unit. The long-term gains are less patient harm and lower rates of employee burnout.[25] Ensuring that physicians have a strong voice in the environment of patient care protects the hospital from litigating violations of the corporate practice of medicine.

THE CAUSE EFFECT

Moving beyond I/O psychology into motivation strategies that will increase hospital workforce reliability without violating the corporate practice of medicine laws, there is an organizational success strategy known as "the cause effect." This effect is a major advantage that health care leaders have, if they choose to capitalize on it. The cause effect centers on employee motivation, rather than talent, in order to make an organization thrive. The corporation's definition of success is central to employee motivation. In health care, the motivation of workers is clearly patient focused. Health care workers, in general, are deeply motivated by patient care. This widespread level of passion in an industry is rare, and hospital leaders can benefit from it using the cause effect. The flip side is the aforementioned moral injury that occurs when employees feel they are working against their deeply held motivations. The cause effect recognizes that employees must buy into the central purpose of the organization.[27]

Let this be a warning to any manager who thinks they can fool their health care workers with public relations and branding stunts. The fabulous e-mail blasts and events in the lobby will not fool those who are touching and talking to patients every day. They will know if their patients are safe and if the leaders value patient safety. If the health care workers continually get the message that the corporation's definition of success is profit based, then the majority of health care workers will not buy into this model of success. As a general rule, health care does not attract profit-focused workers; there are many fields that offer profits with far less physical, emotional, and mentally taxing work than health care. Those who show up on the frontlines of health care are those who are driven by the desire to help patients. To truly motivate health care workers, the organization must be genuine in the "cause" that the organization is aiming to move toward.[27]

An organization certainly has to meet its financial obligations; thus, finances do tie into patient care and safety. If health care workers are to buy into the success of a corporation, the corporation will need to provide a vision of patient safety and care. Any financial success will need to be tied to the vision of patient care, which is supported by the financial vitality of the organization. Successful projects have at their core a palpable cause. Rallying teams around this shared sense of purpose means tapping into their hearts. And when the entire team builds collective identity around a common cause, the project transcends "work" and becomes a mission. Games are changed. Tables are turned. Crises are averted. We call this the cause effect.[27]

A STORY OF ORGANIZATIONAL TURNAROUND

In 2001, Anne Mulcahy stepped up as the proverbial captain of the ship of Xerox. As CEO, she held the responsibility to steer Xerox away from disaster as it careened toward Chapter 11 bankruptcy. The year before she took the wheel as CEO, Xerox had lost $273 million (year 2000), but under her leadership, the company avoided bankruptcy and rebounded to profits ($91 million in 2003).[28]

So how did she do it? How did she turn around a company with over $17 billion in debt and six years of record-breaking losses? She stepped into her role with a defined vision and set out getting her employees to buy into it.[29]

Mulcahy sought honest evaluation and feedback from the employees. She was met with a culture where there was unwillingness to speak up and tell an authority figure the truth about what was needed. Mulcahy found it to be essential to create an environment where employees felt safe in giving honest and constructive feedback while moving toward the vision she laid out: "They have to know that they won't be penalized for speaking up and that their bosses take their suggestions seriously. You can never depend on filtering information up through the company. You have to talk to frontline employees."[28]

Mulcahy saw the need for employees to have a vision of a future that they wanted to buy into. She was approached by employees asking what life after the turnaround would look like. She is quoted as saying, "I would think to myself, 'Why aren't you asking me whether or not we're going to make it?'" Realizing these concerns needed to be met with a road map from the current situation to the place where employees wanted to be, she took the unusual step of writing a fictitious *Wall Street Journal* article describing Xerox in the year 2005. "We outlined the things we hoped to accomplish as though we had already achieved them. We included performance metrics—even quotes from Wall Street analysts. It was really our vision of what we wanted the company to become."[29] She then led the company into an operation that matched the fictitious article. She created a vision that her employees bought into. She sought their input. She created a culture of safety. She turned around the sinking ship.[29]

In keeping with Mulcahy's successful method, this chapter ends with a fictitious memo. As Mulcahy did with the fictitious *Wall Street Journal* article, this memo is written in the future. It tells of a health care corporation that was desperately in need of a turnaround. It is an exercise in imagination and self-evaluation. What does your corporation want to be writing memos about three years from now? Do you want things to keep going as they are going? Or is this something that you would be prouder of?

Memo

Esteemed workers,

Several years ago, we were in a dark time in the history of our institution. Employee burnout was at an all-time high, and patient safety was at an all-time low. This was not because of our knowledge, not because of our skills. Health care can do more now than could even be dreamed of 100 years ago when antibiotics were first invented. Yet, many of you were left without feeling that you had a place at the table.

In this scene, we were hit with the biggest possible challenge, a pandemic. Many of you were struggling with your motivation to show up to work before the pandemic hit. When it did hit, you were asked to work more, to risk more, and to give more than you ever dreamed. The fatigue and pain that you already felt got immeasurably worse.

At this institution, we did not give in. We decided to take this devastating event and use it as an opportunity to build a better institution. We did not tell you what that institution would look like; we asked you what it should look like. Your years of expertise and wisdom shaped our vision into one that would actually deliver effective and safe patient care.

Central to our rebuilding process and the root of our subsequent success was the health of health care workers. We no longer treated health care worker health as an afterthought or pet project. We made it central to our plan. We invested in building a work environment that no one wanted to leave. We invested in safe work schedules. This meant that we hired more employees for schedules that used to be done by less. We did not cut the pay or benefits for anyone. We simply added more people to care for our patients. It cost us more money up front, but we have saved millions by reducing employee turnover and reducing elastic costs related to safety.

We listened to you through safety and workflow initiatives. We now have a healthy and happy workforce. The result is excellent patient care. All of our metrics have improved. Our patient outcomes are the top in the nation. Our patient satisfaction scores are excellent. These improved metrics have made us the institution where patients want to receive care.

With your help, we created a system that expands and contracts depending on the needs of patients. Using your experience, we did this in a way that adds to employees' quality of life. This has made us the institution that employees want to work at. We do not have to pay hundreds of thousands of dollars to recruiters in order to leverage someone to sign a contract that will maximize the amount of work we can get before they leave. Now, health care workers want to work here. We don't have to try to trap them into working here.

All of this has led to a dramatic reduction in lawsuits against the institution. Increased patient safety initiatives have led us to have the lowest malpractice premiums in the nation. Other lawsuits are down as well. We previously had to defend civil rights lawsuits for discriminatory behavior and workplace harassment. Defending these suits one at a time, without implementing meaningful programs to identify and address workplace harassment and discrimination, was costing us hundreds of thousands of dollars in legal fees. It also led to disruptions in our workforce and harmed employees, at a cost that was difficult to calculate. We stopped ignoring the problem, we investigated what was really happening in our institution, and we implemented meaningful systematic change. As a result, there have been no viable suits against us in the last several years. Further, the diversity of employees has improved, and now our work force reflects the community we serve. This has led to higher quality care and better community relationships.

Looking back on how far we have come, it is hard to imagine how you worked in the old environment. You certainly are tenacious. At one time, we relied too much on that tenacity. We relied on it until you were burnt out, depressed, and suicidal. You deserved better. Your patients deserved better.

As your CEO, I am so proud of how far this institution has come. I thank you for your vision, your contribution, your wisdom, and your participation in the process. You are essential in our continued journey to be the gold standard of medicine. I look forward to your ideas going forward. I know we can do this together.

With humility,

Your CEO

CONCLUSION

The corporate practice of medicine restrains corporations and nonphysician interference in medicine in four main ways: by prohibiting business entities from employing physicians to provide medical care; by requiring entities that provide medical services be owned and operated by licensed medical doctors; by prohibiting professional fee splitting between licensed medical professionals and nonlicensed individuals or business entities; and by stating within management services agreements that management fees must be set at fair market value.

Despite this being the letter of the law, the feeling among many physicians is that they are being told by administrators what devices to use, what medications can be prescribed, and how much time they have to discuss the risk, benefits, and alternatives with the patient. Physicians are demoralized by short production line–style office visits. Often underestimated is the mental toll on health care workers when their patients experience serious adverse events. The epidemic of physician and health care worker burnout has an economic cost to the system that should be considered when interpreting existing legislation and promotion of new legislation on the corporate practice of medicine.

The prohibition on the corporate practice of medicine has many exceptions. The interference in the physician-patient relationship has inherent dangers for the patient and physician. Our current system is manifesting the consequences of such interference. It is possible to legislate stricter corporate practice of medicine laws to try and restore protections for physicians and patients. It is also possible to employ nonlegal strategies for safety, motivation, and respect for the physician-patient relationship.

KEY POINTS:

- Generally, the definition of corporate practice of medicine law is the prohibition of corporations from practicing medicine or employing a physician to provide professional medical services.
- The main reason behind corporate practice of medicine law is to avoid divided loyalty and impaired confidence between the interests of a corporation and the needs of a patient.
- Patient safety is central to laws that limit the corporate practice of medicine.
- The corporate practice of medicine restrains corporation and nonphysician interference in medicine in four main ways: by prohibiting business entities from employing physicians to provide medical care; by requiring entities that provide medical services be owned and operated by licensed medical doctors; by prohibiting professional fee splitting between licensed medical professionals and nonlicensed individuals or business entities; and by ensuring that management fees stated within management services agreements are set at fair market value.
- The legislative trend is toward increasing restrictions on the corporate practice of medicine in an effort to protect patient safety.
- Courts have allowed employment contracts between physicians and nonprofit hospitals as a matter of public policy.

- In general, health care workers and the public do not think that hospital corporations are currently safe enough or functioning for the best interest of patients.
- Patient safety is closely related to health care worker well-being.
- Corporate attitudes and systems design strongly influence a culture of safety.
- Health care worker burnout is associated with patient safety. When patients are in danger, health care workers experience burnout.
- Safety culture is promoted by taking a system approach, rather than an individual approach, to safety.
- Industrial organizational psychology has demonstrated that the work-life balance of hospital employees is important for patient safety.
- Corporate organizations can improve patient safety by engaging in evidence-based practices and engaging in culture reform that centers on health care worker well-being.

References:

1. Theodore Roosevelt: I believe in corporations. AZ Quotes. https://www.azquotes.com/quote/1413358. Accessed September 3, 2021.
2. Welk P. The corporate practice of medicine doctrine as a tool for regulating physician-owned physical therapy services. *J Law Commerce*. 2004;23:231.
3. Axelrod J. The future of the corporate practice of medicine doctrine the future of the corporate practice of medicine doctrine. *DePaul J Health Care Law*. 1997;2:103.
4. Brunkow J. 3 Steps to navigate through the corporate practice of medicine. Becker's Hospital Review. 2020. https://www.beckershospitalreview.com/legal-regulatory-issues/3-steps-to-navigate-through-the-corporate-practice-of-medicine.html. Accessed September 3, 2021.
5. Gustavson M, Taylor N. At death's door: Idaho's corporate practice of medicine doctrine. Idaho L Rev 479, 518. Published 2011. https://sbp.senate.ca.gov/sites/sbp.senate.ca.gov/files/At%20Deaths%20Door%20Idahos%20Corporate%20Practice%20of%20Medicine%20Doctrine.pdf. Accessed September 3, 2021.
6. Starr P. *The Social Transformation of American Medicine: The Rise of a Sovereign Profession and the Making of a Vast Industry*. 2nd ed. New York, NY: Basic Books; 1984.
7. *The People v United Medical Service*, 362 Ill 442 (Ill 1936).
8. *Berlin v Sarah Bush Lincoln Health Ctr*, 179 Ill 2d 1 (Ill 1997).
9. *Gupta v Eastern Idaho Tumor Institute, Inc.,* 140 SW3d 747 (Tex App 2004).
10. Facing up to medical error. *BMJ*. 2000;320(7237):A.
11. Reason J. Human error: models and management. *Br Med J*. 2000;320(7237):768–770.
12. Healthcare System. Gallup Historical Trends. https://news.gallup.com/poll/4708/healthcare-system.aspx. Accessed April 3, 2021.
13. Mello MM, Studdert DM, Thomas EJ, Yoon CS, Brennan TA. Who pays for medical errors? An analysis of adverse event costs, the medical liability system, and incentives for patient safety improvement. *J Empir Legal Stud*. 2007;4(4):835–860.
14. Weeks WB, Bagian JP. Making the business case for patient safety. *Jt Comm J Qual Saf*. 2003;29(1):51–54.
15. Dean W, Talbot S, Dean A. Reframing clinician distress: moral injury not burnout. *Fed Pract*. 2019;36(9):400–402.
16. Blanding M. The Economic Cost of Physician Burnout. Harvard Business School: Working Knowledge. 2019. https://hbswk.hbs.edu/item/the-economic-cost-of-physician-burnout. Accessed September 7, 2021.

17. Noseworthy J, Madara J, Cosgrove D, et al. Physician burnout is a public health crisis: a message to our fellow health care CEOs. Health Affairs Blog. Published 2017. https://www.healthaffairs.org/do/10.1377/hblog 20170328.059397/full/. Accessed September 7, 2021.

18. Waterman AD, Garbutt J, Hazel E, et al. The emotional impact of medical errors on practicing physicians in the United States and Canada. *Jt Comm J Qual Patient Saf*. 2007;33(8):467–476.

19. Barroso G. "All models are wrong, but some are useful." George E. P. Box. Marie Skłodowska-Curie Innovative Training Network. https://www.lacan.upc.edu/admoreWeb/2018/05/all-models-are-wrong-but-some-are-useful-george-e-p-box/. Accessed September 7, 2021.

20. Woodward HI, Mytton OT, Lemer C, et al. What have we learned about interventions to reduce medical errors? *Annu Rev Public Health*. 2010;31(1):479–497.

21. Thomas EJ, Sexton JB, Neilands TB, Frankel A, Helmreich RL. The effect of executive walk rounds on nurse safety climate attitudes: a randomized trial of clinical units. *BMC Health Serv Res*. 2005;5(1):28.

22. Pronovost P, Sexton B. Assessing safety culture: guidelines and recommendations. *Qual Saf Health Care*. 2005;14(4):231–233.

23. Sexton B, Thomas E, Helmreich RL. Error, stress, and teamwork in medicine and aviation: cross sectional surveys. *BMJ*. 2000;320(7237):745–749.

24. Industrial and organizational psychology. American Psychological Association. https://www.apa.org/ed/graduate/specialize/industrial. Accessed September 7, 2021.

25. Portoghese I, Galletta M, Coppola RC, Finco G, Campagna M. Burnout and workload among health care workers: the moderating role of job control. *Saf Health Work*. 2014;5(3):152–157.

26. Sonnentag S, Fritz C. Recovery from job stress: the stressor-detachment model as an integrative framework. *J Org Behav*. 2015;36(S1):S72–S103.

27. The cause effect. Deloitte. https://www2.deloitte.com/content/dam/Deloitte/us/Documents/process-and-operations/us-the-cause-effect-book.pdf. Accessed July 17, 2020.

28. The cow in the ditch: how Anne Mulcahy rescued Xerox. Knowledge@Wharton. https://knowledge.wharton.upenn.edu/article/the-cow-in-the-ditch-how-anne-mulcahy-rescued-xerox/. Accessed September 7, 2021.

29. Vollmer L. Anne Mulcahy: the keys to turnaround at Xerox. Stanford Graduate School of Business. https://www.gsb.stanford.edu/insights/anne-mulcahy-keys-turnaround-xerox. Accessed September 7, 2021.

CHAPTER 29

Presumption Laws for Firefighter Cancers

Kenji Saito, MD, JD, FACOEM

INTRODUCTION

A growing number of studies demonstrate that firefighters are exposed to more toxins and have higher rates of cancer relative to the general population.[1,2] Recently, there has been an increase in the number of states adopting cancer presumption laws for firefighters, which most often fall under workers' compensation. Presumptive legislation shifts the burden of proof to the employer; it holds the employer and insurer responsible for disproving that the cancer was unrelated to work as a firefighter. While these laws aim to compensate firefighters for the significant expenses associated with cancer diagnosis and treatment, many first responders are employed by municipalities or governmental divisions, and the financial burden of this legislation on local governments can be significant.[3]

In recognition of the increased risks associated with line-of-duty exposures, federal regulations were passed in 2010 and 2018 to secure funding for health complications in first responders and survivors of the 9/11 terrorist attacks and to develop and maintain a voluntary registry of the incidence of certain cancers in firefighters.[4,5] There is no federal legislation directly addressing firefighter presumption law, and the state laws vary significantly. In an attempt to make these laws more accessible to the public, the First Responder Center for Excellence, which is a nonprofit organization providing education on and developing a research network committed to reducing first responder occupational illness, injury, and death, has summarized the presumptive legislation on their website.[5] Additionally, the International Association of Fire Fighters (IAFF) Division of Occupational Health, Safety, and Medicine developed an information database of the current presumptive disability provisions in the United States and Canada.[6]

Every state in the United States has either passed or considered presumptive legislation for firefighters diagnosed with cancer; a total of 48 states and Washington, DC, have passed legislation, of which 31 states have passed the legislation under workers' compensation (Table 29-1). The two remaining states without laws, Delaware[7] and South Carolina,[8] have bills under review by state legislators. Although nearly all states have passed presumptive laws to compensate firefighters or family members for cancers attributed to occupational exposures, the legislation varies significantly across state lines. Half of the states with presumptive laws cover volunteers, and 45% of states require proof of exposure to carcinogens. Firefighters must serve typically at least five years prior to their cancer diagnosis to be eligible for the presumption, although some

Table 29-1. Data Summarization of All 50 States and Washington, DC

State	Presumptive Law: Type of Code	Cancer Language	Includes Volunteers	Years of Service	Statute of Limitation	Physical Exam Requirements	Rebuttable[a]	Require Proof of Carcinogen Exposure
Alabama	GP	Generic[b]	Yes	3 years	Must be currently employed	Preemployment	Yes	Yes
Alaska	WC		Yes	7 years	5 years[c]	Preemployment + annual exams	Yes ••	Yes
Arizona	WC		No	5 years Full time	15 years, diagnosis before age 65	Preemployment	Yes ••	Yes
Arkansas[d]	RP and GP		No	5 years	Diagnosis before age 68		Yes	Yes
California	WC and RP	Generic	Yes	5 years	10 years[c]		Yes	Yes
Colorado[d]	WC and GP		No	5 years		Preemployment	Yes	No
Connecticut[d]	WC		Yes			Preemployment	Yes	No
Delaware *NOT YET PASSED*	WC	Generic	Yes	5 years	5 years	Preemployment + annual exams	Yes •	Yes
Washington, DC	WC		No	10 years	Must be currently employed	Preemployment + annual exams	Yes	Yes
Florida	GP		No	5 years	10 years		Yes ••	No
Georgia[d]	GP		Yes	1 year	1 year		No	No
Hawaii	WC		Yes	5 years	10 years[c]	Preemployment	Yes	Yes
Idaho	WC		Yes	See Table 29-2	10 years	Preemployment	Yes •	Yes

Illinois	WC and RP	Generic	No	5 years	Must be currently employed	Preemployment	Yes ••	No
Indiana	WC	Generic	No	5 years	5 years		Yes •	Yes
Iowa	RP		No			Preemployment	No	No
Kansas	RP	Generic	No	5 years			Yes	No
Kentucky	GP		Yes	5 years	10 years, death before age 65		Yes •	Yes
Louisiana	GP		Yes	10 years	5 years[c]		Yes	No
Maine	WC		Yes	5 years	10 years, diagnosis before age 70	Preemployment	Yes	No
Maryland	WC		Yes	10 years		Preemployment	No	Yes
Massachusetts	RP		No	5 years	5 years	Preemployment	Yes	No
Michigan[d]	WC		Yes	5 years	Must be currently employed		Yes •	Yes
Minnesota	WC	Generic	No			Preemployment	Yes	No
Mississippi	WC		Yes	10 years	5 years[c]		Yes	No
Missouri	RP		No	5 years (10 years for volunteers)	20 years, diagnosis before age 65	Physical within 5 years of claim	Yes •	Yes
Montana	WC		Yes	see Table 29-2	10 years	Preemployment + annual exams every other year	Yes •	No

(Continued)

Table 29-1. Data Summarization of All 50 States and Washington, DC (Continued)

State	Presumptive Law: Type of Code	Cancer Language	Includes Volunteers	Years of Service	Statute of Limitation	Physical Exam Requirements	Rebuttable[a]	Require Proof of Carcinogen Exposure
Nebraska	GP		No	10 years	3 months	Preemployment	Yes	Yes
Nevada	WC		Yes	5 years	5 years		Yes	Yes
New Hampshire	WC	Generic	Yes	10 years	20 years	Preemployment	Yes •	Yes
New Jersey	WC	Generic	Yes	7 years	20 years, diagnosis before age 75	Preemployment	Yes	Yes
New Mexico	WC		No	See Table 29-2		Preemployment	Yes	No
New York[d]	RP		Yes	5 years	2 years, 5 years for New York City	Preemployment	Yes	No
North Carolina[d]	RP		No				No	No
North Dakota	WC	Generic	No	5 years	2 years if <10 years of service; otherwise, 5 years	Preemployment + periodic exams[f]	Yes •	No
Ohio	WC	Generic	Yes	6 years	20 years, diagnosis before age 70	Preemployment	Yes ••	Yes
Oklahoma	RP	Generic	Yes			Preemployment	Yes	No
Oregon	WC		No	5 years	7 years[g]	Preemployment	Yes •	No
Pennsylvania	WC	Generic	Yes	4 years	600 weeks	Preemployment	Yes	Yes
Rhode Island	GP	Generic	No			Preemployment	Yes	No
South Carolina NOT YET PASSED	WC		Yes	10 years		Preemployment	Yes	No
South Dakota	RP	Generic	No			Preemployment	No	No

State	Provision	Presumption factors	Tobacco use prohibition	Minimum years of service	Time limit after service	Medical exams	Presumption can be rebutted	Applies to cancer
Tennessee	GP	••••	No	5 years	5 years	Preemployment + annual exams with cancer screenings	Yes	Yes
Texas	GP	• •	Yes	5 years	Currently employed	Preemployment	Yes ••	No
Utah	WC	•	Yes	8 years	3 months	Annual exams	Yes •	No
Vermont	WC	••••	Yes	5 years	10 years, diagnosis before age 65	Preemployment + cancer screenings recommended by ACS	Yes •	No
Virginia	WC	••••	Yes	12 years	5 years	Preemployment	Yes	Yes
Washington	WC	•••	No	10 years	5 years[c]	Preemployment	Yes ••	No
West Virginia	WC	••	No	5 years	Diagnosis before age 65		Yes •	No
Wisconsin	GP	••••	No	10 years		Preemployment	Yes •	No
Wyoming	WC	Generic	Yes	10 years	10 years	Preemployment	Yes •	Yes

[a]Presumption can be overcome by a preponderance of evidence:
- Tobacco use ("firefighter or a firefighter's cohabitant has regularly and habitually used tobacco")
- Exposure not linked to cancer ("carcinogen to which the member has demonstrated exposure is not reasonably linked to the disabling cancer")
- Existing cancer diagnosis
- Other (physical fitness and weight, lifestyle, hereditary factors, exposure from other employment or nonemployment activities)

[b]Example of "generic" language: "…exposed agent classified by the International Agency for Research on Cancer or its successor agency as a group 1 or 2A carcinogen."

[c]"…period of three calendar months for each year of requisite service but may not extend more than 60 (or 120) calendar months following the last date of employment."

[d]Alternate source of funding outside of legislation.

[e]Every 5 years during the 1st to 20th year of service; every 3 years beginning at the 21st year of service.

[f]For 1 to 10 years of service, physical exam required every 5 years; for 11 to 20 years of service, every 3 years; and for 21 or more years of service, every year.

[g]Does not apply to prostate cancer if first diagnosed after 55 years of age.

Abbreviations: ACS, American Cancer Society; GP, general provisions; RP, retirement, pension; WC, workers' compensation.

Table 29-2. Required Years of Service by Cancer Diagnosis[9-11]

Type of Cancer	Years of Service
Breast[a]	5
Leukemia	5
Testicular[b]	5
Brain	10
Colorectal	10
Esophageal	10
Mesothelioma	10
Bladder	12
Ureter	12
Kidney	15
Multiple myeloma	15
Non-Hodgkin lymphoma	15

[a]If diagnosed before the age of 40 without a breast cancer genetic predisposition to breast cancer.
[b]If diagnosed before the age of 40 with no evidence of anabolic steroids or human growth hormone use.

states require six to ten years of service to qualify. A few states, namely Idaho,[9] Montana,[10] and New Mexico,[11] require a specific number of service years based on the cancer diagnosis (Table 29-2). All but two of the states have passed presumptive legislation for specific cancer diagnoses, but these laws vary significantly in language and requirements, namely how many and which types of cancers may be covered, qualification criteria, and how long the presumption applies. The top five most commonly listed cancers are prostate cancer, brain cancer, multiple myeloma, leukemia, and non-Hodgkin lymphoma (Table 29-3). Additionally, nearly 60% of states require a preemployment physical showing no evidence of cancer for a claim to be compensable. Furthermore, firefighters are only eligible to submit claims within a limited amount of time from their last year of service; in most states, the presumption expires five or ten years after leaving the fire service (Figure 29-1). Many of the laws include clauses that allow the employer to rebut the claims, especially if the firefighter has had significant exposure to tobacco (21 states), has a cancer that is not linked to carcinogens (three states), has an existing cancer diagnosis (two states), or has other cancer risk factors (physical fitness and weight, lifestyle, hereditary factors, exposure from other employment/nonemployment activities) (Figure 29-2). Variations in the language of these laws and how these differences affect a firefighter's qualifications for compensation will be explored in greater depth later in the chapter.

There are many nuances to firefighter presumptive cancer legislation. This trend toward presumption offers an intriguing glimpse of how public policy becomes regulation and its impact on medical care and cost shifting. In this chapter, we will explore the legal theory of

Table 29-3. **Top 15 Most Commonly Listed Cancers**

Prostate
Brain
Multiple myeloma
Leukemia
Non-Hodgkin lymphoma
Lung (including mesothelioma)
Bladder
Breast
Kidney
Skin
Testicular
Colorectal
Esophageal
Cervical
Thyroid

various evidentiary standards and burdens of proof. We will also compare the types of legal code, which influences the cost and funding sources of those laws. Next, we will discuss specific stipulations for claims to be compensable and how these claims may be denied or rebutted. At the end of the chapter, we will use case studies and clinical vignettes to demonstrate how the qualification criteria, statute of limitations, and rebuttable clauses could be applied to claimants in any state.

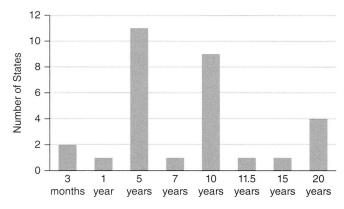

Figure 29-1. Presumption statute of limitations.

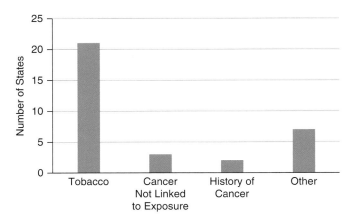

Figure 29-2. Presumption rebuttal by tobacco use, cancer not linked to exposure, history of cancer, or other.

LEGAL THEORY: EXPLAINING EVIDENTIARY STANDARDS AND BURDENS OF PROOF

A standard of proof determines the amount of evidence the plaintiff (person who brings a claim to court) or defendant (party against which the claim is filed) needs to provide in order for the fact finder to reach a particular determination. In almost every legal proceeding, the parties are required to adhere to important rules known as evidentiary standards and burdens of proof. The burden of proof determines which party is responsible for putting forth evidence and the level of evidence they must provide in order to prevail on their claim. This is important to consider in the context of our chapter on firefighter presumption legislation, as it is challenging to prove cancer causation. Previously, firefighters (the plaintiffs) would be responsible for bringing forth enough evidence to prove that their cancer was caused by the occupational exposures associated with firefighting. There are numerous inherent and environmental factors that might increase an individual's risk of developing cancer, so these were particularly difficult cases to argue. Notably, the shift toward presumptive legislation places the burden on the employer to prove that a firefighter's cancer *was not* caused by his or her occupation. Therefore, under the presumption laws, firefighters, as claimants, are at a legal advantage. However, for a firefighter's claim to be considered, they would first carry the burden of proof to present their initial evidence for the claim (e.g., that they meet qualification criteria).

The burden of proof has two components: production and persuasion. First, the firefighter would need to make a claim under the presumption laws, and assuming this would satisfy the burden of production, the case would be allowed to move forward. This burden then automatically shifts to the employer to put forth evidence in the form of witness testimony, documents, or objects to prove that the firefighter's cancer claim is not related to their work. After the employer presents this, the firefighter would then have the opportunity to provide evidence either rebutting the employer's evidence or supporting the firefighter's own arguments. Second, the firefighter must satisfy the burden of persuasion. This burden determines which standard of proof the firefighter must follow in presenting evidence to the judge or jury. Preponderance of the evidence is one type of evidentiary standard used and is clearly stated in some of the states' presumptive laws. Under the preponderance standard, the burden of proof is met when the party with the burden convinces the fact finder that there is a greater than 50% chance that the claim is true. In other words, once the firefighter has successfully put forth an initial claim with evidence, the burden of proof to rebut the claim is met if the employer presents compelling evidence to show that a firefighter's cancer is more likely associated with their history of smoking than their occupational exposures from fighting fires. Some scholars define the preponderance of the evidence standard, in presumptive legislation, as requiring a finding that at least 51% of the evidence favors the defendant's outcome. A majority of states allow the presumption to be rebuttable by a preponderance of evidence, including previous tobacco use or significant exposure, other exposures not linked to cancer, existing cancer diagnoses, or other cancer risk factors, such as physical fitness and weight, lifestyle, hereditary factors, or exposure from other employment or nonemployment activities. While the shift toward presumptive legislation technically gives firefighters the legal advantage in these claims, the imprecise understanding of cancer causation allows the defendants (typically the employers) sufficient opportunity to provide a preponderance of evidence contrary to the firefighter's claims that their cancer is caused by occupational exposures.

COST OF PRESUMPTIVE LEGISLATION

While the goal of presumptive legislation is to support firefighters with a cancer diagnosis, counterarguments to the passage of such laws contend that paying the claims could be cost prohibitive for municipalities. Most presumptive state legislation is covered under workers' compensation; however, many states have presumption laws included in general provisions or retirement/pension legislation. Under workers' compensation, if the municipalities employ the firefighters, they hold the burden of disproving the presumption that work-related exposures were a factor in the development of a firefighter's cancer and are responsible for paying out workers' compensation claims. When the presumption law falls under general provisions, the state is responsible for funding the claims. In the case of retirement/pension laws, the responsible payer varies depending on how the law is written and whether a funding source is attached to the legislation. According to the National Council on Compensation Insurance (NCCI) in a report published in November of 2018, the actual costs of presumptive legislation are unclear at this time: "[the] NCCI generally expects that the enactment of such presumptions will result in increases in workers compensation costs; however, the extent of such increases is difficult to estimate due to significant data limitations."[3] Presumptive cancer legislation offers financial protection to firefighters due to their potential increased occupational exposures to carcinogens, but paying for such claims is expected to increase costs for states, municipalities, and employers.

PAYMENT SOURCES AND PAYOUT ALTERNATIVES

To accommodate such expenses, some states have modified how these claims will be covered. One such alternative is to create a trust fund for paying out benefits. In Arkansas, for example, the state trust fund provides a one-time death benefit worth $150,000 to families of firefighters diagnosed with cancer,[12] whereas North Carolina's Contingency and Emergency Fund provides a $100,000 death benefit to families of deceased firefighters.[13] Michigan created a first responder presumed coverage fund as a separate fund in the state treasury for the purpose of paying benefits provided under the law.[14] New York created the NYS Volunteer Firefighter Enhanced Cancer Disability Benefits Act to provide monetary assistance to volunteer firefighters in the event they are diagnosed with a covered cancer.[15] Other accommodations have been made in Colorado to allow employers to participate in a voluntary firefighter cancer benefits program, which is a health trust that provides benefits to firefighters based on the cancer diagnosis and award level.[16] Connecticut created a relief fund to be used to pay lost wages of firefighters during their treatment for cancers.[17] Georgia passed a bill in 2017 that requires legally organized fire departments to provide sufficient insurance coverage, which has led some municipalities to buy coverage through the Georgia Firefighters' Cancer Benefit Program.[18]

Some states have other methods for limiting claim costs. Georgia, Florida, and Mississippi approved presumptive legislation that caps the payment to firefighters diagnosed with cancer. For example, Georgia's law states that firefighters may receive lump sum payments not exceeding $50,000 during their lifetime.[19] Florida's law provides a one-time payout of $25,000 upon the initial diagnosis of cancer and a continued benefit of at least 42% of the firefighter's most recent annual salary for 10 years after the termination of employment as an alternative to workers' compensation.[20] Mississippi is another state that has adopted a lump-sum payment instead of pursuing workers' compensation coverage; the approved Mississippi First Responders Health and Safety Act, which went into effect on July 1, 2021, allows $35,000 of coverage for each diagnosis depending on the severity of the cancer and life expectancy.[21] Firefighters diagnosed with nonmetastasized cancers may receive $6250 for their diagnosis and may also receive disability benefits at 60% of their monthly salary or $5000 (whichever is less) for the following three years. Volunteers may receive a monthly benefit of $1500 for three years. The combined total of benefits received by any first responder during his or her lifetime may not exceed $50,000. While cancer treatment and management may be expensive, many states have adopted presumptive legislation that provides coverage for some cancer-related costs by creating alternative funding sources or limiting the total benefits paid to firefighters.[21]

QUALIFCATION CRITERIA: LIMITATIONS OF APPLICABILITY AND REBUTTAL CLAUSES

Other cost-saving measures include limitations on the applicability of the presumption and clauses that allow rebuttal under certain circumstances. These are specific eligibility requirements that firefighters must meet in order to qualify for the presumption. Similarly, rebuttable clauses would be statements in the legislation that allow the defendants (employers in the case of workers' compensation) to refute the claims. For example, some states (Illinois,[22] Maryland,[23] Minnesota,[24] and South Dakota[25]) include language that specifies "a firefighter ... who is unable to perform duties in the department by reason of a disabling cancer ... is presumed to have an occupational disease," indicating that the presumption applies only if the firefighter is no longer able to work due to disability or death from cancer. Furthermore, many states limit the number or types of cancers to which the presumption may apply, while other states, such as Ohio, are more generous in their cancer language: "Cancer contracted by a firefighter who has been exposed to agent classified by the International Agency for Research on Cancer or its successor agency as a group 1 or 2A carcinogen."[26] North Carolina,[13] for example, lists only four types of cancer to qualify, whereas Florida[20] specifies that "cancer" can be 1 of 21 unique types of cancer.

Additional restrictions include service requirements, statutes of limitations, age at diagnosis, or physical exam requirements. The service requirements address the concern that firefighters will file claims for cancer diagnoses received early in the course of their service, which may or may not be related to workplace exposures. The latency period, defined as the time interval between exposure and disease onset, can last anywhere from 2 to 57 years.[27] Of note, as researchers continue to improve genetic screening tools and increase their knowledge of epigenetics, cancers are beginning to be detected earlier, which may offer various confounding factors to consider in the context of time-based presumption laws. In most states, these required years of service are defined simply by year, but some states specify the following: the years must be "full-time regularly assigned to hazardous duty" (Arizona[28]), "regularly respond to firefighting emergency call" (Utah[29]), or perform "service 75% of the 2 years immediately preceding his or her disability" (Arkansas[30]). Florida[20] and Kentucky[31] require that the years be continuous or consecutive. By including this specific language, legislators tried to limit claims for cancers that would be less likely related to occupation (i.e., if the firefighter worked only a few hours weekly for five years of service).

The statute of limitations defines presumption coverage for cancers diagnosed within designated periods of time of last active fire service and employment status as a full-time or part-time paid employee. In the context of presumption legislation, many laws state that claims cannot be brought forth after a specified period of time (i.e., they have a statute of limitations). For some exposures, such as gamma rays, radon, or asbestos, the cancer latency can be five to ten years; however, for most exposures, it can take approximately 20 years for cancer to develop and manifest.[32] This may limit the opportunity for firefighters to submit claims for compensation if the latency period of the cancer outlasts the law's statute of limitations. Interestingly, Alaska,[33] California,[34] Hawaii,[35] Louisiana,[36] Mississippi,[21] and Washington[37] qualify the statute of limitations by years of service worked. For example, Alaska law states: "Following termination of service, the presumption established in … this subsection extends to the fire fighter for a period of three calendar months for each year of requisite service but may not extend more than 60 calendar months following the last date of employment."[33]

Limitations on the age at which cancer is diagnosed may reduce the number of claims due to the known correlation between increasing general risk of contracting many diseases with increasing years of life. Arizona,[28] Arkansas,[38] Kentucky,[32] Maine,[39] Missouri,[40] New Jersey,[41] Ohio,[26] Vermont,[42] and West Virginia[43] specify ages before which the cancer must be diagnosed in order for the firefighter to qualify for the presumption.

Additionally, 75% of states have some kind of physical exam requirement. This specification typically stipulates that an exam must have been performed before or during the course of employment that did not show evidence of cancer. Alaska[33] specifies that there must be a preemployment physical, as well as an annual medical exam during each of the first seven years of employment that did not show evidence of the disease. Other states, notably Tennessee[44] and Vermont,[42] are more concerned with the type of physical examination; the annual exams in Tennessee must include cancer screenings for specific types of cancer, and Vermont requires cancer screening evaluations "as recommended by the American Cancer Society based on the age and sex of the firefighter."[44]

The intent of presumptive legislation is to make it easier for firefighters to seek compensation (workers' compensation, disability benefits, or death benefits) for cancers that appear to have arisen out of their exposures in the line of duty. Despite this cultural shift in favor of claimants, legislators integrated language that would limit applicability of claims for cancers unlikely to be caused by their firefighting jobs, thus reducing the costs and burden on the defendants.

PROMINENT CASE LAWS AND CLINICAL VIGNETTES

This chapter reviewed how recent changes in state legislation across the country favor firefighters by shifting the burden of proof to the employers. These legal changes have been attracting media attention for falling short of their intended purposes; despite these laws, firefighters' claims are often denied. Many firefighters have challenged these denials with various outcomes.[45] The following cases demonstrate how litigation of these new laws is playing out.

CASE LAW # 1

Paul Morrison started working as a firefighter for the city of Sanford, Maine, in 1981. In the spring of 2011, he was diagnosed with a cancerous brain tumor, for which he underwent subsequent treatment and recovery. Eventually, he was able to return to work as a full-duty firefighter in March of 2012. Mr. Morrison filed his claim with the Workers' Compensation Board in July of that same year. The court ruled in favor of the firefighter's claim that his cancer was related to occupational exposures and supported the law holding his employer responsible for disproving that his cancer was unrelated to work as a firefighter. However, the city challenged the ruling as beyond the judges' legal authority and that the claimant did not meet statutory criteria for application of the presumption, which was denied. At this point, expert testimony was brought forth regarding the general etiology of Mr. Morrison's particular brain tumor, and the judges concluded that none of the experts were in a position to assess the plaintiff's individual exposure risk from firefighting. They further stated that the evidence on causation was "equipoise," meaning that the presumption was not rebutted: "Accordingly, the [judges] found the presumed facts, including that Mr. Morrison contracted cancer in the course of and as a result of his employment as a firefighter."[46] The city filed further challenges to the ruling, which were denied.

This case is notable for its demonstration of the power of presumption law. Despite the evidence of Mr. Morrison's cancer causation being balanced, namely, that there was not enough compelling data to convince the judge of another more likely cause of his cancer, the ruling was to approve his claim that his cancer "was contracted in the course of and as a result of employment as a firefighter."[46] The case also illustrates how these various state laws may be interpreted in more than one way; thus, it is within the board's rulemaking authority to "fill in the 'gray areas,' bringing practical and appropriate considerations to bear on the operation of the Act."[46]

CASE LAW # 2

Scott Sladek began his career as a firefighter for the city of Philadelphia in 1994, prior to which he had received no diagnoses or treatments for cancer and was deemed in overall good health based on physical examination. In January of 2007, he was diagnosed with malignant melanoma and underwent surgery to remove the lesion. Mr. Sladek filed a petition for workers' compensation benefits in June of 2012, claiming that his melanoma developed resultant of exposure to Group 1 carcinogens while working as a firefighter. The city denied his claim, but the workers' compensation judge granted his petition after further testimony in 2013, which led to a lengthy process of appeals by the city. After various courts weighed in on the case, it was concluded that Mr. Sladek "failed to meet his initial burden to show that his malignant melanoma is a type of cancer caused by the Group 1 carcinogens to which he was exposed in the workplace to establish an occupational disease."[47] The firefighter appealed his case to the Pennsylvania Supreme Court, which ultimately ruled in favor of his petition in 2018. The Pennsylvania Supreme Court further opined that firefighters are responsible for meeting the qualification criteria of the law by showing "that their cancer could be caused by exposure to a known carcinogen" but that the employers remain responsible for proving it was not work related.[47]

The tumultuous course of this firefighter's petition illustrates the inherent ambiguity of pinning cancer causation on specific factors. In this case, there was significant discussion regarding the differences between "general" and "specific" causation. In one expert testimony, it was argued that general causation "tells us that something can cause an outcome," whereas "[s]pecific causation involves an analysis of circumstances and risk factors present in a particular case."[47] The ultimate decision by the courts was that epidemiologic evidence ("general causation") is not sufficient to rebut the legislatively created presumption of compensability, but it is sufficient for presenting evidence of the claimant meeting qualification criteria. In other words, the burden of proof requires the defendant to bring forth very specific risk factors or circumstances of a particular case to meet the preponderance of evidence standard. Some states have accounted for this by specifying the types of evidence that may be brought forth to rebut claims, such as previous tobacco use, existing or previous cancer diagnoses, or other factors such as physical fitness and weight, lifestyle, hereditary factors, and exposure from other employment or nonemployment activities.

CLINICAL VIGNETTE # 1

John is a 69-year-old man from Maine presenting to his primary care clinic with fatigue and a 10-pound weight loss over the past month. His medical history is significant for hypertension and hyperlipidemia managed on an angiotensin-converting enzyme (ACE) inhibitor and a statin. His surgical history is unremarkable, and he has no allergies. Immunizations and cancer screenings are up to date. Regarding social history, John worked as a paid firefighter for 20 years with a local rescue squad. He retired at age 65, lives at home with his wife of 45 years, and eats a well-balanced, low-salt, low-fat diet. He walks his dog twice daily. He denies tobacco or drug use, and drinks one glass of wine on special occasions. His family history is significant for diabetes and hyperlipidemia, but there is no known cancer.

Workup reveals a new diagnosis of lymphoma. Further investigation reveals documented exposures to carbon monoxide, hydrochloric acid, benzene, hydrogen cyanide, and nitrogen dioxide. The patient used protective equipment in compliance with the policies of the Office of the State Fire Marshal in effect during the course of the investigator's or sergeant's employment. Upon review of his chart, he was examined by his primary care physician yearly throughout the course of his employment. None of his physicals showed any evidence of cancer.

"Presumption. If a firefighter who contracts cancer has met the requirements of subsections 3, 6 and 7, there is a rebuttable presumption that the firefighter contracted the cancer in the course of employment as a firefighter and as a result of that employment, that sufficient notice of the cancer has been given and that the disease was not occasioned by any willful act of the firefighter to cause the disease."[39]

The State of Maine requires that firefighters must have undergone a standard, medically acceptable test without evidence of the cancer during the time of employment as a firefighter (subsection 3). Additionally, the claimant must have been employed as a firefighter for five years and, except for an investigator or sergeant in the Office of the State Fire Marshal, regularly responded to firefighting or emergency calls (subsection 6). Finally, to qualify for the presumption, a firefighter must sign a written affidavit declaring that the firefighter's diagnosed cancer is not prevalent among the firefighter's blood-related parents, grandparents, or siblings and that the firefighter has no substantial lifetime exposures to carcinogens that are associated with the firefighter's diagnosed cancer other than exposure through firefighting (subsection 7). Other criteria include the following:

- "Cancer" diagnosis, meaning kidney cancer, non-Hodgkin lymphoma, colon cancer, leukemia, brain cancer, bladder cancer, multiple myeloma, prostate cancer, testicular cancer, or breast cancer
- Must be diagnosed with cancer within 10 years of the firefighter's last active employment as a firefighter or prior to attaining 70 years of age, whichever occurs first
- A representative from the Office of the State Fire Marshal must represent that the investigator or sergeant used protective equipment in compliance with the policies of the Office of the State Fire Marshal in effect during the course of the investigator's or sergeant's employment.[39]

According to the state's criteria, John would qualify for workers' compensation under this presumption law.

- Cost: Who pays for his cancer-related expenses?
  - The employer is responsible for paying unless they can successfully rebut the claim. In this case, we do not know who employed this firefighter, but in many cases, the municipality would be the firefighter's employer and defendant in the claim. Notice that Maine's law does not comment on the type or amount of expenses eligible for payment. Cancer diagnostics and treatments can be very expensive, so there is incentive for employers to avoid these unrestricted costs.
- Limitations of applicability: What if the patient's mother had a history of breast cancer? What if his years of service were not contiguous? What if he waited 12 months to submit the claim and turned age 70?
  - These are all important considerations when reviewing each state's eligibility criteria. In this case, John would have had to sign a written affidavit declaring that his diagnosed cancer is not prevalent among his blood relatives. Since he was diagnosed with lymphoma, not breast cancer, he should still qualify for the presumption. With regard to service specifications, notice that Maine's language is vague relative to other states' legislation; it does not explicitly state that he must have completed his years of service contiguously or that he be full-time regularly assigned to hazardous duty. As for the statute of limitations, this patient would need to submit his claim before his 70th birthday to remain eligible for the presumption.
- Rebuttable clauses: Let us now assume that John is from Alaska and has a remote smoking history of 10 pack-years and an elevated body mass index. According to the laws in Alaska, the employer would be able to rebut this presumption of coverage with a preponderance of evidence.[33] Specifically, it states that "the evidence may include the use of tobacco products, physical fitness and weight, lifestyle, hereditary factors, and exposure from other employment or nonemployment activities."[33] While the intent of the law is to provide coverage for firefighters with increased occupational exposure, this statement provides employers general guidance for the types of evidence that may be used to rebut a firefighter's claims. Due to the prevalence of these other comorbidities and unhealthy lifestyle choices, this clause would make it easier for employers to argue their case. Still, the law states that his cancer would be presumed to be related to his occupation as a firefighter, and thus, the burden of proof remains on the employer to refute the claim for compensation.

CLINICAL VIGNETTE # 2

Susan is a 48-year-old woman from North Carolina presenting to the emergency department with hematemesis, weight loss, and dysphagia. Her medical history and surgical history are unremarkable, and she has no allergies. Susan is a full-time active-duty firefighter and has been working in the field for the past ten years. She denies alcohol, tobacco, or drug use. She is adopted and does not know her family history. A few weeks later, she is diagnosed with esophageal cancer and is scheduled for surgery, followed by chemoradiation.

"When the death of a firefighter occurs as a direct and proximate result of any of the following cancers that are occupationally related to firefighting, that firefighter is presumed to have been killed in the line of duty ... When any covered person is killed in the line of duty, the Industrial Commission shall award a death benefit in the amount of one hundred thousand dollars ($100,000) to be paid to one of the following ... shall be paid from the Contingency and Emergency Fund and such amounts as may be required to pay benefits provided for by this Article are hereby appropriated from said fund for this special purpose."[13]

In its current form, the legislation in North Carolina provides a one-time death benefit payment of $100,000 to family members when the death of a firefighter occurs as a direct and proximate result of any of the following cancers that are occupationally related to firefighting. Those cancers specified in the law include only mesothelioma and testicular, intestinal, and esophageal cancer. The law further states that "in the event of this type of death, the firefighter is presumed to have been killed in the line of duty," which is the justification for such payment. This lump sum payment is supplied by the Contingency and Emergency Fund, which is outlined under the state's general provisions and thus funded by state. Susan is still living, so although the state's presumptive legislation assumes that her disease is related to occupation, only her family qualifies for compensation in the event that she dies from her cancer.

CONCLUSION

Growing evidence demonstrates that fighting fires increases exposure to carcinogens and thus has the potential to increase a firefighter's risk of developing cancer. Recently, there have been significant changes in federal and state regulations to protect and support firefighters with the financial burden of cancer diagnoses and treatments. Although most states have passed presumptive laws to compensate firefighters for cancer attributed to occupational exposures, the legislation varies significantly in coverage, presumption requirements (years of service and physical exams), duration of presumption applicability, and qualifying cancer types. Despite these differences, the presumptive nature of these laws demonstrates increased national concern for occupational exposures and the associations with cancer.

KEY POINTS:

- Firefighters are at increased risk for developing cancer due to occupational exposures.
- Cancer causation is difficult to prove, but recently, legislation has been approved in many states including presumptive measures that shift the burden of proof to the employer.
- There are no federal presumptive laws for firefighters with cancer, and nearly all states have passed some form of these laws.
- The compensation and coverage of presumptive legislation for firefighters with cancer vary significantly depending on the state in which that firefighter resides.

- The presumptive nature of the law shifts the burden of proof to the employer, which gives firefighters the legal advantage in these claims.
- The burden of proof determines which party is responsible for putting forth evidence, and the level of evidence they must provide in order to prevail on their claim is referred to as a "preponderance of evidence."
- Cost is a major concern for opponents of presumptive legislation and defendants (often the employers) in these cases.
- Some states have structured their legislation to pay out these claims through workers' compensation, from the state's coffers or special funds set up for disability and death benefits.
- Firefighters must meet specific criteria in each state to qualify for compensation.
- The qualifications can be ambiguous and open to interpretation. They also vary greatly across state lines and are unique to each state's legislative code.
- Even after meeting all criteria to submit a compensable claim under presumptive legislation, a firefighter's claim may be rebuttable under certain circumstances.

References:

1. Daniels RD. The most popular NIOSH content from 2017. NIOSH Science Blog. Centers for Disease Control and Prevention. Published May 10, 2017. https://blogs.cdc.gov/niosh-science-blog/2017/05/10/ff-cancer-facts/. Accessed April 6, 2021.
2. Leukemia and Lymphoma Society. Firefighters and cancer risk. Published March 21, 2019. https://www.lls.org/managing-your-cancer/firefighters-and-cancer-risk. Accessed April 6, 2021.
3. Racicot F, Spidell B. Presumptive coverage for firefighters and other first responders. NCCI Research Brief. Published November 2018. https://www.ncci.com/Articles/Documents/Insights-Research-Brief-Presumptive-Coverage.pdf. Accessed April 6, 2021.
4. Firefighter Cancer Registry Bill clears Congress. International Association of Fire Chiefs. Published June 22, 2018. https://www.iafc.org/press-releases/press-release/firefighter-cancer-registry-bill-clears-congress. Accessed April 6, 2021.
5. The fire service cancer toolkit. Fire Service Occupational Cancer Alliance. https://www.firstrespondercenter.org/cancer/. Accessed April 6, 2021.
6. Presumptive Health Initiative home. International Association of Fire Fighters. https://www.iaff.org/presumptive-health/#1555251950049-fa213803-8fa7. Accessed April 6, 2021.
7. Senate Bill 126. Delaware General Assembly. Bill Detail: Delaware General Assembly. http://www.legis.delaware.gov/BillDetail/47553. Accessed April 6, 2021.
8. H. 3106 Status Information. 2019-2020 Bill 3106: Firefighter, presumption of certain illnesses. South Carolina Legislature Online. Published April 24, 2019. https://www.scstatehouse.gov/sess123_2019–2020/bills/3106.htm. Accessed April 6, 2021.
9. Idaho Code § 72-438. https://legislature.idaho.gov/statutesrules/idstat/Title72/T72CH4/SECT72-438/. Accessed April 13, 2021.
10. Montana Code Annotated § 39-71-1401. https://leg.mt.gov/bills/mca/title_0390/chapter_0710/part_0140/sections_index.html. Accessed April 13, 2021.
11. New Mexico Statutes Annotated 1978 § 52-3-32. https://nmonesource.com/nmos/nmsa/en/item/4394/index.do#!b/52-3-32. Accessed April 13, 2021.
12. Arkansas Code § 21-5-705. https://law.justia.com/codes/arkansas/2010/title-21/chapter-5/subchapter-7/21-5-705/. Accessed April 13, 2021.

13. North Carolina General Statutes, Chapter 143, Article 2A. https://www.ncleg.gov/EnactedLegislation/Statutes/PDF/ByArticle/Chapter_143/Article_12A.pdf. Accessed April 13, 2021.
14. Michigan Compiled Laws § 418-405. http://www.legislature.mi.gov/(S(a2yyis1vfb3aqvyfvu1bpcak))/mileg.aspx?page=GetObject&objectname=mcl-418-405. Accessed April 13, 2021.
15. New York General Municipal Law §10-205. https://www.nysenate.gov/legislation/laws/GMU/205-CC. Accessed April 13, 2021.
16. Colorado Revised Statutes §29-5-401. https://codes.findlaw.com/co/title-29-government-local/co-rev-st-sect-29-5-401.html. Accessed April 13, 2021.
17. Moran J. Firefighters Cancer Relief Fund and post-traumatic stress legislation. Office of Legislative Research. Published October 16, 2018. https://www.cga.ct.gov/2018/rpt/pdf/2018-R-0277.pdf. Accessed April 6, 2021.
18. Firefighters' Cancer Benefit Program. Georgia Municipal Association. https://www.gacities.com/What-We-Do/Service/Insurance/Firefighters-Cancer-Benefit.aspx. Accessed April 6, 2021.
19. Georgia Code §25-3-23. https://law.justia.com/codes/georgia/2016/title-25/chapter-3/article-2/section-25-3-23/. Accessed April 13, 2021.
20. Florida Statutes §112-1816. https://www.myfloridahouse.gov/Statutes/2019/0112.1816/. Accessed April 13, 2021.
21. Mississippi Code 1972 Annotated § 25-15-405. https://advance.lexis.com/container?config=00JAAzNzhjOTYxNC0wZjRkLTQzNzAtAtYjJlYS1jNjExZWYxZGFhMGYKAFBvZENhdGFsb2cMlW40w5iIH7toHnTBIEP0&crid=98807842-39e1-49e1-a5b8-1e3fc1e3983d&prid=911feb84-39cc-4212-9f23-84fa09dd905a. Accessed April 13, 2021.
22. 40 Illinois Compiled Statutes § 5/4-110.1. https://www.ilga.gov/legislation/ilcs/ilcs4.asp?DocName=004000050HArt%2E+4&ActID=638&ChapterID=9&SeqStart=26400000&SeqEnd=33700000. Accessed April 13, 2021.
23. Maryland Statutes § 9-503. http://mgaleg.maryland.gov/mgawebsite/Laws/StatuteText?article=gle&section=9-503&enactments=False&archived=False. Accessed April 13, 2021.
24. Minnesota Statutes §176-011. https://www.revisor.mn.gov/statutes/cite/176.011#stat.176.011.15. Accessed April 13, 2021.
25. South Dakota Codified Laws § 9-16-3.3. https://sdlegislature.gov/Statutes/Codified_Laws/2036403. Accessed April 13, 2021.
26. Ohio Revised Code § 4123.68. https://codes.ohio.gov/ohio-revised-code/section-4123.68. Accessed April 13, 2021.
27. Howard J. Minimum latency and types or categories of cancer. Published October 12, 2012. https://www.cdc.gov/wtc/pdfs/policies/WTCHP-Minimum-Cancer-Latency-PP-01062015-508.pdf. Accessed April 6, 2021.
28. Arizona Revised Statutes § 23-901.01. https://www.azleg.gov/viewdocument/?docName=https://www.azleg.gov/ars/23/00901-01.htm. Accessed April 13, 2021.
29. Utah Code § 34A-3-113. https://le.utah.gov/xcode/Title34A/Chapter3/34A-3-S113.html?v=C34A-3-S113_2015051220150512. Accessed April 13, 2021.
30. Arkansas Code § 24-10-607. https://law.justia.com/codes/arkansas/2015/title-24/chapter-10/subchapter-6/section-24-10-607/. Accessed April 13, 2021.
31. Kentucky Revised Statutes § 61.315. https://apps.legislature.ky.gov/law/statutes/statute.aspx?id=50252. Accessed April 13, 2021.
32. Evaluation of latent and presumptive periods. Veterans and agent orange: length of presumptive period for association between exposure and respiratory cancer. Published January 1, 1970. https://www.ncbi.nlm.nih.gov/books/NBK215871/. Accessed April 6, 2021.
33. Alaska Statutes § 23-30-121. https://codes.findlaw.com/ak/title-23-labor-and-workers-compensation/ak-st-sect-23-30-121.html. Accessed April 13, 2021.
34. California Statutes § 3212.1. https://leginfo.legislature.ca.gov/faces/codes_displaySection.xhtml?sectionNum=3212.1.&lawCode=LAB. Accessed April 13, 2021.
35. Hawaii Revised Statutes § 386-21.9. https://www.capitol.hawaii.gov/hrscurrent/Vol07_Ch0346-0398/HRS0386/HRS_0386-0021_0009.htm. Accessed April 13, 2021.

36. Louisiana Revised Statutes § 33:2011. http://www.legis.la.gov/Legis/Law.aspx?d=89498. Accessed April 13, 2021.
37. Revised Code of Washington § 51.32.185. https://app.leg.wa.gov/RCW/default.aspx?cite=51.32.185. Accessed April 13, 2021.
38. Arkansas Code § 21-5-705. https://law.justia.com/codes/arkansas/2015/title-21/chapter-5/subchapter-7/section-21-5-705. Accessed April 13, 2021.
39. Maine Revised Statutes §328-B. http://www.mainelegislature.org/legis/statutes/39-a/title39-Asec328-B.html. Accessed April 13, 2021.
40. Missouri House Bill No. 1641. https://house.mo.gov/billtracking/bills181/hlrbillspdf/4971H.01I.pdf. Accessed April 13, 2021.
41. New Jersey § 34:15-31.8. https://lis.njleg.state.nj.us/nxt/gateway.dll?f=templates&fn=default.htm&vid=Publish:10.1048/Enu. Accessed April 13, 2021.
42. 21 Vermont Statutes Annotated § 601. https://legislature.vermont.gov/statutes/section/21/009/00601. Accessed April 13, 2021.
43. West Virginia Code §23-4-1. http://www.wvlegislature.gov/WVCODE/code.cfm?chap=23&art=4#01. Accessed April 13, 2021.
44. Tennessee Code Annotated § 7-51-201. https://law.justia.com/codes/tennessee/2010/title-7/chapter-51/part-2/7-51-201/. Accessed April 13, 2021.
45. Bavis L. Laws intended to protect firefighters who get cancer often lack teeth. NPR. Published January 4, 2019. https://www.npr.org/sections/health-shots/2019/01/04/660701244/laws-intended-to-protect-firefighters-who-get-cancer-often-lack-teeth. Accessed April 14, 2021.
46. Morrison v City of Sanford (Maine 2019), WCB No. 11-005321B, Appellate Division, Case No. App. Div. 17-0017, Decision No. 19-22.
47. *City of Philadelphia Fire Department v Workers' Compensation Appeal Board (Sladek)*, 2018. http://www.pacourts.us/assets/opinions/Supreme/out/j-56-2017mo.pdf#search=%22scott%20sladek%22. Accessed April 14, 2021.
48. Firefighter's Cancer Presumption S-716. Published February 19, 2018. https://njmel.org/wp-content/uploads/2018/02/2018-White-Paper-1.2.20.18.pdf. Accessed April 6, 2021.
49. State laws establishing presumption of firefighter cancer as a result of duty-related exposure. National Volunteer Fire Council. https://www.nvfc.org/state-laws-establishing-presumption-of-firefighter-cancer-as-a-result-of-duty-related-exposure/. Accessed April 6, 2021.
50. The National Institute for Occupational Safety and Health (NIOSH). Centers for Disease Control and Prevention. Published May 25, 2018. https://www.cdc.gov/niosh/. Accessed April 6, 2021.
51. Chemicals, cancer, and you. Agency for Toxic Substances and Disease Registry. https://www.atsdr.cdc.gov/emes/public/docs/Chemicals,%20Cancer,%20and%20You%20FS.pdf. Accessed April 6, 2021.

CHAPTER 30

COVID-19 Pandemic

Victor Waters, MD, JD, FCLM

INTRODUCTION

To date, as of April 2021, the coronavirus disease 2019 (COVID-19) pandemic has resulted in 560,000 deaths in the United States and 2.9 million deaths worldwide.[1] Among patients with COVID-19, cancer is an independent risk for higher mortality rates compared with those without cancer.[2] The pandemic has also caused a sharp reduction in cancer screening and postponement of ongoing or planned therapy, which are contributing factors to non–COVID-19–related cancer deaths. Specifically, chemotherapy, radiation therapy, screening colonoscopies and bronchoscopies, surgeries (diagnostic, therapeutic, or palliative), interventional radiology procedures, needle biopsies, and even basic follow-up blood work and x-rays were delayed, postponed, or canceled. The complete disruption of outpatient and hospital services for prolonged periods in many geographic areas (rural, suburban, and urban) has placed a great deal of stress on health care systems managing cancer patients during the pandemic.[3]

Cancer patients' increased risk for death during COVID-19 was also due to a host of other factors. Cancer patients were reluctant to go to hospitals, outpatient surgical centers, or offices due to fears of contracting COVID-19.[4] Some hospitalized cancer patients were discharged prematurely because of the high demand for beds, resulting in risk for readmissions or even patients' reluctance to be readmitted.[5] Some cancer patients had limited transportation access during "lockdown," and family and friends were reluctant to chaperone.[6] Finally, overly stressed emergency medical services systems resulted in delayed ambulance responses, and ambulances were limited to life-threatening radio-dispatched calls only.[7]

COVID-19 liability, defined as health care workers' risk for liability during the COVID-19 pandemic, is expected to increase significantly in the coming years after COVID-19 because of the following predispositions:

1. General distrust of the medical community.[8]
2. Misinformation about COVID-19 that has caused confusion and a lack of global census.[9]
3. Distrust of the Black and Brown communities toward the medical community. It is well known that communities of color were disproportionately impacted by COVID-19, with more deaths and hospitalizations.[10] Sadly, Dr. Susan Moore, a Black physician diagnosed with severe COVID-19 infection, chronicled her racist treatment by her colleagues. She subsequently died.[11]

4. Lack of timely in-person access to providers, which contributed to breakdowns in communications about results or treatment plans.
5. Use of telemedicine, which has skyrocketed to over 1000% for outpatient visits.[12] Telemedicine certainly has added value during the crisis but has obvious limitations, such as the physician's inability to perform a physical assessment. In addition, it is difficult to build trust and engagement between the physician and patient remotely and to discuss deeply complicated conversations about cancer care, prognosis, and care plans.

LEGAL THEORIES

Medical Negligence

Medical Negligence is committed when a patient received inadequate care from a medical professional. The area of tort law known as negligence involves harm caused by failing to act as a form of carelessness, possibly with extenuating circumstances.[13]

In general, for a lawyer to file a negligence claim, he or she must prove the following four elements[14]:

1. The doctor had a duty of care to the patient.
2. The doctor breeched that duty, failing to conform to a standard.
3. The doctor's conduct is connected or a proximate cause.
4. There is harm to the patient.

The failure to meet the standard of care does not mean "ideal care," "perfect care," or even the care that an average physician would provide. Most courts define it as a "minimal standard," which may be an arguable fact determined by expert medical witnesses on both sides (plaintiff and defendant). A cancer patient's attorney may argue that the standard of care was not met in diagnosis (including underestimating the aggressiveness of the cancer); as a result of delay in care, which created harm; or as a result of a complication during the course of care that was foreseeable and perhaps avoidable.

Wrongful Death Claim

Wrongful death is a form of negligence where the attorney for a family or estate representative files a claim against the physician or hospital for *consortium damages* as a result of their loss of a "loved one."[15] The COVID-19 pandemic has not only destroyed thousands of lives, including those of cancer patients without COVID-19 infection, but families have suffered immensely from lack of access to their love ones during their hospital course and have been often unable to say their goodbyes in the final moments of life. This has resulted in economic hardships, resulting in millions being laid off and unemployed, and an increase in families seeking monetary damages under a wrongful death claim is expected, which includes compensation for burial expenses, pain and suffering, emotional distress, medical treatment cost, and loss of companionship.[15] These are compensatory damages meant to provide restitution for the family member or to make them "whole" financially. It is likely that grieving family members of deceased cancer patients will file claims when they perceive that their loved one's death was facilitated.

Failure of Informed Consent

Informed consent is the written or verbal permission from a patient who is informed of the benefits, risk, and alternatives of a procedure or treatment. Failure to provide informed consent so can result in civil or even criminal liability.[16]

To establish a cause of action or, in other words, to file a claim for damages under the doctrine of lack of informed consent, the plaintiff-attorney must prove three things[17]:

1. Failure to disclose alternatives
2. Reasonable person would have elected not to undergo treatment
3. Harm

Failure to Disclose Alternative

Failure to disclose alternative is defined as follows: "the failure of the person providing the professional treatment or diagnosis to disclose to the patient such alternatives thereto and the reasonably foreseeable risks and benefits involved as a reasonable medical, dental or podiatric practitioner under similar circumstances would have disclosed, in a manner permitting the patient to make a knowledgeable evaluation."[17]

Legally, it is called the "professional standard," which is based on old common law: What does the doctor think is best for the patient to know? Acceptable standards are usually established by state and federal agencies, medical associations, and The Joint Commission.

Under failure to disclose alternative, the standard of care rendered is not at issue. In fact, the physician may have performed the procedure flawlessly but may still be liable under failure of informed consent if a patient suffers harm, such as a postoperative complication that should have been discussed during the informed consent process. The COVID-19 pandemic may have disrupted physicians' ability to properly perform and engage with cancer patients with meaningful conversations about risk, benefits, and alternatives to care. Communicating effectively through masks worn by both physicians and patients can be challenging. The physician may delegate the informed consent process to an allied health professional who is not actually performing the procedure, which increases liability because the patient may not acquire the same level of reasonable understanding of risks and benefits compared to when a physician performs the informed consent process.

COVID-19 IMMUNITY STATUTES

Immunity states were established to mitigate liability for health care workers during the pandemic where many areas of the country hospital census were over capacity with COVID-19 and non–COVID-19 patients. Hospitals expanded medical services to nonclinical sections or built tents. Intensive care unit patients were doubled up. Emergency rooms held admitted patients for several hours to days due to lack of hospital beds and resources. Ancillary services, such as lab, x-ray, computed tomography, and magnetic resonance imaging, could not keep up with demand. This created an enormous strain on health systems and demand for physician services. The immunity statutes were meant to assist in reducing physician liability fears in assisting hospitals and clinics during this crisis. The following is a discussion of principle immunity statutes and their strengths and vulnerabilities. Precedent has not yet been established due to the fact that the pandemic is not over and because filed claims have been delayed or postponed because of COVID-19. It is unclear whether these statutes will safeguard health care workers against liability in the future.

Federal Immunity Statutes

PREP Act

The Public Readiness and Emergency Preparedness (PREP) Act authorizes the secretary of the Department of Health and Human Services (secretary) to issue a PREP Act declaration. The declaration provides immunity from liability (except for willful misconduct) for claims "of loss caused, arising out of, relating to, or resulting from administration or use of countermeasures to diseases, threats and conditions."[18]

The PREP Act provides immunity to liability under certain circumstances; "administration or countermeasure to diseases," meaning providers providing COVID-19 treatments during a declared state of emergency are immune from liability, including patients who die or "of loss". Courts will define the meaning "of loss" and whether this will expand to include any consequential harms to the patient during COVID-19 treatment.

CARES Act

The Coronavirus Aid, Relief, and Economic Security (CARES) Act[19] protects health care professional from liability under federal or state law for any harm caused by an act or omission in the provision of health care services during the COVID-19 public health emergency so long as health care services in response to the public health emergency are performed in a *volunteer* capacity and the act or omission occurs in the course of providing health care services within the scope of the license, registration, or certification and in good faith (see section 3215).[19]

This statute provides immunity from "any harm" (not just "loss" or death) during a declared COVID-19 public health emergency, but it protects only those providers in a "volunteer capacity" and within the "scope of license." Will courts define the statute in a strict or narrow manner? For example, will it apply to a health care worker who providers services at no charge or no physician reimbursement? It is unclear how courts will rule under this statute.

Additionally, it is unclear how courts will define "scope of practice or registration." The COVID-19 pandemic has required assistance of physicians outside their usual and customary services, but this does not mean that a non–surgically trained physician can perform surgical procedures. That would be considered outside their scope of practice. However, physicians have been asked to volunteer to manage inpatient and emergency room services or provide ventilator care management normally assigned to specialists in those areas. It is unclear how courts will rule.

State Immunity Statutes

Twenty states have enacted COVID-19 immunity statutes. Other states, such as California, have immunity statutes that are applicable to any declaration of a state of emergency, including COVID-19.

New York covid immunity statute

Declaration of purpose. A public health emergency that occurs on a statewide basis requires an enormous response from state and federal and local governments working in concert with private and public health care providers in the community. The furnishing of treatment of patients during such a public health emergency is a matter of vital state concern affecting the public health, safety and welfare of all citizens. It is the purpose of this article to promote the public health, safety and welfare of all citizens by broadly protecting the health care facilities and health care professionals in this state from liability that may result from treatment of individuals with COVID-19 under conditions resulting from circumstances associated with the public health emergency.[20]

The New York statute, like many other state statutes, protects health care professionals who treat COVID-19 patients. The question is whether health care professionals include allied health professionals (physician assistants/nurse practitioners) or students in training, such as residents and fellows. Some statutes clearly define health care professionals as including residents and fellows. Others are silent. It is unclear how courts will interpret these statutes.

Federal and state immunity statutes limitations

Most statutes provide clear limitations of the immunity clauses[21]:

1. Willful misconduct
2. Intentional or criminal misconduct
3. Gross negligence
4. Reckless misconduct

PREVENTION

To mitigate risk of liability during the pandemic, health care workers must be vigilant in risk management reduction practices.[22] The following are some practical suggestions:

1. Physicians caring for cancer patients need to make sure that they are communicating effectively with their patients, especially clearly explaining that delays in the patients' care will not impact their overall prognosis. Physicians need to resist the temptation to participate in "blame game" by blaming the hospital or others for delays in care.
2. Clear and accurate documentation is critical. Physicians need to memorialize discussions with the patient and families in medical records, including virtual visits or calls.
3. Discussions involving informed consent for procedures should be documented in medical records. Do not rely on the "4 corners" of an informed consent document. There needs to be a clear picture of what transpired during the informed consent discussion, especially if there are unusual circumstances or difficult conversations.
4. Language barriers need to be managed effectively, preferably using an on-site interpreter for difficult conversations or reviewing an informed consent. Avoid relying on family members for interpreting.

5. Be knowledgeable and empathetic to cultural and racial differences in how cancer patients and families respond to difficult conversations or end-of-life care. Understand that some cultures or races may express anger or even rage. As long as the provider feels safe, allow them to "vent" and express their pain and anguish. Do not escalate the encounter by being defensive, and do not immediately resort to calling security or even police (unless there is a threat).

6. If there is a bad outcome or death that could possibly result in a claim, report it immediately to your indemnity insurance carrier, risk manager, or supervisor. This proactive approach will permit the case to be thoroughly investigated and allow the documentation of unforeseen circumstances during the COVID-19 pandemic that may have contributed to the harm of the patient.

7. Do not avoid conversations with family members or patients should there be a bad outcome. These conversations can result in "closure" for families. It may mitigate anger from family members, which is often a trigger for claims.

8. Be prepared during conversations to "apologize." This is not analogous to "admission" of fault. It is simply acknowledging the patient's or family member's discontent with the service. Avoid casting blame on others.

CLINICAL VIGNETTE # 1

Early during the COVID-19 pandemic (declared state of emergency), a 50-year-old hospital executive presents to an urgent care owned by a hospital with cough and fever. The physician assistant (PA) diagnoses a viral syndrome. The patient returns two days later and is reassessed by the PA with labs and chest x-ray revealing pneumonia. The patient is sent home on antibiotics. COVID-19 testing is unavailable at the urgent care. Two days later, the patient arrives in the emergency room with severe shortness of breath. The patient is intubated and within minutes goes into cardiac arrest and dies. Lab test confirms COVID-19. The family files a wrongful death claim alleging negligence in failing to diagnosis COVID-19 infection.

Is the PA protected under the immunity statute for misdiagnosis during the COVID-19 pandemic?

The question is whether the immunity statutes cover PAs. In some states, the statutes expressly state that PAs fall under the definition of health care provider. Other statutes are silent. If the state's immunity protects the PA, the next question is whether the PA's and supervising physician's "act of omission" by not testing for COVID-19 is protected under federal or state immunity statutes. The answer is possibly. Omission during the treatment of COVID-19 infection is delineated in some statutes. If the PA or supervising physician "volunteered" for services, they could be immune under the federal statutes (CARES Act). If immunity is not granted, the defense can argue "lack of causation" by asserting that even if the patient was diagnosed earlier, there was no indication to admit the patient to the hospital, nor were early therapeutic interventions (e.g., monoclonal antibodies) available.

CLINICAL VIGNETTE # 2

During the declared COVID-19 pandemic, a patient underwent an outpatient needle biopsy for a mass peripherally located in the lung, adjacent to the thorax. Because of its location, the risk of pneumothorax or bleed was ascertained to be low. Nevertheless, when the needle was inserted, it punctured a bronchial vessel, which caused a major hemorrhage requiring prophylactic emergency intubation and blood transfusions. The patient survived and filed a claim under failure of informed consent.

Will the proceduralist be protected under the immunity statutes?

The answer is probably not. Even under an emergency declaration, the immunity statutes do not provide en blanc protection from all liability. The trier of facts would show there is no nexus between the COVID-19 epidemic and outpatient radiology operations. Failure of informed consent theory may succeed. It must be determined whether a reasonable person would expect that they would require lifesaving interventions from a relatively benign procedure where the tumor biopsied is close to the lining of the thorax. Failure of informed consent is a form of battery, and none of the immunity statutes would apply under this theory.

CLINICAL VIGNETTE # 3

A 90-year-old woman fractured her hip, was admitted to a hospital and underwent treatment, and was subsequently admitted to a skilled nursing facility (SNF). The patient developed COVID-19 infection and was readmitted to the hospital but subsequently died from COVID-19 infection. A COVID-19 state of emergency had been declared. The family files a wrongful death claim.

Do the immunity statutes protect the hospital or SNF against liability?

Under state and federal statutes, both the hospital and SNF may be protected under the immunity statutes, but this is disputable. Statutes protect providers who treat COVID-19. It is unclear whether these statutes would apply to a patient who acquires COVID-19 infection during the course of a disease unrelated to COVID-19. Lawsuits are already underway against SNFs with large outbreaks. If the SNF negligently permitted a worker on site and tracing confirmed that the patient contracted the COVID-19 infection from the worker, the SNF may be liable. Even under conditions of a severe staff shortages, courts may not allow staffing shortages as a defense. In fact, courts may determine this as "willful misconduct," which excludes the SNF from immunity protection. If the SNF is owned in part or fully by the hospital, the hospital will be found liable. If the hospital was aware of the SNF outbreak but transferred the patient to the SNF, it may not be protected under the immunity clause because it might be determined to have committed reckless conduct.

CLINICAL VIGNETTE # 4

A 23-year-old man has been diagnosed with testicular cancer with metastatic spread to the lung. The COVID-19 test is negative. The cardiac surgeon needs to perform an open thoracotomy to relieve further mediastinal shifting. The surgery is not designated as urgent or emergent. The surgery is postponed due to the COVID-19 epidemic. The patient subsequently dies shortly afterward. His family files a wrongful death claim alleging negligence due to delay in care.

Is the surgeon protected under the immunity statutes?

Again, courts would have to decide whether COVID-19 immunity statutes can be broadly defined as extending to protect providers who cared for non–COVID-19 patients during the epidemic. Some states expressly provide immunity protection for providers whose care for non–COVID-19 patients was delayed due to the pandemic. In states that are silent regarding immunity for care of non–COVID-19 patients, courts may deny immunity. The next issue is determining whether the delay in care of a palliative procedure accelerated the patient's death and caused preventable pain and suffering.

CONCLUSION

COVID-19–related liability poses a real threat to oncologists, surgeons, and proceduralists over the next several years. Plaintiff-attorneys will test the limits of the immunity statutes.

For now, there is no clear precedent regarding whether courts will broadly or narrowly define immunity statutes. However, it is likely that non–COVID-19 cancer patients whose care has been compromised during the COVID-19 epidemic may succeed in penetrating the immunity protection depending on the state in which the claim is filed. Keep in mind that the immunity statutes do not prevent a plaintiff or representative from filing a claim. They can and will file claims. However, the courts will determine, based on the "trier of facts," whether it is sufficient for a summary judgement under the immunity statutes. For now, providers must apply standards and recommendations according to their specialties. They must carefully follow proper triage protocols, determining the cancer patient's risk as a result of delays. Providers should be meticulous in documentation and communicating with their patients and families. The documentation needs to reflect the tenuous conditions that may have affected directly or indirectly the care of the cancer patient.

KEY POINTS:

- COVID-19 liability is a threat to providers in the care of cancer patients in the near future.
- Multiple predisposing conditions exist in the community that cause distrust and anger toward the medical community.

- Cancer is an independent risk factor for mortality during COVID-19.
- Disruption of outpatient and hospital services has affected cancer diagnosis, therapy, and management of care.
- Federal and state immunity statutes were created to give health care workers liability protection during a declared state of COVID-19 emergency.
- There are limitations to immune statutes, such as willful misconduct or intentional acts or omissions.
- Defendant-attorneys will challenge immunity statutes in seeking relief for damages.
- To mitigate risk against liability during the COVID-19 pandemic, providers must apply risk mitigation reduction strategies to their daily practice.

References:

1. Corona virus maps US and worldwide maps. *New York Times*. https://www.nytimes.com/interactive/2020/us/coronavirus-us-cases.html. Accessed September 8, 2021.
2. de Joode K, Dumoulin DW, Engelen V, et al. Impact of the coronavirus disease 2019 pandemic on cancer treatment: the patients' perspective. *Eur J Cancer*. 2020;136:132–139.
3. Patt D, Gordan L, Diaz M, et al. Impact of COVID-19 on Cancer care: how the Pandemic is delaying cancer care and treatment for American seniors. *JCO Clin Cancer Inform*. 2020;4:1059–1071.
4. COVID fears of may be causing patients to ignore medical emergencies. NPR News. https://www.npr.org/2020/05/06/851173949/covid-19-fears-may-be-causing-people-to-ignore-medical-emergencies. Accessed September 8, 2021.
5. Donnelly JP, Wang XQ, Iwashyna TJ, Prescott HC. Readmission and death after initial hospital discharge among patients with COVID-19 in a large multi-hospital system. *JAMA*. 2021;325(3):304–306.
6. Tsamakis K, Gavriatopoulou M, Schizas D, et al. Oncology during the COVID-19 pandemic: challenges, dilemmas, and the psychosocial impact on cancer patients. *Oncol Lett*. 2020;20(1):441–447.
7. Interim recommendations for emergency medical services (EMS) systems and 911 public safety answering points/emergency communication centers (PSAP/ECCs) in the United States during the coronavirus disease (COVID-19) pandemic. Centers for Disease Control and Prevention. https://www.cdc.gov/coronavirus/2019-ncov/hcp/guidance-for-ems.html. Accessed September 8, 2021.
8. At least 181 public health leaders nationwide have resigned, retired or been fired amid pandemic. KTLA December 14, 2020. https://ktla.com/news/coronavirus/at-least-181-public-health-leaders-nationwide-have-resigned-retired-or-been-fired-amid-pandemic/. Accessed September 8, 2021.
9. Commentary: erosion of trust threatens essential element of practicing medicine. Modern Healthcare. March 9, 2019. https://www.modernhealthcare.com/opinion-editorial/commentary-erosion-trust-threatens-essential-element-practicing-medicine. Accessed September 8, 2021.
10. Disparities in COVID illnesses. Centers for Disease Control and Prevention. https://www.cdc.gov/coronavirus/2019-ncov/community/health-equity/racial-ethnic-disparities/increased-risk-illness.html#:~:text=The%20highest%20percent%20of%20COVID,within%20the%20total%20U.S.%20population. Accessed September 8, 2021.
11. Black doctors die of COVID after complaining of racist treatment. *New York Times*. December 12, 2020. https://www.nytimes.com/2020/12/23/us/susan-moore-black-doctor-indiana.html. Accessed September 8, 2021.
12. Murez C. Health care after covid: the rise of telemedicine. *US News and World Report*. January 5, 2021. https://www.usnews.com/news/health-news/articles/2021-01-05/health-care-after-covid-the-rise-of-telemedicine. Accessed September 8, 2021.
13. Garner BA. *Black's Law Dictionary*. 11th ed. Eagan, MN: Thomson West; 2019.
14. Negligence elements. FindLaw. https://www.findlaw.com/injury/accident-injury-law/elements-of-a-negligence-case.html. Accessed September 8, 2021.

15. Wrongful death. NYC Bar. https://www.nycbar.org/get-legal-help/article/personal-injury-and-accidents/wrongful-death/. Accessed September 8, 2021.
16. *Cobbs v Grant*, 8 Cal 3d 229 (1972).
17. NY PBH L § 2805-d (1).
18. Public Readiness and Emergency Preparedness Act. US Department of Health and Human Services. https://www.phe.gov/Preparedness/legal/prepact/Pages/default.aspx. Accessed September 8, 2021.
19. CARES Act, S.3548, 116th Congress (2019-2020). https://www.congress.gov/bill/116th-congress/senate-bill/3548. Accesses September 8, 2021.
20. NY Covid Immunity Statutes. New York S 7506 Signed Chapter 56.
21. Standards of medical conduct. What are they and why are they so important. Relias Media. https://medicalacademy.com/product/law-for-docs/. Accessed September 8, 2021.
22. Law-4-Docs.com. Medical Malpractice CME Course. Victor Waters, MD, JD, FCLM, President and CEO.

Index

NOTE: A *t* following a page number indicates tabular material, and *f* following a page number indicates a figure.